April 1985: First International Conference on AIDS is held in Atlanta, Georgia. ■ Larry Kramer's "The Normal Heart" premieres, one of the first plays to deal with AIDS.

July 1985. Official announcement that movie star Rock Hudson has AIDS and the first story about Ryan White's exclusion from school in Kokomo, Indiana appears on network television.

October 1985: Rock Hudson dies of AIDS.

AIDS DEATH TOLL PASSES 12,000.

June 1986: At the Paris AIDS Conference, Samuel Broder, then director of the United States Public Health Service, reports on preliminary ZDV trials and ddC and ddI laboratory experiments and says, **"I believe AIDS is curable."**

October 1986: U.S. Surgeon General C. Everett Koop issues a landmark report on the AIDS epidemic that calls for public health measures and sex education.

AIDS DEATH TOLL PASSES 27,000.

February 1987: Liberace, age 67, dies of AIDS.

March 1987: Zidovudine (ZDV or AZT), the first HIV-reverse transcriptase-inhibiting drug, is approved for experimental use by the U.S. Food and Drug Administration (FDA). FDA creates a category of drugs that could be sold **before** approval, if they appear safe and show minimal signs of effectiveness.

June 1987: First Presidential Advisory Commission on AIDS created by President Ronald Reagan. ■ Citing public health concerns, the United States bars HIV-infected immigrants and travelers from entering the country.

July 1987: Broadway director Michael Bennett ("A Chorus Line," "Dreamgirls") dies of AIDS at 44.

August 1987: The Ray family home is burned because they have three HIV-infected children who want to attend the local school.

October 1987: U.S. scientists begin preliminary tests of the first experimental HIV vaccine on non-HIV-infected volunteers. ■ Publication of *And the Band Played On,* Randy Shilt's definitive chronicle of the AIDS epidemic.

February 1988: Presidential Advisory Committee states that the nation's blood banking industry response to HIV in the blood supply was **unnecessarily slow.**

August 1988: Tacoma, Washington—First syringe/needle exchange started in the United States.

December 1988: AIDS DEATH TOLL PASSES 60,000.

December 1, 1988: First World AIDS Day.

February 1989: First zidovudine HIV-resistant mutants reported to the CDC.

June 1989: The FDA approves aerosolized pentamidine for the prevention of PCP, a major cause of death among AIDS patients.

December 1989: Kimberly Bergalis is diagnosed with AIDS. She was the first, and beginning 1998, the only case of becoming HIV-infected from a health care worker, her dentist. This case made worldwide headlines.

April 1990: Hemophiliac Ryan White, 18, dies from AIDS, spurring a U.S. Congressional movement to provide funds to cities hardest hit by the disease.

May 1990: FDA approves the use of zidovudine for pediatric AIDS cases, 3 years after approval for use in adults.

June 1990: AIDS DEATH TOLL REACHES FIRST 100,000.

August 1990: FDA approves first HIV-2 testing kit.

June 1991: Ten years into the epidemic, the CDC reports that 1 million Americans are infected with HIV. At this point, half the 500,000 people in the western hemisphere with AIDS have died.

October 1991: Magic Johnson announces he is infected with the AIDS virus. ■ FDA approves a second anti-AIDS drug, ddI. ■ The World Health Organization estimates that nearly 10 million people worldwide are infected with HIV.

December 1991: AIDS DEATH TOLL PASSES 150,000.

March 1992: EIA testing kit for HIV-2 becomes available for clinical use in the United States.

April 1992: Tennis player Arthur Ashe confirms that he has AIDS. He probably contracted the virus via a blood transfusion during a heart-bypass operation.

May 1992: Montagnier and Gallo agree that the viruses they found were the same and originally came from Montagnier's lab.

June 1992: British scientists predict that over the next 15 years AIDS will cut Uganda's projected population growth rate by 20%. ■ The reverse transcriptase-inhibiting drug, ddC, is approved by the FDA. ■ All donated blood in the United States must be tested for HIV-2.

July 1992: The first published reports of a combination drug treatment for AIDS. ■About 30 cases of non-HIV AIDS are reported at the Eighth International AIDS Conference in Amsterdam. By November 1992, 80 cases of non-HIV AIDS have been reported. ■ United States Congress passes Public Health Law 102-321 banning the use of federal funds for needle exchange programs. ■ **CDC announces that as many as 650,000 to 900,000 Americans are HIV-infected and 0.3% or 1 in 300 Americans are HIV-positive.**

October 1992: Harvard Global AIDS Policy Commission estimates that by the year 2000, worldwide there will be between 38 million and 110 million adult/adolescent and 10 million pediatric HIV infections. There will also be about 24 million AIDS cases.

January 1993: The CDC begins the use of a new definition of an AIDS case. Anyone who is HIV-positive and has a T4 cell count of **less than 200/μL of blood has AIDS.** The impact of the new definition is an 111% increase in new cases diagnosed in 1993 over 1992. ■ Ballet dancer Rudolf Nureyev dies of AIDS at 54. ■ **CDC announces that AIDS has become the number one killer of people ages 25 to 44 in the United States.**

February 1993: Arthur Ashe dies of AIDS. He was the first black male to win a Wimbledon title, in 1975.

March 1993: AIDS DEATH TOLL REACHES 200,000.

April 1993: The British/French "Concorde" 3-year trial study on the use of zidovudine (called AZT) in HIV-diseased people shows no evidence that zidovudine therapy delays the onset of AIDS.

May 1993: FDA approves the use/sale of the female condom.

June 1993: Donna Shalala, U.S. Secretary of Health and Human Services, asks the Institute of Medicine to determine who was responsible for HIV in the United States blood supply that infected so many hemophiliacs. ■ First AIDS Day of Compassion in the United States, June 21. ■ Kristine Gebbie is appointed as first U.S. AIDS Policy Director; she resigns on August 2, 1994. ■ The Berlin World AIDS Conference acknowledges a low point in **hope**. Research findings are mostly negative; nucleoside analog monotherapy is declared noneffective. The **hope** early on was that HIV would, like polio, be defeated, but HIV turned out to be more like a cancer, stubbornly resistant to the ingenuity of scientists.

July 1993: HIV/AIDS research budget is increased for 1994 by 21% to $1.3 billion and service programs for HIV/AIDS are increased by 66% to $579 million.

December 1993: Post offices begin selling 29-cent stamps showing the red ribbon of AIDS awareness. ■ The year ends without the production of any significant new HIV/AIDS drugs and without an HIV/AIDS vaccine. ■ **There are 105,990 adult/adolescent and 968 pediatric AIDS cases diagnosed for 1993, the largest number for any given year through 1997.**

January 1994: Donna Shalala, U.S. Secretary of Health and Human Services, begins selecting members for a National Task Force on AIDS Drug Development. Over 50,000 people are involved in HIV/AIDS research/medical health care workforce.

February 1994: National Institutes of Health announces results of ACTG protocol 076, indicating that the use of zidovudine in a select group of HIV-infected pregnant women reduces the risk of perinatal (newborn) HIV infection by two thirds.

April 1994: World champion figure skater John Curry, who won an Olympic gold medal in 1976, dies of AIDS at 44.

AIDS DEATH TOLL PASSES 250,000.

May 1994: Five volunteers in the government's principal HIV-subunit vaccine study become HIV-infected. Scientists still do not understand why

Continued on inside back cover

ACQUIRED IMMUNE DEFICIENCY SYNDROME

Biological, Medical, Social, and Legal Issues

Third Edition

GERALD J. STINE, PH.D.

University of North Florida, Jacksonville

PRENTICE HALL, *Upper Saddle River, New Jersey 07458*

Library of Congress Cataloging–in–Publication Data

Stine, Gerald James.
   Acquired immune deficiency syndrome : biological, medical, social.
and legal issues / Gerald J. Stine. — 3rd ed.
      p.   cm.
   Includes bibliographical references and index.
   ISBN 0-13-789991-2
   1. AIDS (Disease)   I. Title.
   [DNLM: 1. Acquired Immunodeficiency Syndrome.   2. AIDS-Related
Opportunistic Infections.   WC 503 S859a 1997]
RC607.A26S75   1998
362. 1'69792—DC21
DNLM/DLC
for Library of Congress   97-42639
                                                                    CIP

Executive Editor: *David Kendric Brake*
Editor: *Linda Schreiber*
Manufacturing Manager: *Trudy Pisciotti*
Total Concept Coordinator: *Kimberly P. Karpovich*
Cover Designer: *Joe Sengotta*
Cover Illustration: *Laura J. Edwards*
Image Copyright © 1997 PhotoDisc, Inc.

About the Cover: Triple-drug "cocktails" have revolutionized the treatment of HIV and
been credited for dramatic recoveries and increased lifespans for AIDS patients. They have
been proven to effectively drive down the amount of HIV in the bloodstream thus decreasing
the "viral load." Though the rewards are high, participating in one of these therapies
does exact a price. Patients must take dozens of pills a day, some that must be taken every
two hours, some three times a day, some after eating particular foods, some on an empty
stomach, etc. The cover of the third edition of *Acquired Immune Deficiency Syndrome:
Biological, Medical, Social, and Legal Issues* depicts the overwhelming drug regimen for a
patient battling HIV.

 ©1998, 1996, 1993 by Prentice-Hall, Inc.
Simon & Schuster/A Viacom Company
Upper Saddle River, New Jersey 07458

Printed in the United States of America

10   9   8   7   6   5   4   3   2   1

ISBN 0-13-789991-2

Prentice-Hall International (UK) Limited, *London*
Prentice-Hall of Australia Pty. Limited, *Sydney*
Prentice-Hall Canada Inc., *Toronto*
Prentice-Hall Hispanoamericana, S.A., *Mexico*
Prentice-Hall of India Private Limited, *New Delhi*
Prentice-Hall of Japan, Inc., *Tokyo*
Simon & Schuster Asia Pte. Ltd., *Singapore*
Editora Prentice-Hall do Brasil, Ltda., *Rio de Janeiro*

This book, as with my six other HIV/AIDS college-level textbooks,
is also dedicated to
those who have died of AIDS,
those who have HIV disease,
and to those who must prevent the spread of this plague—

EVERYONE, EVERYWHERE.

To date, I have never been more positive about the future for those who are HIV-infected in the United States and other developed nations. The use of anti-HIV drugs in combination has led to a significant reduction in AIDS-related deaths and reductions in opportunistic infections. These events, along with new insight into the biology and pathology of HIV that may lead to a preventive vaccine, provide a shining light against a stark history of the first 16 years of this pandemic.

Unfortunately, the high cost of anti-HIV drugs makes them unavailable for widespread distribution in underdeveloped nations. But hope and help must begin somewhere—someone must first benefit before others can. Let us pull together so that **help,** not just hope, will be available to **all** who need it!

The Author

Contents in Brief

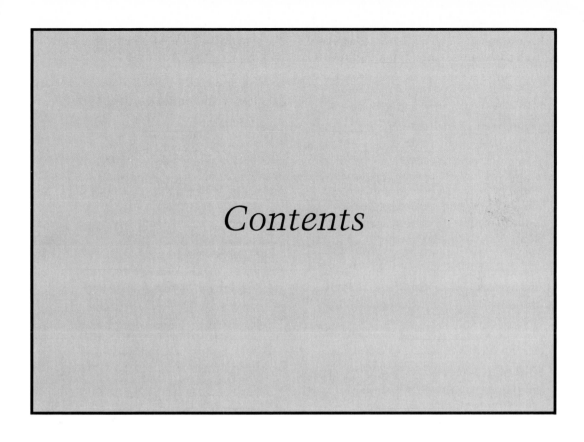

Contents

14 Counseling for HIV Testing, HIV Disease, and AIDS 439

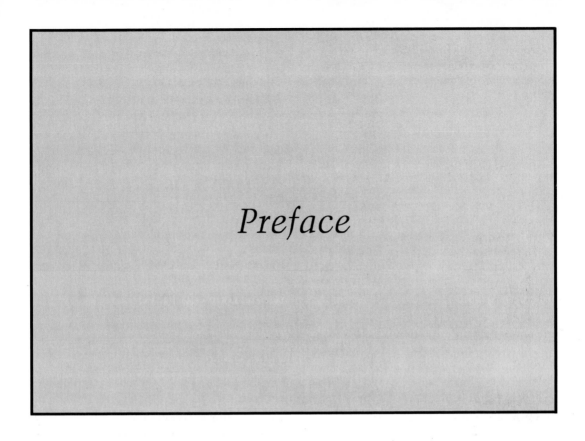

Preface

WHAT IS AIDS?

AIDS is defined primarily by a severe immune deficiency, and is distinguished from virtually every other disease in history by the fact that it has no constant, specific symptoms. Once the immune system has begun to malfunction, a broad spectrum of health complications can set in. AIDS (or Acquired Immune Deficiency Syndrome) is an umbrella term for any or all of 26 known diseases and their symptoms. When a person has any of these 26 microbial or viral caused opportunistic infections, and also tests positive for antibodies to HIV, he or she is diagnosed with AIDS. An AIDS diagnosis is also given to HIV-positive people with a T4 cell count of less than 200/μL of blood.

The history of AIDS is a human affair and is part of a cultural process of attempting to come to terms with a new and often terrifying series of events—of young people dying before their time, of the intermingling of sex and death—in a period in which the world itself is changing before our eyes.

The social meaning of the history of AIDS intimately touches upon ideas about sexuality, social responsibility, individual privacy, health, and the prospect of living a normal life span. Understanding how to respond to AIDS and how to think about this pandemic, is important not only for what it reveals about the ways in which health policy is created in the United States and elsewhere, but also for what it implies about the human ability to meet the challenge of future emerging diseases and long-standing public health problems. The HIV/AIDS pandemic is a current and long-term public health problem worldwide.

LESSONS LEARNED

From the lessons of history it is difficult to conceptualize how the AIDS epidemic will be halted, let alone reversed, in the absence of a **cheap curative drug or a cheap and effective preventative vaccine.** The syphilis epidemic at the early part of the century displayed a similar kind of epidemiology to the present-day AIDS epidemic. The campaigns which were initiated then closely paralleled those in place at present for AIDS. There were vigorous educational programs to reduce sexual high-risk behavior, which were targeted at brothels and prostitutes as well as at military recruits to the United States Army. Scare tactics were spread through the use of posters, pamphlets and radio—today it is television. Serological testing became mandatory before marriages could be licensed in certain states of the USA. But these measures had little appreciable effect on the expansion of the syphilis epidemic. It was only the advent of a cheap, safe, and effective drug, penicillin, which eventually brought the epidemic under control. **BUT** the bacterium (a spirochete) does not change or mutate as rapidly as the AIDS virus. There are mutant HIV in the human population for drugs that have yet to be tested and a highly effective preventive vaccine may not be a reality for HIV!

One lesson learned from HIV/AIDS, is that any disease that is occurring in a distant part of the globe may be in the United States, in your state or in your town, tomorrow. Twenty or even 15 years ago one would not have expected to read that statement.

The advent of miracle drugs and vaccines that conquered the plagues of polio, smallpox, and measles led many people—including scientists—to believe that the age of killer diseases was coming to an end.

The AIDS epidemic changed that perception, and best-selling nonfiction book *The Hot Zone* graphically illustrates how an exotic killer called the Ebola virus—carried into Virginia in 1989 by 450 imported research monkeys—came close to breaking loose in this country. In the hit film *Outbreak*, Dustin Hoffman plays a doctor battling a deadly virus that neither medicine nor the U.S. government can handle. Today, the Centers for Disease Control and Prevention are rethinking their position on the possibility of new plagues occurring in our lifetimes!

To place the HIV/AIDS pandemic in perspective, consider Michael Creighton's *The Andromeda Strain*. The essence of this story revolves around the release of an unidentified and untreatable lethal strain of bacteria into the human population. With a few changes—substituting HIV for bacterium, adjusting the time of death after infection, and describing how one dies from the disease—Creighton could have been writing about HIV/AIDS. But with HIV/AIDS, the onset of a real human tragedy, we are learning about our social contradictions, our strengths and our weaknesses, and we are questioning whether this is a morally acceptable disease. How long will it take for this to become a socially acceptable disease?

AIDS: THE WORST-CASE SCENARIO

As presented in this book, the reader will note the ability of HIV to cause a slow, progressive, and permanent disease. Thus, with no recovery, no loss of infectivity, no development of either individual or group immunity, there is at present, no known biological mechanism which can stop the continuing expansion of the disease unless an effective vaccine were to come about, and at present there is no feasible design for such an effective vaccine. The progressive increase in the pool of HIV can, in theory, only lead to an exponential increase in the number of individuals who will become infected until eventually the majority of the sexually active population will be infected unless interventions are at least moderately successful.

It is **because** this scenario may become reality and **because** people worldwide are becoming HIV-infected every few seconds and dying of AIDS each minute, and **because** together we must try to prevent the further spread of HIV, that this text continues to be updated.

This text reviews important aspects of HIV infection, HIV disease, and the acquired immune deficiency syndrome. It presents a balanced review of factual information about the biological, medical, social, economic, and legal aspects of this modern-day pandemic.

The intricacy of the HIV/AIDS pandemic has unfolded over the last 17 years. Many of the details of basic research, applied biology, medicine, and social unrest are presented in an attempt to convey the few victories and many setbacks within this ongoing saga. Medical and social anecdotes help to convey a sense of the HIV/AIDS tragedy worldwide. The history of the disease describes how the virus is and is not transmitted. Throughout the text there is a special focus on risk behaviors and risk situations involved in HIV transmission and the means to prevent its transmission. The number of social issues raised by this disease are mind-boggling. Many of these issues are presented—some as open-ended questions for class discussions. Such questions help the student reflect on what he or she has read.

PURPOSE

The purpose of this text is to present an understandable scientific explanation of what has been learned about HIV/AIDS over the last 17 years. In addition, it is particularly important to provide students with a conceptual framework of the issues raised by the HIV/AIDS pandemic so that they will be better able to deal with the challenges posed by this disease. Clearly, this pandemic poses new and unforeseen problems with no quick biological solutions. Only through reason can we respond in a socially acceptable fashion.

Because there is a constant stream of new information to be interpreted and shared, a new edition will be published every 2 years. What has been learned and what must still be learned to bring HIV infection, HIV disease, and AIDS under control is valuable information to most, if not all, of us.

Text Use

This text is intended for use in college-level courses on AIDS and as a supplemental HIV/AIDS resource in medical and nursing schools, in colleges of allied health sciences, in psychology department courses on human sexuality and human behavior, in courses on sexually transmitted diseases, in summer teachers programs, in the training of AIDS counselors, in state-mandated AIDS education

courses for health care workers, and for physicians who need a ready source of information on how to prevent HIV infection, HIV disease and its progression to AIDS, and types of therapy available. This text is suitable in those cases where information and education about the various aspects of HIV infection, disease, and AIDS are either wanted or required.

During the 17 years since HIV/AIDS was defined as a new disease, more manpower and money has been poured into HIV/AIDS research than into any other disease in history. Information on the AIDS virus has accumulated at an unprecedented pace. Since the discovery of the AIDS virus in 1982–1983, scientists have learned much about how it functions and how it affects the immune system. More was learned about the AIDS virus in the first 6 years after its discovery than had been learned about the polio virus in the first 40 years of the polio epidemic. During the first 6 years of AIDS research, the virus's genetic material was cloned, its structure ascertained, and individual viral genes identified. In fact, so many billions of dollars have been spent on HIV/AIDS that many now believe that HIV/AIDS research has taken away much-needed resources from other diseases that kill many times more people per year than does AIDS.

TEXT OVERVIEW

Because so much of the HIV/AIDS pandemic has been based on the manipulation of distorted scientific fact, it is necessary to counter these distortions and myths by presenting the most consistent, reproducible, and scientifically acceptable facts as possible. Therefore, this text offers answers to questions many people have about the AIDS virus and how their immune systems are affected by it. Covered herein are the activity of the immune system with respect to HIV disease, where the virus might have come from, how it is transmitted, who is most likely to become infected, viral prevalence (geographical distribution of the number of people infected and those expressing HIV disease and AIDS), possible means of preventing infection, signs and symptoms of

HIV disease and AIDS, chronological definitions of AIDS, the opportunistic infections most often associated with AIDS, FDA-approved and nonapproved drugs and their effectiveness, the potential for a vaccine to the AIDS virus, the tests available to detect HIV infection, the accuracy of these tests, their cost, availability, and confidentiality. The last four text chapters present the essentials of pre- and post-HIV test counseling and the social, economic, and legal issues associated with HIV disease and AIDS. These chapters deal with the fear of HIV infection, the social reaction of the uninfected toward the HIV-infected, the economic burden, and acts of discrimination and the laws in place to protect HIV/AIDS persons.

The majority of references herein are dated between 1987 and 1997. Every state in the United States has HIV-infected people and reported people diagnosed with AIDS. The World Health Organization (WHO) reports that of 209 countries reporting to it, 194 have reported diagnosed cases of AIDS through 1997. The virus is truly pandemic and now threatens most of the human population. Yet it is a preventable disorder, and the steps to prevention are presented in Chapter 9.

Organization of the Text

Chapter 1 presents information on the discovery of the disease and naming of the illness. Chapter 2 discusses the cause of AIDS and the possible origin of the AIDS virus. Chapter 3 presents the biological characteristics of the virus. Chapter 4 presents the drugs in use to prevent HIV reproduction. Chapter 5 discusses the human immune system as it relates to HIV disease and the loss of the immune system's function. Chapter 6 presents the various opportunistic diseases and forms of cancer associated with HIV disease and AIDS. Chapter 7 discusses the clinical profile of biological indicators of HIV disease and AIDS. Chapter 8 presents the means by which HIV is most efficiently transmitted among humans. Chapter 9 details the most effective means to date of preventing HIV infection. Chapter 10 gives the incidence of HIV infections, HIV disease, and AIDS cases among selected behavioral at-risk persons for HIV infection in the United States. Chapter 11 presents the prevalence and problems of HIV disease in women, children, and teenagers. Chapter 12 covers the prevalence of HIV infection and AIDS cases outside the United States. Chapter 13 presents those tests most often used to detect the presence of HIV, biological shortcomings of the tests, the confidentiality or lack of confidentiality before and after test results, and costs. Chapter 14 describes the counseling process for HIV testing, HIV disease, and AIDS. Chapter 15 offers insight to the many social ramifications of having HIV disease or AIDS, human attitudes, and behaviors. Chapter 16 offers a look at the economics of the AIDS industry and Chapter 17 reviews the legal aspects of the AIDS pandemic. There is also a glossary of terms and index and a list of telephone numbers to federal, state, and other groups that offer information and help with all aspects of the HIV/AIDS pandemic.

Special Features

Each chapter contains chapter concepts, a summary, review questions, and references. Answers to questions appear at the back of the book. Chapters also contain definitions for new terms as they are introduced, illustrations, photographs, and tables. All 17 chapters contain boxed information. **Some of the chapters contain highlighted points of view, points of information, cases in point, sidebars, soundoff, and pro and con discussions.** They illustrate and emphasize important events and information about HIV infection, HIV disease, and AIDS. At certain places in the text, discussion statements are provided. Instructors may wish to entertain class discussions in these areas.

As science educators, it is our job to expose our students to the new concepts in biology that are shaping humanity's future. To do that, we must expose them to new vocabulary, new methodologies, new information and new ideas. It is my hope that this text will help in this endeavor.

IN APPRECIATION

The help of the following organizations or people is most deeply appreciated: The Centers for Disease Control and Prevention (CDC), Atlanta, Georgia, for use of slides and literature produced in their *National Surveillance Report* and the *Morbidity and Mortality Weekly Report*; Mara Lavitt and *The New Haven Register* for information on William Bluette; from the CDC, Richard Salik and Patricia Sweeney (Surveillance Branch); Robin Moseley, Patricia Fleming, Todd Webber (Division of HIV/AIDS Prevention), and Eleanor Holland (AIDS Clinical Trial Reference Specialist); E. E. Buff, Biological Administrator, and Barry Bennett, head of Retroviral Testing Services, for their permission and guidance on photographing HIV testing procedures at the Florida Health and Rehabilitation Office of Laboratories Services, Jacksonville, Florida; Denise Reddington, Department of Health and Human Services, Washington D.C., and Regan Alberta of PANOS Institute for their help in obtaining data on the economics of HIV/AIDS worldwide; Russ Havlak of the Infectious Disease Unit, CDC, Atlanta, Georgia; personnel of the National Institute for Allergy and Infectious Diseases, the National Center for Health Statistics, Brookwood Center for Children with AIDS in New York, the George Washington AIDS Policy Center in Washington, D.C., the National Institutes for Health, Hoffman-LaRoche Co., Abbott Laboratories, the Pharm-aceutical Mfg. Association, the National Cancer Institute, Pan American Health Organization, and the Office of Technological Assessment; Teresa M. St. John, University of North Florida for illustrations; the individuals who have contributed photographs; the text reviewers whose work has been greatly appreciated; Larry Monette, who spent countless hours word processing this manuscript; Guy Selander, M.D., who, over the years, has shared his medical journals with me; James Alderman, Eileen Brady, Mary Davis, Signe Evans, Paul Mosley, Ricky Moyer, Sarah Philips, and Barbara Tuck—reference/research librarians at the University of North Florida; Marie Cimmino for out-of-state library research; and to my special family, wife Delores and children Sherri and Garrett, who helped with proofreading and demonstrated a great deal of patience and understanding and gave up family weekends so the text could be completed on time.

This book has benefited from the critical evaluation of the following reviewers:

♦ Dr. Paul R. Elliott, Florida State University
♦ Dr. Robert Fulton, University of Minnesota
♦ Dr. Robert M. Kitchin, University of Wyoming
♦ Dr. Richard J. McCloskey, Boise State University
♦ Dr. Wayne B. Merkley, Drake University
♦ Dr. Linda L. Williford Pifer, University of Tennessee
♦ Dr. Bernard P. Sagik, Drexel University
♦ Professor James D. Slack, Cleveland State University
♦ Dr. Carl F. Ware, University of California, Riverside
♦ Dr. Phyllis K. Williams, Sinclair Community College
♦ Dr. Charles Wood, University of Kansas

A test bank of multiple-choice questions is available free of charge for those who adopt this text for class use. E-mail Linda Schreiber at: Linda_Schreiber@prenhall.com or via mail, Linda Schreiber, Prentice Hall, 1208 East Broadway, Suite 110, Tempe, Arizona 85282.

Dr. Stine is available for HIV/AIDS presentations, peer-related training sessions, and as a consultant to school systems who wish to provide HIV/AIDS education. Telephone 904-641-8979.

Gerald J. Stine, Ph.D.

"THE FACE OF AIDS"

It is two boys, ages 10 and 12, caring for their mother, who is dying from AIDS. The boys get themselves off to school in the morning, make dinner for their mother after school, carry her to the tub to bathe her, softly towel dry her body, which is covered with sores, then help her into bed. How do you go to school and compete academically when your mother is home dying, your family is broke, and you are afraid to tell anyone about the problem?

It is a young gay man in Orange County, California, who is having difficulty breathing. At the local hospital, he is diagnosed with pneumocystic carinii pneumonia (one of the characteristic infections afflicting people with AIDS) and is told, "We don't take care of this kind of pneumonia here." Packed into a car for a 6-hour drive to San Francisco, he's given an oxygen tank — only the oxygen runs out after 4 hours. Arriving at the emergency room at 2 a.m., in a city with no friends or family, he can barely breathe. Three months later he is dead.

It is a young woman who is knitting a scarf for her 2-year-old daughter. She said "I want to leave some legacy for her." She did not yet know her daughter was HIV-positive and most likely would not live long enough to understand the legacy. Most likely the daughter would die before her mother.

It is a child born to one of the 80,000 or so women in New York City who are injection drug users. The child is delivered in central Harlem, a region where 40% of the women receive late or no prenatal care, where the infant mortality rate is three times the national average, and where the main hospital recently suffered from a shortage of penicillin for a year and a half because it could not pay its bills. Initially the baby undergoes withdrawal from a heroin addiction inherited from her mother. Then 5 months later, the child becomes ill with persistent diarrhea. At the hospital they discover that she's not sick with one of the typical poverty-related infectious diseases that plague malnourished inner-city infants. No, the child has AIDS — and with parents unable to care for her, hospitals too crowded to board her, and foster agencies unable to place her, no one knows where or how this child will endure what promises to be a brief, sickly life.

It is about a 25-year-old male who looks 40 less than a year after his AIDS diagnosis. When he first tested HIV-positive, he decided to kill himself when his T4 cell count dropped to 100. When it did, he prepared his last meal, said goodbye to close friends, and bought a handgun. After dinner he put on his favorite cassette, raised the gun—but could not end his life. What now, he asks, this was my ace in the hole!

It is a young man who lives in Miami, and he's not ready to come home. He wants to remain independent. Eventually he will come home. His family must be prepared to care for him and to deal with all the issues they will face. His mother is a high school teacher, but she has never told anyone about her son. She says when he comes home it will be impossible to hide the fact that he has AIDS. "I am not sure how the community and our friends are going to respond."

For 1997 through the year 2000 and beyond, the Face of AIDS, due to the successful use of AIDS drug cocktail therapy, takes on a new and different look—of GUILT. Many who have recovered, even from their death beds, and feel "new" again, feel guilty because many are still dying and many do not have access to these drugs.

It is about establishing new relationships, giving up disability insurance, finding employment, and experiencing a life they thought they had lost.

It is THE FEAR THAT ALL THIS MAY BE JUST SHORT TERM—THAT THE VIRUS WILL WIN IN THE END!—This is a Face of AIDS made possible because science has provided new drug therapies!

The Face of AIDS is surely around us. It is a disease that invites commentary, requires research, and demands intervention. Inevitably linking sex and death, passion and politics, it continues to generate controversy. Appearing as a new and lethal infectious disease, at a time when the biomedical establishment in the United States has shifted its focus to chronic disease, AIDS has called into question many of the premises of the biomedical profession.

Whatever we do now, the die is already cast for many millions of people. The HIV/AIDS epidemic will exact an enormous toll. What is at stake is the possibility of shaping the future course of the pandemic, of modulating the suffering that inevitably will occur as a result of the infections that already exist. An epidemiological catastrophe is unavoidable. What can be limited are the dimensions of the catastrophe.

Introduction: Brief Histories of Other Global Epidemics, World AIDS Conferences, Overview of HIV/AIDS, and the AIDS Quilt

TEST OF YOUR CURRENT KNOWLEDGE

Before reading this book, review and answer the following statements about HIV infection and AIDS and answer either True or False to test your current knowledge:

♦ Infection by HIV can be prevented.

♦ Worldwide, the virus is primarily spread through heterosexual contact.

♦ Asymptomatic infected persons can infect others.

♦ High HIV infection risk is associated with having many sexual partners.

♦ HIV is fragile and easily destroyed by environmental agents when outside the human body.

♦ Casual contact does not spread HIV.

♦ HIV is not transmitted to humans via insects.

♦ The current risk of acquiring HIV via blood transfusions in the United States is low.

♦ Children can safely attend school with a classmate who is HIV-infected or has AIDS.

♦ Even without using precautions, health care workers are at a low risk for acquiring HIV infection.

♦ There is no cure for HIV disease or AIDS.

♦ In the United States about 60% of all persons expressing AIDS have died; worldwide it is over 80%.

♦ AIDS may be close to 100% lethal—sooner or later a person who expresses AIDS dies prematurely.

♦ It is believed that 90% to 95% of those infected with HIV will eventually progress to AIDS.

♦ There are people who are genetically resistant to HIV infection.

All of the preceding statements are true. Information concerning these statistics and answers to other questions that you may have can be found within.

> It was the best of times, it was the worst of times, it was the age of wisdom, it was the age of foolishness, it was the epoch of belief, it was the epoch of incredulity, it was the season of Light, it was the season of Darkness, it was the spring of hope, it was the winter of despair. . .
>
> Charles Dickens, *A Tale of Two Cities*

Nothing in recent history has so challenged our reliance on modern science nor emphasized our vulnerability before nature. We have lived with the acquired immune deficiency syndrome (AIDS) epidemic, witnessing its paradoxes every day. People living with the human immunodeficiency virus live with the fear,

pain, and uncertainty of the disease; they also endure prejudice, scorn, and rejection. **This must change!**

HISTORY OF GLOBAL EPIDEMICS

There has never been a time in human history when disease did not exist. The history of epidemics dates at least as far back as 1157 BC to the death of the Egyptian pharaoh, Ramses V, from smallpox. Over the centuries, this extraordinarily contagious virus spread around the world, changing the course of history time and again. It killed 2,000 Romans a day in the 2nd century AD, more than 2 million Aztecs during the 1520 conquest by Cortez, and some 600,000 Europeans a year from the 16th through the 18th centuries. Three out of four people who survived the high fever, convulsions, and painful rash were left deeply scarred and sometimes blind. Because victims' skin looked as if it had been scalded, smallpox was

--------- **POINT OF INFORMATION I.1** ---------

INFECTIOUS DISEASE PARADIGM

Most new infections are **not** caused by truly new pathogens. They are caused by microorganisms (bacteria, fungi, protozoa, and helminths) and viruses that have been present for hundreds or thousands of years, but they are newly recognized and named because of recently developed techniques to identify them. Human activities drive the emergence of disease and a variety of social, economic, political, cultural, climatic, technological, and environmental factors can shape the pattern of a disease and influence its emergence into populations. For example, travel can greatly affect the emergence of disease and human migrations have been the main source of epidemics throughout history. Trade caravans, religious pilgrimages, and military campaigns facilitated the speed of plague, smallpox, cholera, and now AIDS. Global travel is a fact of modern life and, equally so, the continued evolution of microorganisms and viruses; therefore, seemingly new infections will continue to emerge, and known infections will change in distribution, frequency, and severity.

DISEASES CAUSED BY VIRUSES AND MICROORGANISMS HAVE HAD 3 BILLION YEARS TO EVOLVE—WE SHOULD NOT EXPECT TO CONQUER THEM EASILY!

--------- **POINT OF INFORMATION I.2** ---------

SMALLPOX—A BIOLOGICAL WEAPON?

Smallpox may have been the most useful weapon of biological warfare in history. European colonialists repeatedly took advantage of the special susceptibility of the Amerindian population, deliberately spreading the deadly virus among the natives who were successfully defending their rights to the lands and resources of the Americas. For example, in 1763 Sir Jeffrey Amherst, commander in chief of all British forces in North America, was having great difficulty controlling the Pontiac Indians in the Western Territories. At Amherst's insistence, blankets inoculated with live smallpox viruses were distributed to the Pontiac, obliterating the tribe. The deliberately induced epidemic quickly spread to the northwest, claiming large numbers of Sioux and Plains Indians, crossed the Rockies and inflicted huge death tolls among Native Americans from south California all the way north to the Arctic Circle tribes of Alaska. This devastation was cited in the official WHO history of smallpox [FENNER, F., et al. (1988). *Smallpox and Its Eradication.* Geneva: World Health Organization].

known as the **"invisible fire."** Even now, malaria in underdeveloped countries afflicts 300 million people, killing about 2.1 million each year. The problem is compounded by development of drug-resistant malarial strains of protozoa. **Thus epidemics are not new to humankind, but the fear they impose on each generation is.**

Major recorded pandemics (global) and epidemics (regional) that have devastated large populations are described in Table I-1.

The 1970s witnessed the emergence of Lyme disease (1975), Legionnaires disease (1976), and toxic shock syndrome (1978). In the 1980s, the human immunodeficiency virus (HIV) and three new human herpes viruses (HHV 6, 7, and 8) were identified. In 1994, a physician in Gallup, New Mexico, was called to care for a man who had collapsed at a funeral. Soon, several others in New Mexico had also suffered from sudden respiratory failure.

As victims contracted the disease, they went from seemingly perfect health to flu-like symptoms, to a horrific state where their lungs began to fill with blood. Most of them died.

Within a few weeks, the Centers for Disease Control and Prevention identified this killer: **hantavirus**—a rodent-borne organism that had infected many GIs during the Korean War and killed hundreds. But the Korean type of hantavirus causes death through kidney failure. Somehow the hantavirus had found its way to the United States and mutated into a virus that invades the lungs.

The outbreak of hantavirus occurred first in 1993 in Arizona, Colorado, New Mexico, and Utah. Beginning 1998, 208 people have been infected in 26 states with the rodent-borne (deermouse) virus and 98 of these people have died of acute respiratory distress. There is no vaccine for this virus. In mid-1994 there was an outbreak of necrotizing fasciitis (fash-e-i-tis)—tissue destruction caused by a tissue-invasive strain of Group A streptococcus, a bacterium. This bacterium is a deadly variant strain of the Group A streptococcus that causes "strep throat." The infected may die from bacterial shock, disseminated blood coagulation (clotting), or respiratory or renal (kidney) failure. Also, in September of 1994, health authorities in Brisbane, Australia were suddenly confronted

with 11 dead horses and the death of their trainer. The killing agent was identified within 2 weeks. It is a new virus called **equine morbillivirus** that causes a fatal respiratory disease. Although nonhuman morbilliviruses have been associated with new and emerging animal diseases, no new human morbillivirus has been reported since the 10th century, when measles was described [Cause of fatal outbreak in horses and humans traced. (1995). *Science*, 268 (32):94–97]. Overall the virus has killed 13 of 25 infected horses and one of the two humans who became infected. This outbreak is an isolated event; no additional infections have been identified. The virus in this case was eliminated by the death of the infected. But where did the virus come from? Where will it show up next and under what conditions? The natural host of the virus has not been identified as of the beginning of 1998. This virus causes the cells lining the blood vessels to clump, creating holes in the vessel walls that allow fluid leakage into the lungs. The horses and the human drowned in their own fluids.

Although emerging viruses may contain novel mutations or represent gradual evolution, more often they emerge because of changes in behavior or the environment whereby they are introduced to a new host. Viruses that are pathogenic in novel human and nonhuman hosts include Marburg and Ebola viruses; hantaviruses; human immunodeficiency virus; Lassa virus; dolphin, porpoise, and phocine morbilliviruses; feline immunodeficiency virus; and bovine spongiform encephalopathy agent, which in 1996 threatened the possible destruction of the entire cow population of Europe causing economic loss of billions of dollars and a major unemployment problem. And, there are the **rotaviruses**. Rotaviruses are detected in 20% to 70% of fecal specimens from children hospitalized with acute diarrhea, and in developing countries they cause about 870,000 deaths each year. Even in the United States, rotavirus is associated with 3% of all hospitalizations of children younger than 5 years old, which translates to 55,000 to 70,000 hospitalizations per year, with medical and indirect costs in excess of $1 billion. Efforts to prevent disease by improving water or sanitation seem unlikely to succeed, because all children in developed and developing countries become infected with rotavirus in

TABLE 1-1 Plague in History

Disease	Dates	Place	Number Killed	Causative Organism	Time to Prevention/Cure (in years)
Measles	from 430 BC	Greece/Rome/World	Millions	Paramyxovirus	1,712
Bubonic Plague	1347–1351	Europe/Asia/Africa	75 million	Pasteurella pestis	580
Cholera	1826–1837	New Jersey	900,000	Vibrio cholerae	75
	1849	United Kingdom	53,293		
	1947	Egypt	11,755		
Tuberculosis	1930–1949	United States	1,000,000	Mycobacterium tuberculosis	85
Malaria	1954–1970		150,000		
	1847–1875	Africa/India	20 million +	Plasmodia	100
Scarlet Fever	1861–1870	United Kingdom	972 per million people	Beta-Hemolytic streptococci	45–44
Polio	1921–1970	North America	37,000	Polio viruses Types I, II, III	30–50
Typhus	1917–1921	Russia	2,500,000	Rickettsias	25
Influenza	1918–1919	U.S./Europe	21,640,000	Influenza virus	57
Small Pox	from 1157 BC	Europe (middle ages)	Many millions	Smallpox virus	2,390
	1926–1930	India	423,000		
Gonorrhea	from 590 BC / 1921–1992	United States	57,477	Neisseria gonorrhoeae	1,832
Yellow Fever	from AD / 1986–1988	Nigeria	10,000	Arbovirus	488
AIDS	1981–1998	United States (estimated)	Deaths 440,000 — Cases 715,000	Human Immunodeficiency Virus	Treatments but no cure
	1981–1998	World (estimated)	9,000,000 / 10,000,000		

4

———— BOX I.1 ————

OTHER LETHAL VIRUSES IN OUR TIME

Richard Preston, in his 1994 book *The Hot Zone* describes the progression of illness as the Ebola virus kills humans:

Ebola...triggers a creeping, spotty necrosis that spreads through all the internal organs. The liver bulges up and turns yellow, begins to liquefy, and then it cracks apart.... The kidneys become jammed with blood clots and dead cells, and cease functioning. As the kidneys fail, the blood becomes toxic with urine. The spleen turns into a single huge, hard blood clot the size of a baseball. The intestines may fill upon completely with blood. The lining of the gut dies and sloughs off into the bowels and is defecated along with large amounts of blood.

The Ebola virus resists all drug therapy to date and kills up to 80% or more of those infected within 1 to 3 weeks after infection. (HIV kills over 90%—it is slower but more lethal)

HISTORY

There have been seven confirmed outbreaks of Ebola. The first was in 1976 when Belgian doctors discovered the virus at a hospital in northern Zaire; it was named Ebola Zaire after the Zairian river flowing through the region. There were two more outbreaks in 1979, one in Zaire and one in southern Sudan. The fourth outbreak occurred once more in Zaire, in a city named Kikwit, a city of 600,000 people, in May of 1995. It struck again in December of 1995 in Gozon, Ivory Coast, again in February 1996 in Mayibout, Gabon, and again in November 1996 in Johannesburg, South Africa. And, each time the virus quickly ran its course of human destruction and disappeared. The result of the new Ebola epidemics was 357 confirmed cases of infection of which 268 have died. In 1989, a strain of Ebola virus appeared in Reston, Virginia, just a short distance from Washington, DC. One hundred monkeys had arrived at the Reston Primate Quarantine Unit from the coastal forests of the Philippines on October 4. Two monkeys were dead on arrival and 10 more died during the next few days. Contrary to all expectations, the illness spread to the unit's non-Philippine monkeys. Samples of monkey tissue were sent to the U.S.

Army Medical Research Institute of Infectious Diseases for examination. Their tests proved positive for Ebola Zaire. The investigation quickly became a potentially volatile political crisis. The quarantine unit was a hot zone containing an organism classified as "biosafety level four": one for which no cure or vaccine existed.

In what has to be considered as an extraordinary piece of luck, this strain of Ebola virus, even though it appeared identical to the lethal form of Ebola Zaire, was harmless to humans. As it appeared to be spread among the monkeys via the air, if that virus was the lethal form of Ebola, the consequences for this heavily populated area of the Eastern Coast would have been unimaginably horrific.

Class Discussion: In what ways would the entire United States and other countries have been affected?

ORIGIN AND TRANSMISSION

Beginning 1998, a natural host of the Ebola virus has not been identified, though similar viruses are carried by monkeys and rodents. With respect to transmission, Ebola is believed to be spread primarily through an exchange of body fluids and secretions, not casual contact. Most of those infected with Ebola have high fevers and bleed to death from hemorrhaging. There is no treatment or vaccine. Peter Piot said the Zairian hospital where he discovered Ebola in 1976 had 120 beds and only three syringes to inject 300 to 600 patients per day, sometimes for weeks on end. That same year, 274 of 300 infected people died in an Ebola outbreak in one Zairian village. Because Ebola is lethal so quickly, it is ill-suited to sustain an epidemic. **It kills the infected so quickly they don't have an opportunity to transmit the virus to others.** This is why in each of the seven outbreaks in population-dense areas the epidemics were short-lived.

SOME OTHER LETHAL VIRUSES THAT INFECT HUMANS

Ebola is just one of a number of viruses to have emerged from the jungle in the past few decades; others include **Lassa** and **Marburg** viruses in Africa; **Sabía**, **Junin**, and **Machupo** viruses in South America; in 1995 a virus, yet to be named,

———— BOX I.1 *(continued)* ————

was found, in Brazil, to cause lung destruction and death; and the AIDS virus. HIV probably originated in Africa, but unlike Ebola, it is ideally suited to spread around the globe. The HIV-infected can remain symptom-free for years, which provides the opportunity for them to infect others.

Are there other viruses as dangerous as HIV—or even more dangerous—lurking on the edge of civilization? That's the question that haunts public health officials. In the most recent science fiction-like laboratory scare on August 8, 1994, a scientist at the Yale Arbovirus Research Unit became infected with Sabia. The newly emerging insect-borne virus that had been dis-

covered in Brazil only 2 years earlier. The scientist inhaled virus material from a leaking plastic centrifuge tube. An inquiry by the Centers for Disease Control and Prevention (CDC) charged the researcher with misconduct and the unit with poor emergency response protocols.

[HORTON, RICHARD. (1995). *Infection: The Global Threat.* New York: Reviews April 6, 24–28].

Class Question: Should the public be informed about the dangers of research on viruses lethal to humans before it is allowed to begin?, to continue?

---

the first 3 to 5 years of life. A high priority has therefore been placed on the generation of a safe and effective vaccine.

Some 29 newly identified disease-causing agents have emerged over the past 25 years, and 6 old diseases are re-emerging: TB, diphtheria, cholera, dengue fever, yellow fever, and bubonic plague. The world is not becoming a safer place in which to live. More people are crowding into cities and humans continue to intrude into once remote areas. Clearly some diseases are more lethal than others and AIDS may be the most lethal of all "new" diseases to strike humans in the 20th century.

SILENT TRAVELERS

In 1962, Sir MacFarlane Burnet, the 1960 Nobel Prize recipient for his work on immunological tolerance, wrote, ". . . one can think of the middle of the 20th century as the end of one of the most important social events in history, **the virtual elimination of the infectious disease as a significant factor in social life.**" This statement represents the complacency that developed in the United States and some other countries in regard to threats to the human race posed by the microbial world. More recently, Joshua Lederberg, president of the Rockefeller University from 1978 to 1990, wrote, "The ravaging epidemic of AIDS has shocked the world ... **We will face similar catastrophes again** . . . We have too many illusions

that we can . . . govern the remaining vital kingdoms, the microbes, that remain our competitors of last resort for domination of the planet." This statement represents a more realistic assessment of the current situation, by recognizing the fact that improvements in sanitation and introduction of antimicrobial agents and vaccines **have failed to eliminate the health risks from exposure to infectious agents**.

In *Harrison's Principles of Internal Medicine*, which was published a little more than a decade ago, Margaret Winker wrote that "infectious diseases are more easily prevented and more easily cured than any other major group of disorders. . . ." A new disease called "acquired deficiency of cell-mediated immunity in young homosexual men" occupied less than a column of text. "Slim's disease," recognized possibly as early as 1952, did not warrant an entry, but the dramatic decline in tuberculosis seen during the previous decade was noted to have "leveled off." This complacency allowed a greater focus on heart disease and cancer. Ten years later, cardiovascular disease mortality has declined, and much of the public knows that high cholesterol and blood pressure should be controlled. **Infectious disease, meanwhile, has climbed to the third leading cause of death in the United States.**

Since the 1980s, we have come to view infectious diseases with a humbler eye. The victories of a quarter century ago ring hollow as AIDS ravages, enterococci (disease-causing bacteria) become resistant to all standard treatments, and the once easily treated pneumococcus demonstrates antimicrobial drug resistance. Unknown diseases develop with uncomforting frequency, and the Ebola virus has been identified outside the confines of Zaire. Once considered unique and isolated, these events penetrate every corner of the globe. As was recognized in 1892 when the first international sanitary convention on cholera was adopted, infectious diseases cannot be observed, battled, or understood street by street or country by country. A global approach is necessary [WINKER, M.A., et al. (1996). Infectious diseases: a global approach to a global problem. *JAMA*, 275:245–246].

Infectious diseases are still mankind's leading causes of death, killing about half of the 52 million people worldwide who die every year. We tend to forget that long-known infections such as TB, measles, malaria, infant diarrhea, and respiratory infections remain at the top of the list. They are most dangerous in developing nations, but some of them are now re-emerging in the United States and other industrialized countries.

Far from being invulnerable, humans are in fact at the mercy of innumerable microscopic agents that can erupt at any time by mutating (changing) into a virulent form, crossing a species barrier, or escaping from an environmental niche.

There have been some great achievements in the battle against these microbes. Yet the only complete victory over any infectious disease so far has been the eradication of smallpox. However, one of the early achievements in the approaching millennium will be the global eradication of poliomyelitis. Polio eradication will eliminate disease, reduce disability, and produce direct savings of at least $1.5 billion per year [HULL, HARRY. (1997). Pax Polio. *Science*, 275:40–41]. And during 1998, a new malaria vaccine shown to be 80% effective in small-scale testing will be field tested in Africa. Malaria kills 1 in 5 children in Africa, Southeast Asia, and Central America.

["Emerging Infectious Diseases: Reduce the Risk" was the theme in the United States for World Health Day, April 7, 1997. The day focused on challenges associated with emerg-ing, re-emerging, and drug-resistant infections. Infectious diseases remain the world's leading cause of death.]**

VIRUS ASSOCIATED WITH CANCERS AND OTHER KNOWN DISEASES

In the mid- to late 1980s, numerous correlations were discovered between viruses and various types of cancers. For example, Epstein-Barr virus was associated with nasopharyngeal carcinoma and B-cell lymphoma, hepatitis B virus with liver cancer, and human papillomavirus with cervical cancer. Now, a decade later, scientists are finding out that viruses may also play a role in an array of other diseases, like atherosclerosis and diabetes, as well as such mental disorders as schizophrenia. Additional connections will be made between viruses and many types of diseases in the future because virologists are turning their attention more and more to diseases to which there is no known cause.

AIDS: ITS PLACE IN HISTORY

As the statistics on AIDS cases mounted, its identity as an inescapable plague seemed confirmed. It appeared to mimic the frightening epidemics of the past: cholera, yellow fever, leprosy, syphilis, and the Black Death. The history of AIDS—the history that seemed relevant to understanding the new pandemic—would be the history of the epidemics of the past. Medical history suddenly gained new social relevance; policy analysts, lawyers, and journalists all wanted to know whether past epidemics could provide some clues to the current crisis. How had societies attempted to deal with epidemics in the past? The contemporary meaning of past plagues was read in the face of AIDS.

The AIDS pandemic is certainly one of the defining events of our time. There are stories to be told from it, stories of the people infected and affected by it—the well, the ill, the dying, and the survivors. And there are the stories of scientific discovery, of the human immunodeficiency virus (HIV) and viral mechanisms, and of genetic mysteries being understood. And then there are stories of scientific politics, claims and counterclaims, and the manipulating that goes on in the stratosphere of high-level science.

"A third of the world died," wrote Jean Froissart at the end of the 14th century, when medieval medicine had little to offer against the Black Death. Now, at the end of the 20th century, we see modern science registering its progress about a plague of our own time.

AIDS is the most dramatic, pervasive, and tragic pandemic in recent history. So deep an impression has the AIDS epidemic made on public perceptions that according to a Louis Harris poll in 1994, almost 30% of the population now believes that the "greatest threat to human life" is AIDS or some other kind of plague. The HIV/AIDS pandemic consists of two parts: one medical, the other social. HIV/AIDS infection has provoked a reassessment of society's approaches to public health strategy, health care resource allocation, medical research, and sexual behavior. Fear and discrimination have affected virtually every aspect of our culture. Both the medical challenge and, in particular, the social challenge will continue in the foreseeable future. Arthur Ashe, a world-class tennis player, so feared discrimination against himself and family that he lived with AIDS for $3^{1}/_{2}$ years before he was forced to reveal he had AIDS (Figure I-1).

Fear and Ignorance About AIDS and Other Pandemics

The fear of HIV infection and the ignorance about its causes have created bizarre behavior and at times barbaric practices, strange rituals, and the attempt to isolate those afflicted.

The Black Plague during its most destructive time killed over 500 people a day. Instead of being concerned about providing care to the victims, people spent their time deciding how deep to dig the graves so that none of the horrid fumes would come up and infect others. It was determined that a grave should be six feet deep; and that is exactly how deep it is today. Plague victims were herded together into cathedrals to die or to pray for faith healing to save them. In 14th century Germany and Switzerland, the Christians blamed the Jews for

FIGURE I-1 Arthur Ashe—Winner of Two United States Tennis Championships. On April 8, 1992 Ashe announced that he had AIDS. He died on February 6, 1993 at age 49. He became infected with HIV from a blood transfusion during heart bypass surgery in 1983. In 1988 his right hand suddenly became numb. Brain surgery revealed a brain abscess caused by toxoplasmosis. He asked two questions, "Why do bad things happen to good people?" and "Is the world a friendly place?" Ashe was the United States Davis Cup Captain for 5 years and supported the NCAA Proposition 42 academic requirements for athletes. In 1975 he became the first black to win a Wimbledon men's title. After learning that he had AIDS, Ashe completed his third book, *A Road to Glory*, a three-volume history of black athletes in the United States. (*Photograph courtesy of AP/Wide World Photos*)

the outbreak of bubonic plague, believing that the Jews were poisoning the water—the very same water that the Jews were drinking. As a result, whole communities of Jews were slaughtered. And in the 1400s and 1500s, when syphilis was spreading across the world killing thousands, the Italians called it the French disease. Of course, the French called it the Italian disease. In the 1930s, cholera was considered a punishment for people unwilling to change their lives—the poor and the immoral. In New York the Irish were blamed. In the early 20th century, polio in America was believed to be caused by Italian immigrants.

Deaths from Disease: Polio, Smallpox, Measles, and Bubonic Plague

Four agents of disease, the poliovirus, smallpox virus, measles virus, and the bubonic plague bacterium are responsible for hundreds of millions of human deaths throughout history. The population of the indigenous Indians of Central and South America dropped from an estimated 130 million to about 1.6 million, more as a result of measles and plague than from war. In the 19th century measles has been held to have been responsible for the total annihilation of the Indian population of the island of Tierra del Fuego. Plague swept through Europe in the 14th century destroying a quarter of Europe's population. Between 1600 and 1650 the population of Italy actually fell from 13.1 million to 11.4 million. In Venice, an average of 600 bodies were collected daily on barges. More than 50,000 Venetians died in the plague of 1630-1631, leaving a population smaller than at any time during the 15th century. The most recent outbreak of bubonic plague occurred in India in August of 1994.

The smallpox and polio viruses may well go back to the early beginnings of humans but would have mostly been concealed by the enhanced susceptibility of those infected to more common (or more recognizable) infections. Childhood leukemia, apparently newly emergent in the 1950s, was similarly an artifact of the widespread use of antibiotics for the treatment of the infections from which leukemic people previously died.

Worldwide, smallpox killed over 100 million people by 1725. Smallpox is the only viral disease ever eradicated. The World Health Organization says that the polio virus may also be eliminated from the human population early in the next century, if not sooner. The smallpox death of Egyptian pharaoh Ramses V in 1157 B.C. is the first known. Invading armies then spread smallpox through Africa and Europe. The Spanish brought it to Mexico. Edward Jenner discovered a virus related to smallpox and created a vaccine in the 1870s. Only humans got smallpox. It disappeared after a global vaccination campaign in the 1960s. The last known natural case was in Somalia in 1977.

Influenza

Each year as winter approaches, millions of shots of influenza (flu) vaccine are given, mainly to people who are especially susceptible to the virus (the very young, the elderly, asthmatics, and diabetics). The vaccine is a cocktail of recent influenza A and B strains and affords some protection against genetic changes in these vaccine strains. Nevertheless, in recent history thousands have died from influenza infection; in the 1957–1958 epidemic, for instance, 1 in 300 over age 65 died. There is evidence that the flu virus has been with us since 430 B.C. But in 1890 in China, the duck-borne virus crossed over into swine, then into humans, causing thousands of deaths. This epidemic was followed by severe flu epidemics in 1900, 1918 (the Spanish flu), 1957 (the Asian flu), and 1968 (the Hong Kong flu). The flu epidemic of 1918 and 1919 caused between 20 and 50 million deaths worldwide. Six hundred thousand people died in the United States during this brief interval at an economic cost of $100 billion. This virus was antigenically similar to the swine virus and it appears to have disappeared from the human population following the 1918–1919 pandemic. This virus is, however, still carried in the swine population with an occasional crossover into humans without person-to-person transmission. Why such widespread transmission of the swine virus among humans has not reoccurred is not known—and that in itself is fearful! It could happen again, even though there is a vaccine. During the epidemic of 1918, in San Francisco, all citizens were required to wear masks. One form of therapy was "cabbage baths." People did not jump into a tub with some cooked cabbage; they ate the cabbage and urinated into the tub. The flu victims then got into the tub. There may have been a positive side to the bath because once you got out, a distance was created between you and other people. In this way, the baths may have helped stop person-to-person transmission.

The incidence of influenza-related deaths in the United States currently ranges from about 10,000 in years with low influenza activity to more than 40,000 in more severe influenza epidemics [Researchers seek new weapon against flu. (1997). *Science*, 275:756; Influenza 1994–1995: Now's the time to prepare. (1994). *J. Resp. Dis.*, 15:675].

Tuberculosis, Hepatitis B, and Malaria

In 1937, 112,000 Americans contracted tuberculosis and 70,000 died. About one billion people worldwide have died from Mycobacterium tuberculosis (a bacterium 1/25,000th of an inch long) since 1970. One in three people worldwide carry this organism! Currently, about 10 million people in the United States are infected with TB, but only 5% develop the disease. In 1997, over 2 million adults worldwide died of hepatitis B and of the 44 million children who contracted measles, 1.5 million died. Four thousand people die every day from malaria. Parents and children quietly cope; the ill were and are served, not shunned—that is, until the HIV/AIDS epidemic. The nine leading causes of death due to bacterial, protozoal or viral infections are given in Table I-2.

OVERVIEW ON HIV/AIDS

What Is AIDS?

AIDS is defined primarily by severe immune deficiency, and is distinguished from virtually every other disease in history by the fact that it has no constant, specific symptoms. Once the immune system has begun to malfunction, a broad spectrum of health complications can set in. AIDS is an umbrella term for any or all

TABLE I-2 Microbes Causing Most Deaths Worldwide, 1997

Infectious disease	Cause	Annual Deaths
Acute respiratory infections (mostly pneumonia)	Bacterial or viral	4,400,000
Diarrheal diseases	Bacterial or viral	3,200,000
Tuberculosis	Bacterial	3,100,000
Hepatitis B	Viral	2,000,000
Malaria	Protozoan	3100,000
Measles	Viral	1,500,000
Neonatal tetanus	Bacterial	600,000
AIDS	Viral	1,000,000
Pertussis (whooping cough)	Bacterial	360,000

Sources: World Health Organization; Harvard School of Public Health.

of some 26 known diseases and symptoms. When a person has any of these diseases or has a T4 lymphocyte count of less than 200/μL of blood and also tests positive for antibodies to HIV, an AIDS diagnosis is given.

Who Are the Most Likely to Become HIV-Infected?

When all things are held equal, the most important identifying variable is income. Regardless of race, orientation, or language, those in the lower economic brackets are more likely to become HIV-infected. As the pandemic spreads, it is becoming more of a disease that can affect any person regardless of sexual preference or race, but in particular it is becoming more of a disease of the poor, the group within any society that has inadequate access to health care. As the pandemic increases globally, it is becoming more of a disease of the underdeveloped nations. **And where HIV is becoming more a disease of heterosexuals, it is also becoming a disease of women, because transmission to women from heterosexual contact is easier than for men** (see Chapter 11). Also, remember that women are disproportionately represented among those living in poverty anywhere in the world.

The impact of this pandemic is unique. Unlike malaria or polio, previous modern pandemics, it mostly affects young and middle-aged adults. This is not only the sexually most

WHY ALL THE FUSS ABOUT HIV/AIDS?

So it is now, after 17 years, killing **1 million** people a year worldwide. But what of the other diseases, and how many people are they killing each year? Respiratory infections, **over 4 million**; diarrheal diseases, **over 3 million**; TB, **over 3 million**; hepatitis B infection, **over 2 million**; measles, **about 1.5 million**; malaria, **over 2 million**; and there are about **12 to 15 million** who die each year from cardiovascular diseases! **So, why is HIV/AIDS recognized or believed to be a larger threat?**

First, this virus is mainly transmitted during sexual intercourse. Since few human societies talk openly and honestly about sex, this makes this disease difficult to discuss; and since sex is a very private activity, it makes the transmission of HIV very difficult to control.

Second, it has an extraordinary capacity for change and rapid global spread. Through 1998, an estimated 9 million people will have died of AIDS worldwide; by the end of the century this figure is expected to be at least 11 million. Malaria, TB, heart disease, cancer: no other disease is spreading or growing at this rate. And in spite of HIV/AIDS campaigns in most countries, there is little evidence so far of any slowdown in the **spread** of the epidemic. By the end of the century, over 40 million people are expected to have been infected by HIV.

Third, there is a long asymptomatic period between infection and illness. On average, it takes about 10 to 12 years for someone infected with HIV to develop AIDS. During this time, the HIV-infected will show few if any recognizable symptoms, but he or she will be able to infect other people.

This long asymptomatic period is **rare in human infectious diseases**. The long asymptomatic period that occurs between cause and effect has, for years, made it difficult to persuade individuals or governments to take the pandemic seriously. People **dying** today represent those infected 10 to 20 years ago; the results of anything

we do now to reduce transmission will not be apparent until the next century.

Fourth, HIV/AIDS is more serious than many more common diseases **because of the age groups it attacks**. Some diseases—measles and diarrhoea, for example—affect mainly **infants and children**; others, such as heart disease and cancer, **affect mainly the old**. But because HIV is predominantly transmitted sexually, AIDS mainly kills people in **their 20s through their 40s**. A major increase in deaths among these age groups, the most productive section of society, presents a much greater impact socially and economically than deaths that occur among children or old people would have.

Fifth, in the past, plagues were often marked by their lack of discrimination, by the way in which they killed large numbers of people with little regard for race, wealth, sex, or religion. **But AIDS was different from the beginning.** It immediately presented a **political as much as a public-health problem**. Homosexuals, who until this pandemic had been mostly closeted in the United States, were suddenly at the heart of a health crisis as profound as any in modern American history.

Sixth, with respect to therapy, HIV disease/AIDS requires the use of some of the most **expensive** and **toxic drugs** in medical history.

So why all the fuss about HIV/AIDS? It is caused by a **unique virus** that **changes itself faster** than a rumor making the gossip column of a tabloid. It is lethal, it is transmitted, most often sexually, it affects people in their reproductive and most productive years, it is exceptionally expensive to treat, it defies our best scientists who are working to create a vaccine for preventing infection and transmission, and it is a disease that has severely stigmatized those who have it. And lastly, it has awakened our most primal fear, that of dying a horrible death caused by unknown agents—**this new virus means there are others in waiting.**

HIV HAS BUT ONE REQUIREMENT TO CONTINUE ITS PRESENCE ON EARTH: A HUMAN HOST!

active years for individuals, but also their prime productive and reproductive years. Thus the impact of HIV/AIDS is demographic, economic, political, and social. HIV/AIDS is a disease of human groups and its demographic and social impacts multiply from the infected individual to the group. In the most affected areas, infant, child, and adult mortality is rising and life expectancy at birth is declining rapidly. The cost of medical care for each infected person overwhelms individuals and households.

Acquired Immune Deficiency Syndrome (AIDS), first identified in 1981, is the final stage of a viral infection caused by the Human Immunodeficiency Virus (HIV). Medical experts recognize two strains: HIV-1, discovered in 1983, which is generally accepted as the cause of most AIDS cases throughout the world; and HIV-2, discovered in West Africa in 1986 and later found in some former Portuguese colonies elsewhere and in Europe. **HIV is a retrovirus: a virus that inserts—probably for life—its genetic material into the genetic material of the host cells at the time of the infection**. Inasmuch as the ability to remove genetic material from cells is beyond the capability of current medical science, the infection may be said to be **incurable**. AIDS is characterized by a profound loss of cell-mediated immune function and the depletion of a special kind of white blood cell called a **CD4 or T4 lymphocyte**.

AIDS: A CAUSE OF DEATH

AIDS is now the seventh leading cause of death among 1- to 4-year-olds, sixth among 15- to 24-year-olds, and second among 25- to 44-year-olds in the United States.

There is the expectation that parents will die before their children. Because of the HIV/AIDS epidemic, it is not working out that way for many thousands of parents. They are watching their children die in the prime of life.

The facts on HIV infection, disease, and AIDS that are presented in the following chapters, when understood, clearly place the responsibility for avoiding HIV infection on *YOU*. You must assess your lifestyle; if you choose not to be abstinent, you must know about your sexual partner and you must practice safer sex. **Never think that you are immune to HIV infection.**

June 5, 1997 marked the beginning of the 16th year of the AIDS pandemic. No cure has been found and, although AIDS is now christened the "manageable illness," people who are sick must make endless compromises to this disease. The AIDS pandemic forces people to face their mortality daily, for months and years.

FIRST REPORTS ON AIDS CASES IN THE UNITED STATES

On June 5, 1981, the first cases of the illness now known as acquired immunodeficiency syndrome were reported from Los Angeles in five young homosexual men diagnosed with *Pneumocystis carinii* pneumonia and other opportunistic infections.

Initially, AIDS appeared among homosexual males; most frequently those who had many sex partners. Further study of the gay population led to the conclusion that the agent responsible for AIDS was being transmitted through sexual activities. In 1982, cases of AIDS were reported among hemophiliacs, people who had received blood transfusions, and injection drug users. These reports all had one thing in common—an exchange of body fluids, in particular blood or semen, was involved. In January 1983, the first cases of AIDS in heterosexuals were documented. Two females, both sexual partners of IDUs, became AIDS patients. This was clear evidence that the infectious agent could be transmitted from male to female as well as from male to male. Later in 1983, cases of AIDS were reported in Central Africa, but with a difference. The vast majority of African AIDS cases were among heterosexuals **who did *not* use injection drugs**. These data supported the earlier findings from the American homosexual population: that AIDS is primarily a sexually transmitted disease. And the risk for contracting AIDS increased with the number of sex partners one had and the sexual behaviors of those partners. Thus early empirical observations on which kinds of social behavior placed one at greatest risk of acquiring AIDS were later supported by surveillance surveys, testing, and analysis.

THE EDUCATIONAL COMMUNITY

Like most complex problems, the AIDS epidemic poses special problems for educators. One of the most disturbing is discrimination against the HIV-infected. People worldwide have from the very beginning of the AIDS pandemic learned to **categorize**, **rationalize**, **stigmatize**, and "**persecutize**" those with HIV disease and AIDS. Perhaps the worst display of stigmatization and discrimination occurs against children, especially those of school age. Guidelines from the U.S. Surgeon General, federal and state health officials, and the medical community have not calmed the fears of misinformed parents. Many stories have made headlines and television news concerning children who have been barred from attending school. While the courts can order admission, they cannot assure peer and adult acceptance. Persuasion must come through a better understanding of the disease. Parents can be reassured through reminders that HIV/AIDS is not transmitted by casual contact. Students must also be educated about HIV/AIDS. The following Gallup Poll results (Table I-3), although taken in 1988, are about what one would still find true in 1997.

Since the latter half of the 1980s, schools throughout the United States have been offering education programs to teach adolescents about human immunodeficiency virus (HIV) infection. Beginning 1997, 40 states required HIV/AIDS education for adolescents (40 states offered some HIV/AIDS education in their elementary schools). However, the effect of such programs on HIV-related knowledge and behavior among adolescents is largely unknown.

------- POINT OF VIEW I.2 -------

SILENCE = DEATH: SILENCE AND STIGMA

The silence comes because we are talking about sex, we are talking about needles and injection drug use—things we are not good at talking about as a community. But silence is also perpetuating this pandemic, and it must be talked about everywhere, by everyone! By the time former president Ronald Reagan gave his **first** speech on the AIDS crisis in America, hundreds of thousands of Americans were HIV-infected, 36,000 men, women, and children had been diagnosed with AIDS, and over 25,000 had died of AIDS—the year, 1987!

TABLE I-3 1988 Gallup Poll Results on Age Related HIV/AIDS School Education

	National Totals %	Public School Parents %	Non-Public School Parents %

The Gallup Poll asked those who favored having public schools developed an HIV education program (90% of all respondents) the following questions:

At what age should students begin participating in an HIV education program?

Under 5 years	6	5	11
5–9 years	40	43	42
10–12 years	40	39	32
13–15 years	10	11	13
16 years or older	1	1	1
Don't know	3	1	1

Should public schools teach what is called "safer sex" for HIV prevention? (This was understood to mean teaching about the use of condoms.)

Should	78	81	72
Should not	16	16	25
Don't know	6	3	3

Source: 20th Annual Gallup Poll on the Public's Attitudes Toward the Public Schools.

WORLD INTERNATIONAL AIDS CONFERENCES

The International AIDS Conference has been the timepiece of the pandemic. The venue, content, style, and mood of each meeting temporarily freezes in time the state of the worldwide HIV/AIDS pandemic.

In 1983, there were relatively so few groups involved with HIV/AIDS research that they could stay in contact by telephone. As the virus spread many countries became involved in HIV/AIDS research and clinical care. International, national and state meetings were formed as a way to exchange new information. The international meetings continue to receive the most press coverage. Since the first international AIDS conference in 1985, the conferences have grown in size to the point that scientists are questioning their usefulness. As of 1994, the International Conference on AIDS will be held every 2 years. Some idea of the size increase can be gained by comparing the first and eleventh meetings:

The First International Conference on AIDS, Atlanta, 1985:

♦ Number of AIDS cases 9,608, USA
♦ Number of deaths 4,712, USA
♦ Number of Delegates 2,000

The Eleventh International Conference on AIDS, Vancouver, British Columbia, July 7–12, 1996:

♦ Number of AIDS cases: 554,000 USA
♦ Number of Deaths: 339,000 USA
♦ Number of Delegates: 14,137

The Eleventh International Conference on AIDS took place under the banner, One World–One Hope. The deep pessimism that held stage during the Tenth International Conference on AIDS in 1994, because researchers appeared to be far from producing effective HIV drugs for therapy or a preventive vaccine, gave way to a kind of euphoric optimism at the Eleventh Conference, spurred on by (**1**) the latest successful clinical trial results using combination drug therapies to block HIV replication, (**2**) the announcement of large reductions of HIV (viral load) in the blood of HIV-infected people using new drugs called protease inhibitors (Figure I-2), and (**3**) Robert Gallo's announcement of evidence showing that a newly discovered chemokine receptor plays a crucial role in HIV's ability to infect macrophage and T4 cells. Gallo's hope is that this work will lead to the development of inexpensive, synthetic blockers of chemokine receptors that can be used for HIV therapy with little to no side effects. Peter Piot, head

FIGURE I-2   Dr. David Ho, Eleventh International HIV/AIDS Conference, Vancouver, BC, July 11, 1996. Dr. Ho, a leading AIDS researcher from the Diamond AIDS Research Centre in New York is speaking about the recent success in reducing viral load using protease inhibitors and combination drug therapy. His pioneering efforts, using new HIV/AIDS drugs, have helped lift a death sentence—for a few years at least, and perhaps longer—on tens of thousands of AIDS sufferers. He asked the question, **"Can HIV be eradicated from the body?"** With this single question based on his research, he **galvanized** the AIDS community. David Da-i Ho was *Time's* Man of the Year for 1996. (*Photograph courtesy of REUTERS/Jeff Vinnick/Archive Photos*)

——— BOX I.2 ———

MARY D. FISHER SPEAKS ABOUT AIDS AT THE 1992 REPUBLICAN NATIONAL CONVENTION (Figure I–3)

I bear a message of challenge, not self-congratulation. I want your attention, not your applause. I would never have asked to be HIV-positive. But I believe that in all things there is a good purpose, and so I stand before you, and before the nation, gladly.

The reality of AIDS is brutally clear. Two hundred thousand Americans are dead or dying; a million more are infected. Worldwide, 40 million, or 60 million, or 100 million infections will be counted in the coming few years. But despite science and research, White House meetings and congressional hearings, despite good intentions and bold initiatives, campaign slogans, and hopeful promises—despite it all, it's the epidemic which is winning tonight.

In the context of an election year, I ask you—here, in this great hall, or listening in the quiet of your home—to recognize that the AIDS virus is not a political creature. It does not care whether you are Democrat or Republican. It does not ask whether you are black or white, male or female, gay or straight, young or old.

Tonight, I represent an AIDS community whose members have been reluctantly drafted from every segment of American society. Though I am white, and a mother, I am one with a black infant struggling with tubes in a Philadelphia hospital. Though I am female, and contracted this disease in marriage, and enjoy the warm support of my family, I am one with the lonely gay man sheltering a flickering candle from the cold wind of his family's rejection.

This is not a distant threat; it is a present danger. The rate of infection is increasing fastest among women and children. Largely unknown a decade ago, AIDS is the third leading killer of

FIGURE I-3 Mary Fisher, age 44, addressed the delegates at the 1992 Republican National Convention. Fisher, previously diagnosed with AIDS, called the disease a "present danger" that leaves no one safe. She also called for compassion in place of ignorance and silence. She said, **"The virus asks only one question: Are you human?"** (*Photograph courtesy of REUTERS/ Steven Jaffe/Archive Photos*)

young adult Americans today—but it won't be third for long. Because, unlike other diseases, this one travels. Adolescents don't give each other cancer or heart disease because they believe they are in love. But HIV is different. And we have helped it along—we have killed each other—with our ignorance, our prejudice, and our silence.

We may take refuge in our stereotypes, but we cannot hide there for long. Because HIV asks only one thing of those it attacks: Are you human? And in this is the right question: Are you human?

Because people with HIV have not entered some alien state of being. They are human. They have not earned cruelty and they do not deserve meanness. They don't benefit from being isolated or treated as outcasts. Every one of them is exactly what God made: a person. Not evil, deserving our judgment; not victims, longing for our pity. People. Ready for support and worthy of our compassion.

My call to the nation is a plea for awareness. If you believe you are safe, you are in danger. Because I was not hemophiliac, I was not at risk. Because I did not inject drugs, I was not at risk. My father has devoted much of his lifetime to guarding against another holocaust. He is part of the generation who heard Pastor Neimoller come out of the Nazi death camps to say, "They came after the Jews and I was not a Jew, so I did not protest. They came after the Trade Unionists, and I was not a Trade Unionist, so I did not protest. They came after the Roman Catholics, and I was not a Roman Catholic, so I did not protest. Then they came after me, and there was no one left to protest."

The lesson history teaches is this: If you believe you are safe, you are at risk. If you do not

——————— **BOX I.2** (*continued*) ———————

see this killer stalking your children, look again. There is no family or community, no race or religion, no place left in America that is safe. Until we genuinely embrace this message, we are a nation at risk.

Tonight, HIV marches resolutely towards AIDS in more than a million American homes, littering its pathway with the bodies of the young. Young men. Young women. Young parents. Young children. One of the families is mine. If it is true that HIV inevitably turns to AIDS, then my children will inevitably turn to orphans.

My family has been a rock of support. My 84-year-old father, who has pursued the healing of the nations, will not accept the premise that he cannot heal his daughter. My mother has refused to be broken; she still calls at midnight to tell wonderful jokes that make us laugh. Sisters and friends, and my brother Philip (whose birthday is today)—all have helped carry me over the hardest places. I am blessed, rich and deeply blessed, to have such a family.

But not all of you have been so blessed. You are HIV seropositive but dare not say it. You have lost loved ones, but you dare not whisper the word AIDS. You weep silently, you grieve alone.

I have a message for you: It is not you who should feel shame. It is we. We who tolerate ignorance and practice prejudice, we who have taught you to fear. We must lift our shroud of silence, making it safe for you to reach out for compassion. It is our task to seek safety for our children, not in quiet denial, but in effective action.

Some day our children will be grown. My son Max, now four, will take the measure of his mother; my son Zachary, now two, will sort through his memories. I may not be here to hear their judgments, but I know already what I hope they are.

I want my children to know that their mother was not a victim. She was a messenger. I do not want them to think, as I once did, that courage is the absence of fear; I want them to know that courage is the strength to act wisely when most we are afraid. I want them to have the courage to step forward when called by their nation, or their Party, and give leadership, no matter what the personal cost. I ask no more of you than I ask of myself, or my children.

To the millions of you who are grieving, who are frightened, who have suffered the ravages of AIDS firsthand: Have courage and you will find comfort.

To the millions who are strong, I issue the plea: Set aside prejudice and politics to make room for compassion and sound policy.

To my children, I make this pledge:
I will not give in, Zachary, because I draw my courage from you. Your silly giggle gives me hope. Your gentle prayers give me strength. And you, my child, give me reason to say to America, "You are at risk."

And I will not rest, Max, until I have done all I can to make your world safe. I will seek a place where intimacy is not the prelude to suffering.

I will not hurry to leave you, my children. But when I go, pray that you will not suffer shame on my account.

To all within the sound of my voice, I appeal: Learn with me the lessons of history and grace, so my children will not be afraid to say the word AIDS when I am gone. Then their children, and yours, may not need to whisper it at all.

God bless the children, and bless us all—and good night.

---

of UNAIDS, said "nobody can call AIDS an inevitably fatal, incurable disease anymore." Implying that AIDS is curable at the moment, however, is wishful thinking rather than scientific fact. During the 7 days of this meeting an estimated 60,000 people became HIV-infected worldwide and 24,932 died of AIDS (Figure I-4).

The Twelfth International Conference on AIDS, will take place in Geneva, Switzerland on June 28–July 3, 1998.

THE AIDS MEMORIAL QUILT

The purpose of the quilt is to educate. The "AIDS Quilt" is made up of individual fabric

FIGURE I-4 Peter Piot of Belgium, Director of the United Nations Program on AIDS (UNAIDS), addressing a news conference on upcoming anti-AIDS vaccine trials in Brazil and Thailand during 1997. (*Photograph courtesy of Archive Photos*)

ered an area larger than two football fields and it took less than 2 hours to read all the names. In 1992 it took 60 hours. By mid-1994, the quilt contained over 28,000 panels bearing over 40,000 names, required over 30 acres to lay out and weighed 28 tons. As of mid-1996 the quilt weighed 45 tons with 45,000 panels about 77,000 names. Displayed in its entirety, it will stretch the length of 12 football fields. It is the largest piece of folk art in the world and continues to increase in size daily. The quilt was the idea of Cleve Jones, of San Francisco, who in 1985 feared AIDS would become known for the number of people it killed. He wanted a way of remembering the people, who were, in many cases, his friends. There are about 50 miles of seams and 26 miles of canvas edging. There are panels from each of the 50 states. Each day new panels arrive from across the United States and 29 foreign countries to be added to the quilt (Figure I-5). For those left behind, the panels represent an expression of love and a sign of grief—a part of the healing process (Figure I-6). A few of the well-known people who have died of AIDS are seen in Figures I-7 through I-10.

panels, each the size of a grave, measuring three feet by six feet, stitched together. In October 1987, the AIDS quilt was first put on display on the mall in Washington, D.C. At that time it contained 1,920 panels and cov-

FIGURE I-5 Photograph taken of a section of the quilt in July of 1991.

FIGURE I-6 A photograph of a single panel of the quilt taken in July of 1991.

Portions of the quilt tour in major cities. Donations made for viewing the quilt are being used to support local Names Project chapters and their staffs.

Each panel has its own story. The stories are told by those who make the panels for their lost friends, lovers, parents, and children. The complete quilt was displayed in Washington, D.C., October 11–13, 1996 for the last time—it is too large to view again as a whole. It took 10 boxcars and a freight train to transport this work of art to the nation's capital.

Decade of Remembrance

People nationwide celebrated the 10th anniversary of the AIDS Quilt on July 21, 1997.

For more information about the Names Project's AIDS Memorial Quilt, call (415) 882-5500 or write: The NAMES Project Foundation, 310 Townsend St., Suite 310, San Francisco, CA 94107.

For information about your state chapter, contact the Names Project coordinator at (201) 888-1790.

WORLD AIDS DAY

December 1, 1988 was the first acclaimed *World AIDS Day* (WAD). The slogan was *"Join the Worldwide Effort."* World AIDS Day is a day set aside to pay tribute to those who have AIDS and to those who have died of AIDS. Its purpose is to increase our awareness of AIDS. The first WAD did not attract much attention outside the gay community. In 1989, the slogan was *"Our Lives, Our World—Lets Take Care of Each Other."* Artists got together and held the first annual *Day Without Art* to coincide with World AIDS Day. For the second annual Day Without Art/World AIDS Day on December 1, 1990, at least 3,000 art organizations in the United States were involved. They included the Smithsonian Institution as well as small American art galleries and art galleries in Canada, England, France, and The Netherlands.

The second annual Day Without Art/World AIDS Day was commemorated by shrouded sculptures, darkened marquees, and exhibits depicting the loss of life to HIV infection and AIDS. At 8 PM on December 1, 1990, the Manhattan and San Francisco skylines were dimmed for 15 minutes. On Broadway, the marquees were darkened for 1 minute and 23 cable TV stations as well as broadcasts in England, Canada, and Australia were interrupted with a 1-minute announcement about AIDS. (Slogan was "Women and AIDS")

The third annual Day Without Art/World AIDS Day, 1991, was the largest AIDS event ever. The slogan was "Sharing the Challenge." It was intended to underline the global nature of the pandemic and to foster awareness that only by pooling efforts, resources, and imagination can hope prevail against the common threat. Many more people, businesses, and industries became in-

FIGURE I-7 Brad Davis, Film Star (center). Voted best actor by the Foreign Press Associations Golden Globes Awards (1979) for his work in *Midnight Express*. The film was the story of an American imprisoned in Turkey. Brad became HIV-infected through drug use, was diagnosed with AIDS in 1985, and died at age 41 in 1991. (*Photograph courtesy of AP/Wide World Photos*)

volved for the first time. World AIDS Day 1992 adopted the slogan "A Community Commitment." The slogan for World AIDS Day 1993 was "A Time to Act." Topics covered were: fighting denial, discrimination, and complacency; bridging the resource gap; reducing women's vulnerability to infection; prevention; and providing humane care. The slogan for 1994 was "The Global Challenge; AIDS and the Family." World AIDS Day 1995 carried the slogan "Shared Rights, Shares Responsibilities." The meaning is that all people – men, women, children, the poor, minorities, migrants, refugees, sex workers, drug injectors, gay men – have the right to be able to avoid infection, the right to health care if sick with AIDS, and the right to be treated with dignity and without discrimination. For 1996, the slogan was "One World. One Hope." For information on World AIDS Day 1997, write 108 Leonard Street, 13th Floor, New York, NY 10013 or call (212) 513-0303, or world AIDS Day Public Information Office, WHO-GPA, 1211 Geneva 27, Switzerland.

THE WORLD HEALTH ORGANIZATION

The World Health Organization (WHO) has established a global program on HIV infection and AIDS. The program has three objectives: to prevent new HIV infections, to provide support and care to those already infected, and to link international efforts in the fight against HIV infection and AIDS. Beginning 1998, the WHO estimated there will be about 10 million AIDS cases and some 35 million cases of HIV infection worldwide. By the end of 1996, there were 29 million HIV infections and 8 million AIDS cases. Michael Merson, past director of the WHO's Global Program on AIDS, said in a recent interview, "It is very unlikely that the

FIGURE I-8   Rock Hudson, Movie and Television Star. A Hollywood legend and undisclosed homosexual. He was the first major public figure to reveal he had AIDS. The conventional wisdom, expressed by journalist Randy Shilts in 1987 (Figure I-9) is **"that there were two clear phases to the disease in the United States: there was AIDS before Rock Hudson and AIDS after."** This common observation has been confirmed by others who also note that Hudson's 1985 disclosure that he was suffering from AIDS—rather than a change in the character of the epidemic or the introduction of new, substantive information about AIDS—led to a permanent increase in media attention to the disease. Hudson died in 1985 at age 59. (*Photograph courtesy of AP/Wide World Photos*)

global prevalence of HIV infection will stabilize or level off for at least several decades." The WHO estimates that 10 million children and 30 to 40 million adults will be HIV-infected by the year 2000. Merson added, "The global balance of HIV infection is rapidly tipping toward the developing countries. In 1985, somewhere around 50% of the world's total infections, we estimated, were in developing countries. But now we estimate that by the year 2000, 75% to 80% will be in developing countries and by the year 2010, as many as 90%."

In 1995 the United Nations Secretary-General chose Peter Piot to begin a joint United Program on AIDS (UNAIDS). Piot's job is to coordinate actions and reduce dupli-

FIGURE I-10 Wladziu Valentino (Lee) Liberace, Internationally Known Pianist and Entertainer. Died of AIDS February 4, 1987 at the age of 67. (*Photograph courtesy of AP/Wide World Photos*)

FIGURE I-9 Randy Shilts, author of "And The Band Played On" (Viking Penguin Press, 1987), died of AIDS February 17, 1994. (*Photograph courtesy of AP/Wide World Photos*)

cation among the six co-sponsors of UNAIDS: United Nations Children's Fund (UNICEF), the United Nations Development Programme (UNDP), the United Nations Educational, Scientific and Cultural Organization (UNESCO), the United Nations Population Fund (UNFPA), the World Bank, and WHO.

BREAKTHROUGHS OFFER NEW HOPE!

"And hope is brightest when it dawns from fears."—Sir Walter Scott, 1771–1832

Through 1995, the diagnoses of AIDS was a devastating death sentence. Those seeking to treat it seldom uttered the words "AIDS" and "hope" in the same sentence. What a differ-

ence a year can make! In 1996 and through 1997, those terms have become inextricably linked in the minds of researchers and patients. And while the new optimism must be tempered with numerous caveats, 1996 ushered in a series of stunning breakthroughs, both in AIDS treatment and in basic research on HIV.

THERAPY

On the therapeutic side, new drugs called **protease inhibitors** can now dramatically reduce HIV levels in the blood when taken alone or with other antiviral compounds. At the same time, polypeptide molecules called **chemokines** have been unveiled as potent foes of HIV. To enter cells, HIV must bind to cell surface proteins that normally serve as receptors for the chemokines—and people born with defective receptors are immune to HIV infection. This work offers new insight into the pathogenesis of the disease and may one day blossom into new treatment or even vaccines. The years 1998 and 1999 should reveal a new era of hope and success in the fight against HIV/AIDS.

THE FUTURE

The history of HIV/AIDS is one of remarkable scientific achievement. Never in the history of man has so much been learned about so complex an illness in so short a time. We moved into the 1990s with hope and the determination to find better therapies and a vaccine. The task is formidable but it has to be done and it will be accomplished. The evolving story of the HIV/AIDS epidemic has been one of the major medical news events of the past 17 years. It is getting hard to imagine medicine without HIV/AIDS. But we must be careful not to blame this disease on our already failing health care system. As the National Commission on AIDS said:

> The AIDS epidemic did not leave 37 million or more Americans without ways to finance medical care, but it did dramatize their plight. This epidemic did not cause the problems of homelessness—but it has expanded it and made it more visible. The epidemic did not cause the collapse of the health care system— but it has accelerated the disintegration of our public hospitals and intensified their financing problems. The AIDS epidemic did not directly augment problems of substance abuse—but it has made the need for drug treatment for all who request it a matter of urgent national priority.

HIV/AIDS is a truly persistent global epidemic and will require a proportionate response to bring it to heel. It will be the plague of our lifetimes—and probably that of our children's lives as well. **We already have children age 17 and younger who don't know what an HIV-free world is. They were born into this epidemic.** To survive this epidemic, society must prevent the faces from becoming faceless. The chapters on HIV infection, HIV disease, and AIDS in this book will help bring widespread information on the virus into focus. The information within these chapters should also help eliminate many of the myths and irrational fears, or FRAID (fear of AIDS), generated by this disease. There is much work to be done by both scientists and society.

Perhaps a borrowed anecdote says it best:

> As the old man walked the beach at dawn, he noticed a young woman ahead of him picking up starfish and flinging them into the sea. Finally catching up with the youth, he asked her why she was doing this. The answer was that the stranded starfish would die if left to the morning sun.
>
> "But the beach goes on for miles and there are millions of starfish," countered the old man. "How can your effort make any difference?"
>
> The young woman looked at the starfish in her hand and threw it to safety in the waves. "It makes a difference to this one," she said.

(Adapted from *The Unexpected Universe* by Loren Eiseley. Copyright 1969, Harcourt Brace, New York)

Too easily can we become overwhelmed by the enormity of the AIDS pandemic. The numbers of patients and their constant needs have caused many to become paralyzed into inactivity and lulled into indifference. Like the old man, many ask "Why bother?"

For the sake of every individual living with HIV, we must focus on what each one of us can do. Each person can make a difference. Believing this, we are empowered to cope with the larger whole. **WE MUST NOT LET AIDS DICTATE THAT 49 IS OLD AGE AND AGE 39 OUR LIFE EXPECTANCY.**

TOLL-FREE NATIONAL AIDS HOTLINE

♦ For the English-language service (open 24 hours a day, 7 days a week), call 1-800-342-AIDS (2437).

♦ The Spanish service (open from 8 AM to 2 AM, 7 days a week) can be reached at 1-800-344-SIDA (7432).

♦ A TTY service for the hearing impaired is available from 10 AM to 10 PM Monday through Friday at 1-800-243-7889.

- National AIDS Clearinghouse, 1-800-458-5231.
- National HIV Telephone Consultation Service for Health Care Professionals, (800) 933-3413, San Francisco General Hospital, Bldg. 80, Ward 83, Room 314, San Francisco, CA 94110.
- HIV/AIDS Treatment Information Service, (800) HIV-0440 (448-0440), 9 AM- to 7 PM Eastern time, Monday-Friday. (800) 243-7012 Teletype number for the hearing-impaired, 9 AM- to 5 PM Eastern time, Monday-Friday, Box 6303, Rockville, MD 20849-6303.
- AIDS Clinical Trials Information Service, (800) TRIALS-A 874-2572, 9 AM-7 PM Eastern time, Monday-Friday. Information on clinical trials of AIDS therapies.
- National Gay and Lesbian Task Force AIDS Information Hotline (800) 221-7044.
- Gay Men's Health Crisis AIDS Hot Line, (212) 807-6655.
- National HIV/AIDS Education & Training Centers Program, (301) 443-6364, Fax: (301) 443-9887.
- AIDS National Interfaith Network, (202) 546-0807, Fax: (202) 546-5103, 110 Maryland Ave., NE, Room 504, Washington, DC 20002.
- National Hemophilia Foundation, (212) 219-8180, 110 Greene St., Suite 303, New York, NY 10012.
- Pediatric AIDS Foundation, (310) 395-9051.
- National Pediatric HIV Resource Center, 1 (800) 362-0071.
- AIDSLINE via the National Library of Medicine. Free access via Grateful Med, obtained from NLM at (800) 638-8480.
- National Institute on Drug Abuse Hotline, (800) 662-HELP (4357).
- National Sexually Transmitted Diseases Hotline (800) 227-8922.
- American Civil Liberties Union Guide to local chapters, 202-544-1076.
- AIDS Policy and Law, (215) 784-0860.
- National Conference of State Legislatures HIV, STD and Adolescent Health Project, (303) 830-2200.
- United States Conference of Mayors, (202) 293-2352.

- Centers for Disease Control and Prevention, Public Inquiry, (404) 639-3534.
- Food and Drug Administration, Office of Public Affairs, (301) 443-3285.
- American Red Cross, Office of HIV/AIDS Education, 1 (800) 375-2040.
- World Health Organization, (202) 861-4354.

COMPUTER SITES

- AIDS Treatment Data Network, (800) 734-7104, 611 Broadway, Suite 613, New York, NY 10012. http://health.nyam.org:8000/public_html/net work/index:html, e-mail: AIDSTreatD@AOL. COM. A home page on the internet for people with AIDS and their caregivers, it provides information on approved and experimental treatments for AIDS-related conditions. It also publishes a quarterly directory of clinical trials on HIV and AIDS, in English and Spanish.
- AMA HIV/AIDS Information Center, World Wide Web site (http://www.ama-assn.org) offers clinical updates, news, and information on social and policy questions. Cosponsored by Glaxo Wellcome Inc.
- Gay Men's Health Crisis (GMHC), Site on the World Wide Web (http://www.gmhc.org) provides on-line forums hosted by GMHC representatives.

For additional help you may wish to consult with your college or community library. They may have access to the following AIDS-related data bases:

- Aidsline—90,000 references to journals, books, and audiovisuals
- Aidstrials—information on 500 clinic trials of drugs and vaccines
- Aidsdrugs—a dictionary of drugs and experimental chemicals and biological agents against the virus
- Dirline—lists over 2,300 organizations and services that provide public information on HIV disease and AIDS

TOLL-FREE STATE AIDS HOTLINES

For information about HIV-specific resources and counseling and testing services, call your state AIDS hotline:

Alabama	800-228-0469	Montana	800-233-6668
Alaska	800-478-2437	Nebraska	800-782-2437
Arizona	800-548-4695	Nevada	800-842-2437
Arkansas	501-661-2133	New Hampshire	800-324-2437
California (No.)	800-367-2437	New Jersey	800-624-2377
California (So.)	800-922-2437	New Mexico	800-545-2437
Colorado	800-252-2437	New York	800-541-2437
Connecticut	800-342-2437	North Carolina	800-733-7301
Delaware	800-422-0429	North Dakota	800-472-2180
District of Columbia	202-332-2437	Ohio	800-332-2437
Florida	800-352-2437	Oklahoma	800-535-2437
Georgia	800-551-2728	Oregon	800-777-2437
Hawaii	800-922-1313	Pennsylvania	800-662-6080
Idaho	208-345-2277	Puerto Rico	800-765-1010
Illinois	800-243-2437	Rhode Island	800-726-3010
Indiana	800-848-2437	South Carolina	800-322-2437
Iowa	800-445-2437	South Dakota	800-592-1861
Kansas	800-232-0040	Tennessee	800-525-2437
Kentucky	800-654-2437	Texas	800-299-2437
Louisiana	800-922-4379	Utah	800-366-2437
Maine	800-851-2437	Vermont	800-882-2437
Maryland	800-638-6252	Virginia	800-533-4148
Massachusetts	800-235-2331	Virgin Islands	800-773-2437
Michigan	800-827-2437	Washington	800-272-2437
Minnesota	800-248-2437	West Virginia	800-642-8244
Mississippi	800-537-0851	Wisconsin	800-334-2437
Missouri	800-533-2437	Wyoming	800-327-3577

ACQUIRED IMMUNE DEFICIENCY SYNDROME
AIDS

What do we know about AIDS? The next 17 chapters will present the many faces of the AIDS pandemic in the United States and other countries. Unlike people, the AIDS virus (HIV) does not discriminate; and it appears that most humans are susceptible to HIV infection, its suppression of the human immune system, and the consequences that follow. The viral infection that leads to AIDS is the most lethal, the most feared, and the most socially isolating of all the sexually transmitted diseases. **We must, as a people, fight against AIDS, not against each other** (Figure P-1).

FIGURE P-1 The Loneliness of AIDS. Skip Bluette, diagnosed with AIDS July 1986, died July 1988. He suffered the indignity of having to lie to a dentist to get treatment. He suffered the ignorance of nurses afraid to touch him. He suffered the loss of his greatest pleasures—discos, gourmet meals, movies, and sex with men. Family was vital to Skip. So vital that on July 17, the day he died, their presence was his final wish.

Skip Bluette wanted his story told. Photographer Mara Lavitt interviewed and photographed him during the last 8 months of his life. Portions of Lavitt's article, which appeared in *The New Haven Register*, are presented in the following chapters. (*By permission of Mara Lavitt and* The New Haven Register)

Acquired Immune Deficiency Syndrome: Discovering Its Cause

CHAPTER CONCEPTS

♦ AIDS is a syndrome, not a single disease.

♦ The first cases of AIDS-related *Pneumocystis carinii* pneumonia (PCP) were reported by the Centers for Disease Control and Prevention (CDC) in June of 1981; the first case of Kaposi's sarcoma in July 1981.

♦ Luc Montagnier discovered the AIDS virus in 1983.

♦ The first CDC definition of AIDS was presented in 1982 and expanded in 1983, 1985, and 1987, and again on January 1, 1993.

The letters A, I, D, S (AIDS) are an acronym for Acquired Immune Deficiency Syndrome.

A = acquired	=	a virus received from someone else
I = immune	=	a protection against disease-causing microorganisms
D = deficiency	=	a loss of this protection
S = syndrome	=	a group of signs and symptoms that together define AIDS as a human disease

AIDS: A DISEASE OR A SYNDROME?

AIDS has been presented in journals, non-science magazines, newspaper articles, and on television as a disease. But a disease is a pathological condition with a single identifiable cause. As we learned from the days of Louis Pasteur and Robert Koch, there is a single identifiable organism or agent for each infectious disease.

AIDS patients may have many diseases. Most AIDS patients have more than one disease at any given time. Each disease produces its own signs and symptoms. Collectively, the diseases that are expressed in an AIDS patient are referred to as a **syndrome.** The number of different diseases an AIDS patient has and the severity of their expression reflects the functioning of that person's immune system.

Between 1982 and 1983, the agent that destroys an essential portion of the human immune system was identified by French scientists as a virus. From that point on there was a specific infectious agent associated with the cause of AIDS. The symptoms of viral-induced AIDS can begin **only** after one has been infected with a specific virus. This virus is now called the *H*uman *I*mmunodeficiency *V*irus (HIV). The specific viral induced disease is referred to specifically as HIV/AIDS because there are other reasons for a suppressed immune system, like congenital inherited immune deficiencies, exposure to radiation, alkylating agents, corticosteroids, certain forms of cancer and cancer chemotherapy, that also produce AIDS-like symptoms. *Because individuals can express AIDS for reasons other than becoming HIV-infected, unless stated otherwise all information herein will refer only to AIDS caused by HIV and referred to as HIV/AIDS.*

Over time the AIDS virus depletes a subset of Lymphocytes called T4 helper cells, that are essential in the proliferation of cells necessary to cell-mediated immunity and in the production of antibodies (Figure 1-1). Thus, cell-mediated immunity and antibodies are critical components of the human immune system. Without the ability to produce a sufficient number of immune specific cells and immune specific antibodies, the body is vulnerable to a large variety of infections caused by organisms and viruses that normally do not cause human disease. It is these infections that create the symptoms and progression of illnesses that eventually kill AIDS patients. Thus AIDS begins with HIV infection. Technically it can be called **HIV disease** or **HIV T4 helper cell dis-**ease, but the popular press, scientists, and others still refer to HIV disease as AIDS. But, AIDS is the end stage of chronic HIV infection. AIDS is not transmitted, the virus is. People do not die of AIDS per se. They die of opportunistic infections, cancers, and organ failures brought on by a failed immune system.

It is believed that eventually almost everyone who is **correctly** diagnosed with HIV/AIDS will die. But all who become HIV-infected may not progress to AIDS. Estimates are that some 5% of the HIV-infected population will not progress to AIDS. This implies that there is a percentage of the population that is resistant to HIV-associated immune system suppression. In mid-1996, a gene for HIV resistance was identified! (see Chapter 4).

Naming the Disease

Early in 1981, Michael Gottlieb had identified a new syndrome that seemed to target gay men. Each of the cases was different, but **all had one thing in common: whatever was making the men sick had singled out the T cells for destruction**. Eventually the body's battered defenses couldn't shake off even the most harmless microbial intruder. The men were dying from what doctors termed opportunistic infections, such as *Pneumocystis* **pneumonia** which attacks the lungs, and **toxoplasmosis**, which often ravages the brain.

In June of 1981, the Centers for Disease Control and Prevention (CDC) first reported on diseases occurring in gay men that previously had only been found to occur in people whose immune systems were suppressed by drugs or disease [*Morbidity and Mortality Weekly Report (MMWR)*, 1981].

The report stated that five young men in Los Angeles had been diagnosed with *Pneumocystis carinii* pneumonia (PCP) in three different hospitals. Because cases of PCP occurred almost exclusively in immune suppressed patients, five new cases in one city at one time were termed by the report as unusual. The report also suggested "an association between some aspects of homosexual life-style or disease acquired through sexual contact and PCP in this population. Based on clinical examination of each of these cases, the

FIGURE 1-1 Normal Human T Lymphocytes, Monocytes, and Macrophages. Scanning electron micrograph of monocytes, macrophages, and a T4 lymphocyte, magnified 9,000 times. These white blood cells are the targets of HIV infection. Note that the T4 lymphocyte (round cell, at the center) is adhered to a flattened macrophage. (*Photograph courtesy of Dr. M. A. Gonda, Program Resources, Inc., NCI-Frederick Cancer Research Facility. Reprinted from Gonda*, Natural History, *95:78-81, 1986, with permission from* Natural History.)

possibility of a cellular immune dysfunction related to a common exposure might also be involved."

In July 1981, the CDC (*MMWR*, 1981) reported that an uncommon cancer, *Kaposi's sarcoma* (KS), had been diagnosed in 26 gay men who lived in New York City and California. This was also an unusual finding because KS, when

it occurred, was usually found in **older** men of Hebrew or Italian ancestry. The sudden and dramatic increase in pneumonia cases, all of which were caused by a widespread but generally harmless fungus, *P. carinii*, indicated that an infectious form of immune deficiency was on the increase. This immune deficiency disease, initially called GRID for Gay-Related Immune Deficiency, was noted to be quickly spreading in the homosexual community, among users of injection drugs, and among blood transfusion recipients. This new mysterious and lethal illness appeared to be associated with one's lifestyle. These early cases of immune deficiency heralded the beginning of an epidemic of a previously unknown illness. By 1982 and 1983, the disease was reported in adult heterosexuals and children and was subsequently called AIDS.

DISCOVERY OF THE AIDS VIRUS

There was no shortage of ideas on what caused AIDS. It was believed by some to be an act of God, a religious curse or penalty against the homosexual for practicing a biblically unacceptable lifestyle that included drugs, alcohol, and sexual promiscuity. The reverend Billy Graham said "AIDS is a judgement of God." Jerry Falwell stated that AIDS is God's punishment, the scripture is clear, "we do reap it in our flesh when we violate the laws of God." Some believed AIDS was due to sperm exposure to amyl nitrate, a stimulant used by some homosexuals to heighten sexual pleasure (Gallo, 1987). Others believed there was no specific infectious agent. They believed that certain people who *excessively stressed their immune systems* experienced immune system failure, and before it could recover, other infections killed them. But many scientists who had expertise in analyzing the sudden onset of "new" human diseases felt the cause of this form of human immune deficiency was an infectious agent. They believed that the agent was transmitted through sexual intercourse, blood, or blood products and from mother to fetus. They also believed that this agent which led to the loss of T cells was smaller than a bacterium or fungus because it passed through a filter normally used to remove those microorganisms. It turned out after further studies that this agent fit the profile of a virus.

In January of 1983, Luc Montagnier (Mont-tan-ya) and colleagues at the Pasteur Institute in Paris isolated the AIDS virus (Hobson et al., 1991). In May of that year, they published the first report on a T cell retrovirus found in a patient with **lymphadenopathy** (lim-fad-eh-nop-ah-thee), or swollen lymph glands. Lymphadenopathy is one of the early signs in patients progressing toward AIDS. The French scientist (Figure 1-2) named this virus **lymphadenopathy**-associated virus (LAV) (Barre-Sinoussi et al., 1983).

Naming the AIDS Viruses: HIV-1, HIV-2

During the search for the AIDS virus, several investigators isolated the virus but gave it different names. For example, Robert Gallo (Figure 1-3) named the virus HTLV III (For the Third Human T Cell Lymphotropic Virus). Because the collection of names given this virus created some confusion, the Human

FIGURE 1-2 Luc Montagnier, from the Pasteur Institute in Paris. He and colleagues discovered the human immunodeficiency virus (HIV), the cause of AIDS. In October 1997, he moved to the United States. He accepted an endowed professorship at Queens College, New York to run a new AIDS research institute. *(Photograph courtesy of AP/Wide World Photos)*

Retrovirus Sub-committee of the Committee on the Taxonomy of Viruses reduced all of the names to one: **human immunodeficiency virus** or **HIV**. This term has now been accepted for use worldwide.

In 1985, a second type of HIV was discovered in West African prostitutes. It was named HIV type 2 or **HIV-2**. The first confirmed case of HIV-2 infection in the United States was reported in late 1987 in a West African woman with AIDS. By December 1990, 16 additional cases of HIV-2 infection were reported to the CDC (*MMWR*, 1990). Beginning 1997, a total of 71 HIV-2 infections have been reported from 16 states of the United States. Of the 71 infected persons, 54 are black and 42 are male. Forty-nine were born in West Africa, 9 in the

FIGURE 1-3 Robert Gallo, Director, Institute of Human Virology. *(Photograph courtesy of AP/Wide World Photos)*

be direct genetic descendants of each other (Marlink, 1996). Clinically, what has been learned about HIV-1 appears to apply to HIV-2, except that HIV-2 appears to be less harmful (cytopathic) to the cells of the immune system, and it reproduces more slowly than HIV-1.

Unless stated otherwise, all references to HIV in this book refer to HIV-1.

DEFINING THE ILLNESS: AIDS SURVEILLANCE

Data gathered from AIDS patients between 1981 and the end of 1983 showed there were 2,042 AIDS cases reported and 63% of them had died. All demonstrated a loss of T4 lymphocytes, and all died with severe opportunistic infections. Opportunistic infections are caused by organisms and viruses that are normally present but do **not** cause disease unless the immune system is damaged. Clearly there was an immediate need for a name and definition for this disease so that a rational surveillance program could begin.

Definitions of AIDS for Surveillance Purposes

The initial objective of AIDS surveillance was to describe the epidemic in terms of time, place, and individuals and to recognize immediately changes in rate and pattern in the spread of AIDS. Early surveillance was done to gather data in order to generate information of value in planning control programs. Because a *cellular deficiency of the human immune system* was found in every AIDS patient, along with an assortment of other signs and symptoms of disease, and because the infection was *acquired* from the action of some environmental agent, it was named **AIDS** for **Acquired Immune Deficiency Syndrome.**

In order to establish surveillance, a system for monitoring where and when AIDS cases occurred and a workable definition had to be developed. The definition had to be *sensitive* enough to detect every possible AIDS patient while at the same time *specific* enough to exclude those who may have AIDS-like symptoms, but were not infected by the AIDS virus.

United States (including 3 infants born to mothers of unspecified nationality), and 3 in Europe. The region of origin was not identified for 10 of the persons, although 4 of them had a malaria-antibody profile consistent with residence in West Africa. Twelve have developed AIDS-defining conditions and six have died. These case counts represent minimal estimates because completeness of reporting has not been assessed; reporting varies from state to state according to state policy.

The earliest evidence to date of an individual exposed to HIV-2 comes from a case report on an infection most likely occuring in Guinea Bissau in the 1960s. Earlier extensive serosurveys in West Africa are rare or nonexistent. In genetic terms, HIV-2 is much more closely related to the SIV group of viruses than to HIV-1. Both HIV-2 and HIV-1 may have been derived from ancestral SIV variants that were from distinct regions and species and do not appear to

In 1982, there was no *single characteristic* of AIDS that would allow for a useful definition for surveillance purposes. Because immunological testing was essentially unavailable, the first AIDS surveillance definition was based on the clinical description of symptoms. The *first* of many criteria for the diagnosis of AIDS were: (**1**) the presence of a reliably diagnosed disease at least moderately predictive of cellular immune deficiency; and (**2**) the absence of an underlying cause for the immune deficiency or for reduced resistance to the disease (*MMWR*, 1982). Because the symptoms varied greatly among individuals, **this was a poor first definition**.

Arbitrary AIDS Definitions

The initial definition of AIDS was thus an arbitrary one, reflecting the partial knowledge of the clinical consequences that prevailed at the time. Various systems for classifying HIV-related illnesses have been devised since 1982 to take into account increasing knowledge about the spectrum of those illnesses. But the definition of AIDS has remained largely unchanged, partly for epidemiological reasons: a standard definition of AIDS makes it easier to monitor the incidence of the disease over time. Had the whole picture of HIV infection and its clinical consequences been known in 1982, the term **"AIDS"** would never have been coined. Instead, we would refer to the various stages of **"HIV disease"** (or perhaps, following an older tradition, "Gottlieb's disease," after Mike Gottlieb, who first described it).

The 1982 definition was modified in 1983 to include new diseases then found in AIDS patients. With this modification, AIDS became reportable to the Centers for Disease Control and Prevention (CDC) in every state. In 1985, additional diseases were included in the AIDS case definition. Those diseases were disseminated histoplasmosis, chronic isosporiasis, and some of the non-Hodgkin's lymphomas (a form of cancer).

Part of the 1982 through 1985 AIDS case definitions was the description of patients with AIDS-related complex (ARC). The symptoms of ARC included swollen lymph nodes (lymphadenopathy), weight loss, loss of appetite, fever, rashes, night sweats, and fatigue. But ARC patients did not appear to have opportunistic infections, and because HIV antibody testing was not widely available, their antibody status was unknown. By 1987, the need for a mid-AIDS classification was unnecessary. Antibody tests were available and much more was known about the onset of opportunistic infections. Thus the CDC dropped ARC from their 1987 AIDS definition. Extrapulmonary tuberculosis, HIV encephalopathy (brain disease), HIV wasting syndrome, presumptive *Pneumocystis carinii* pneumonia (PCP), and esophageal candidiasis (both fungal infections) were added to the definition (Table 1-1). For AIDS diagnoses in children, multiple or recurrent bacterial infections were added.

Broadly speaking, the term *AIDS* may be understood as referring to the onset of life-threatening illnesses as a result of HIV disease that results from an HIV infection. AIDS is the end stage of a disease process which may have been developing for 5, 10, 15 or more years, for most of which time the infected person will have been well and quite possibly unaware that he or she has been infected.

Thus the number of AIDS cases reported from 1987 through 1992 reflects the revisions of the initial surveillance case definition. One major drawback to all of the CDC AIDS definitions is the fact that through 1992, the Social Security Administration (SSA) used the CDC AIDS definition to determine disability. But all the definitions were primarily based on symptoms and opportunistic infections in men. Therefore, about 65% of women with HIV/AIDS symptoms were excluded from SSA benefits. They were excluded because of failure to be diagnosed with AIDS by the CDC AIDS definition (Sprecher, 1991).

Impact of the 1993 Expanded AIDS Case Definition— On January 1, 1993, the newest definition of AIDS was put into the surveillance network. The reason for the new CDC definition was that epidemiologists felt the 1987 definition failed to reflect the true magnitude of the pandemic. In particular, it failed to address AIDS in women. In addition, those with T4 counts under $200/\mu L$ of blood are most likely to be severely ill or disabled and in greatest need of medical and social services. With the

TABLE 1-1 1987 CDC Definition of AIDS

ADULT

A. Without laboratory evidence for HIV infection:
  • Lymphoma of brain (<60 years of age)
  • Lymphoid interstitial pneumonitis (<13 years of age)
B. With laboratory evidence for HIV infection:
  • Disseminated coccidioidomycosis
  • HIV encephalopathy
  • Isosporiasis (persisting > 1 month)
  • Lymphoma of brain (any age)
  • Non-Hodgkin's lymphoma (B cell or undifferentiated)
  • Recurrent Salmonella septicemia
  • Extrapulmonary tuberculosis
  • HIV-wasting syndrome
  • Recurrent bacterial infections (<13 years of age)
  • Disseminated histoplasmosis

PEDIATRIC

Children with AIDS may have infectious diseases that are not covered by the adult CDC AIDS definitions. Thus children under 15 months are classified separately from older children because passive maternal antibodies may be present.

To Be HIV-Infected, Children Under 15 Months Must:

1. Show HIV in blood and tissues.
2. Show evidence of humoral and acquired immune deficiency and have one or more opportunistic infections associated with AIDS.
3. Show other symptoms meeting the CDC definition of AIDS.

To Be HIV-Infected, Children Between 16 Months and 12 Years Must:

1. Show 1 and 3 above.
2. Show HIV antibodies.

This definition was updated on January 1, 1993 to include all persons with a T4 cell count of less than 200/μL of blood. See text for additional details.

(Adapted from Roger J. Pomerantz, M.D., "The Chameleon Called AIDS," Harvard Medical School, 1988.)

new AIDS definition, these people are eligible earlier in their illness for federal and state medical and social assistance programs.

CDC revised the classification system for HIV infection to emphasize the clinical importance of the T4 lymphocyte count in the categorization of HIV-related clinical conditions. Consistent with this revised classification system, CDC has expanded the AIDS surveillance case definition to include all HIV-infected persons who have less than 200 T4 lymphocytes/μL of blood, or a T4 lymphocyte percent less than 14% of total lymphocytes (Table 1-2). In addition to retaining the 23 clinical conditions in the 1987 AIDS surveillance case definition, the expanded definition includes (**1**) pulmonary tuberculosis, (**2**) invasive cervical cancer, and (**3**) recurrent pneumonia in persons with documented HIV infection (Table 1-3). This expanded definition requires laboratory evidence for HIV infection in persons with less than 200 T4 lymphocytes/μL or with one of the added clinical conditions. The objectives of these changes are to simplify the classification of HIV infection and the AIDS case reporting process, to be consistent with standards of medical care for HIV-infected persons, to better categorize HIV- related morbidity, and to reflect more accurately the number of persons with severe HIV-related immunosuppression who are at highest risk for severe HIV-related morbidity and most in need of close medical follow-up. The addition of the three clinical conditions reflects their documented or po-

TABLE 1-2 T4 Lymphocyte Counts Related to Percentages of Total Lymphocytes

T4 Cell Category	T4 Cells/μL	Percent T4 Cells of Total Lymphocytes
(1)	≥ 500	≥ 29
(2)	200–499	14–28
(3)	<200	<14

1. Normal adult T4 cell count ranges from 900 to 1,200 T4 cells/μL of blood.

2. The equivalences of T4 cells to percent of total lymphocytes were derived from analyses of more than 15,500 lymphocyte subset determinations from seven different sources: one multistate study of diseases in HIV-infected adolescents and adults, and six laboratories (two commercial, one research, and three university-based). The six laboratories are involved in proficiency testing programs for lymphocyte subset determinations.

(Adapted from *MMWR*, 1993.)

TABLE 1-3 List of 26 Conditions in the AIDS Surveillance Case Definition

- Candidiasis of bronchi, trachea, or lungs
- Candidiasis, esophageal
- Cervical cancer, invasive[a]
- Coccidioidomycosis, Disseminated or extrapulmonary
- Cryptococcosis, extrapulmonary
- Cryptosporidiosis, chronic intestinal (>1 month duration)
- Cytomegalovirus disease (other than liver, spleen, or nodes)
- Cytomegalovirus retinitis (with loss of vision)
- HIV encephalopathy
- Herpes simplex: chronic ulcer(s) (>1 month duration); or bronchitis, pneumonitis, or esophagitis
- Histoplasmosis, disseminated or extrapulmonary
- Isosporiasis, chronic intestinal (>1 month duration)
- Kaposi's sarcoma
- Lymphoma, Burkitt's (or equivalent term)
- Lymphoma, immunoblastic (or equivalent term)
- Lymphoma, primary in brain
- *Mycobacterium avium complex* or *M. kansasii,* disseminated or extrapulmonary
- *Mycobacterium tuberculosis,* disseminated or extrapulmonary
- *Mycobacterium tuberculosis,* any site (pulmonary[a] or extrapulmonary)
- *Mycobacterium,* other species or unidentified species, disseminated or extrapulmonary
- *Pneumocystis carinii* pneumonia
- Pneumonia, recurrent[a]
- Progressive multifocal leukoencephalopathy
- Salmonella septicemia, recurrent
- Toxoplasmosis of brain
- Wasting syndrome due to HIV

[a]Added in the 1993 expansion of the AIDS surveillance case definition.
(Adapted from the CDC, Atlanta, Georgia.)

Of the 106,618 Adult/Adolescent AIDS cases reported in 1993, 57,574 (54%) were reported based on conditions added to the definition in 1993; and 49,044 (46%) were reported based on pre-1993 defined conditions (Table 1-4). Of the 57,574 cases reported based on 1993-added conditions, 52,392 persons (91%) had severe HIV-related immunosuppression only; 4,030 (7%), pulmonary tuberculosis (TB); 1,151 (2%), recurrent pneumonia; and 576 (1%), invasive cervical cancer (19 persons were reported with more than one of these opportunistic illnesses). A substantial increase in the number of reported AIDS cases occurred in all regions of the United States. Of areas reporting more than 250 cases, the proportion of cases based on the 1993-added criteria ranged from 35% in North Carolina ($n = 1,353$) to 71% in Colorado ($n = 1,323$).

When compared to 1992 data the increase in reported cases in 1993 was greater among females (151%) than among males (105%). Proportionate increases were greater among blacks and Hispanics than among whites. The largest increases in case reporting occurred among persons aged 13–19 years and 20–24 years; in these age groups, a greater proportion of cases were reported among women (35% and 29%, respectively) and were attributed to heterosexual transmission (22% and 18%, respectively).

Compared with homosexual/bisexual men, proportionate increases in case reporting were greater among heterosexual injecting-drug users (IDUs) and among persons reportedly infected through heterosexual contact.

tential importance in the HIV epidemic. Invasive cervical cancer is included on the basis of an epidemiological link between HIV infection and cervical dysplasia, and reports that HIV speeds the progression of both cervical dysplasia and cancer. From January 1, 1993 through December 1993, 5,729 new AIDS cases were reported based on the presence of one of the three clinical conditions.

The expanded AIDS surveillance case definition has had a substantial impact on the number of reported cases in 1993.

TABLE 1-4 AIDS Cases by Race/Ethnicity Reported for 1996, United States

Race/Ethnic Group	AIDS Cases	Percentage of Cases
White	26,291	38
Black	28,413	41
Hispanic	12,996	18.9
Asian/Pacific Islander	563	0.8
American Indian	210	0.3
Total	68,473[a]	100

[a]Pediatric AIDS cases for 1996, 678; Total 1996, 69,151.

Women, blacks, heterosexual IDUs, and persons with hemophilia were more likely than others to be reported with 1993-added conditions. Most of these differences were attributable to reports of the three opportunistic illnesses added in 1993; of 5,729 persons reported with a 1993-added opportunistic illness, 26% were women, 48% were heterosexual IDUs, and 63% were black. The number of Hispanics reported under the 1993-added criteria reflected reports from Puerto Rico: 38% of the 3,173 reports from Puerto Rico were based on the 1993-added criteria, compared with 54% of the 15,145 cases among Hispanics from other areas.

The pediatric AIDS surveillance case definition was **not** changed in 1993. During 1993, 990 children aged <13 years were reported with AIDS, an increase of 21% compared with the 783 cases reported in 1992. In 1994, for the first time, pediatric AIDS cases exceeded 1,000 (1,090). For 1995, there were 800 AIDS cases and for 1996, 678. Collectively, since 1990, 50% were female, and most were either black (55%) or Hispanic (27%) and were infected through perinatal HIV transmission (93%). New York, Puerto Rico, and Florida reported 51% of the pediatric AIDS cases.

If all of the approximately 1 million persons in the United States with HIV infection were diagnosed and their immune status known, it is estimated that 120,000–190,000 persons who do not have AIDS-indicator diseases would be found to have T4 lymphocyte counts $< 200/\mu L$ **(in March 1992 the CDC reduced the number of HIV-infected in the United States to between 650,000 and 900,000).** However, since not all of these persons are aware of their HIV infection status, and of those who are, not all have had an immunological evaluation, the immediate impact on the number of AIDS cases will be considerably less. Under the 1987 AIDS surveillance criteria, approximately 49,106 AIDS cases were reported in 1992, but 106,618 were reported for 1993. In 1994, there were 80,691 new AIDS cases. For 1995, the number of new cases was 74,180. For 1996 the number of new AIDS cases was 69,151 and about the same for 1997.

Revised AIDS Definition Creates Backlog

The effects of the expanded surveillance definition was greatest in 1993 because of the backlog in number of persons who fit the new AIDS definition. Once most of these cases are reported through 1997, the yearly incidence should fall off to between 55,000 and 65,000 cases a year into the year 2000. Finally, the expanded HIV classification system and the AIDS surveillance case definition have been developed for use in conducting public health surveillance. They were not developed to determine whether any statutory or other legal requirements for entitlement to federal disability or other benefits are met.

The revised surveillance case definition does not alter the criteria used by the Social Security Administration in evaluating claims based on HIV infection under the Social Security disability insurance and Supplemental Security Income programs. The Social Security Administration has recently proposed a new method for the evaluation of HIV infection and criteria to determine eligibility for disability. Other organizations and agencies providing medical and social services should develop eligibility criteria appropriate with the services provided and local needs (*MMWR*, 1993).

Problems Stemming from Changing the AIDS Definition for Surveillance Purposes

Each time the definition of AIDS has been altered by the CDC, it has led to an increase in the number of AIDS cases. In 1985, the change in definition led to a 2% increase over what would have been diagnosed prior to the change. The 1987 change led to a 35% increase in new AIDS cases per year over that expected using the 1985 definition. The 1993 change resulted in a 52% increase in AIDS cases over that expected for 1993. Such rapid changes alters the baseline from which future predictions are made and makes the interpretations of trends in incidence and characteristic of cases difficult to process. For the first time because of the 1993 AIDS definition, one could be diagnosed with AIDS and remain symptom-free for years (become HIV positive and have a T4 cell count of less than 200).

SUMMARY

Much continues to be written about HIV/ AIDS. Some of it, especially in lay articles, has been less than accurate and has led to public confusion and fear. **HIV infection is not AIDS. HIV infection is now referred to as HIV disease. AIDS is a syndrome of many diseases,** each resulting from an opportunistic agent or cancer cell that multiplies in humans who are immunosuppressed. The new 1993 CDC AIDS definition will allow, over the long term, earlier access to federal and state medical and social services for HIV-infected individuals.

REVIEW QUESTIONS

(Answers to the Review Questions are on page 575.)

1. The letters A, I, D, and S are an acronym for?
2. Is AIDS a single disease? Explain.
3. When was the AIDS virus discovered and by whom?
4. In what year did CDC first report on a strange new disease which later was named AIDS?
5. Name one acronym for HIV.
6. How many times has CDC changed and expanded the definition of AIDS? In what years?

7. Why did the CDC do away with the ARC definition?
8. What is one major advantage of the new CDC AIDS definition for the HIV-infected?

REFERENCES

BARRE-SINOUSSI, FRANCOISE, et al. (1983). Isolation of a T-lymphocyte retrovirus from a patient at risk for acquired immune deficiency syndrome (AIDS). *Science,* 220:868–871.

GALLO, ROBERT C. (1987). The AIDS virus. *Sci. Am.,* 256:47–56.

HOBSON, SIMON WAIN, et al. (1991). LAV revisited: Origins of the early HIV-1 isolates from Institut Pasteur. *Science,* 252:961–965.

MARLINK, RICHARD, (1996), Lessons from the second AIDS virus HIV-2. *AIDS,* 10:689–699.

Morbidity and Mortality Weekly Report. (1981). Pneumocystis pneumonia—Los Angeles, 30:250–252.

Morbidity and Mortality Weekly Report. (1982). Update on acquired immune deficiency syndrome (AIDS)—United States, 31:507–508, 513–514.

Morbidity and Mortality Weekly Report. (1990). Surveillance for HIV-2 infection in blood donors—United States, 1987–1989, 39:829–831.

Morbidity and Mortality Weekly Report. (1993). 1993 Revised classification system for HIV infection and expanded surveillance case definition for AIDS among adolescents and adults, 41:1–19.

Morbidity and Mortality Weekly Report. (1994). Update: Impact of the expanded AIDS surveillance case definition for adolescents and adults on case reporting—United States, 1993, 43:160–170.

SPRECHER, LORRIE. (1991). Women with AIDS: Dead but not disabled. *The Positive Woman,* 1:4.

Origin of HIV: An Opportunistic Virus

- AIDS is not caused by HIV infection.
- AIDS is caused by HIV infection.
- An unbroken chain of HIV transmission has been established between those infected and the newly infected.

THE CAUSE OF AIDS: THE HUMAN IMMUNODEFICIENCY VIRUS

The unexpected appearance and accelerated spread of an unknown lethal disease soon raised several important questions: **What** is causing the disease? **Where** did it come from? **How** does the causative agent function? **What** are the characteristics of the agent? These four questions will be answered.

This section has a subtitle which implies that AIDS is the result of HIV infection. There are a relatively small number of scientists and non-scientists as of this writing who claim that HIV does **not** cause AIDS. For a balanced HIV/AIDS presentation, this claim will be presented first.

HIV Does Not Cause AIDS: A Minority Point of View

Peter Duesberg is perhaps the most vocal in his concern that the scientific community is investigating the wrong causative agent. Duesberg is a molecular biologist at the University of California at Berkeley and a member of the National Academy of Sciences. Duesberg has advanced his anti-HIV/AIDS hypothesis at great expense to himself. He states that "I have been excommunicated by the retrovirus-AIDS

————— BOX 2.1 —————

SEX AND HIV DO NOT CAUSE AIDS!

Medical Doctor Puts His Life on the Line to Prove It.

On October 28, 1993, Robert Willner held a press conference at a North Carolina hotel, during which he jabbed his finger with a bloody needle he had just stuck into a man who said he was infected with HIV. Willner is a physician who recently had his medical license revoked in Florida for, among other infractions, claiming to have cured an AIDS patient with ozone infusions. He is also the author of a book, *Deadly Deception: The Proof that SEX and HIV Absolutely DO NOT CAUSE AIDS*. He insists that jabbing himself with the bloody needle, which he describes as "an act of intelligence," was not meant to sell books. "I'm interested in proving to people that there isn't one shred of scientific evidence that HIV causes any disease".

USA Today, October 3, 1994, carried a full-page advertisement to promote the selling of Willner's book. A full-page ad in this newspaper, regardless of location, if carried nationally costs $57,500. **Question for class discussion:** Did *USA Today* management provide socially responsible advertisement or did money talk and responsibility walk? What is the potential medical downside of this advertisement?

The scientific journal *Science* (1994; 226:1642–1649) presented a series of six articles by Jon Cohen concerning the *question* of whether HIV causes AIDS. The articles are a balanced review of the scientific facts as they relate to the question.

Robert Willner died April 15, 1995 from an apparent heart attack.

community with noninvitations to meetings, noncitations in the literature and nonrenewals of my research grants, which is the highest price an experimental scientist can pay for his convictions."

In 1971, he co-discovered cancer-causing genes in viruses. In the March 1987 issue of *Cancer Research,* Duesberg published "Retroviruses as Carcinogens and Pathogens: Expectations and Reality." The article provoked wide-based scientific discussion and received a lot of popular press coverage. Duesberg argues that there is no evidence that HIV causes AIDS. He has published additional articles in *Science* (1988) and in the *Proceedings of the National Academy of Sciences* (1989) stating that HIV is not the cause of AIDS. In May of 1992, Duesberg was the featured speaker at an alternative AIDS conference, "AIDS: A Different View," promoted by homeopathic physician Martien Brands. The week of meetings was spent giving new interpretations to some of the data used to establish HIV as the causative agent of AIDS. In short, Duesberg suggests that there is no single causative agent, that the disease is due to one's **"lifestyle."** He marshals arguments to support his theory that, in the

United States and probably in Europe, AIDS is a collection of noninfectious deficiencies predominantly associated with drug use, malnutrition, parasitic infections, and other specific risks.

Duesberg believes that the tests which detect HIV antibodies are useless. In the June 1988 issue of *Discovery* he said, "If somebody told me today that I was antibody positive, I wouldn't worry one second. I wouldn't take Valium. I wouldn't write my will. All I would say is that my immune system seems to work. I have antibodies to a virus. I am protected."

In June 1990, Weiss and Jaffe wrote a critical refutation of Duesberg's theory that HIV cannot be the cause of AIDS. Duesberg's response suggested that he was unaware of published data that clearly answer the questions he raises concerning HIV involvement in AIDS. For example, one of Duesberg's major points is that no one has yet shown that hemophiliacs infected with HIV progress to AIDS. The data on matched groups of homosexual males and hemophiliacs which show that *only* those infected with HIV develop AIDS have been available for a number of years. (Weiss et al., 1990).

Duesberg's arguments and disagreements with the vast majority of prominent scientists who have researched the causal agent of AIDS are many. But they pale when placed next to the overwhelming evidence which leaves no doubt in the opinion of most scientists that HIV causes AIDS (see Andrews, 1995; Cohen, 1995; Moore, 1996).

Based on an August 1992 report in *Newsweek*, a father discussed his decision, based on Duesberg's claims, to counsel his infected hemophiliac son to avoid zidovudine (ZDV) treatment. This situation is similar to what happened when desperate cancer patients followed the advice of a credentialed academician who recommended vitamin therapy as the cure for cancer. Based on this advice, some people failed to undergo truly effective therapy. **Questions**: Is Duesberg's opinion on this issue inadvertently harmful to humans? To the scientific process? Will the use of his idea, that HIV does not cause AIDS, provide a course of action that will stop the Acquired Immune Deficiency Syndrome?

Duesberg's Belief That HIV Does Not Cause AIDS Continues

In 1996, Duesberg's book, *Inventing the AIDS Virus,* was published. Through 1997, Duesberg still insisted that HIV does not cause AIDS. He believes that HIV is just another opportunistic agent like those that cause other opportunistic diseases (Duesberg, 1993, 1995a, 1995b; Moore, 1996). With each new scientific report, it becomes more difficult for Duesberg to maintain his position. However, he remains unconvinced that HIV causes AIDS regardless of the reports that newborn infants with HIV got HIV *only* from HIV-infected mothers and progress to AIDS while noninfected newborns from the same mothers do not progress to AIDS and that some 50% of HIV-infected hemophiliacs have developed AIDS yet **no** HIV-negative hemophiliac has ever developed AIDS (Darby et al., 1995; Levy, 1995; Sullivan et al., 1995). In addition, Duesberg claims that the drug AZT (Zidovudine) causes AIDS—then what does he make of the AIDS Clinical Trials Group (ACTG) Protocol 076 that demonstrated AZT treatment of women during pregnancy and de-livery reduced transmission from mother to infant from 25% in the placebo-treated mothers to 8% in those who received AZT (Connor et al., 1994)?

For those who wish to read more on the rebuttal of Duesberg's arguments, read the study reporting on the death rate among HIV-positive and HIV-negative British hemophilia patients (Baum, 1995; Darby et al., 1995; Editorial, 1995).

In Defense of Duesberg

In defense of Duesberg, Buianoukas (1995) writes that "We at HEAL (Health Education AIDS Liaison) maintain that what is called AIDS is no more complicated than a recreational drug–fear–medical drug disease syndrome which, with the exception of acute medical care, is out of the purview of orthodox medicine." Robert Root-Bernstein authored "Rethinking AIDS" in 1993. This book attempts to support Duesberg's hypothesis that there is no link between HIV and AIDS. His main thesis is that scientists do not have the necessary information to conclude that HIV causes AIDS. He believes, first, that the right studies on the cause of immunosuppression have not been done and, second, that there need not be a common thread (such as the virus) associated with this new disease, no common denominator such as a causative transmissible agent, but on the other hand he does not rule out the case for a single infectious organism that has yet to be identified.

In 1993, Britain's *Sunday Times* took the Duesberg claim that HIV does not cause AIDS to a new level by runing a series of articles disclaiming HIV as the cause of AIDS. The *Sunday Times* continued to run these articles throughout 1994 (Dickson, 1994; Karpas, 1994). In mid-1994, Kary Mullis (recipient of the Nobel prize in chemistry for his invention of the polymerase chain reaction—see chapter 12 for explanation) joined Duesberg and the *Sunday Times* by saying, "the idea that HIV was the 'probable cause of AIDS' was not a scientifically proven fact, nor, indeed, was there any clear evidence that AIDS was spread through sexual contact. I think we [spread] retroviruses by our lungs, not by our genitals." Mullis continued by saying, "it is not a scientific fact, or even a supposed fact, that HIV is the probable cause of AIDS." Mullis is unrepentant in the face of those who complained his ideas were undermining the activities of AIDS health-workers around the world. Critics of Mullis state that he has limited knowledge of HIV/AIDS and no scientific authority to speak on the cause of AIDS (Dickson, 1994).

Mullis himself appeared unfazed by such criticisms. His main concern was that the efforts of "a lot of talented people in the medical profession had been diverted" by misconceptions about HIV.

A Member of the United States Government Enters the Dispute

In March 1995, a letter was sent to eight government scientists and officials who influence AIDS research and policies, in which freshman Representative Gil Gutknecht (R-MN) questions the "HIV = AIDS hypothesis and its inability or effective treatment." His query echoes the arguments of Peter Duesberg. Gutknecht's initial inquiry asks whether recreational drug use and anti-HIV drugs might be the true cause of AIDS and questions whether AIDS is contagious.

Gutknecht's staffers think the federal AIDS effort—based on the conclusion that HIV causes AIDS—"will be seen as the greatest scandal in American history and will make Watergate look like a no-fault divorce" (Stone, 1995).

Talk Show Host Claims AIDS Is a Myth—October 1996, Fort Lauderdale, Florida—A talk show host and two medical professionals have been proclaiming over the airwaves on Miami's WLQY-AM, probably South Florida's most popular Haitian radio station, that AIDS is a myth, and have been urging listeners, an estimated 155,000 Haitians, to discontinue medication and refuse treatment.

The commentators told the *Sun-Sentinel* of Fort Lauderdale that they have ample proof that AIDS does not exist and that the health care industry made it up to increase business. People should stop taking AIDS drugs and wearing condoms, they said in interviews for the article.

"We are not spreading lies. What we are saying are facts," said Henri-Claude Saint-Fleur, a North Miami Beach psychologist who was educated in France. "I'm happy to tell people the truth. I know lots of people who stopped taking their AIDS medication and are living well."

HIV/AIDS counselors say Haitian patients from at least four treatment centers have stopped seeing doctors because of the show.

Class Discussion: Comment on the radio station's right to provide air time to promote this theme "AIDS IS A MYTH." Do the commentators have a right to tell people to stop taking their medications? Are they liable for such advice? Should they be liable?

Evidence That HIV Causes AIDS

It has been firmly established that there is a high correlation between HIV infection and the development of AIDS. With respect to establishing HIV as the causative agent of AIDS, let's look at the evidence:

1. The virus has now been identified in virtually all AIDS patients tested; in over 90% of those with pre-AIDS symptoms (formerly called AIDS related complex or ARC), that is, individuals who are HIV-positive and have symptoms of HIV disease; and in individuals who are HIV-positive but appear to be healthy.

2. The virus has been identified by electron microscopy inside and on the surface of T4 cells in HIV-positive and AIDS patients (Figure 2-1A,B).

3. Recent work of Bruce Patterson and Steven Wolinsky has shown that the genetic material of HIV (HIV-DNA) can be found in as many as 1 in 10 blood lymphocytes of persons with HIV disease (Cohen, 1993).

4. Antibodies against the virus, viral antigens, and HIV RNA have been found in HIV-positive and AIDS patients.

5. There is an absolute chronological association between the emergence of AIDS and the appearance of HIV in humans worldwide.

6. There is a chronological association of HIV-positive individuals who progress to AIDS. People who are truly HIV-negative, and without the need for chemotherapy or radiation treat-

THE UNITED STATES GOVERNMENT CREATED HIV

Leonard Horowitz, a past medical advisor to dental and medical supply companies, turned author, claims the United States government is responsible for creating HIV and the Ebola virus! In a speech at the Capital Mall, Washington, D.C., on Labor Day weekend, 1996, Horowitz stated that, "the problem I [Horowitz] had was reconciling the fact that the dentist [David Acer, the Florida dentist who stands accused of infecting his patients with HIV], though a psychopath, was no fool. And he held in his possession one of the most incriminating documents I had ever seen. A 1970 Department of Defense Appropriations request for $10 million for the development of immune system ravaging viruses for germ warfare. In fact, the document, which I lay before you today, reads like this:

Within the next 5 to 10 years, it would probably be possible to make a new infective microorganism which could differ in certain important aspects from any known disease-causing organisms. Most important of

these is that it might be refractory to the immunological and therapeutic processes upon which we depend to maintain our relative freedom from infectious disease. . . . A research program to explore the feasibility of this could be completed in approximately 5 years at a total cost of $10 billion. . . . It is a highly controversial issue and there are many who believe such research should not be undertaken lest it lead to yet another method of massive killing of large populations.

So Dr. Acer created a crime, a mystery, that couldn't be solved, without implicating the government and causing a larger mystery to be investigated. That is, the origin of AIDS and Ebola—the subject of my last three years of research, and why I have come before you today."

Class Discussion: Is this a feasible scenario? If **Yes**, on what factual evidence do you base this conclusion. If **No**, why not?

---

ments, do not demonstrate HIV antibodies and never demonstrate AIDS. For example, prior to 1985, 75% to 90% of hemophiliacs in the United States tested HIV-positive. They became HIV-infected because the virus was present in blood factor VIII concentrates self-administered by hemophiliacs to clot their blood. In addition, the use of blood donor prepared blood factor VIII concentrates

prior to 1985 has been linked to HIV infections wherever the bloodconcentrate was used. Over half of these HIV-infected individuals have developed AIDS and 56% have died from it.

7. Hemophiliacs from low- and high-risk behavior groups were equally infected from HIV-contaminated blood factor VIII concentrates.

8. The virus is found in HIV-positive and AIDS

THE RELATIONSHIP BETWEEN THE HUMAN IMMUNODEFICIENCY VIRUS AND THE ACQUIRED IMMUNODEFICIENCY SYNDROME

Each time Peter Duesberg publishes an article claiming that HIV does not cause AIDS, the phone lines at the National Institute of Allergy and Infectious Diseases (NIAID), at the Centers for Disease Control and Prevention, and at AIDS-related research centers across the United States ring for days; nonstop. In order to answer the critics of the HIV-AIDS relationship, the NIAID published a detailed 61-page report ("The Relationship Between the Human Immunodeficiency Virus and the Acquired Immunodeficiency Syndrome") outlining and discussing the data that leaves no doubt in the HIV/AIDS Scientific Community that HIV is the causative agent (NIAID, 1995).

FIGURE 2-1 Viral Replication in Human Lymphocytes. Scanning electron micrograph of HIV-infected human T4 lymphocyte. **A**, A single cell infected with HIV showing virus particles and microvilli on the cell surface (magnified 7,000 times). **B**, Enlargement of a portion of the mountain-like cell surface in (**A**) showing multiple virus particles budding out of the cell surface (magnified 20,000 times). As each HIV exits the cell, it leaves a hole in the cell membrane. (*Photograph courtesy of K. Nagashima, Program Resources, Inc., NCI-Frederick Cancer Research Facility*)

patients but not in healthy low behavioral risk individuals.

9. With the exception of persons who had their immune systems suppressed due to genetic causes or by drug therapy, prior to the appearance of the virus, there were no known AIDS-like cases. The virus has been isolated worldwide—but only where there are HIV-positive people and AIDS patients.

10. An HIV-positive identical twin born to an HIV-positive mother developed AIDS, but the HIV-negative twin did not.

11. Only HIV-positive mothers transmit HIV into their fetuses and only these HIV-positive newborns progress to AIDS. HIV-negative newborns from HIV-positive mothers **DO NOT** get AIDS!

12. Drugs developed specifically to inhibit the replication and/or maturation of HIV, thereby lowering the level of HIV found in HIV infected people, have delayed the onset of HIV disease and, for HIV infected pregnant women, have **decreased** the birth of HIV infected infants by 66%.

13. **IF** HIV does not cause AIDS, how do we scientifically explain the positive effects of drugs used to affect the early and late stages in the life cycle of HIV that have lowered viral load to unmeasurable levels in the blood of those with HIV disease and AIDS and have virtually restored life for those at death's door and who are now back at work!

14. Finally, there have been numerous reports in the literature on HIV-infected individuals (homosexual, bisexual, and heterosexual) transmitting the virus to their sexual partners, both eventually dying of AIDS. *The unbroken chain of HIV transmission between prostitutes and their customers, between injection drug users sharing the same syringe, from infected mothers to their unborn fetuses, and so on all lead to the inescapable conclusion that HIV does cause AIDS.*

In short, Koch's Postulates have been satisfied:

HIV disease meets all four criteria!

1. The causative agent must be found in all cases of the disease. (**It is.**)
2. It must be isolated from the host and grown in pure culture. (**It was.**)
3. It must reproduce the original disease when introduced into a susceptible host. (**It does.**)
4. It must be found in the experimental host so infected. (**It is.**)

Thus the identification of HIV as the causative agent of AIDS is now firmly accepted by scientists worldwide.

Question for Class Discussion: You have just read some of the evidence for and against HIV being the cause of AIDS. Assuming you agree with the vast majority of HIV/AIDS investigators worldwide, that HIV does cause AIDS, do you think there comes a time at which dissenters forfeit their right to make claims on other people's time and trouble by the poverty of their arguments and by the wasted effort and exasperation they have caused?

NOW discuss the value of the dissenter.

NOW discuss the danger of the dissenter's information or claims.

ORIGIN OF HIV: THE AIDS VIRUS

More than virtually any other disease, AIDS has generated myths and far-fetched theories about its origin, its causes, and even its very existence. These are probably linked to fear and denial prompted by a virus which is fatal, incurable, and sexually transmitted—and can infect people for years before they show any signs of illness.

Why Do Scientists Want to Know Where HIV Originated?

The object of determining the origin of the AIDS virus is to gain insight into how the virus may have evolved the unique set of characteristics that enable it to destroy the human immune system. Such information will offer valuable clues as to how rapidly the virus is evolving and how to combat it and perhaps help prevent future viral plagues.

If, for example, HIV is a new virus, say less than 30 years old, the many different varieties of HIV now infecting people worldwide prob-

ably evolved from a common ancestor sometime after World War II. And new varieties can be expected to continue evolving at what would be a frightening pace for several more decades, possibly producing new strains of the virus that are even more dangerous than those now infecting people. This could mean that vaccines now being developed based on current virus strains may not be useful in 10 to 20 years. But, should the known strains of the virus prove to be hundreds or thousands of years old, it might be possible that the current types of HIVs are in a state of global balance and they would not be expected to offer scientists any shocking evolutionary surprises in the future.

Ideas on the Origin of HIV, UFOs, Biological Warfare, and Cats

Fear stimulates the imagination. Out of human fear have come some rather strange explanations for the origin of the AIDS virus. Early reports had unidentified flying objects (UFOs) crashing to Earth and releasing a "new organism" that would wipe out humanity.

There have been frequent reports in the Soviet press linking AIDS with American biological warfare research. The Soviets agreed in August 1987 to stop these reports (Holder, 1988). There are also reports of extremism, as in the case of Illinois State Representative Douglas Huff of Chicago who told the *Los Angeles Times* that he gave over $500 from his office allowance fund to a local official of the Black Hebrew sect to help the group investigate its claim that Israel and South Africa created the AIDS virus in a laboratory in South Africa. Huff said AIDS is "**clearly an ethnic weapon, a biological weapon**" designed specifically to attack nonwhites (*CDC Weekly*, 1988).

Still another myth to surface is that the AIDS virus came from domestic cats. Because of its similarities to human AIDS, feline immunodeficiency virus has been called "feline AIDS." The cat retrovirus may damage cats' immune systems leaving the animals vulnerable to opportunistic infections *or* it may cause feline leukemia. However, the cat virus has never been shown to cause a disease in humans.

The origin of HIV has been attributed to

HIV-contaminated polio, smallpox, hepatitis and tetanus vaccines, the African green monkey, African people, their cattle, pigs, and sheep—and the CIA. With respect to the use of HIV-contaminated vaccines, a number of recent articles suggest that early monkey kidney cultures used to produce the polio vaccine carried HIV. Review of the literature offers *no* evidence that this occurred. And the argument for the safety of the polio vaccine lies in the absence of any AIDS-related diseases among the hundreds of millions of persons vaccinated worldwide (Koprowski, 1992).

Now over 17 years (1981–1998) into the AIDS epidemic, researchers are still baffled by the question: Where did the AIDS virus come from? AIDS is now known to be caused by two human immunodeficiency viruses, HIV-1 and HIV-2. The former, the cause of most AIDS cases worldwide, *appears to have spread from Central Africa; while the latter has so far been confined mainly to West Africa and the islands off its coast.* Several theories have been proposed to explain the origins of the AIDS epidemic. Most have been speculative rather than verifiable; and several have caused offense, particularly those which refer to sexual practices with monkey blood (Gilks, 1991). Charles Gilks (1992) states that HIV may have entered the human population by the direct inoculation of malaria-HIV-infected blood into human prisoner-volunteers. **The problem with this theory is that it is not testable so it, like others, will remain an unproven theory proposed to explain the origin of HIV/AIDS.**

At the Fifth International Conference on AIDS in Montreal (1989), Vanessa Hirsch and colleagues presented evidence that a virus isolated from a species of West African monkey, the Sooty Mangabey (an ash-colored monkey), may have infected humans 20 to 30 years ago. They believe this virus subsequently *evolved into HIV-2.* Hirsch et al. studied a virus known as the simian immunodeficiency virus (SIVsm) that infects both wild and captive sooty mangabey monkeys. They molecularly cloned and sequenced the DNA of the virus and constructed an evolutionary tree of the several known primate immuno-deficiency viruses. This tree showed SIVsm to be more closely re-

lated to HIV-2 than to HIV-1.

Gerald Meyers of Los Alamos National Laboratory states that SIVsm and HIV are so closely related that when HIV-2 is found in a human, it may be the sooty mangabey virus. However, HIV-1, that causes AIDS, does not sufficiently resemble HIV-2 or SIVsm, thus HIV-1 probably did not evolve from SIVsm/ HIV-2. **Still, the prevailing theory is that humans were first infected through direct contact with HIV-infected primates. The primate to human scenario is easier to accept than humans infecting primates.** Humans have hunted, handled, and even eaten primates for thousands of years. Recent laboratory accidents have shown that SIV can infect humans. Even though at the moment, no identifiable disease has been associated with the SIV/human infections, such accidents have demonstrated the potential for cross-species transmission of HIV-related viruses. Why not believe the same for the origin of HIV-1?

There also remains the possibility that HIV has been present but remained an obscure virus in the human population for a long time before it was recognized as a lethal agent, similar perhaps to the polio virus which surely existed in the human population for years prior to its being discovered as the cause of the polio epidemic of 1894. After all, there is ample evidence that primates, historically, have harbored lentiviruses (the class that includes SIV and HIV). Why should humans be any exception?

Adam Carr (*AIDS in Australia*, 1992) writes that the most widely accepted view on the origin of HIV is that the virus is endemic to a remote part of central Africa, possibly in the mountains of eastern Zaire, and that it began to spread to other parts of Africa only after the area had been penetrated by Europeans in the twentieth century.

In colonial Africa, it is quite possible that a low but persistent level of AIDS cases could have gone unnoticed by the poorly developed health services of the time. In the 1970s, when rapid urbanization and its attendant social changes began in Zaire and neighboring countries, the epidemic began to accelerate and come to the attention of health authorities. By this time it would have begun to spread to other countries. Tourists, soldiers (there were thousands of Cuban troops in neighboring Angola in the mid-1970s), guest workers, and other travelers would have taken the virus to Europe, the Caribbean, and North America. **The first documented case of AIDS in Europe was seen in a Danish surgeon who had worked in Zaire. She died in 1976.**

Discussion of the African origins of HIV has caused controversy. Some African governments protested at suggestions that Africa was "responsible" for the AIDS epidemic, and even denied that AIDS was a problem in their countries. For most of the 1980s, the military government of Zaire would not allow outsiders to investigate the spread of AIDS and did not report AIDS cases to the World Health Organization. Some Africans denounced "racist" Western media for reporting AIDS as an African plague. Carr states that "by 1990, when it was obvious to all that HIV infection was tragically widespread in central, southern, and eastern Africa, this controversy had largely ended. HIV infection is far too widespread in Africa to be the result of recent importation from outside; the African epidemic clearly precedes the Western one." **Regardless, where HIV/AIDS arose is irrelevant to medical science—when and how HIV entered the human population is relevant.**

In summary, there are at least three possible origins of the AIDS virus: (1) it is a human-made virus, perhaps from a germ warfare laboratory; (2) it originated in the animal world and crossed over into humans; and (3) HIV has existed in small isolated human populations for a long time and, given the right set of conditions, it escaped into the larger population. Computer modeling of DNA sequence in HIV and SIVsm suggests that HIV evolved within the last 100 years. So, for now, the question remains: Is AIDS a new disease or an old disease which was late being recognized—so late that we will never know its true source of origin, the origin of HIV?

An additional question to where HIV came from is whether it has always caused disease. From the study of human history, as it relates to human disease, scientists have numerous examples that show that as human habits change, new diseases emerge. Regardless of whether HIV is old or new, history will show that social changes, however small or sudden, have most likely hastened the spread of HIV. In the 1960s, war, tourism, and commercial trucking forced the outside world on Africa's once isolated villages. At the same time, drought and industrialization prompted mass migrations from the countryside into newly teeming cities. Western monogamy had never been common in Africa, but as the French medical historian Mirko Grmek notes in his book, *History of AIDS* (1990), urbanization shattered social structures that had long contained sexual behavior. Prostitution exploded, and venereal disease flourished. Hypodermic needles came into wide use during the same period, creating yet another mode of infection. Did these trends actually turn a chronic but relatively benign infection into a killer? The evidence is circumstantial, but it's hard to discount.

Whatever the forces are that brought us AIDS, they can surely bring other diseases. By encroaching on rain forests and wilderness areas, humans are placing themselves in ever-closer contact with animal species and their deadly parasites. Activities, from irrigation to the construction of dams and cities, can expose humans to new diseases by expanding the range of the rodents or insects that carry them. Stephen Morse, a Rockefeller virologist, studies the movement of microbes among populations and species. He worries that human activities are speeding the flow of viral traffic. More than a dozen new diseases have shown up in humans since the 1960s, nearly all of them the result of once exotic parasites exploiting new opportunities. (Certain of these new disease-causing agents, for example, the Ebola virus, are discussed in Box I.1.)

The Difference Between HIV, HIV Disease, and AIDS

It is important for people to understand the distinction between the terms HIV, HIV disease, and AIDS. There is an immense difference between being infected with HIV, expressing various kinds of diseases because of the continued presence of HIV (HIV disease), and being diagnosed as having AIDS.

HIV is the term for the virus that damages the immune system. The continued presence of HIV may eventually cripple the body's ability to fight off opportunistic diseases referred to collectively as HIV disease. AIDS is the end result of HIV disease. People with HIV disease are diagnosed as having AIDS if they are HIV-positive and develop one or more of some 26 diseases or conditions such as *Pneumocystis carinii* pneumonia (PCP), Kaposi's sarcoma, pulmonary tuberculosis, invasive cervical cancer, recurrent pneumonia, or demonstrate a T4 lymphocyte cell count of less than $200/\mu L$ of blood.

Many more people, in any country, are infected with HIV or are in some stage of HIV disease than have developed AIDS. Many HIV-infected people can live 10 years or longer without experiencing illness.

SUMMARY

The AIDS virus was discovered and reported on by Luc Montagnier of France in 1983. Identifying the virus that caused the immunosuppression that caused AIDS allowed for AIDS surveillance definitions that began in 1982. The recent recognition of non-HIV AIDS cases is not unexpected and can be explained. **There is no new threat of another AIDS-causing biological agent.**

REVIEW QUESTIONS

(Answers to the Review Questions are on page 575.)

1. What may be the strongest nonlaboratory evidence for saying that AIDS is caused by an environmental agent?

2. Where might HIV have originated and where did the first HIV infections appear?

REFERENCES

ANDREWS, CHARLA. (1995). "The Duesberg Phenomenon." What does it mean? *Science,* 267:157.

BAUM, RUDY. (1995). HIV link to AIDS strengthened by epidemiological study. *Chem. Eng. News,* 74:26.

BUIANOUCKAS, FRANCIS. (1995). HIV, an illusion. *Nature,* 375:197.

CDC Weekly. (1988). Extremists seek to blame AIDS on Jews. July: 11.

COHEN, JON. (1993). Keystone's blunt message: 'It's the Virus, Stupid'. *Science,* 260:292–293.

CONNOR, EDWARD. (1994). Reduction of maternal infant transmission of HIV with zidovudine treatment (ACTG 076). *N. Engl. J. Med.,* 331:1173–1180.

CULLITON, BARBARA J. (1992). The mysterious virus called "Isn't." *Nature,* 358:619.

DARBY, SARAH, et al. (1995). Mortality before and after HIV infection in the complete UK population of haemophiliacs. *Nature,* 377:79–82.

DICKSON, DAVID. (1994). Critic still lays blame for AIDS on lifestyle, not HIV. *Nature,* 369:434.

DUESBERG, PETER H. (1990). Duesberg replies [to the charges of Weiss and Jaffe]. *Nature,* 346:788.

DUESBERG, PETER H. (1993). HIV and AIDS. *Science,* 260:1705–1708.

DUESBERG, PETER H. (1995a). The Duesberg Phenomenon: Duesberg and other voices. *Science,* 267:313.

DUESBERG, PETER H. (1995b). Duesberg on AIDS causation: the culprit is noncontagious risk factors. *The Scientist,* 9:12.

EDITORIAL. (1995). More conviction on HIV and AIDS. *Nature,* 377:1.

GILKS, CHARLES. (1991). AIDS, monkeys and malaria. *Nature,* 354:262.

GILKS, CHARLES. (1992). AIDS and malaria experiments. *Nature,* 355:305.

GRMEK, MIRKO. (1990). *History of AIDS: Emergence and Orgin of a Modern Pandomic.* Princeton, NJ: Princeton University Press.

HOLDER, CONSTANCE. (1988). Curbing Soviet disinformation. *Science,* 242:665.

KARPAS, ABRAHAM. (1994). AIDS plagued by journalists. *Nature,* 368:387.

KOPROWSKI, HILARY. (1992). AIDS and the polio vaccine. *Science,* 257:1024–1026.

LEVY, JAY. (1995). *HIV and the Pathogenesis of AIDS.* Washington, DC: ASM Press, 359 pp.

MOORE, JOHN. (1996). À Duesberg, adieu! *Nature,* 380:293–294.

NATIONAL INSTITUTE OF ALLERGY AND INFECTIOUS DISEASES. (1995). The relationship between the human immunodeficiency virus and the acquired immunodeficiency syndrome. *National Institutes of Health,* 1–61.

ROOT-BERNSTEIN, ROBERT. (1993). *Rethinking AIDS.* New York: Free Press, 512 pp.

STONE, RICHARD. (1995). Congressman uncovers the HIV conspiracy. *Science,* 268:191.

SULLIVAN, JOHN, et al. (1995). HIV and AIDS. *Nature,* 378:10.

WEISS, ROBIN A., et al. (1990). Duesberg, HIV and AIDS. *Nature,* 345:659–660.

CHAPTER
3

Biological Characteristics: Genes and Genotypes of HIV

CHAPTER CONCEPTS

♦ Retroviruses are grouped into three families: oncoviruses, lentiviruses, and foamy viruses.

♦ HIV is a lentivirus.

♦ HIV RNA produces HIV DNA which integrates into host cell to become a **proviral** DNA.

♦ HIV contains **nine genes**; its three major structural genes are GAG-POL-ENV.

♦ Six HIV genes regulate HIV reproduction and at least one gene influences infection.

♦ HIV undergoes rapid genetic changes within infected people.

♦ The reverse transcriptase enzyme is highly error prone.

♦ HIV causes immunological suppression by destroying T4 helper cells.

♦ HIV is classified into major (M) and outlier (O) genetic subtypes.

Viruses are microscopic particles of biological material, so small that they can be seen only with electron microscopes. A virus consists solely of a strip of genetic material (nucleic acid) within a protein or fatty (lipid) coat.

Viruses are parasitic organisms; they live inside the cells of their host animal or plant, and **can reproduce themselves only by forcing the host cell to make viral copies.** The new virus leaves the host cell and infects other similar cells. By damaging or killing these cells, some viruses cause diseases in the host animal or plant. Genetically, viruses are the simplest forms of "**life-like agents**" ; the genetic blueprint for the structure of the **human immunodeficiency virus (HIV)** is 100,000 times smaller than that contained in a human cell. The complete sequence of 9,749 nucleotides which form the genetic code for HIV has been identified and their arrangement sequenced (mapped).

Scientists have produced a great deal of information about the human immunodeficiency virus over a relatively short time. The immediate involvement of so many scientists followed by the rapid identification of the causative agent of AIDS is unequaled in the history of medical science. More is known about HIV than about the viruses that cause such long-standing human diseases as polio, measles, yellow fever, hepatitis, flu, and the common cold. Humankind is very fortunate that HIV entered the human population as a pathogen in the mid to late 1970s. By then scientists had discovered and begun to exploit the molecular aspects of biology. Molecular methodologies necessary to begin the immediate study of HIV were in place to define and refine our knowledge of viruses and, in particular, learn about HIV.

RETROVIRUSES

There are three subfamilies of retroviruses, two of which are associated with human disease: **oncoviruses** (cancer-causing—of which HTLV-I and -II are members) and **lentiviruses** or slow viruses of which HIV-1 and HIV-2 are members. **Spumavirus** is the third group but is not known to be associated with human disease. As a lentivirus, HIV has genetic and morphologic similarities to other animal lentiviruses such as those infecting cats (feline immunodeficiency virus), sheep (visna virus), goats (caprine arthritis-encephalitis virus), and nonhuman primates (simian immunodeficiency virus).

The retroviruses and in particular the lentiviruses have presumably been present for thousands of years. Modern sociodemographic changes and other human factors have allowed rapid mutating lentiviruses, such as HIV, to find new niches and host populations in which to reproduce. Now let us review some of the characteristics of the AIDS virus, HIV.

HUMAN IMMUNODEFICIENCY VIRUS (HIV)

HIV is a retrovirus (Figure 3-1). Retroviruses are so named because they **REVERSE** the usual flow of genetic information within the host cell. In all living cells, normal gene expression results from the genetic information of DNA being copied into RNA (Figure 3-2). The RNA is translated into a specific cellular protein. In all living cell types, the directions for protein synthesis come from the species' genetic information contained in its DNA:

$$DNA \rightarrow RNA \rightarrow Protein\ Synthesis$$

In brief, retrovirus RNA is copied, using its reverse transcriptase enzyme, into a complementary single strand of DNA (Figure 3-3). The single-strand retroviral DNA is then copied into double-stranded retroviral DNA (this replication occurs in the cell's cytoplasm). At this point the viral DNA has been made according to the instructions in the retroviral RNA. This retroviral DNA migrates into the host cell nucleus and becomes integrated (inserted) into the host cell DNA. It is now a **provirus** (Figure 3-4). From this point on, the infection is irreversible—the viral genes are now a part of the cells genetic information. In this respect, HIV can be considered as an acquired dominant genetic disease! A provirus, like the "mole" in a John LeCarre spy novel, may hide for years before doing its specific job. But for HIV, there is evidence that in some human cells the provirus begins to produce new copies of HIV RNA immediately after becoming a provirus or shortly thereafter.

Before the HIV provirus's genes can be expressed, RNA copies of them that can be read by the host cell's protein-making machinery must be produced. This is done by **transcription**. Transcription is accomplished by the cell's own enzymes. But the process cannot start until the cell's RNA polymerase is activated by various molecular switches located in two DNA regions near the ends of the provirus: the **long terminal repeats**. This requirement is reminiscent of the need of many genes in multicellular organisms to be "turned on" or "off" by proteins that bind specifically to controlling sequences.

Some of the cellular signaling proteins that bind to HIV's long terminal repeats are members of an important family of proteins known as NF-kB/Rel. Present in virtually all human cells, these regulatory proteins in-

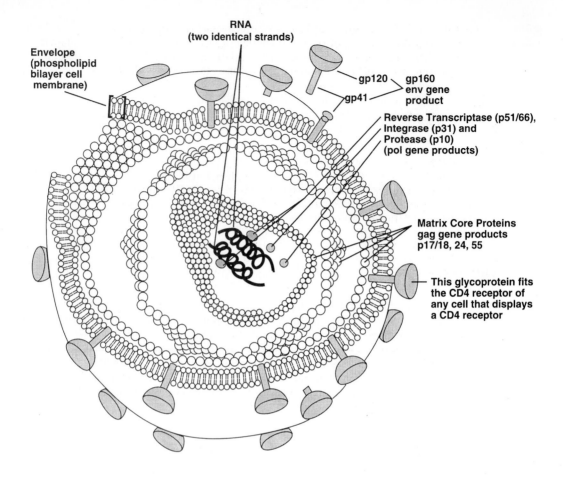

RNA
(two identical strands)

Envelope
(phospholipid
bilayer cell
membrane)

gp120
gp41

gp160
env gene
product

Reverse Transcriptase (p51/66),
Integrase (p31) and
Protease (p10)
(pol gene products)

Matrix Core Proteins
gag gene products
p17/18, 24, 55

This glycoprotein fits
the CD4 receptor of
any cell that displays
a CD4 receptor

crease the transcriptional activity (production of RNA) of many genes. Significantly, cells increase production of some protein members of this family when they are stimulated by foreign proteins or by hormones that control the immune system. It appears that HIV utilizes the NF-kB/Rel proteins resulting from activation of immune cells to boost its own transcription!

Production of Viral RNA Strands or RNA Transcripts

Within the host cell nucleus, proviral DNA, when activated, produces new strands of HIV RNA. Some of the RNA strands behave like messenger RNA, producing proteins essential for the production of HIV. Other RNA strands become encased within the viral core proteins to become the new viruses (Figure 3-4). Whether the transcribed RNA strands become mRNA or RNA strands for new viruses depends on whether or not the newly synthesized RNA strands undergo complex processing. RNA processing means that after the RNA is produced, some of it is cut into segments by cellular emzymes and then reassociated or **spliced** into a length of RNA suitable for protein synthesis. The RNA strands that are spliced become the mRNA used in protein synthesis. The unspliced RNA strands serve as new viral strands that are encased in their protein coats (capsids) to become new viruses that bud out of the cell (Figure 3-5).

Two distinct phases of transcription follow the infection of an individual cell by HIV. In

FIGURE 3-1 Human Immunodeficiency Virus. It infect cells by a process of membrane fusion that is mediated by its envelope glycoproteins (gp120-gp41, or Env) and is generally triggered by the interaction of gp120 with 2 cellular components: CD4 and a coreceptor belonging to the chemokine receptor family. The virus is a sphere measuring 1,000 A or 1/10,000 mm in diameter. The truncated cone-shaped core in a spherical envelope is the dominant feature. In this diagram the virus has been sectioned to better visualize its internal structure. The membrane of HIV is derived from the host cell. HIV gains the membrane while "budding" out or exiting the cell. Each free HIV leaves a hole in the cell membrane. The membrane, acquired from its host cell, consists of two lipid (fat) layers impregnated with some human proteins, for example Class I and Class II human lymphocyte antigen complexes important for controlling the immune response. The external viral membrane also contains molecules of viral glycoproteins (**gp**)— a sugar chain attached to protein. Each glycoprotein appears as a spike in the membrane. Each spike consists of two parts: **gp41** which extends through the membrane; and **gp120** which extends from the end of gp41 to the outside and beyond the membrane (the numbers 41 and 120 represent the mass of —> *as a footnote* the individual gps in thousands of daltons. As a complete unit, gp41 plus gp120 is called gp160. These two membrane or **envelope** proteins play a crucial role in binding HIV to CD4 protein molecules found in the membranes of several types of immune system cells. The gp160 precursor is cleaved into envelope (gp120) and transmembrane (gp41) proteins in the cell's Golgi compartment. The HIV envelope complex is transported via vesicles to patches in the outer cell membrane. Full-length HIV RNA is complexed with capsid proteins and the nucleocapsid is transferred to the cell surface membrane at envelope-containing sites. The binding of gp to CD4 receptors makes such immune system cells vulnerable to infection. Other HIV proteins are located and described in this figure. *Entering a host*

Within the cone-shaped core there are two identical strands of viral genomic RNA, each coupled to a molecule of transfer RNA (tRNA) that serves as a primer for reverse transcription of viral RNA into viral DNA. HIV RNA is 9,749 nucleotide bases long. Also present with the RNA are an **integrase**, a **protease**, and a **ribonuclease enzyme**. The released virus is processed internally by HIV protease to form the characteristic dense lentivirus core. Most HIV appear to have initiated DNA synthesis prior to completion of budding and maturation. Actual maturation of HIV takes place after it buds out of the cell (see Figure 4-11). *life cyc.?*

the first or early phase, RNA strands or transcripts produced in the cell's nucleus are snipped into multiple copies of shorter sequences by cellular splicing enzymes. When they reach the cytoplasm, they are only about 2,000 nucleotides in length. These early-phase short transcripts encode only the virus's **regulatory proteins**; the structural genes that constitute the rest of the genome are among the parts that are left behind. In the second or late phase, two new size classes of RNA— long (unspliced) transcripts of 9,749 nucleotides making up the new viral genome and medium-length (singly spliced) transcripts of some 4,500 nucleotides—move out of the nucleus and into the cytoplasm. The 4,500 nucleotide transcripts encode HIV's structural and enzymatic proteins (Greene, 1993). The life cycle of HIV, from infection to new virus, takes from 8 to 16 hours.

Experimental results reported by Somasundaran et al. (1988) showed that when lymphoid cell lines or peripheral blood lymphocytes were infected with a laboratory strain of HIV, up to 2.5 million copies of the viral RNA were produced by cells; and within 3 days

Prior to 1970, cell biologists thought that genetic information flowed only in one direction:

In 1970 the reverse transcriptase enzyme (RT) was found in a virus. These viruses became known as retroviruses.

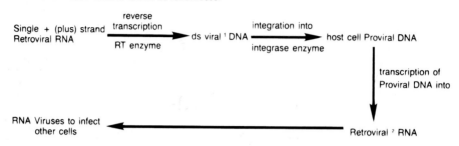

^{1}ds = Double stranded DNA

^{2}If the RNA transcripted is spliced, RNA base sequences are rearranged. This RNA = messenger RNA and is used to make retroviral protein. If RNA transcripted is not spliced, it becomes the RNA genome of the new virus.

FIGURE 3-2   Human and Retroviral Flow of Genetic Information. The general directional flow of genetic information in all living species is from DNA, where the information is stored, into RNA, which serves as a messenger for the construction of proteins which are the cells' functional molecules. This unidirectional flow of genetic information has been referred to as the "central dogma' of molecular biology. In the 1960s, Howard Temin and colleagues discovered an enzyme that copied RNA into DNA, a reverse of what was normally expected, thus the name *reverse transcriptase*.

of infection, up to 40% of the total protein synthesized by the cells was viral protein. This is an unprecedented takeover for a retrovirus which typically makes only modest amounts of RNA and protein.

Much of what HIV does after entering the host cell or while integrated as a retroprovirus depends on the activity of the retroviral genes.

BASIC GENETIC STRUCTURE OF RETROVIRAL GENOMES

The first retrovirus was isolated from a sarcoma (a cancer) in chickens by Peyton Rous in 1911 and named the Rous sarcoma virus. The basic genetic structure of the Rous sarcoma virus and all animal retroviruses is the same. They all con-

tain retroviral RNA sequences that code for the **same three genes** abbreviated GAG, POL, and ENV. Flanking each end of the retroviral genome is a sequence of similar nucleotides called long terminal repeats or redundancies (LTRs).

$$5' = \underset{\text{LTR}}{\underline{\qquad}} \frac{\text{GAG \quad POL \quad ENV}}{} \underset{\text{LTR}}{\underline{\qquad}} = 3'$$

Some of the animal retroviruses such as the Rous sarcoma virus contain an additional **onc** or **oncogene** that, along with its LTRs, causes a rapid form of cancer in chickens which kills them in 1 to 2 weeks after infection. Without the *onc* gene the virus causes a *slow progressive cancer.*

FIGURE 3-3 Proposed Production and Function of Retroviral Provirus. Note the reverse transcriptase enzyme has three functions: **(1)** to act as an RNA-dependent DNA polymerase transcribing single-strand DNA from viral RNA; **(2)** to demonstrate RNase H activity (RNase H is a subunit of the RT enzyme) by hydrolyzing the retroviral RNA off the RNA–DNA complex; and **(3)** to act as a DNA-dependent polymerase and transcribe the second DNA strand complementary to the first DNA strand. The process of viral RNA transcription is complex. When completed, the viral RNA gives rise to the formation of either linear or circular molecules of proviral DNA. Each end of the provirus contains an identical long series of terminal-repeating nucleotides or LTRs. LTRs are not a part of the viral genome. Although retroviral DNA integration is considered to be the normal route for RNA virus reproduction, retroviral reproduction may occur without proviral integration (see Figure 3-4).

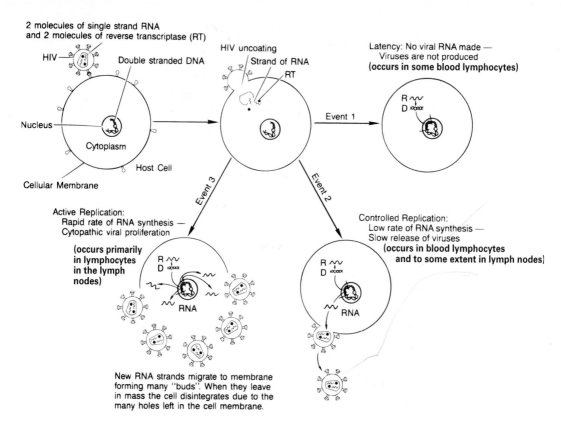

FIGURE 3-4 Proposed Reproductive Cycle for HIV. After cellular infection, HIV may have three choices with regard to its reproduction. The choice for reproduction occurs after the virus enters the cell's cytoplasm and its RNA is exposed to the cell's environment. *In all three choices, single-stranded HIV retroviral RNA is first transcribed into single-stranded retroviral DNA.* This ss DNA is then transcribed into a double stranded molecule that may begin producing HIV RNA, some used for production of virus proteins and others to be incorporated into the mature virus. As the virus accumulate, they move to the cell membrane, become imbedded, and when the cell ruptures it releases the membrane- enveloped viruses. The most common route for retroviruses, the ds DNA migrates to the host cell nucleus, circularizes, and becomes integrated (inserted) into the cellular DNA. Occasionally the retroviral DNA is transcribed and new viruses exit through the membrane. Choice 3 is similar to Choice 2 except it takes immunogenetic stimulation to activate the steady production of virions which exit through the cell membrane. Evidence for the use of all three choices has been found in vivo for HIV. (See text for further details on retroviral reproduction.)

Steps in viral replication

1. Attachment
2. Uncoating
3. Reverse transcription of single strand RNA
4. DNA synthesis of second strand
5. Migration to nucleus
6. Integration
7. Viral transcription
8. RNA nuclear transport
9. Protein synthesis
10. RNA packaging and virion assembly
11. Viral proteins move into cell membrane
12. Release of virus
13. Maturation completed

FIGURE 3-5 Life Cycle of HIV. After fusion of viral and cellular membranes, the inner part of HIV, called the **core**, is delivered into the cell cytoplasm. Uncoating of the core occurs, releasing two identical RNA strands, accompanying structural proteins and enzymes necessary for HIV replication. HIV RNA is then copied into HIV DNA which is then transported into the cell's nucleus for insertion into the host cell's DNA. This feature of the virus life cycle is essential for the spread of HIV in vivo, because it allows infection of nondividing cells such as terminally differentiated macrophages and nondividing T4 lymphocytes. Because, at any given time most T4 cells in the body are resting, and because macrophages are the other main viral target in vivo, this ability is **essential**! There is still some confusion as to whether HIV becomes a latent infection once HIV DNA becomes inserted or integrated into the host DNA. Evidence from 1994 and 1995 indicates that whether HIV is latent depends on the tissue that one is investigating. For example, in the T4 lymphocytes within the lymph nodes HIV is constantly being replicated, while some T4 lymphocytes in the blood carry HIV in the latent state. Depending on cell type, T4 or macrophage, chemokine coreceptors CXCR4 (FUSIN) and/or CC-CKR-5 are used by HIV to enter T4 and macrophage cells. (See Chapter 5 for details on chemokine receptors and HIV cell entry.)

Retroviral Genome of HIV

What sets the HIV genome apart from all other known retroviruses is the number of genes in HIV and the apparent complexity of their interactions in regulating the expression of the GAG-POL-ENV genes (Figure 3-6).

***The Nine Genes of HIV*—** The HIV genome contains at least nine recognizable genes. As can be seen in Table 3-1, five of the nine genes are involved in regulating the expression of the GAG-POL-ENV genes.

The letters **GAG** stand for group-specific antigens (proteins) that make up the viral nucleocapsid. The GAG gene codes for internal structural proteins, the production of the dense cylindrical core proteins (**p24**, a nucleoid

shell protein with a molecular weight of 24,000; and several internal proteins, p7, p15, p17, and p55) which have been visualized by electron microscopy. The GAG gene has the ability to direct the formation of virus-like particles when all other major genes (POL and ENV) are absent. It is only when the GAG gene is nonfunctional that retroviruses (HIV) lose their capacity to bud out of a host cell. Because of these observations, the GAG protein has been designated the virus particle-making machine (Wills et al., 1991).

The **POL** gene codes for HIV enzymes, protease (p10), the virus-associated polymerase (reverse transcriptase) that is active in two forms, p51 or p66, and endonuclease (integrase, p31) enzymes. The integrase enzyme

FIGURE 3-6 Genome of HIV. Nine of the genes making up the HIV genome have been identified. They are positioned as shown. Six of these genes are involved in a complex set of interactions that modify the regulation of the GAG-POL-ENV genes. Five are essential for HIV replication and six control reproduction (see text for details). The maxtrix protein, p17, forms the outer shell of the core of HIV, lining the inner surface of the viral membrane. Key functions of p17 protein are: orchestrates HIV assembly, directs gag p55 protein to host cell membrane, interacts with transmembrane protein, gp41, to retain envelope coded proteins within HIV and contains, a nuclear localization signal that directs HIV RNA integration complex to the nucleus of infected cells. **This feature permits HIV to infect nondividing cells, a distinguishing feature of HIV** (Matthews et al., 1994).

TABLE 3-1 Genes of the HIV-1

Name(s)	Molecular M	
GAG (group antigen)	p17	
	p24	
	p7	
POL (polymerase)	p10	
	p32	
	p66, p	
ENV (envelope)	gp120	
	gp41	
tat (transactivator protein)[a]	p14	
rev (differential regulator of expression of virus protein)	p19	Protein; Transport of spliced/unspliced RNA from nucleus to cytoplasm
vif (virus infectivity factor)	p23	Required for ineffectivity as cell-free virus
nef (negative regulator) factor)	p27	Retards HIV replication
vpr (virus protein R)	?	Triggers cells steroid production to produce HIV
vpu (virus protein U)	p16	Required for efficient viral replication and release-budding

[a] Transactivator gene—the product of their genes influences the function of genes some distance away.

cuts the cell's DNA and inserts the HIV DNA. Evidence from retroviral deletion studies shows that the loss of LTRs on the 3' side of the POL gene stops viral DNA integration into the host genome. However, nonintegrated DNA, without its LTRs and integrase enzyme, can still produce new viruses. This clearly demonstrates that viral DNA integration is not essential for viral multiplication even though integration is the normal course of events (Dimmrock et al., 1987).

The regulation of HIV transcription appears to be intimately related to the onset of HIV disease and AIDS. Thus interruption or inactivation of the POL gene would appear to have therapeutic effects (Kato et al., 1991).

The ENV gene codes for HIV surface proteins, two major envelope glycoproteins (gp120, located on the external "spikes" of HIV and gp41, the transmembrane protein that attaches gp120 to the surface of HIV) that become embeded throughout the host cell membrane, which ultimately becomes the **envelope** that surrounds the virus as it "buds" out (Figure 3-7). Studies on how HIV kills cells have revealed at least one way that the enve-

lope glycoproteins enhance T helper cell death. The envelope glycoproteins cause the formation of **syncytia; that is, healthy T cells fuse to each other forming a group around a single HIV-infected T4 cell.** Individual T cells within these syncytia lose their immune function (Figure 3-8). Starting with a single HIV-infected T4 helper cell, as many as 500 *uninfected* T4 helper cells can fuse into a single syncytium. Continued creation of these syncytia could deplete a T4 cell population.

Several studies have demonstrated that the appearance of syncytium-inducing (SI) HIV strains during the chronic phase of HIV disease heralds an abrupt loss of T4 lymphocytes and a clinical progression of the disease. Although the SI phenotype is detected in many patients with AIDS, it has also been isolated from individuals who have not gone on to an early development of AIDS. However, the marked decrease in the T4 lymphocyte counts after shifting from non-SI (NSI) to SI strains as well as the negative effect SI strains have on primary HIV infection suggests that their appearance may not be just a consequence, but the actual cause of immune system alterations (Torres et al., 1996).

Mature form

Budding particles

FIGURE 3-7 Budding and Mature Retroviruses. This is a photograph of HIV taken by electron microscopy. Note the difference between the free or mature HIV and those that are just budding out through the membrane of a T4 helper cell. This cell came from an HIV-infected hemophiliac. Closely observing the mature HIV, one can make out the core protein area surrounded by the cell's membrane (virus envelope). (*Courtesy CDC, Atlanta*)

It should be noted that the T4 lymphocyte level in an 18-month-old child is approximately 2,500/μL and T4 numbers decrease from this age on with average numbers in 15- to 50-year-olds at 900 to 1,200/μL, respectively.

The Six Genes of HIV That Control HIV Reproduction— Collectively, the six additional HIV genes tat, rev, nef (regulatory genes) and vif, vpu, vpr (auxiliary genes) working together with the host cell's machinery actually control the reproductive retroviral cycle: adhesion of HIV to a cell, penetration of the

cell, uncoating of HIV genome, reverse transcription of the RNA genome producing proviral DNA and immediate production of new viral RNA, or the integration of the provirus and later viral multiplication. The six genes allow for the entire reproductive scenario to occur in 12 to 24 hours in growing cells.

Gene Sequence— The HIV proviral genome has been well characterized with regard to gene location and sequence (Figure 3-6), but the function of each gene is not completely understood. The genes for producing regulatory proteins can be grouped into two classes: genes that produce proteins essential for HIV replication (*tat* and *rev*), and genes that produce proteins that perform accessory functions that enhance replication and/or infectivity (**vif, nef, vpr,** and **vpu**) (Rosen, 1991).

Gene Function— The entire genome is 9,749 nucleotides in length. Each end of the proviral genome contains an identical long sequence of nucleotides, the long terminal repeats. Although these LTRs are not considered to be genes of the HIV genome, they do contain regulatory nucleotide sequences that help the five regulatory genes control GAG-POL-ENV gene expression (Figure 3-6). For example, it is known that the **vif** gene is associated with the infectious activity of the virus. Vif may also be involved in viral replication, but it does not appear to influence the production of GAG-POL-ENV proteins.

The **tat** gene is essential for HIV replication (Parada et al., 1996). It is one of the first vital genes to be transcribed. The tat gene produces a transactivator protein, meaning that the gene produces a protein that exerts its effect on viral replication from a distance rather than interacting with genes adjacent to *tat* or their gene product. *Tat* contains two coding regions or exons—areas that contain genetic information for producing a diffusible protein—which, through the help of the LTR sequences, increases the expression of HIV genes thereby increasing the production of new virus particles. Tat protein consists of 86 amino acids and binds to cadmium or zinc. The tat protein interacts with a short nucleotide sequence called TAR located within the 5′ LTR region of HIV mes-

FIGURE 3-8   Formation of T4 Helper Cell Syncytia. A single infected T4 helper cell can fuse with as many as 500 uninfected T4 helper cells. The formation of syncytia lead to a loss or depletion of T4 helper cells from the immune system. (*Courtesy of Dr. Tom Folks, National Institute of Allergy and Infectious Diseases*)

senger RNA (mRNA) transcripts (Matsuya et al., 1990). Once that tat protein binds to the TAR sequence, transcription of the provirus by cellular RNA polymerase II accelerates at least 1,000-fold.

The **rev** gene (regulator of expression of viral protein) also contains two exons that together code for a 116-amino acid protein. What the *rev* gene does is selectively increase the synthesis of HIV structural proteins in the latter stages of HIV disease, thereby maximizing the production of new viruses. It does this by regulating splicing of the HIV RNA transcript (cutting out nucleotide sequences that exist between exons and bringing the exons together) and transporting spliced and unspliced RNAs from the nucleus to the cytoplasm (Patrusky, 1992; Fritz et al., 1995).

The **nef** gene (negative regulator protein) produces a protein that is maintained in the cell cytoplasm next to the nuclear membrane. It is believed **nef** functions by making the cell more capable of producing HIV. Several antigenic forms of nef protein have been found which suggest multiple activities of nef within

HIV-infected cells (Kohleisen et al., 1992; Sagg et al., 1995).

The functions of the **vpr** gene, which codes for a 96-amino acid viral protein R, which is associated with the transport of cytoplasmic viral DNA into the nucleus. Vpr is also involved in steroid production which in turn helps produce HIV, is required for the efficient assembly or release of new HIV viruses, and stops T4 cell division. Vif is necessary for complete reverse transcriptions of viral RNA into viral DNA. Vpu codes for a viral protein U that destroys the CD4 protein within the T4 lymphocyte, thus helping HIV to bud out of the cell. All three genes (vif, vpr, and vpu) appear to be necessary for HIV to cause disease.

Of the HIV regulatory proteins, Tat, Rev, and Nef are termed **early** proteins, because their production results from the cutting and splicing of full-length HIV mRNA; Vif, Vpu, and Vpr are termed **late** proteins, since their production results from unspliced or single-spliced mRNA.

Genetic Stability of Species— The individual or collective characteristics (phenotypes) of any virus, cell, or multicelled organism depend on the expression of their genes and the interaction of gene products within a given environment. From a biological point of view, changes in phenotype (observable characteristics) that are inheritable are by definition genetic changes. Such changes occur due to changes in the hereditary material. Changes in hereditary material may occur by nucleotide addition, substitution, and deletion. These changes are referred to as **genetic mutations**. Genetic mutations provide biological heterogeneity and genetic diversity (similarity as a species but dissimilarity with regard to certain characteristics). Genetic diversity results from slow but ever-present mutations that alter the phenotype. Investigations on the rate at which genetic mutations occur in living species indicate that DNA is a stable molecule with relatively low mutation rates for any given gene. Because of low mutation rates within the DNA of a species' gene pool (all of the genes that can be found in the DNA of a species) and selection pressures by a slowly changing environment, species evolution is constant but very slow.

Genetic mutations in the strain of an organism or virus produce genetic and phenotype **variants** (different members) of that strain. Regardless of the rate at which mutations occur, they are genetic mistakes—they are not intentional, they just happen by chance. Most mutations or genetic mistakes either make no difference to an organism or virus (silent mutations) or they cause a change. **Few genetic mistakes within a stable environment improve the species. After all, the species arrived at this point in time via genetic and environmental selection pressures—those with the best constellation of genes survived to reproduce those genes.** In species that produce large numbers of offspring, genetic mistakes that are lethal or lead to an early death are of little consequence to the species. A genetic mistake that improves the chance of survival and reproduction is retained.

Genetic Stability of HIV— A virus like HIV can produce many thousands of replicas within a single cell. Genetic mistakes during viral replication produce variant HIVs. In biological economic terms, HIV replicas are in-

expensive to make. Even if most of these mutant HIV replicas are inactive or throwaway copies, it makes little if any difference to the HIV per se. However, if a few HIV replicas received environmentally advantageous mutant genes, these HIV mutants would survive as well as or better than the parent HIVs. **Both parent HIV and mutant HIV can reproduce in the same cell and exchange genes.** Over time, if only the mutant or variant HIVs were transmitted to other people and undergo still further genetic changes, these variant HIVs could, with sufficient accumulative genetic changes, become a new subtype of HIV—for example, an HIV-3 strain.

Investigations of some of the *RNA* viruses revealed relatively high mutation rates. Thus some of the RNA viruses are our best examples of evolution in **"real"** time. Because of their high error rate during replication they show, as expected, both high genetic diversity and biological heterogeneity in their host, and a rate of evolution about a million times faster than DNA-based organisms (Nowak, 1990). The human immunodeficiency virus in particular fits this category. Heterogeneity of HIV is reflected by: (**1**) the difference in the kinds of cells variant HIV infects; (**2**) the way different HIV mutants replicate; and (**3**) the way different variants of HIV harm infected cells.

It is now known that HIV is capable of enormous genetic flexibility, which gives rise to drug resistance, escape from immune responses and failure of vaccination attempts. What is not known are the factors contributing to viral diversity in individual infections. Clearly the high error rate of the reverse transcriptase (because this enzme lacks a 3′ to 5′ exonuclease proofreading ability, i.e., it cannot correct mistakes once made) and the high turnover rate in infected cells generate vast numbers of different virus mutants. The diversity of newly produced variants, however, is shaped by a combination of mutation, recombinations of HIV RNA, and selection forces. The main selective forces that have been proposed to drive HIV diversity are the immune response, cell tropism, (cell types most likely to attract HIV) and random activation of infected cells. At the time of sero-

THE MALARIA PARASITE CAN MIX AND MATCH ITS GENES TO STAY AHEAD OF THE HUMAN IMMUNE SYSTEM

Among the greatest forces that have shaped human history are the infectious diseases. To date only one has been totally eradicated—smallpox. Over time, the United States Public Health Department (USPHD) promised the eradication of several others but failed. The reasons are many, some political, others social, and some biological, like viral or parasite resistance to various drugs and/or having the ability to stay continuously one step ahead of the human immune system's ability to search and destroy the invading virus or parasite. Of course the most recent example of human immune system failure to cope occurs with HIV infection. But **to best appreciate how a parasite can puzzle the human immune system, let's look at how the parasite** *Plasmodium falciparium* **(plas-mo-de-um fal-sip-a-rum) switches its proteins to vary its appearance to our immune system.** And as a result the immune system fails to bring malarial infection under control. First, the USPHD and World Health Organization (WHO) thought they could eradicate malaria using DDT to kill off the mosquitoes carrying the parasite and transmitting it among people and with the use of the drug chloroquine to treat persons already infected. Over time, these mosquitoes became resistant to both DDT and chloroquine! Malaria is now re-emerging as one of the most important infections in the world. Each year about a half *billion* people develop the disease and one to two million die of it—most are young children. In 1994 and 1995, there was great hope that a prepared malarial vaccine would work—it didn't. But scientists continue to unravel how the parasite escapes the immune system, such work will allow for the production of a preventive vaccine by the year 2000. Collectively, in 1995, four research papers that appeared in the journal *Cell* (*82*: 1–4, 77–87, 89–90, 101–110) and two papers that appeared in *The Proceedings of the National Academy of Sciences* (*92*: 5749–5753, 5793–5797) reveal how the malarial parasite switches the kinds of proteins it uses to make up its outer membrane so that the body must continually make new and different antibodies against each of these proteins. The investigators in the cited papers found a large number of variability genes that this single cell parasite rearranges to generate any of millions of different changes in its proteins with which the immune system must cope (Nowak, 1995).

As the amazing story unfolds, the parasite begins by infecting human red blood cells (RBCs). The damaged RBC should be transported to the spleen where such cells are destroyed as would be the malarial parasite. But this does not happen. The parasite turns on the genes necessary to produce a protein that, when exported to the membrane surface of the damaged RBC, acts as a receptor or attachment site that anchors the RBC to the inner surface of blood vessels. The attachment stops the journey of damaged RBCs to the spleen. The parasite now has the time to reproduce. As soon as the immune system makes antibody against the anchoring receptors, the parasite rearranges some of its 150 variation genes to produce still other receptor or anchoring proteins **(antigenic variation)**. Now that these variation genes have been identified. There is renewed hope that a preventative vaccine is in the immediate future. It is possible that most all human viruses and parasites are capable of antigenic variation to some degree and in different manners.

conversion a person may carry a homogeneous virus population, but then diversification occurs as HIV infects many different cell types and tissues in the body (Bonhoeffer et al., 1995).

For further information on HIV evolution, diversity, and HIV disease progression, see Chapter 7, Box 7.2.

GENETIC MUTATION

One mechanism for producing HIV variants or HIV mutants results from a **highly error-prone reverse transcriptase** (RT) enzyme of HIV. Preston and colleagues (1988) found that HIV transcriptase makes at least one error (mutation) in each HIV genome per round of replication in a cell! Other investigators say that reverse transcriptase, on average, introduces a mutation once in every 2,000 nucleotides or about five mutations per round of replication! This unusually high rate of nucleotide misincorporation (substitution, addition, and deletion) as proviral DNA is being made by RT is responsible for generating the genetic diversity and heterogeneity found among the isolates of HIV. In short, the high error rate in producing proviral DNA means that each HIV-infected cell will carry variant or mutant HIV, most of which will be genetically unique (Vartanian et al., 1992). **This high rate of mutation underlies HIV's remarkable ability to become resistant to drug therapies.**

GENETIC RECOMBINATION IN HIV

HIV carries two identical RNA molecules that can individually undergo genetic mutation. They are joined together in parallel at one end (5′ end). This RNA strand relationship makes it possible for genetic (RNA) recombination between these two strands and with other RNA strands in the area. Genetic recombination among and between these RNA strands contributes to the remarkable genetic variability of HIV. Thus as new RNA copies accumulate in the host cell cytoplasm, they recombine with each other (exchange parts or participate in RNA strand switching), producing new varieties of HIV (Levy, 1988).

Completing the Picture on Producing HIV Genetic Variability

Both mutation and recombination contribute, perhaps equally, to the variety of HIV subtypes. Recombination also appears responsible for the rapid emergence of certain subtypes within group M. Subtypes A, B, C, and D are distinct throughout their genomes. But type E, prevalent in southeast Asia and India and thought to be particularly capable of transmission heterosexually, appears to be a **recombinant of a primordial E with part of the long terminal repeat (LTR) sequences and the gp120 envelope gene of subtype A.** Identical recombination breakpoints were found in five type E isolates,

four from Thailand and one from the Central African Republic.

At least one of every 10 HIV patient isolates are intersubtype recombinants. The true incidence is unknown, as the isolates studied were not obtained at random, nor were genomes completely sequenced. Some strains may be multiple recombinants; the early Zairian isolate HIV-1 MAL is an A/D recombinant. Some HIV recombinants have been spread worldwide as, for example, the recombinant African subtype G was responsible for a large hospital outbreak in Russia following the use of inadequately sterilized needles.

Recombination is probably facilitated by geographic intermixing of subtypes, co-infection of an individual with different subtypes, and co-infection of cells with different susceptibilities for different subtypes (Laurence, 1997).

Michael Saag and colleagues (1988) examined the generation of molecular variation of HIV by sequential HIV isolates from two chronically infected people. They found 39 distinguishable but highly related genomes (HIV variants). **These results indicate that HIV heterogeneity occurs rapidly in infected individuals; and that a large number of genetically distinguishable but related HIVs rapidly evolve in parallel and coexist during chronic infection.** That is, whenever a drug or the immune response successfully attacks one variant, another arises in its place. Pools of related genetic variants are often referred to as **quasispecies** (Delwart et al., 1993; Diaz et al., 1997).

Additional evidence indicates that some HIV genetic variants demonstrate a preference (tropism) as to the cell type they infect. This means that one genetic change may allow the virus to enter cells that were once immune to the virus. The rapid genetic change which results in altered viral products makes it very difficult to design a vaccine or drug that will be effective against all HIV variants. To date, HIV drug-resistant mutants have been found for all FDA-approved nucleoside and non-nucleoside analogs and protease inhibitors used in the treatment of HIV-infected people and AIDS patients! (Chapter 4 presents a discussion of currently used drug therapies for HIV/AIDS.)

HIV Antigenic Variation— This is the product of the mutations that occur in the GAG-POL-ENV genes. Immunological investigations on GAG and POL gene proteins show that these two genes are relatively stable. That is, although mutant GAG and POL gene proteins have been found in different viral isolates, the amount of variation for these gene products appears to be minimal. Antibodies are made against the GAG-POL-ENV gene proteins, but it is the antibodies made against the ENV gene protein that appear to be the most important. These antibodies neutralize the envelope glycoproteins that seem to be an essential part of HIV's infecting process. However, it is the ENV gene that is subject to frequent mutations, producing HIV with different envelope glycoproteins within a given individual. Some HIV strains cannot infect certain CD4 cell lines due to a genetic change that has altered the virus-CD4 binding/fusion reaction (Putney et al., 1990). For example, some HIV variants that can enter T cell lymphocytes cannot enter macrophage and vice versa, yet both use the CD4 binding site. AIDS investigators Mayer-Cheng, E.V. Fenyo, K. Dehurst, and N. Tersmette report that virus isolates obtained from patients with advanced AIDS contain HIV that is more cytopathic than the HIV isolated earlier in the course of the disease and that these more cytopathic strains of HIV have demonstrated host cell tropism. HIV isolated from asymptomatic people normally infects CD4 + lymphocytes and CD4 + monocytes, but the more cytopathic HIV is capable of infecting and replicating in a variety of non-CD4 cell types in the brain, gastrointestinal tract, kidney, and other tissues (Nowak et al., 1991).

It now appears that **HIV can constantly change its surface antigenic composition, thereby allowing it to escape antibody neutralization.** This immune selection of HIV mutants allows the virus to persist in the presence of an immune response. This immune selection viral phenomenon is not new. It is what the influenza virus does yearly so that last year's vaccine will not protect people from this year's variation. However, HIV differs from viruses such as influenza. Influenza and other viruses do not have an RNA to DNA replication step so they are not as mutable as the retroviruses.

Because of the error-prone reverse transcriptase enzyme used by the retroviruses, the possibility of genetic change far exceeds that for any other known nonretroviral human pathological virus.

DISTINCT GENOTYPES (SUBTYPES) OF HIV-1 WORLDWIDE BASED ON ENV AND GAG PROTEINS

Because HIV proteins change so rapidly, it is hard to destroy or neutralize them with a single drug or single vaccine. In order to better understand globally circulating strains of HIV, HIV investigators have placed, based on the genetic diversity, the various HIV strains into two major groups, **M**, for the **main** HIV genotypes found in different populations and **O** for HIV genotypes that are significantly different from those in the **M** group.

Group M Subtypes

There are 10 subtypes or clades of group M: A, B, C, D, E, F, G, H, I, and J (Table 3-2). The M subtypes have been analyzed with respect to the differences between them based on the variations found in their GAG and ENV proteins (Robertson et al., 1995).

Eight of 10 different M subtypes or clades (A through H) and O have been globally mapped (geographically located) by Deborah Brix and colleagues (1996) in Figure 3-9. This figure demonstrates the dissemination of the different subtypes from 1990 through 1996. Clearly, subtype B predominates in North America. The explosive epidemic in Southeast Asia is chiefly attributable to subtype E. There are ample documented introductions of subtype E from endemic areas into the United States and the Western Hemisphere.

International Genetic Subtypes

Numerous groups have shown an increase in intermixing of HIV genetic subtypes in multiple international locales. HIV subtypes A, B, C, D, F, and G have appeared throughout Europe; B, F, and C have been found in Brazil; one-third of new infections in Germany are

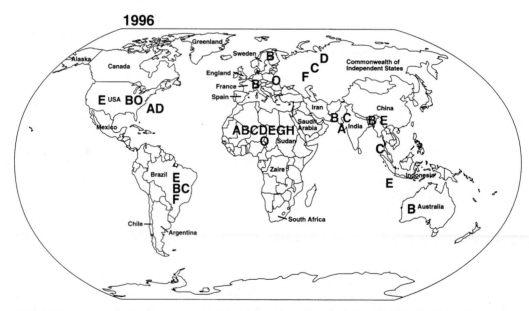

FIGURE 3–9 Global Distribution of the Eight **M** Subtypes and **O** in 1990 and 1996. A total of 10 M subtypes are known (see text for details). Clearly this global map shows that HIV subtypes are **no** longer continent based—all subtypes are now present on all continents (*AIDS Clinical Care*, 1996). The worldwide spread of viral subtypes makes it clear that a **world vaccine** will be required, that is, one that is not subtype specific. None appears to be on the horizon, although large-scale trials with existing envelope vaccines are under way in some developing countries.

non-B; 15% of infections in a New York City hospital are non-B; increasingly, E is found among injecting drug users in Thailand, from 24% subtype E in 1991 to 44% in 1995, and among heterosexual risk groups, a change from 86% subtype E in 1991 to 98% in 1995; and group O has been detected in seven African countries, France, Spain, and in the United States, as well as M/O dual infections. In South Africa, there is spreading of subtypes B and D throughout the homosexual population and C/E throughout the heterosexual cohorts studied. The impact of this is an increasing spread of non-B subtypes into previous "B" areas, which has significant implications for vaccine development.

HIV RNA Recombination

Recombination, the intermixing of viral RNA strands, mediated by HIV reverse transcriptase leads to abrupt and extensive genomic shifts, which generates increased diversity and may lead to increased fitness for HIV. Researchers have shown that HIV E and G are not distinct subtypes, but rather represent recombinant viruses between subtype E and G with subtype A. Infection of a chimpanzee with a second HIV strain from a different subtype resulted in recombinants between the two strains. The impact of recombination is highly relevant for vaccine development and demonstrates a need for cross-protection among subtypes and raising the concern of recombination increasing infectivity or enhancing immune escape (Brix et al., 1996).

Robertson and colleagues (1995) also reported that eight of the group M subtypes appear to have been involved in recombination with each other, giving rise to genetic hybrids. These studies raise questions of whether a vaccine that works against one of the subtypes, will work against a subtype hybrid. Gerald Meyers has been tracking HIV variants for several years. To do this he has sequenced the nucleotides of the GAG gene. From his analysis he has found five major genotypes of HIV subtypes worldwide. Each genotype differs from the other by about 35%. Other families of subtypes are likely to appear over time. Meyers believes that all five families arose from a common viral HIV source and the differentiation of one HIV into another began around 1960 (Goldman, 1992). Two of the five families have been found in Thailand. One family, genotype E, infects heterosexuals almost exclusively. According to Luis Soto-Ramirez and colleagues (1996) subtype E grows more efficiently than other HIV subtypes in Langerhans' cells which are found on the surface of the vagina and represent an initial cell contact for source of HIV infection. Genotype B and E are found in injection drug users (Moore, 1994). Joost Louwagie and colleagues (1993) sequenced the GAG gene from 55 international HIV isolates from people in 12 countries on four continents. Their work resulted in finding seven separate and distinct HIV genotypes A, B, C, D, E, F, and G mentioned above. None of these genotypes were contained within the physical boundaries of one country. Genotype B was found globally. Genotypes A and D were found in a broad east to west belt across sub-Saharan Africa from Senegal to Kenya. Genotype C was found in a north-to-south pattern in Africa.

Worldwide, at least these 10 genetic subtypes exist, based on **envelope genetic sequence** (A → J) and **each subtype** differs at the nucleotide level from any other subtype by as much

TABLE 3-2 Worldwide Distribution of the More Dominant HIV-1 Subtypes (Clades)

Region	Predominant Subtype(s)
U.S.	B
Asia	E, C
South America	B
Africa	A, C, D
Europe	B
Southeast Asia	B
India	C

It is important to recognize that the classification of HIV into subtypes is provisional and only reflects those isolates that happen to have been collected and characterized. Moreover, since current classification is primarily based on parts of *env* or *gag*, proteins, the degree to which taxonomies using these areas of the genome accurately reflect viral evolution remains uncertain. Therefore, present taxonomic classifications will likely be modified as more viral isolates are characterized and our understanding of HIV variation and evolution increases (Hu et al., 1996). **Also see Figure 3–9.**

MYSTERIES OF HIV SUBTYPES

Two epidemiologic mysteries have eluded HIV/AIDS researchers for years. The **first** is why heterosexual intercourse has accounted for approximately 10% of HIV transmission in the United States and Western Europe to date, but more than 90% of HIV transmission in Asia and Africa.

The **second** mystery has centered around a subtype B HIV epidemic among injection drug users in Thailand. This epidemic began in the mid-1980s, and plateaued with less than 100,000 people infected. Several years later, however, a subtype E HIV epidemic took hold in Thailand. This epidemic has exploded among heterosexuals, with over a million people already infected. Most surprising, perhaps, is that subtype B—while present in Thailand, India, and several African countries—has not caused heterosexual epidemics in those places.

Although differences in the rate of heterosexual transmission may also be due to factors such as sexual behavior and the presence of other sexually transmitted diseases, none of these considerations has yet adequately accounted for the widespread heterosexual epidemics in Asia and Africa. Investigators have begun to focus on how biologic characteristics of the individual subtypes might also play a role. These findings about subtype cellular affinities do not suggest that subtype B cannot be transmitted heterosexually— it is throughout the United States and elsewhere. The point is that subtype B seems to be transmitted through vaginal intercourse far less efficiently than the subtypes that predominate in Asia and Africa. It has been shown that Langerhans' cells are located in specific areas, such as the vagina, cervix, and penile foreskin. They do not appear to localize in the rectal or colon mucus membranes. Experiments with HIV-infected Langerhans' cells and uninfected T4 cells showed that HIV-infected Langerhans' cells readily formed clusters and syncytia with T4 cells, resulting in efficient cell-to-cell transmission. It was also demonstrated that during the cell-to-cell interaction, Langerhans' cells not only effectively infect T4 cells but also activate them, resulting in enhanced virus replication (UNAIDS, 1997). Thus, the enhanced efficiency of subtype E to attach to Langerhans' cells may help account for the explosive heterosexual spread of the epidemic in countries such as Thailand, while the heterosexual epidemic in the industrialized world has thus far remained at a comparatively low rate (Essex, 1996).

as 35%. Envelope sequences of isolates within a subtype can vary genetically by as much as 15%. Although there are geographic patterns of strain prevalence, multiple strains are found in many countries. A **single sequence envelope subtype** B is dominant in the United States, probably related to a strong **founder effect** (the initial subtype to become established in the United States). Subtype D, found almost exclusively in Africa's Lake Victoria region (Rwanda, Uganda, and Tanzania), appears to be the most rapidly lethal. Subtype E is found almost exclusively among heterosexual HIV-infected persons.

Group O Subtypes

Group O contains at least 30 genetically different subtypes of HIV. Group O subtypes are referred to as "**outlier**" because their RNA base sequence is only 50%, similar to the known genotypes of the M group. The O variants have been known since 1987 but have been found mainly in Cameroon, Gabon, and surrounding west African countries that, to date, have only been marginally affected by AIDS. Group O viruses were of concern primarily because their divergence from group M was sufficient to miss their detection by ELISA HIV testing. (The ELISA test is discussed in Chapter 13.) Beginning 1998, only two cases of HIV subtype O infection have been reported in the United States. This subtype was found in a Los Angeles county woman and a Maryland woman; both came into the United States from Africa (*MMWR*, 1996). HIV subtype O is not routinely tested for in the United States.

The rapid evolution of HIV families of variants has researchers abandoning hopes of developing a single vaccine effective against all variants. It may be feasible to concoct multiple-strain cocktail vaccines like those used in the flu vaccinations. (There are three major flu virus families.)

SUMMARY

HIV is a retrovirus. It has RNA for its genetic material and carries reverse transcriptase enzyme for making DNA from its RNA. HIV, using its enzyme, copies its genetic information from RNA into DNA which becomes integrated into host cell DNA and may remain silent for years, or until such time as it is activated into producing new HIV. HIV contains at least nine genes; three of them, GAG-POL-ENV, are basic to all animal retroviruses. The six additional genes are involved in the infection process and regulate the production of products from the three genes. HIV, because of its error-prone reverse transcriptase enzyme, mutates at an unusually high rate. With time, many mutant HIV variants can be found within a single HIV-infected person. A vaccine against one mutant HIV may not work against a second—like the vaccines made yearly against different mutant influenza viruses.

REVIEW QUESTIONS

(*Answers to the Review Questions are on page 575.*)

1. Why is HIV called a retrovirus?

2. What are the three major genes common to all retroviruses? How many additional genes does HIV have?

3. Why are retroviruses, and HIV in particular, believed to be genetically unstable? Give two reasons for your answer.

4. What is believed to be the major reason for the high rate of genetic mutations in HIV production?

REFERENCES

AIDS Clinical Care. (1996). Freeze frame: a picture of the pandemic in 1996. 8:82,85.

BONHOEFFER, SEBASTIAN, et al. (1995). Causes of HIV diversity. *Nature,* 376:125.

BRIX, DEBORAH, et al. (1996). Summary of track A: Basic science. *AIDS,* 10 (suppl. 3): S85–S106.

COHEN, MITCHELL, et al. (1994). When bugs outsmart drugs. *Patient Care,* 28:135–146.

DELWART, ERIC, et al. (1993). Genetic relationships determined by a DNA heteroduplex mobility assay: Analysis of HIV envGenes. *Science,* 262:1257–1262.

DIAZ, RICARDO, et al. (1997). Divergence of HIV quasispecies in an epidemiology cluster. *AIDS,* 11:415–422.

DIMMROCK, N.J., and PRIMROSE, S.B. (1987). *Introduction to Modern Virology,* 3rd ed. Oxford: Blackwell Scientific Publications.

ESSEX, MAX. (1996). Deciphering the mysteries of subtypes: communities of color, Spring/Summer: *Harvard AIDS Rev.,* 18–19.

FIELDS, BERNARD. (1994). AIDS: Time to turn to basic science. *Nature,* 369:95–96.

FISCHL, MARGARET. (1984). Combination retroviral therapy for HIV infection. *Hosp. Pract.,* 29:43–48.

FRITZ, CHRISTIAN, et al. (1995). A human nucleoprotein-like protein that specifically interacts with HIV-Rev. *Nature,* 376:530–533.

GOLDMAN, ERIK L. (1992). HIV-1 appears to have at least 5 distinct subtypes. *Fam. Pract. News,* 22:9.

GREENE, WARNER. (1993). AIDS and the immune system. *Sci. Am.,* 269:99–105.

HU, DALE, et al. (1996). The emerging genetic diversity of HIV. *JAMA,* 275:210–216.

KOHLEISEN, MARKUS, et al. (1992). Cellular localization of Nef expressed in persistently HIV-1 infected low-producer astrocytes. *AIDS,* 6:1427–1436.

LAURENCE, JEFFREY. (1997). HIV vaccine conundrum. *Aids Reader,* 7:1–2,27.

LENNOX, JEFFREY, (1995). Approaches to gene therapy. *International AIDS Society—USA,* 3:13–16.

LEVY, JAY A. (1988). Mysteries of HIV: Challenges for therapy and prevention. *Nature,* 333:519–522.

LOUWAGIE, JOOST, et al. (1993). Phylogenetic analysis of GAG genes from 70 international HIV-1 isolates provides evidence for multiple genotypes. *AIDS,* 7:769–780.

MATSUYA, HIROAKI, et al. (1990). Molecular targets for AIDS therapy. *Science,* 249:1533–1543.

MATTHEWS, STEPHEN, et al. (1994). Structural similarity between p17 matrix protein of HIV and interferon-2. *Nature,* 370:666–668.

MOORE, JOHN, et al. (1994). The who and why of HIV vaccine trials. *Nature,* 372:313–314.

Morbidity and Mortality Weekly Report. (1993). Nosocomial enterococci resistant to vancomycin—United States, 1989–1993, 42:597:599.

Morbidity and Mortality Weekly Report. (1996). Identification of HIV-1 group O infection–Los Angeles County, California. 45:561–565.

NOWAK, MARTIN A. (1990). HIV mutation rate. *Nature,* 347:522.

NOWAK, MARTIN A., et al. (1991). Antigenic diversity thresholds and the development of AIDS. *Science,* 254:963–969.

NOWAK, RACHEL. (1995). How the parasite disguises itself. *Science,* 269:755.

PATRUSKY, BEN. (1992). The Intron story. *Mosaic,* 23:20–33.

PRESTON, BRADLEY D., et al. (1988). Fidelity of HIV-1 reverse transcriptase. *Science,* 242:1168–1171.

PUTNEY, SCOTT D., et al. (1990). Antigenic variation in HIV. *AIDS,* 4:S129–S136.

ROBERTSON, DAVID, et al. (1995). Recombination in HIV-1. *Nature,* 374:124–126.

ROSEN, CRAIG A. (1991). Regulation of HIV gene expression by RNA-protein interactions. *Trends Genet.,* 7:9–14.

SAAG, MICHAEL S., et al. (1988). Extensive variation of human immunodeficiency virus Type-1 *in vivo. Nature,* 334:440–444.

SAGG, MICHAEL S., et al. (1995). Improving the management of HIV disease. *Advanced Causes in HIV Pathogenesis,* pp. 1–30. February 25, Swissotel, Atlanta (Michael Sagg Program Chair).

SOMASUNDARAN, M., et al. (1988). Unexpectedly high levels of HIV-1 RNA and protein synthesis in a cytocidal infection. *Science,* 242:1554–1557.

SOTO-RAMIREZ, LUIS, et al. (1996). HIV-Langerhans' cell tropism associated with heterosexual transmission of HIV. *Science,* 271:1291–1293.

TORRES, YOLANDA, et al. (1996). Cytokine network and HIV syncytium-inducing phenotype shift. *AIDS,* 10:1053–1055.

UNAIDS. (1997). Inplications of HIV variability for transmission: Scientific and policy issues. *AIDS,* 11:1–15.

VARTANIAN, JEAN-PIERRE, et al. (1992). High-resolution structure of an HIV-1 quasispecies: Identification of novel coding sequences. *AIDS,* 6:1095–1098.

WILLS, JOHN W., et al. (1991). Form, function and use of retroviral Gag protein. *AIDS,* 5:639–654.

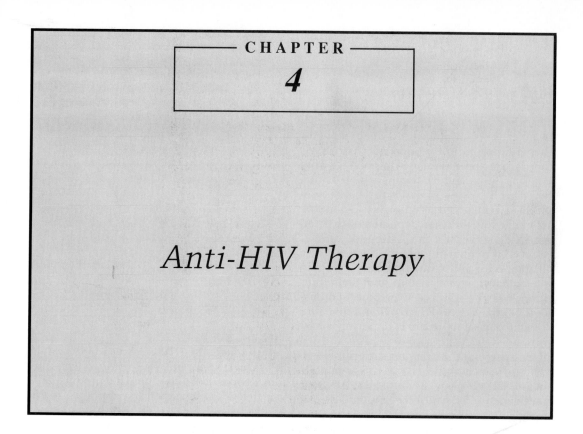

CHAPTER

4

Anti-HIV Therapy

CHAPTER CONCEPTS

♦ There may not be a cure for HIV disease.

♦ From March 1987 through 1997, 11 anti-HIV drugs received FDA approval.

♦ There are no anti-HIV drugs free of clinical side effects.

♦ All nucleoside analogs work by inhibiting the HIV reverse transcriptase enzyme which functions **early** in the HIV life cycle.

♦ All protease inhibitors work by inhibiting the HIV protease enzyme from its function **late** in the HIV life cycle.

♦ Viral load is the number of HIV RNA strands found at any one time in human plasma.

♦ Viral load is associated with HIV disease progression.

♦ Viral load is associated with perinatal HIV transmission.

♦ Pediatric anti-HIV therapy is in a state of confusion.

♦ Scientists do not expect the production of an effective anti-HIV vaccine before the year 2005.

We are constantly humbled by the devastation that something so small, HIV, can cast upon something so large, a human (Box 4.1, Figure 4-1). This chapter provides no final answers; there is no curative therapy, no truly outstanding therapies (drugs that benefit all HIV-infected without major side effects) against HIV, and, with the limited number of **expensive** anti-HIV drugs that are available, debate continues about the details on the standard of care for HIV/AIDS patients. Because some 90% to 95% of HIV-infected people develop AIDS, and because 90% of all **new** HIV infections are occurring in developing nations, an **inexpensive**, **easily taken**, environmentally tolerant, effective HIV-directed therapy is essential. Physicians need a drug that works against HIV as antibiotics once worked against a large variety of disease-causing bacteria. (See Point of Information 4.1.)

GOALS FOR ANTI-HIV THERAPY

The ideal solution would be to prevent HIV from causing an infection. Then anti-HIV therapies would not be necessary. However, there are no means available to stop HIV from entering the body and infecting a limited number of cell types—primarily those cells displaying CD4 antigen receptor sites. Following HIV infection, there is a depletion of cells carrying CD4, especially the T lymphocyte (T4) cells of the human immune system. (See Chapter 5 for an explanation of cell types in the human immune system and their function.) With T4 cell loss, over time immunological response is lost. Loss of immunological response leads to a variety of opportunistic infections (OIs). The suppression of the immune system and increasing susceptibility to OIs and cancers give HIV/AIDS a multidimensional pathology. Because HIV/AIDS is a multidimensional syndrome, it is unlikely that a single drug will provide adequate treatment or a cure (Box 4.2, Figure 4-2).

An ideal goal for HIV drug investigators would be to find a drug that excises all HIV proviruses from the cell's DNA. It is very unlikely that this kind of drug will soon, if ever, be available. Alternatively, the elimination of all HIV-infected cells might be of comparable benefit, as long as irreplaceable cells are not lost through the process. In essence, this is the goal that the human immune system sets for itself, yet falls short of reaching, in the vast majority of HIV-infected individuals.

In the absence of a curative weapon (Box 4.3, Figure 4-3), therapies must be designed to prevent the spread of the virus in the body. Some of these anti-HIV therapies are presented in this chapter.

Can HIV Infection Be Cured?: NEVER SAY NEVER

An effective cure means cleansing the body of the HIV. To find a cure, HIV incorporation into human DNA and subsequent reproduction of new virus must be understood. Without

interference, the **HIV provirus** will remain in host-cell DNA for life. The provirus can, at any time, become activated to mass produce HIV which leads to cell death and eventually to the individual's death. As of this writing, there is no way to prevent either the proviral state or proviral activation. However, with the use of combination anti-HIV drug therapy to suppress HIV replication, scientists now believe that if HIV replication can be suppressed long enough, all HIV-infected cells will die off and there will be a cure (see Point of View 4.5).

ANTI-HIV DRUGS HAVING FDA APPROVAL

The **gold standard** for determining the efficacy (effectiveness) of a new treatment is that it alters the disease in a way that is beneficial to the patient. Therefore, the end points most often used in clinical trials of therapies for a chronic disease such as HIV include prolongation of life or the time to a significant disease complication.

But, studies using these end points require large numbers of patients and/or the passage of considerable amounts of time. **Surrogate markers** (i.e., physiological measurements that serve as substitutes for these major clini-

———— **BOX 4.1** ————

DRUG THERAPY FOR WILLIAM "SKIP" BLUETTE

William "Skip" Bluette (continued from page 25) 3 weeks before he died. Treatment to maintain Skip was failing—the multiple opportunistic infections were defeating the best medicine had to offer.

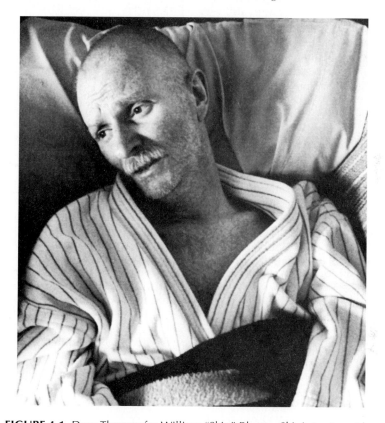

FIGURE 4-1 Drug Therapy for William "Skip" Bluette. Skip's treatment included amphotericin B, an anti-fungal drug, to combat meningitis. Starting in July 1986, he had to visit one of the hospital's clinics at least once a week to receive his treatments, which were given over several hours. Skip started taking zidovudine, a drug known to slow the progress of the disease, during the summer of 1987. Unfortunately, zidovudine also made it difficult for his body to produce blood cells. Skip stopped taking zidovudine when this occurred. In June of 1988, Skip started cleaning out his closets. He said it was part of the dying process to give belongings away "so you know where they're going." Partly, in jest, he said he wanted his ashes scattered on 42nd Street in New York—he thought that's where he got AIDS.

He was hospitalized July 5, 1988. It was presumed that he had *Pneumocystis carinii* pneumonia, which Skip called "the killer." His breathing and speaking were labored. He had inflammation of the pancreas, for which he received morphine, and his kidneys began to fail. (*By permission of Mara Lavitt and* The New Haven Register)

THE BEGINNING OF ANTIBIOTIC THERAPY

Prior to the advent of antibiotics, drugs used to kill disease-causing bacteria, the United States Public Health Department and physicians nationwide did the best they could to save lives by using some rather inventive techniques that worked. One such device **created in 1943** was the **Fever Box**. It was used to cure syphilis and gonorrhea caused by the bacteria *Treponema pallidum* and *Neisseria gonorrhea*, respectively. The Fever Box was used to cure people of these two sexually transmitted diseases in Jacksonville, Florida and Chicago, Illinois.

In Jacksonville's health clinic, infected people were placed in a Fever Box containing light bulbs inside a cabinet. Body temperature was increased to 106°F and an arsenic solution was injected into the bloodstream. This method shortened treatment time for syphilis from 18 months to 48 hours.

Surgeon General Thomas H. Parran Jr. inspected the clinic in December 1943, along with Florida Senator Spessard Holland. Parran predicted the Jacksonville treatment center would become the prototype for similar clinics all across America. Before this could happen, **antibiotics** against these and other diseases were discovered.

THE DISCOVERY

In the spring of 1942. A young woman was dying of blood poisoning in the Yale-New Haven Hospital after experiencing complications following a miscarriage. With her fever raging at 106°F, her doctors decided to gamble on a last-ditch measure—a new experimental drug. A courier from the Merck Pharmaceutical Company arrived carrying a brown paper bag. It contained 5.5 grams of crystalline penicillin—about a teaspoonful—representing half the wartime supply then available in the United States. The drug was passed through a filter for purification and dissolved in a saline solution for intravenous injection. Penicillin, in development for 14 years, was about to be tried in a human being.

The penicillin targeted in on the *Streptococcus* organisms causing septicema and collapsed their cell walls in much the same way that a pin deflates a balloon. By midnight, her temperature had fallen from 106°F to 100°F; by morning, it was down to normal for the first time in a month. She made a full recovery. Her month-long hospital-ization cost $10 a day; the penicillin that cleansed her blood of bacteria was free.

WHERE DID THIS ANTIBIOTIC COME FROM?

In 1928, a rare airborne fungus, *Penicillium notatum*, came in through the open window of Alexander Fleming's London research lab and landed on an agar plate containing a culture of bacteria. The fungus killed the bacteria, a very significant event, but it required 10 years to produce enough of the drug to prove that it destroyed disease-causing bacteria in animals. Nazi bombing raids had relocated the historic quest for a human antibiotic from Oxford, England to America.

FROM THE MIRACLE TO AIDS

This woman's miracle began the modern war on disease. Overnight, doctors became optimists. Dr. Lewis Thomas, the distinguished medical essayist, would later note, "The realization that disease could be turned around by treatment was a totally new idea in 1942." Soon, penicillin and its 200 cousins the "wonder drugs," had proven that medicine could control most bacterial diseases.

And yet …

Spring, 1993: Anthony Fauci, MD, Director of the National Institute of Allergy and Infectious Diseases at the National Institutes of Health (NIH), was born in 1940. Today, Fauci is the leader of the U.S. war on AIDS, the virus-caused disease that is beyond cure by penicillin—and so far, all other drugs (Breo, 1993).

The discovery of penicillin and numerous other antibiotics led us into a false sense of security—"we met the enemy and they are ours." Perhaps it would be better to say, we have met the enemy and they are us. Because of the wonder drugs, attention to basic research on the real issues of how bacteria, protozoa, and viruses cause disease and why they cause a disease in humans or other species was diverted to other things of importance. Mechanisms of pathogeneicity were for the most part neglected in the grand scheme of things. AIDS has brought the need for basic research back into focus as no other event has over the last 40 to 50 years.

VIGIL FOR WILLIAM "SKIP" BLUETTE

The vigil for William "Skip" Bluette (continued from page 69) 48 hours before he died. Time and therapy were running out on Skip. His last wish was to have his sisters Arlene and Nancy near when he died and they were there. On July 15, 1988 the doctors told Nancy and her mother that Skip's kidneys had failed—this time Skip would not recover. He died on July 17. He was 42 years old.

FIGURE 4-2 The Vigil for William "Skip" Bluette. The Bluette family rallied around Skip from the moment they found out he had AIDS. In April 1988, his mother had a heart attack but she survived it.

Skip celebrated his 42nd birthday on May 18; it was his second birthday since his diagnosis. (*By permission of Mara Lavitt and* The New Haven Register)

cal events) can eliminate this problem if their validity and correlation with clinical outcome can be confirmed. The use of surrogates has the potential to shorten the duration of clinical trials and expedite the development of new therapies.

The T4 or CD4+ immune cell number is the best studied and most commonly used surrogate for clinical efficacy of anti-HIV therapies. It is imperfect, however, because changes in T4 cell number per microliter of blood are only partially explained by the therapy. And, T4 cell counts exhibit a high degree of day-to-day variation in individuals, and methods used to count these cells are difficult to standardize.

From March of 1987 through the end of 1997, 11 anti-HIV drugs have received United States FDA approval for use in persons infected with HIV (Table 4-1).

Five of the 11 FDA-approved anti-HIV drugs are nucleoside (nuk-lee-o-side) analogs (each drug resembles one of the four nucleosides that are used in making DNA) and two are nonnucleosides. All seven are reverse transcriptase

———— BOX 4.3 ————

WILLIAM "SKIP" BLUETTE: MAY 18, 1946–JULY 17, 1988

FIGURE 4-3   Free of Pain—One with the Universe—William "Skip" Bluette. On July 20, 1988 Skip's body was cremated. There was a memorial service. On July 21, Skip's ashes were buried in Evergreen Cemetery. (*By permission of Mara Lavitt and* The New Haven Register)

inhibitors. The other four drugs are HIV-protease (pro-tee-ace) inhibitors.

FDA-APPROVED NUCLEOSIDE ANALOG REVERSE TRANSCRIPTASE INHIBITORS

All of the known mechanisms by which HIV impairs the human immune system depend on HIV reproduction. Therefore, the development of anti-HIV replication drugs would appear to be a positive **first step** in controlling HIV reproduction.

Each of the five nucleoside analogs (Figure 4-5) on entering an HIV-infected cell interferes with the virus' ability to replicate itself (Figure 4-6). That is, **when any of the five nucleoside analogs are incorporated into a strand of HIV DNA being newly synthesized, it stops further synthesis of that DNA strand**. The nucleoside analog stops the HIV enzyme, reverse transcriptase, from joining the next nucleoside into position. The five FDA-approved nucleoside analogs are all members of the family of 2′,3′-dideoxynucleoside analogs. By name they are **zidovudine** (ZDV), often **mistakenly called AZT (3′-azido-2′,3′-deoxythymidine)**,

THE END OF AIDS?

This title was placed in $2^3/4$-inch block print on the December 2, 1996 cover of *Newsweek* Magazine (Figure 4-4)! In print $3/8$ inch high over to the left side it said, "**not yet—but new drugs offer hope.**" But then, of the many, many thousands of people who walk by the newsstands or read *Newsweek*, how many ever see the small print when such bold print declares "**THE END OF AIDS**." Clearly, sensationalism sells copy, but what of the **media's moral responsibility**? How many seeing this cover message decided to change their HIV preventive behavior? How many decided that their energies were no longer needed in the fight against AIDS? How many felt their financial, emotional, and physical contributions are no longer necessary? In short, it is **noble** to offer **hope**, but **irresponsible** to offer or suggest myth! Let's **hope** this cover will become a reality soon, but wait until it does before making such questionable promises in a lay publication for millions of readers.

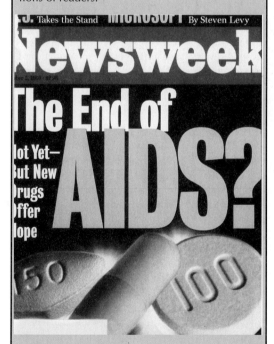

FIGURE 4-4 AIDS CURE? Although this bold suggestion was premature for 1996, the new anti-HIV drugs have given the HIV-infected great hope—they can now contemplate a future.

trade name **Retrovir**; **didanosine** or **ddI** (**2′,3′-dideoxyinosine**), trade name **VIDEX**; **dideoxycytosine**, zalcitabine or **ddC** (**2′,3′-dideoxycytosine**), trade name **HIVID**; **stavudine** or **d4T**, trade name **Zerit**; and **lamivudine** or **3TC**, trade name **Epivir** (Table 4-1).

Focus on Zidovudine (ZDV), Dideoxyinosine (ddI), Dideoxycytosine (ddC), Stavudine (d4T), and Lamivudine (3TC)

Each of the five drugs (Figure 4-5) has limited effectiveness as a **monotherapy**. The principal limitations are: 1) they are not 100% effective in stopping HIV reverse transcriptase from making HIV DNA; 2) positive clinical effects are short term, they are not sustained; 3) each drug has its own set of toxic side effects; and 4) individually they do not delay the onset of AIDS.

Side Effects

Each of the five reverse transcriptase inhibitors (RTIs) is associated with severe to moderate side effects. For example, zidovudine causes anemia (lowered blood cell count), nausea, headache, and lethargy and inhibits mitochondrial DNA replication in humans (de Martino et al., 1995); didanosine causes peripheral neuropathy (PN) (a burning pain in hands and feet) and pancreatitis (a dangerous swelling of the pancreas) and is very hard to take by people with poor appetites; zalcitabine causes PN and mouth ulcers; stavudine causes PN; and lamivudine causes hair loss and PN.

SELECTION OF HIV DRUG-RESISTANT MUTANTS

HIV reverse transcriptase, the enzyme that copies (transcribes) HIV RNA into HIV DNA, is **unable to edit transcription errors during nucleic acid replication** (Roberts et al., 1988). Because there is no repair or correction of mistakes (as occurs in human cells), there are about one to five mutations in each new replicated HIV DNA HIV RNA strand (Coffin, 1995). This means, that **each new virus** is dif-

TABLE 4-1   Anti-HIV Therapy: Nucleoside Analogs and Protease Inhibitors

Name	FDA Approved	Usual Daily Dosage	Cost/Day[a]
Nucleoside analogs (reverse transcriptase inhibitors)			
Zidovudine (AZT, ZDV; Retrovir)	March 1987	600 mg	$14.00
Didanosine (ddI; Videx)	October 1991	200–400 mg	$3.34
Zalcitabine (ddC; Hivid)	June 1994	2.25 mg	$7.50
Stavudine (d4T; Zerit)	June 1994	60–80 mg	$8.80
Lamivudine (3TC; Epivir)	November 1995	300 mg	$6.22
Abacavir (1592)	? (Glaxo Wellcome/Vertex)	—	Phase III
Non-nucleoside compounds (nonnucleoside reverse transcriptase inhibitors)			
Nevirapine (Viramune)	June 1996	400 mg	$6.88
Delavirdine (Rescriptor)	April 1997	1.2 g	$7.40
DMP 266 (Sustiva)	?(Merck)		
Protease inhibitor drugs[b]			
Saquinavir (Invirase)	December 1995 (Hoffman-La Roche)	1.2 g	$21.60
Ritonavir (Norvir)	March 1996 (Abbott)	1.2 g	$16.15
Indinavir (Crixivan)	March 1996 (Merck)	1.6 g	$16.39
Nelfinavir (Viracept)	March 1997 (Agouron)	2.25 g	$18.58
ABT-378	Expected January 1998 (Abbott)	—	Phase III testing
VX-478	? (Glaxo Wellcome/Vertex)	—	Phase III testing

[a]Cost is based on wholesale price of 100-pill bottle or largest size available as listed in 1995 Red Book or based on information from the manufacturer.

[b]Saquinavir, ritonavir, indinavir, and nelfinavir are FDA approved. Saquinavir, ritonavir, and indinavir were approved in 97, 72, and 42 days, respectively.

Telephone numbers for information concerning the use of the individual protease inhibitors are:

Saquinavir/Invirase	Hoffman-La Roche Inc./800-526-6367
Ritonavir/Norvir	Abbott Labs/800-633-9110
Indinavir/Crixivan	Merck & Co./800-672-6372
Nelfinavir/Viracept	Agouron/888-847-2237
VX-478/—	Glaxo Wellcome Inc./800-722-9292

ferent from most of the other HIV that is being produced! And, new virus is being produced at a rate of 1 billion to 10 billion per day! Coupled with the high rate of viral production is the production of between 10^4 and 10^5 (10 thousand and 100 thousand) new HIV mutants each day in one person. Thus, virtually all possible mutations, and perhaps many combinations of mutations, are generated in each patient daily (Ho et al., 1995; Wain-Hobson, 1995; Wei et al., 1995; Hu et al., 1996; Mayers, 1996). It is not surprising, therefore, that HIV emerges with reduced drug sensitivity under the selective pressure of antiretroviral therapy. Such strains are referred to as **drug-resistant** mutants. In fact, mutations that confer resistance to nucleoside analog reverse transcriptase inhibitors, non-nucleoside reverse transcriptase inhibitors, and protease inhibitors **have all been identified in persons who have never been treated with antiretroviral drugs** (Tables 4-2 and 4-3). The **first** zidovudine-resistant HIV was reported in 1989. Thus, with the wider use of antiretrovirals, pretreatment resistance will probably occur with increasing frequency.

It is clear that the appearance of drug-resistant HIV is a function of the number of HIV replication cycles that take place during infection, and that combination therapy that suppresses HIV replication to undetectable levels can delay or prevent the emergence of resistant strains (Figure 4-7). Abundant evidence has linked the presence of HIV drug resistance to therapy failure (Moyle, 1995).

DOES SOCIETY WANT MIRACLE DRUGS FOR HIV?: THE NEW TREATMENTS COULD MAKE THE PANDEMIC WORSE!

The drug penicillin cured syphilis and gonorrhea, and many experts confidently predicted that these diseases would soon be eradicated forever.

But both diseases are caused by bacteria and their transmission is caused by human behavior, namely unprotected sex with multiple partners. Scientists at the time (1940s and 1950s) reasoned that if effective treatment was available, people would return to the risky behavior that spread the diseases, leading to unintended consequences. For example, because of the success in curing a variety of sexually transmitted diseases (STDs) using penicillin, the government virtually stopped educational programs on STDs, and the sexual revolution, spurred at least in part by a belief that STDs were now curable, created new opportunities for STD-causing microbes to spread.

By the early 1980s, 2.5 million Americans were contracting gonorrhea every year, and syphilis ranked as the third most common infectious disease in the nation. Things came full circle when the casual use of antibiotics produced drug-resistant strains of gonorrhea that literally destroyed penicillin and rendered other antibiotics useless.

While antibiotics are indeed miracle drugs that have saved millions of lives, in the end these treatments ultimately helped spread and strengthen the bacteria that cause some of the worst STDs.

Relative to treating HIV, studies indicate that when drugs called protease inhibitors are used with other drugs, such as ZDV and 3TC, they can reduce HIV to unmeasurable amounts in the blood of many infected people.

But this news, a triumph for medicine, is a mixed blessing for medical ecology. It could turn out that what happened with penicillin and its use in other STDs could apply equally to HIV. One nightmarish scenario circulating among scientists is that triple-combination therapy—resistant HIV could render the AIDS epidemic more intractable than it already is.

That nightmare is based on three factors. **First**, HIV mutates more quickly than any other known virus, and strains have evolved that evade every drug, including protease inhibitors, and many drug combinations. **Second**, the new combination therapies are extraordinarily expensive and difficult to take. Some drugs must be taken on an empty stomach several times a day with up to a quart of water. Others cause terrible side effects. And, if people do not take the drugs correctly and on time (compliance), the chance of developing resistance to the combination cocktail is greatly enhanced. And if they infect another person, that person may be drug-resistant from the start. **Third**, AIDS prevention efforts have faltered, especially in the most afflicted communities. AIDS is exploding in Third World countries and in the United States among poor and minority people, especially women. Also, the gay male population is undergoing a widely documented "**second wave**" of infections. If the potential for death has not been enough to compel people to practice safer sex, what might happen when that threat lessens? Unfortunately, no one really knows what is going to happen—until it has happened!

Class Discussion: What do you think should be done to eliminate the problem as presented?

During 10 years of a person's infection, HIV can undergo as **much genetic change (mutations)** as humans might experience in the course of millions of years, which makes it extremely **difficult to develop treatments** that have **long-term effectiveness** (*Scientific American*, August 1995).

In summary, the frequency of genetically variant HIV within an HIV population is influenced by the mutation rate, fitness of the mutant to survive, the size of the available HIV pool for genetic recombination, and the number of HIV replication cycles.

The Demise of Monotherapy

The use of one anti-HIV RTI drug at a time (monotherapy) leads to HIV drug-resistant mutants to a clinical end point such that David Cooper, an AIDS-drug therapy researcher declared 1995 the year of the "**demise of monotherapy for HIV and the ascendancy of**

FIGURE 4-5 Structure of Five FDA-Approved Nucleoside Analog Drugs Which Inhibit HIV Replication. These nucleoside analog agents competitively inhibit deoxynucleoside triphosphates (part of the HIV proviral DNA chain) when incorporated by HIV reverse transcriptase, causing DNA chain termination. Azidothymidine triphosphate (AZT-TP) competes with deoxythymidine triphosphate (dTTP), dideoxycytidine triphosphate (ddC-TP) competes with deoxycytidine triphosphate (dCTP), and dideoxyinosine (ddI) is converted to dideoxyadenosine triphosphate (ddA-TP), which competes with deoxyadenosine triphosphate (dATP). Stavudine (d4T) competes with deoxythymidine triphosphate (dTTP). Lamivudine (3TC) competes with deoxycytidine triphosphate (dCTP).

combination drug therapy" (Simberkoff, 1996; Stephenson, 1996).

HOW COMBINATION DRUG THERAPY CAN REDUCE THE CHANCE OF HIV DRUG RESISTANCE

Combination drug therapy works because a single strand of RNA, the genetic material of HIV, must be multiply mutant, that is, it must carry a genetic change or become resistant to **each** new drug used. So, the greater number of drugs used, each capable of stopping HIV replication by interfering with the function of reverse transcriptase, the greater the number of genetic changes that must occur in a single RNA strand of the virus. For reasons of explanation, say that the **chance of change** in one gene of HIV for resistance to a single drug occurs in **ONE** RNA strand during the production of 100,000 (100 thousand) or 1×10^5 such strands. **This is a reasonable figure!** Then to have a second gene mutation occur in that **same** single strand for resistance to a second drug, again at 1×10^5 means that only one RNA strand in 10,000,000,000 (10 billion) or 1×10^{10} would carry both genetic changes. For three separate gene mutations occurring in one RNA strand

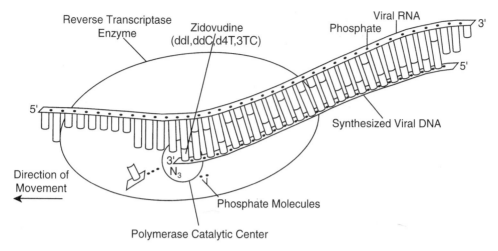

FIGURE 4-6 Incorporation of Nucleoside Analog Preventing HIV Replication. Zidovudine (ZDV) is a synthetic thymidine analog that is widely used in the treatment of HIV disease and AIDS. HIV-RT is 100 times more sensitive to ZDV inhibition than is the **human transcriptase**. The incorporation of zidovudine-triphosphate into HIV DNA by the action of HIV reverse transcriptase terminates DNA chain extension because polymerization or the incorporation of the next nucleotide adjacent to the azide (N_3) group cannot occur. Similar blockage of DNA replication occurs when ddl, ddC, d4T, or 3TC are used. All five nucleoside analogs terminate reverse transcriptase activity.

——————— **POINT OF INFORMATION 4.2** ———————

THE DRUG DEVELOPMENT AND APPROVAL PROCESS

In the United States, the drug discovery and FDA approval currently takes an average of 12 to 15 years and costs about $500 million (from the laboratory to the drugstore). In 1996, Merck & Co. claims to have spent **$1 billion** over 10 years to bring the protease inhibitor **Crixivan** to market! The clinical trial process for a drug usually includes $3\frac{1}{2}$ years of preclinical testing using laboratory and animal studies and 6 years of studies (clinical trials) in humans. **Phase I** includes 20 to 80 healthy volunteers and takes about a year to **test the drug's safety. Phase II** takes about 2 years and involves 100 to 300 persons with the disease to **assess the drug's effectiveness** and to look for side effects. **Phase III** of clinical trials lasts about 3 years and includes 1,000 to 3,000 patients to **verify effectiveness** and **identify adverse reactions of a drug**. Since 1989 the FDA has allowed phases I and II to be combined to shorten the approval process

on new medicines for serious and life-threatening diseases. It now takes about 19 months for a drug to go through the review process for approval by the FDA. About **one in five medicines** that begin a clinical trial is **approved** for consumer use.

In 1996, 79 companies turned out 122 medicines and vaccines for AIDS and AIDS-related conditions. This is in addition to 42 HIV and HIV-related FDA-approved medicines already on the market.

The most difficult part of presenting anti-HIV therapies to the public is the analysis of the incredible amount of new information continuously coming out in the scientific literature and attempting to make sense out of some very contradictory findings!

(*The Drug Development and Approval Process*, Pharmaceutical Manufacturers Association, November 1996)

TABLE 4-2 Genetic Alterations of Nucleotides Associated with the Use of Nucleoside and Non-nucleoside Anti-HIV Drugs

Reverse Transcriptase Inhibitor	Codon Mutations in the Reverse Transcriptase Gene[a]
Nucleoside	
Zidovudine (ZDV)	41, 67, 70, 215, 219
Didanosine (ddI)	65, 74, 75, 184
Zalcitabine (ddC)	65, 69, 74, 75, 184
Lamivudine (3TC)	184, 75
Stavudine (d4T)	75 (rare), 184
Abacavir (1592)	65, 74, 115, 184
Non-nucleoside	
Nevirapine	103, 106, 108, 181, 188, 190
Liviride	103, 181
Delavirdine	181, 236
DMP-266	100, 108, 179, 181

[a]Cross-resistance is a common feature when using these drugs.
(Source: Vella et al., 1996; Vella, 1997)

TABLE 4-3 Genetic Alterations of Nucleotides Associated with the Use of Protease Inhibitor Anti-HIV Drugs

Protease Inhibitor	Codon Mutations in the Protease Gene[a]
Saquinavir	10, 48, 63, 71, 90
Ritonavir	20, 33, 36, 46, 54, 71, 82, 84, 90
Indinavir	10, 20, 24, 46, 54, 63, 64, 82, 84, 90
Nelfinavir	10, 30, 35, 36, 46, 62, 63, 71, 77, 84, 88
141W94 (under development)	10, 46, 47, 50, 84

[a]Cross-resistance has been shown in all four FDA protease inhibitors. For example, persons on saquinavir and who developed resistant mutation **48** eventually develop mutation **82** for resistance to indinavir and ritonavir. **It is now clear that in many people combination drug therapy fails not because of the development of drug resistance, as no genetic HIV drug resistance types were found, but because of poor drug absorption by their bodies and/or poor adherence to their drug-taking schedule.**
(Source: Vella et al., 1996; Vella, 1997)

then, it would be $(1 \times 10^5) \times (1 \times 10^5) \times (1 \times 10^5)$ or only one RNA strand out of 1,000,000,000,000,000 (one thousand trillion) would carry a resistance to all three drugs at the same time. But as small as this number is, because 1 billion to 10 billion genetically different RNA strands are produced each day in one individual, and because individual RNA strands can ex-

FIGURE 4-7 Production of HIV. Each dark hole in the T4 cell membrane represents the emergence of one new HIV that came off the membrane and is loose in the body. Each T4 cell produces about 250 HIV before it becomes nonfunctional. Each HIV in this photograph is genetically different from any other HIV being released from this T4 cell and most likely genetically different from any other HIV in the body. (*Source: The CDC, Atlanta, GA*)

change genes (a process called recombination), strains of HIV resistant to three drug combinations have appeared! This is why it is so important to **slow** the replication of HIV—fewer rounds of replication mean fewer RNA strands, thus fewer possibilities of producing HIV that are resistant to AIDS drug cocktails! Current AIDS drug cocktails, especially those using one or more protease inhibitors, quickly and significantly reduce HIV replication—this is why people on these combination therapies must take them **on schedule**, in prescribed doses, and maybe for the rest of their lives!

Best Choices for Combination Therapy?

Data from a variety of sources, notably the ATCG 175 and the European/Australian Delta studies showed that using nucleoside analog combination therapy can increase and maintain T4 cell count, reduce **viral load**, and reduce clinical HIV disease progression. The best tolerated combinations are: zidovudine/didanosine, zidovudine/lamivudine, and zidovudine/zalcitabine. Combinations to avoid are stavudine/zalcitabine and didanosine/zalcitabine (Ruiz et al., 1996; Saag et al., 1996; Staszewski et al., 1996; Volberding, 1996). Adding a protease inhibitor to the above two-drug combinations has resulted in sustained suppression of HIV replication!

Problems in Drug Selection

Recent studies have shown that each HIV-infected T4 cell produces about 250 new HIV. Collectively sufficient numbers of T4 cells and other cells carrying the CD4 protein (macrophage, etc.) are infected to produce say 10 billion HIV per day. Now, if there were a significantly large number of effective drugs available and if their use was carefully scheduled, theoretically HIV disease could become just another chronic illness. **But**, there is a problem of **cross-resistance**—HIV resistant to one drug have been found to be resistant to similar drugs (see Tables 4-2 and 4-3). Because of cross-resistance, new drugs will have to be found to stay ahead of HIV's ability to become resistant to them.

——— POINT OF VIEW 4.4 ———

THE HURDLE PARADIGM

For ease in understanding, each drug might be looked at as a hurdle that HIV must overcome to cause harm. A hurdle two tiers high makes it twice as difficult for HIV to overcome and hurdles three tiers high, four tiers high, and so on, make it increasingly difficult for HIV to gain resistance to all the drugs at one time. But, given time, if HIV is allowed to replicate its RNA at the **exceptional speed** that it does, HIV will eventually appear that can overcome the hurdle, that is, become resistant, regardless of how many drugs one adds to the cocktail within reason of **safe human consumption**. Remember there are limits as to how many of these toxic drugs one can safely tolerate!

SLOWING THE EMERGENCE OF VIRAL RESISTANT STRAINS

Widespread use of nucleoside HIV reverse transcriptase inhibitors, even in combination, have **incompletely suppressed viral replication and this has led to the emergence of resistant HIV strains, increasing the risk of *transmission* of drug-resistant HIV.** But recent (1996/1997) use of combinations of protease inhibitors and reverse transcriptase inhibitors **slow viral replication sufficiently to prevent the generation of drug-resistant HIV**, increasing the asymptomatic period and extending the lives of people with AIDS!

VIRAL LOAD: ITS RELATIONSHIP TO HIV DISEASE AND AIDS

Viral load refers to the number of HIV RNA strands in the plasma or serum of HIV-infected persons (a discussion of HIV RNA production is provided in Chapter 3; also see referenced material, Jurriaans et al., 1994 and Henrard et al., 1995). Methods now exist to quantitate the amount of HIV RNA in the blood plasma or serum of HIV-infected people. (**Plasma** is a transparent yellow fluid that makes up about 55% of blood volume. **Removing** fibrinogen and blood clotting factors from plasma results in **serum**.)

Viral load measurements are a useful surrogate marker that can provide therapeutic guidance during all stages of HIV disease, including the clinically asymptomatic period, es-

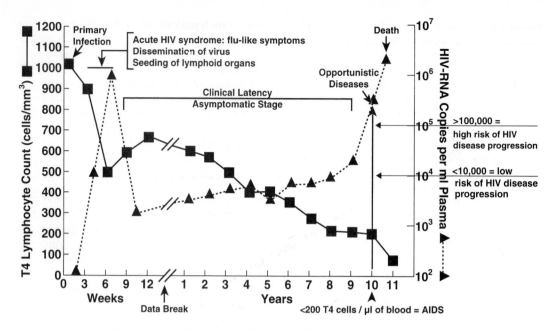

FIGURE 4-8 Clinical Course of HIV Disease as Related to T4 Cell Count and Level (number) of HIV-RNA Copies (viral load) in Plasma. During primary infection (the time period between infection and development of HIV antibody), HIV RNA levels spike (*triangles*) and HIV disseminates (*spreads*) throughout the body. This is followed by an abrupt drop in measurable HIV RNA in the blood (probably due to the production of HIV antibody), followed by a steady rise in HIV RNA until death. Over these same time periods, there is a continuous loss of T4 cells (*squares*). Note that the asymptomatic stage can be quite long—on average about 10 to 12 years, at which time T4 cell counts drop and HIV RNA copies increase to levels where there is high risk of opportunistic infections.

pecially when the T4 cell count is maintained at levels close to normal.

When Is Viral RNA Found in the Plasma

HIV RNA strands are present during all stages of the disease, and the viral load increases with more advanced disease (Piatak et al., 1993; Saksela et al., 1994). Following infection with HIV, there is usually a rapid, transient increase of HIV proteins and RNA followed by a lengthy period of viral RNA replication at lower but measurable amounts (Figure 4-8). In well-characterized groups with known dates of HIV seroconversion, a high viral load immediately after seroconversion (Mellors et al., 1995) and at 3 years after seroconversion (Jurriaans et al.,

1994) appear to be strong predictors of HIV disease progression. However, for most patients with asymptomatic HIV infection, the time of the primary infection is unknown. The levels of viral load prior to the diagnosis are also unknown. In order to determine the predictive value of an isolated viral load measurement under these circumstances, John and colleagues (1996) developed a mathematical model to predict the time to symptomatic disease based on viral load measurements in **untreated patients** with asymptomatic HIV infection and T4 cell counts greater than 500/mL of blood.

Their analysis, based on their mathematical model, suggests that the initial viral load after seroconversion is predictive of the rate of progression of disease, as was shown experimen-

TABLE 4-4 Decimal, Exponent, and Logarithms

Decimal Number	Exponential Form	Log_{10} Value
100,000,000	10^8	8
10,000,000	10^7	7
1,000,000	10^6	6
100,000	10^5	5
10,000	10^4	4
1,000	10^3	3
100	10^2	2

Each number is a 10-fold change from the previous one.

tally by Mellors et al. (1995) and Henrard et al. (1995). Their data show that in the absence of antiretroviral treatment, persons with a viral load of 10^5 (100,000) copies/mL serum may begin **progression to AIDS** (PTA) in less than 3 years and people with a viral load half a log higher (at 500,000) may begin PTA in less than 1 year. [See Table 4-4. A **log** just means a 10-fold difference. For example, an increase in viral load, say from 1,000 to 10,000 (1×10^3 to 1×10^4), is one log. A decrease from 100,000 to 1,000 is a **two-log reduction**. Thus a **one-log** increase or reduction in viral load means that the viral load has increased or decreased by 90%; a **two-log** increase or reduction is a 99% change; a **three-log** increase or reduction is a 99.9% increase or reduction, and so on.] **In contrast**, people with a viral load of $10^{4.5}$ (50,000) have about 2 years and may have up to 8 years before beginning PTA. People with a viral load of 10^4 (10,000) RNA copies/mL have about 3 years and may have up to 19 years before beginning PTA. The rate of change of the viral load was also an important predictor of HIV disease progression; the time since seroconversion had only a minor effect. A knowledge of **both** variables may provide a more accurate prediction than either variable alone. The cumulative viral load over time is a function of both the initial viral load and the rate of change of viral load (how fast are new HIV being made) and may thus be a sensitive measure of the progression of disease. This may be particularly useful for asymptomatic untreated patients with high T4 cell counts when the values of other surrogate markers are usually within normal limits. In patients at advanced stages of disease, and in treated patients, the rates of change of viral load may be more com-

plex. In such patients using T4 cell counts may provide better information than viral load for long-term outcomes such as the incidence of new AIDS-defining illnesses or survival, but viral load changes should be more useful in determining the worth of antiretroviral treatment and guiding therapeutic changes.

USE OF NON-NUCLEOSIDE ANALOG REVERSE TRANSCRIPTASE INHIBITORS

The mechanism of action of **non-nucleoside reverse transcriptase inhibitors (NNRTIs)** is distinct from that of nucleoside analogues. Nucleoside RT inhibitors constrain, or stop, HIV replication by their incorporation into the elongating strand of viral DNA, causing chain termination. In contrast, NNRTIs **are not incorporated** into viral DNA but inhibit HIV replication directly by binding noncompetitively to RT. NNRTIs at first blush appear to offer hope. All four tested did inhibit the RT-HIV enzyme (atevirdine, delvaridine, loviridine, and nevirapine). But this inhibition was **short-lived** because HIV-resistant mutants for each of the non-nucleoside RTI were found within weeks of their use (Table 4-2). Combination therapies using, for example, zidovudine and nevirapine, have shown some success but it turned out that various drug combinations do not extend survival time. But they do extend the asymptomatic period! The FDA approved nevirapine (Viramune) for market in June of 1996.

FDA-APPROVED PROTEASE INHIBITORS

The clinical use of the five FDA-approved nucleoside analog inhibitors of reverse transcriptase, which function **early** in the HIV life cycle, is limited by toxic side effects and the emergence of HIV mutants that resist these drugs. Recall from Chapter 3 that some HIV genes code for reverse transcriptase (RT) integrase and protease enzymes. Later on in the reproductive cycle of HIV a specific protease is required to process the precursor GAG and POL polyproteins into mature HIV components, GAG proteins and the enzymes integrase and protease (Figure 4-9) (Erickson et al., 1990). If

DETERMINATION OF VIRAL LOAD AND QUESTIONS PEOPLE ASK

New viral load blood tests have been developed that help show how much HIV is in the blood. Through 1997 only one has been licensed by the FDA. Not all doctors order viral load tests because not all insurance companies pay for them. However, as viral load tests become more widely available, insurance coverage will be there.

The amount of HIV in a patient's blood is important, especially since only about 2% of HIV is in circulating blood. The other 98% is in the lymph system and other body tissue. A low level indicates the disease is stable and a high level may mean treatment should begin or be changed.

AVAILABLE VIRAL LOAD TESTS

Three types have been developed: through 1997 only one has received FDA approval, Amplicors Q-PCR (quantitative polymerase chain reaction, Figure 13[5). The other two tests are the bDNA (branch-chain DNA, Figure 13-7) and NASBA (nucleic acid sequence-based amplification). All three measure the amount of HIV RNA present in the blood of HIV-infected patients. Test results are usually given per milliliter (mL) of blood. Because each HIV carries two copies of RNA, if there are 100,000 copies of HIV RNA it means there are 50,000 copies of the virus present.

RESULTS OF VIRAL LOAD TESTS

Results of viral load tests can range from almost zero to over a million; low numbers mean fewer viruses in the blood and less active disease; high numbers mean more active disease.

The three tests usually give similar results. However, if the patient's viral load is very low, the bDNA may not detect the HIV RNA. Newer versions of all tests may be more accurate and more sensitive. In general, it is best to stay with one type of test for consistency.

RELEVANCE OF VIRAL LOAD TESTING

The test is new and researchers are still trying to decide on the important values for viral load. In general, though, results can be interpreted as follows:

HIV Viral Load Result	Interpretation
5×10^3 (5000) or fewer	correlates with at least a 5-year survival
10^4 (10,000) or fewer copies per mm³ of plasma	Indicates low risk for disease progression
10,000 to 10^5 (100,000) copies per mm³ of plasma	Medium risk
Over 100,000 copies per mm³ of plasma	High risk

Viral load numbers will depend on the viral load test used. For example, a 25,000 RNA strand number determined using a branched DNA (bDNA) test might be read as 50,000 RNA strands using Amplicors' FDA-approved PCR-RT (polymerase chain reaction-reverse transcriptase) test and higher or lower numbers using other HIV RNA testing procedures. Overall however, the lower the viral load, the better. But no single test of any type gives a complete picture of health. Trends over time are important, as are nutrition, physical condition, psychological outlook, and other factors. Current viral load tests can now detect as few as 20 RNA strands/mm³ of plasma.

TYPICAL QUESTIONS ABOUT VIRAL LOAD

1. **What is the cost of a viral load test? Does insurance pay for it?** Beginning 1998, a viral load test cost between $100 and $200. Some insurance policies pay for the test.

2. **If a viral load test result was 12,000 and 6 months later it is 18,000, is the change important?** Viral load may rise and fall without any change in health. The rule of thumb is that viral load change is not significant unless it more than doubles.

3. **How often should viral load be measured?** Measuring viral load every 4 months, at the same time T4 cells are measured, has been suggested.

FIGURE 4-9 Chemical Structures of the Protease Inhibitors. (*Source: Hammer, 1996*) protease is missing or inactive, noninfectious HIV are produced. Therefore, inhibitors of protease enzyme function represents an **alternative** strategy to the inhibition of reverse transcriptase in the treatment of HIV infection.

As research progressed, scientists found that HIV protease is distinctly different from human protease enzymes, so a drug that blocks HIV protease should not affect human normal cell function. This means that HIV protease blockers are specific to HIV protease and that reduces dangerous side effects of protease-inhibiting drugs. Beginning 1997, some 20 HIV protease-inhibiting drugs were under study; six are in classical trials, and four (**saquinavir**, **ritonavir**, **indinavir**, and **nelfinavir**) received the fastest FDA drug approval ever granted by the agency (Figure 4-9). **PROBLEM: AT LEAST 15% OF PEOPLE MUST GIVE UP PROTEASE INHIBITORS BECAUSE OF SEVERE SIDE EFFECTS. AND, ABOUT 15% OF PEOPLE DO *NOT* RESPOND TO PROTEASE INHIBITORS.**

Structure and Function of HIV Protease

Following production of the HIV proteins, the core structure of HIV assembles at the cell membrane. A matrix protein, p17, appears to specify the site of assembly by associating with the cytoplasmic portion of the transmembrane envelope protein gp41. A packaging signal identifies which viral RNA transcripts (messages for making HIV proteins) are to be included into HIV. The assembled HIV core buds through the cell membrane, thus acquiring a lipid envelope complete with envelope proteins. Maturation of the new HIV requires cleavage by HIV protease of the long Gag and Gag-Pol proteins, which occurs during or shortly after HIV budding.

HIV protease, then, is an enzyme required for cutting long lengths of HIV protein into the individual functional proteins found in infectious HIV. The **protease inhibitors** made up of a small number of amino acids (up to 15) bind to the protease active site and inhibit the activity of the enzyme. This inhibition prevents cleavage of the long HIV proteins, resulting in the formation of immature noninfectious viral particles.

VIRAL CONSTRAINTS THAT MAY LEAD TO HIV ELIMINATION FROM THE BODY

John Guatelli (1997) states that a **mathematical model** of HIV replication in human cells indicates that when HIV production is blocked by anti-HIV therapy, the initial large decrease in plasma HIV RNA concentration allows the following conclusions. Each day, approximately 10^{10} (10 billion) HIV are produced and cleared from the body. The "**lifetime**" of a single HIV in the plasma is 12 hours. The life time of a productively infected cell is about 3 days. There are, according to Alan Perelson of Los Alamos National Laboratories, between **1 billion** and **1 trillion** HIV-infected cells in the body producing HIV. The initial decrease in plasma virus induced by anti-HIV therapy continues for about 2 weeks and typically yields a 100-fold drop (e.g., from 100,000 to 1,000) in plasma HIV RNA concentration. The remaining 1% of plasma HIV concentration decreases at a much slower rate. HIV loss in this **second phase** is characterized by an HIV "life time" of 2 to 4 weeks. Overall, the loss of HIV with time suggests the mathematical possibility of the elimination of all HIV after 3+ years of anti-HIV therapy. This model challenges the dogma that an HIV infection can never be completely cleared from the body.

HIV protease is made up of two units, each unit consisting of 99 amino acids, with two aspartyl residues at the base of the active site serving as the target for most of the protease inhibitors under investigation. Protease has two important functions. **First**, it cuts itself loose from other components of the virus by a process known as autocatalysis (self-releasing). **Second**, protease cuts long inactive proteins of HIV into a number of smaller active proteins (Figure 4-10). Each of these smaller proteins, when liberated plays a vital role in viral reproduction and maturation. One of the released proteins is **reverse transcriptase (RT)**, which is required for HIV to reproduce. Any drug capable of blocking protease will also indirectly inhibit the production of RT.

Other proteins help organize various HIV components (proteins and nucleic acid) into a mature, infectious HIV (Figure 4-11). Electron

———— BOX 4.4 ————

PROTEASE INHIBITORS: EXTENDING LIFE; THE DOWNSIDE OF THIS GIFT—RECOVERY??

THE LAZARUS EFFECT: A RETURN TO FUNCTIONAL STATUS!

In November of 1995, one man in his late forties wrote his obituary—he had been fighting off HIV disease, then AIDS, for over 13 years. In another case, the man's T cell count was zero. He was on oxygen and morphine. Funeral arrangements are made, and his friends and family were on a death vigil. They are but two examples of several hundred men, all under the age of 50, who had given up hope—they believed they were a short step away from death. Some ran up huge debts— maxed out all their credit cards and gave lavish gifts. Some regretted the way they had lived or not lived to this point, some became very angry, some made peace with themselves and others, but **all** felt death was imminent. **Then it happened**—the first results of combination therapies using nucleoside and non-nucleoside reverse transcriptase inhibitors **dropped viral load counts** and then, a few months later, the protease inhibitors used alone or in combination with two or three of the nucleoside or non-nucleoside reverse transcriptase drugs dropped viral load counts to **unmeasurable** or **undetectable** levels in people with HIV disease and AIDS patients. **And**, those with significantly lowered viral loads demonstrated **surprising recovery—their T4 cells rebounded, in some cases from below 200 back up to, or approaching, normal!** These "**AIDS cocktails**," as the combination therapies were soon called, gave people with AIDS, for the first time since the beginning of the pandemic in the United States in 1981, a new chance at a productive life.

CAN THERE BE A DOWNSIDE TO SUCH A MIRACLE?

Of course the most tragic downside is the fact that not all who would benefit from the **drug cocktail** can afford it—But that is not the issue that is relevant to the question per se. No, this question pertains to a downside, if any, for people who have access to these drugs.

WHAT KIND OF PROBLEMS EXIST?

Guilt

Many who now feel "new" again feel **guilty** because these drugs are not available to all who need them—the poor and the uninsured in the United States and those in underdeveloped nations.

Re-establishing Relationships

Depending on how long and how severe the illness, the affected became more or less isolated—even "best" friends stopped calling or dropping by. Some who also had AIDS died, while some were too sick to care or mourn them; but now that they have recovered? **WHAT NOW? During 1997, 150,000 to 250,000 people in the United States were on protease inhibitors. These drugs are not yet available to the other 500,000 to 600,000 HIV-infected in the United States. To date they are unavailable in developing nations.**

Ability to Work Again—Loss of Disability Pay!

Disability insurance has been a **cocoon of safety** for many now experiencing "new" life. Traditionally, people with AIDS received disability checks until death. But suddenly it is not so certain that that is going to be the case. People who were expected to die are going to be coming back. Nobody is prepared for this. Now that drug cocktails have extended life expectancies, it is expected that these people will be re-evaluated and lose their disability payments. They will have to go back to work.

Across the United States, AIDS groups are deluged with calls from patients who are excited, confused, or frightened about the prospect of ending disability status and returning to work. In Miami, a psychologist has begun weekly seminars on resumé-writing and job interviews for AIDS patients who have not worked in years. At AIDS Project Los Angeles, coun-

———— **BOX 4.4** (*continued*) ————

selors field 100 calls each week on return-to-work issues.

AIDS patients face a barrage of challenges as they think about rejoining the work force. Job skills sometimes have atrophied. Old careers do not seem fulfilling anymore after a brush with death. Potential employers may not want to hire someone with a costly disease, even though federal law bars discrimination against people with AIDS. And without clear knowledge of the new drugs' staying power, some patients fear that a return to work could be premature, leaving them in dire shape if protease inhibitors fail them and they lose their jobs once again.

Dilemmas of Returning to Work: Two Examples

1. A 38-year-old software engineer shudders to think about the myriad new technologies he must master if he is to resume work. He used to be a star computer programmer, deluged with consulting assignments. Then AIDS forced him to go on long-term disability.

"I'm going to need new software, new tools, new products" to be a success once more. He estimates that retraining courses will cost $10,000; where will the money come from?

2. He considered taking a part-time job at a friend's hat-embroidery shop but decided against it, in part for fear of jeopardizing his government benefits, and also because he isn't sure how long his health will hold up. **"The biggest downside of this disease is that you stop being a dependable person,"** he says. "I couldn't be sure that I would be there every day. That's very hard to acknowledge."

PREVENTION DOWNSIDE

From mid-1996 into 1998, optimism is high on the medical advances using AIDS cocktail therapy. Though researchers applaud recent drug and immunology findings, many worry about the implications. Treatment successes may create a false sense of security, and lead to complacency in prevention efforts. If we are close to a cure, people may say, why bother with politically sensitive issues like needle exchange programs, distribution of free condoms, sex education programs in our schools, and so on. But the therapy is not available to the majority of HIV-infected, even in the developed countries like the United States. What of the other 30+ million HIV-infected worldwide? If too many glowing promises are made too soon—before treatment is available for all, or most of the world—people may revert back to unsafe sex and other behaviors that will increase their risk of becoming HIV-infected. **No, it is not yet time to stop teaching and providing preventive measures!**

POLITICAL DOWNSIDE

As scientists dare ask whether HIV eradication may be possible in some people in the near future (2 to 5 years), the press may be promising more than the scientists can deliver, but the press can and does influence political will. If the political will to fight this disease **weakens** due to the **premature declaration of victory**, this may be the greatest downside of all!

HIV is not yet a chronic disease and has not yet been eradicated from anyone, despite reductions in viral load to **undetectable** levels for over 2 years in some cases.

---

photography of HIV-infected T cells treated with a protease inhibitor shows continued budding of viruses off the cell surface, but these viruses are immature and deformed if HIV protease does not free the necessary HIV proteins so that they can function (Laurence, 1996).

The Four Protease Inhibitors in Use

1. Saquinavir (Invirase)—Saquinavir was the first protease inhibitor (PI) that FDA approved

for use in combination with nucleoside analog drugs in persons with advanced HIV disease. At the time of approval, there were no clinical trial data on survival or progression of HIV disease using saquinavir (Nightingale, 1996).

Immunological and viral test responses confirm that saquinavir has anti-HIV activity at the current dose of 600 mg three times a day, both as monotherapy and in combination with nucleoside analogs. An important feature is that saquinavir appears to be well tolerated with no

A. Why HIV Protease is Essential for HIV Replication

Protease Cutting Sites

Individual Amino Acids

Long Lengths of Inactive Viral Polyprotein

Units of Protease that Cut the Polyprotein into Individual Active Proteins

Protease   Protease   Protease   Protease

A Different Active Protein From Each Separate Length of Polyprotein

(1)   (2)   (3)   (4)

B. How HIV Protease Inhibitors Inhibit Viral Protease Function

Protease

Protease Inhibitor (Drug)

A Protease Inhibitor Binds to the Cutting Site of the Protease. The Inactivited or Blocked Protease Cannot Cut the Polyprotein.

FIGURE 4-10 Protease and Protease Inhibitors. **A**, The function of HIV protease is to release the individual replication enzymes, core proteins, and envelope proteins so that HIV can develop into mature, infective HIV. **B**, Blocking the production of these essential HIV proteins using protease inhibitors produces immature, noninfective HIV. The action (cutting of protein lengths into active HIV components) of HIV protease occurs during and just after HIV buds out of the cell!

reports of serious adverse effects (moderate diarrhea and nausea) related to therapy. Although HIV mutants to saquinavir have been identified, saquinavir mutants appear to develop more slowly and at a lower frequency than with other HIV mutants to anti-HIV drugs (Jacobsen et al., 1995). The available oral formulation of saquinavir has poor absorption (limited bioavailability) and it is hoped that further development may improve this aspect.

Saquinavir is the least potent of the four FDA-approved protease inhibitors. In people who have not yet taken zidovudine (ZDV), it lowered plasma HIV RNA by only 0.2 log at 16 weeks, compared with 0.6 log for ZDV; but both agents in combination gave a 1.0-log decrease along with an average rise of 70 T4 cells/mm³. Data derived from AIDS Clinical Trials Group (ACTG) protocol 229 showed that saquinavir (600 mg 3 times a day) plus

FIGURE 4-11 Representation of HIV Assembly. During the budding process, the viral Gag and Gag-Pol polyproteins assemble at the cell membrane together with viral RNA to form immature HIV. These polyproteins are then cleaved by the HIV-coded protease enzyme to provide the structural and functional (enzyme) proteins essential to form the **mature**, infectious viral core. (*Adapted from Vella, 1995*)

ZDV or ddC had no significant impact on either viral load or T4 cell count at 16 weeks in ZDV-experienced patients, while all three drugs taken together produced a 0.5-log decrease in HIV RNA and a mean 30-cell increase in the T4 count (Laurence, 1996).

2. Ritonavir (Norvir)—Ritonavir is the second PI to be FDA approved. When used as a monotherapy in HIV-infected persons with a T4 count above 50, it produced a 2-log mean decrease in HIV RNA at 6 weeks. However, viral load returned to their original numbers except in those persons who received doses of at least 600 mg twice a day. In these persons there was a 1-log reduction of HIV RNA at 32 weeks and T4 cell counts increased to 150.

The use of ritonavir in **combination** was even more potent when given at 600 mg twice a day for 2 weeks, followed by addition of ZDV (200 mg three times a day) and ddC; in 22 patients a striking 2.5-log drop in HIV RNA sustained for 20 weeks, with a mean increase in T4 cells of 100. Treatment-related side effects were relatively mild; they included nausea and elevations in cholesterol and triglyceride levels (Danner et al., 1995; Markowitz et al., 1995; Laurence, 1996).

In one ritonavir study, involving nearly 1,100 patients, 13% died or suffered further progression of severe AIDS compared with 27% of patients receiving a placebo. In terms of death alone, the death rate was 4.8% among 543 patients who received ritonavir compared to 8.4% among 547 patients who received a placebo.

3. Indinavir (Crixivan)—This protease is perhaps the most potent of the three FDA-approved protease inhibitors. As a monotherapy (600 mg four times a day), it produced a 2-log drop in HIV RNA at 6 weeks and a 1.5-log drop at 24 weeks in persons who were not exposed to ZDV. Indinavir plus ZDV in combination produced a 2.5-log drop in HIV RNA out to 24 weeks. This drop in viral load was equivalent to the ritonavir + ZDV + ddC triple combination described above (Laurence, 1996).

4. Nelfinavir (Viracept)—Nelfinavir has been evaluated at doses similar to the previous three protease inhibitors. At those concentrations, the side effects include diarrhea, dizziness, fatigue, and headaches. It reduces viral load by 1 log for at least 28 days.

GUIDELINES AND RECOMMENDATIONS FOR THE USE OF ANTIRETROVIRAL AGENTS IN HIV-INFECTED ADULTS AND ADOLESCENTS

The Department of Human Services published a draft guideline from a 32-member panel for the use of antiretroviral agents on June 19, 1997. On June 25, a week later, members of the International AIDS Society—USA Panel published, *Antiretroviral Therapy for HIV Infection in 1997* (Carpenter et al., 1997). Both publications advise the earlier, more aggressive use of antiretroviral therapy, offering therapy to all persons with HIV RNA levels greater than 5,000 to 10,000 copies/mL of plasma regardless of their T4 cell count, discourage the use of a fourth drug to the current three drug combinations, and say that

treatment with only two drug combinations is **less than optimal**. The British HIV Association also published a set of similar guidelines (British Guidelines Coordinating Committee, 1997).

The reason for updated antiretroviral therapy is because of newly acquired knowledge about HIV pathogenesis (how HIV causes disease) and the results of the effective use of combination drug therapies through 1996 and early 1997. It is hoped that these guidelines, which now set a **standard of care**, will move insurance companies to pay for treatments.

————————— POINT OF INFORMATION 4.4 —————————

CURRENT PROBLEMS USING COMBINATION THERAPY

First, DURATION: Many patients ask how long they will have to continue combination therapy? But why would they ask this—it's keeping them alive. But, the combinations often involve taking 20 to 50 or more pills a day that must be swallowed according to a rigid schedule that would tax even the most compulsive individual. The timing centers around an empty stomach, and the drugs often cause severe irritation of the stomach. In one case, a patient had to discontinue therapy after 26 weeks because of gastrointestinal intolerance. The viral load went from **undetectable to 98,600 copies/mL** and the T4 cell count fell from 307 to 227/mm³ within 2 weeks! Pills rule life! (See Figure 4-12.)

FIGURE 4-12 Patient Compliance. People with HIV disease and AIDS may take 20, 30, or more different drugs daily, depending on their prescribed medications for the various opportunistic infections and combinations of drugs necessary for anti-HIV therapy. The patient's drug intake, when this photograph was taken, numbered 28 different pills daily.

———— **BOX 4.5** ————

THE NEW AIDS DRUGS: TIMING* IS CRUCIAL

Doctors are deciding that some people should not have access to new anti-HIV drugs because of the complex drug regimen to which HIV and AIDS patients must adhere. Failure to stick to the strict schedule could make the virus resistant to treatment and cause a potential health risk by creating drug-resistant strains of the disease. Here is how one patient described his daily medication schedule:

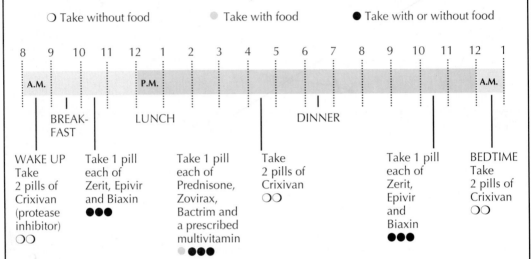

○ Take without food   ● Take with food   ● Take with or without food

| 8 | 9 | 10 | 11 | 12 | 1 | 2 | 3 | 4 | 5 | 6 | 7 | 8 | 9 | 10 | 11 | 12 | 1 |

A.M.   P.M.   A.M.

BREAK-
FAST   LUNCH   DINNER

WAKE UP
Take
2 pills of
Crixivan
(protease
inhibitor)
○○

Take 1 pill
each of
Zerit, Epivir
and Biaxin
●●●

Take 1 pill
each of
Prednisone,
Zovirax,
Bactrim and
a prescribed
multivitamin
●●●●

Take
2 pills of
Crixivan
○○

Take 1 pill
each of
Zerit,
Epivir
and
Biaxin
●●●

BEDTIME
Take
2 pills of
Crixivan
○○

*AIDS combination therapy regimens are arguably the most demanding of any in medicine. Every day must be choreographed to coordinate such basic activities as working, eating, and sleeping with the consumption of a score of pills and liters of water. One patient takes 72 pills daily.

Some drugs require fasting; others must be taken with high-fat meals. Some are taken once a day, some twice, and some three times.

It is a rigorous treatment routine that wreaks havoc on already difficult lives.

One patient, who swallows 16 pills a day, said it took him months to devise a schedule that did not leave him hungry. Now he starts his day with a protease inhibitor, washed down with several glasses of water. Then he has to wait an hour for breakfast.

Between breakfast and lunch, he takes three more pills, and he must eat lunch by 2 P.M. so his stomach can be empty enough for his next protease inhibitor dose at 4:30 P.M. Then he must eat dinner by 6 P.M. to have a full stomach for the next round of drugs. His final challenge is to stay awake to take his last protease inhibitor at 12:30 A.M.

This patient said, "It's a good thing I can actually feel it prolonging my life, because the whole thing is so hard, especially with HIV, which makes you really forgetful."

For most patients, the drugs are also an unwelcome, unending remainder—with side effects like nausea, diarrhea, and kidney stones—that they have HIV (Source: *New York Times*, 3/2/97).

QUESTIONS: How can people high on drugs or those with AIDS dementia or those just too ill to function remember to take their drugs on time? in the proper sequence? or with the proper diet? How many have access to the proper diet, fat vs. non-fatty foods at given times?

STATEMENT: In some large cities like New York, some 75% of HIV/AIDS patients are on **protease inhibitors**. Not to be compliant (that is, taking the medication as prescribed, without failure) is to allow HIV to replicate and give rise to protease inhibitor mutants that may otherwise not occur! Such mutants will then be transmitted to other so, many doctors say they have an ethical responsibility to withhold drug cocktails from some patients after judging them, not as people, but rather as compliant or noncompliant patients.

CLASS DISCUSSION: Is this a moral decision? Why? Why not?

Second, COMPLIANCE—The Achilles Heel of Anti-HIV Therapy: Skipping only a few pills can trigger the emergence of drug-resistant strains of HIV. Such a development could create a worse problem than the initial infection because the resistant virus could overwhelm the individual taking the drugs and anyone else to whom the individual transmitted the virus.

There is a present danger that the behavior of underdosing (not taking enough) or partial compliance (taking the protease inhibitor when they feel like it) or patients who modify their dosage regimens—**to extend their prescription**—may create HIV strains resistant to all currently available drugs. This would lead to an even more devastating AIDS pandemic! The major reason given by 202 HIV-positive people on combination anti-HIV therapy was, **I FORGOT!** (33%). Clearly, the degree of compliance to therapy affects treatment outcome.

Third, COSTS: AIDS is a disease of poverty. The majority of HIV-infected in the United States and worldwide will **never** get a first dose of a protease inhibitor or an AIDS cocktail. The cost **just** for a protease inhibitor is between $12,000 and $20,000 per year! The cost to treat the 800,000 or so Americans would run about $6 billion a year!! Larry Kramer, a co-founder of Gay Men's Health Crises, states that the cost of his drugs to combat AIDS, **which do not include a protease**, amounts to about $19,000 a year; this does not include visits to his doctor or the batteries of blood tests that he routinely requires. And he is asymptomatic. A *New York Times* article in 1997 estimated that drugs for someone with symptomatic AIDS cost about $70,000 a year; in response, a New York University adjunct law professor and gay-rights advocate, wrote a letter to the editor saying that his drugs cost $84,000 a year using protease inhibitors; the annual drug cost can exceed $150,000. At these prices, how many of the nation's 650,000 to 900,000 HIV-infected will be able to afford proper HIV therapy? **AT THESE PRICES PEOPLE HAVE TO CHOOSE WHETHER TO PAY RENT, BUY FOOD, OR PAY FOR THEIR MEDICINE—SOME CHOICE!**

Fourth, SIDE EFFECTS: Because of the short time period from development to approval, many of the drug interaction studies with the protease inhibitors are unpublished or have yet to be performed; therefore, it is difficult to make rational decisions about how to use many of those drugs when using protease inhibitors. Since people with advanced HIV disease use perhaps as many as 15 drugs for the treatment of opportunistic infections and for the treatment of HIV itself and the psychiatric problems that arise with a chronic fatal disease, significant drug interactions resulting in toxic effects are unavoidable.

For practicing clinicians it is more important than ever that **before adding a protease inhibitor to the therapeutic regimen**, the prescriber reviews the drug list of the patient. It is crucial to understand how those drugs are eliminated (renal vs. hepatic, and, if hepatic, conjugation vs. oxidation), so as to make rational choices about those drugs by altering doses as necessary to reduce the likelihood of toxic effects or loss of efficacy. For example, by May of 1997, 83 cases of anti-HIV protease inhibitor therapy-induced **diabetes** was reported to the CDC. All four FDA-approved PIs were involved. The average time of onset was 76 days after beginning treatment. At that time about 150,000 people were on protease inhibitors. There is, at the moment, a rather long list of drugs that should either **not be taken or taken in reduced amounts** when taking a protease inhibitor (Flexner, 1996; Gerber, 1996).

POINT OF VIEW 4.6

CURRENT DRUG/PATIENT REGIMENS MAY CALL FOR A SPECIALIST

Through 1997, there were 11 anti-HIV drugs for use in combination drug AIDS cocktails. Using these drugs, in three-at-a-time combinations, a physician has 1,331 (11^3) prescription options available for any one person. **WHAT TO CHOOSE?—THAT IS THE QUESTION.** Thus, the complexity of today's drug regimens may call for specialist care, analogous to the need for an oncologist to manage complex cancer chemotherapy. In the past it was felt HIV patients could be managed by primary care providers, but today these patients may be better served in the care of specialized physicians.

Protease Inhibitor Side Effects

Saquinavir—Compared to nucleoside analog drugs, **saquinavir** when used alone or with other **non-protease** inhibitor drugs seems to have few side effects. In studies, the most common side effects, occurring in very few people, were rash, diarrhea, stomach discomfort, and nausea.

Ritonavir—Used alone, ritonavir blocks a pathway in the liver that is often used to clear drugs from the body. This affects the way other medications are processed in the body, causing drugs to get backed up in the liver. Of the three PIs, ritonavir is the most problematic for patient safety and tolerability, particularly during the first weeks of therapy. Common side effects are diarrhea, nausea, vomiting, anorexia, headaches, fatigue, and taste disturbances (Deeks et al., 1997). Ritonavir, when used with saquinavir, significantly slows saquinavir metabolism resulting in possible overdosing. Other protease inhibitor interactions, when used in combination, must be studied (Merry et al., 1997).

Indinavir—The most common side effects of indinavir are kidney stones and the temporary elevation of a liver enzyme called bilirubin.

Nelfinavir—The most frequent side effect of nelfinavir is diarrhea.

In summary, the protease inhibitors may cause side effects that have not yet been seen because the number of people using them is relatively small at this point in time. For example, it was recently determined that indinavir and nelfinavir increased plasma concentrations of birth control contraceptives, yet ritonavir **significantly** decreased their levels. All four protease inhibitors interact with and **inhibit** the liver cytochrome P450 enzymes, especially CYP3A. These human cytochrome enzymes are **essential** for metabolizing a large variety of drugs to their nontoxic levels and forms. Because of this effect, many of the medications used in the overall care of HIV-infected people have to be stopped or have their dosage modified, or substitute drugs must be tried.

HIV Resistance to Protease Inhibitors

HIV resistance to all four PIs has been found in clinical trials. The development of HIV resistance to PIs is a major concern (Table 4-3). For example, recent studies (Schmit et al., 1996) found that long-term (1 year) use of **ritonavir** is associated with the production of at least nine different mutations that make HIV resistant to ritonavir. These ritonavir-resistant mutants also demonstrated cross-resistance to **indinavir** and **saquinavir**. John Mellors (1996) reported that within 12 to 24 weeks after **indinavir** therapy, at least 10 different HIV-resistant indinavir mutations occurred and five HIV saquinavir-resistant mutations occurred with the use of the individual drugs. **Cross-resistance to ritonavir occurred in at least 19 isolates of HIV-resistant indinavir mutants.**

Rapid Production of HIV Protease Inhibitor Mutations

The high rate of viral replication found throughout the course of HIV infection and the high frequency of virus mutations occurring during each replication cycle, due to the lack of RNA proofreading or correction mechanisms, are the basis for the emergence of drug-resistant variants under the selective pressure of antiretroviral drugs. In fact, a **Darwinian** model can be applied to HIV dynamics, with the continuous production of genetically different HIV (variants) and the continuous selection of the **fittest** virus.

Unfortunately, with daily production of billions of HIV, and a mutation rate that produces thousands of new mutants each day, **it is likely that any single mutation already exists before any drug is introduced**.

Because resistant variants may exist before treatment is initiated and may evolve (become greater in number) under selective pressure, anti-HIV therapy can address viral resistance in three ways: 1) maximize the suppression of viral replication, the fewer rounds of HIV replication, the fewer HIV mutations possible; 2) use combination drugs requiring HIV to create multiple drug mutations for resistance; and 3) force the emergence of HIV variants with slower replication or decreased virulence.

———— BOX 4.6 ————

CAN COMBINATION THERAPY USING NUCLEOSIDE ANALOGS WITH PROTEASE INHIBITORS CURE HIV DISEASE?

Using a protease inhibitor along with two other nucleoside analogs has created a guarded sense of optimism that a **cure** just might be possible in the near future. There are, however, many, many more skeptics of this belief than believers. To date, physicians marvel at the drop in viral load, to unmeasurable levels, in people who were very sick and their return to a more reasonable quality of life. **The question is, can the viral load be kept that low, and what will happen to the body with that kind of treatment?** There is a real possibility that the therapy will prove too toxic to continue for very long. Or that HIV may find hiding places in the body from which it can eventually reproduce.

But if combination therapy can help people with long-standing HIV infections, it could do even more for those who have just contracted the virus. But, finding people with new HIV infections is not easy; most do not get tested that quickly. But in July 1996, David Ho and colleagues of Aaron Diamond AIDS Research Center found 12 men who had been infected with HIV for no more than 90 days. The men were put on combination therapy and HIV became unmeasurable in their blood's lymph tissues and semen! The ultimate test is to take some of the patients off their medication and see whether HIV increases in their blood. In late 1996, one recovering AIDS patient in San Francisco had no measurable HIV in his blood for the 89 weeks he was on the protease inhibitor-AIDS cocktail. **He** decided to stop the drug therapy; **the virus became measurable within 1 week**.

Also in 1996, Katherine Luzuriaga from the University of Massachusetts, Worcester, described how she and her co-workers treated a twin baby boy and girl with three anti-HIV drugs after they showed signs of infection at 10 weeks of age. The drug combination soon drove HIV RNA in the blood down to undetectable levels. Their levels of antibodies against the virus also steadily declined, another signal that the drugs worked.

But after 16 months of treatment, one child's blood suddenly tested positive for HIV RNA. Since then, the researchers have used a different drug combination to reduce viral load. But these two cases highlight the fact that the new drugs have yet to cure anyone of HIV infection—and it is still unclear whether they will.

The work of Ashley Haase and colleagues (1997) has shown that a 6-month, three-drug combination, eliminated 99% of HIV in tonsils and lymph nodes of 10 HIV-infected people. Their fear, however, is that HIV may be hiding out in brain and other sheltered body tissues. Perhaps a larger problem in eliminating HIV from the body is that of eliminating slow dividing or resting cells that carry HIV in the **proviral** states, that is, HIV DNA integrated within the cells DNA. Such cells may be important reserves of nondeletable HIV that can at some given time become activated and produce HIV (Chun et al., 1997).

David Ho, based on a computer model, predicted that HIV suppression to HIV disappearance would take as long as $2^1/_2$ to 3 years of drug-related HIV suppression before the few remaining infected cells died out, eliminating the remaining virus. The AIDS cocktail may not provide the light at the end of the tunnel, but for now, at least, it has lengthened the tunnel for those with AIDS. **THE AIDS COCKTAIL IS NOT A CURE, A MORNING-AFTER-A-CARELESS-NIGHT PILL, AND IT IS NOT A REASON TO ABANDON SAFER SEX PRACTICES!**

USING THE CURE WORD PREMATURELY CAN CAUSE PROBLEMS: HOPE VS. HYPE

Carelessly using the cure word as it was used during the Eleventh International Conference on AIDS, which received a great deal of television and press coverage, may lull government and medical officials into believing a cure is close and affect government-based funding for continued research. In addition, people may say, why bother with politically sensitive activities such as condom promotion, sex education in schools, or disease-prevention programs for illicit drug users. Let's not invest further in trials of protective vaginal products or genetically engineered vaccines and current safer sex behavior may decline.

AIDS DEATHS DECREASING IN THE UNITED STATES

The number of people reported to have died from AIDS in 1996 decreased 23% nationally, when compared to the number who died in 1995. AIDS deaths fell by 30% in New York City, and by 37% in Connecticut. Florida, which ranks second nationally with respect to numbers of AIDS children and third for adult/adolescent AIDS cases, experienced a 25% drop in AIDS deaths. The number of deaths declined in each of the four regions of the United States (Northeast, 15%; South, 8%; Midwest, 11%; and West, 16%). The number of AIDS deaths also declined among all racial/ethnic groups (non-Hispanic whites, 28%; non-Hispanic blacks, 10%; Hispanics, 16%; Asians/Pacific Islanders, 6%; and American Indians/Alaskan Natives, 32%) and among men (22%) and women (7%). During 1996, HIV infection dropped to the second leading cause of death among persons aged 25 to 44 years. The drop in AIDS deaths is a direct reflection of better overall access to new drugs and overall beneficial health care for those who have HIV disease and those with AIDS.

CAUTION—The use of anti-HIV combination drug therapy from 1996 into 1998 has given thousands of very ill people an unexpected, much im-proved **quality** of life. However, while powerful new drug combinations are delaying disease and death, they have serious limitations, and clinicians and patients who ignore these shortcomings do so at their peril. For example, the new drug therapies **do not** allow the immune system to recover even when the virus can be suppressed. Researchers have spelled out just how distant the goal is of completely rebuilding a full range of immune responses in a HIV-damaged person. Late in 1997, three disconcerting facts came to light. **FIRST**, using new more sensitive RNA tests, 133 people of 151 people (88%) who previously had **no measurable HIV, had measurable HIV** using the new test procedures. **SECOND, the increase in T4 cells** that usually occurs after using combination drug therapy results from a redistribution rather than a regeneration of new T4 cells. That is, T4 cells that are being held in the lymph nodes and other tissues are released into the bloodstream, increasing the number present in the blood (Autran et al., 1997). **THIRD**, in September 1997 at the 37th Interscience Infectious Disease Conference, Steven Deeks reported anti-HIV combination drug therapy **failed to significantly reduce viral load in 53% of people taking the drugs** outside of a clinical trial setting.

Protease Inhibitor HIV Resistance Lessons Learned

Data obtained from indinavir, ritonavir, saquinavir, and nelfinavir studies show a dose-dependent delay in the emergence of resistance. This is the most important property of protease inhibitors that distinguishes them from nucleoside reverse transcriptase inhibitors. Higher doses of nucleosides do not delay resistance or provide a greater effect, but rather increase toxicity. **With increased dose of the protease inhibitors, a more durable reduction in viral RNA response and a delay in resistance are achieved without greater toxicity** (Mellors, 1996).

It appears, based on clinical trial data, that the best way to avoid resistance is to take the drug on time, and not to skip doses. Taking PIs in combination with other anti-HIV drugs has been shown to slow down the development of HIV PI resistance. Researchers have been very clear about one thing: at this point in time, one cannot stop taking a protease inhibitor once started.

Summary

Anti-HIV therapy becomes more complicated with the approval of each new anti-HIV drug (Figure 4-13). Just a few years ago (1990/1991) the only anti-HIV therapy was ZDV or nothing, depending on the patient's disease stage. At that time, the ZDV/ddC and ZDV/ddI combinations were considered alternatives for initial therapy, but there were no data to support their use. By early 1997, five nucleoside analogs, four protease inhibitors, and two non-nucleoside RTI had received FDA approval. Still, the end point of the entire arsenal of anti-HIV therapy is premature death. But, for the first time there are some drugs that offer con-

> # DRAMATIC HEALTH IMPROVEMENTS AMONG AIDS PATIENTS CAUSE A SHIFT IN UNITED STATES HEALTH CARE POLICIES
>
> Powerful new AIDS cocktail (combination therapy) treatments have had dramatic results for thousands of patients, reducing the need for hospital and hospice care. This, in turn, had led some hospitals to consider downsizing their AIDS wards. At the same time, doctors and outpatient clinics are reporting increased demand for HIV-related services. Many physicians now say they are taking care of problems in the office that they used to have to treat in the hospital. Hospices have also reported that fewer AIDS patients are seeking end-of-life care, and patients who do choose hospices are waiting longer to enter them, so stays are shorter. Overall, AIDS health care costs are going down nationwide, and the patients are living longer.
>
> ## THE PRICE FOR SUCCESS: AIDS SOCIAL SERVICE PROVIDERS
>
> Over the last 12 years, an army of AIDS social service providers have been dedicating their lives to caring for people with HIV disease and AIDS. But now their world has changed. With new med-
>
> ications restoring some people to robust health, pressure is building to shift funds away from social services like transportation, housing, and counseling and into drugs and treatment.
>
> In December 1996, Laurie McGinley (*Wall Street Journal*) wrote that Cleve Jones, founder of the AIDS quilt, got a warm reception in October as he walked to the podium of a Washington, D.C. hotel to speak to AIDS social service providers. But his message sent a chill through the audience.
>
> Mr. Jones, who had almost died of AIDS, was now strong thanks to advanced AIDS medication. His message was that drugs, research, and treatment—not social services—should be the priority for public and private funds.
>
> "My point was, 'AIDS Inc., I want you out of business,' " he says. "Some people wanted to string me up."
>
> At press time, the gap between the AIDS social service providers and those favoring increased funding for therapy at the expense of social services continues to grow. There may not be an **acceptable** resolution by the opposing forces to this problem.

siderable promise for the clinical management of HIV infection. Unlike nucleoside analogs, protease inhibitors have no requirement for metabolic activation and are active in a wider range of cell types. In addition, protease inhibitors are well tolerated and are suitable for combination therapy with all current nucleoside analog reverse transcriptase inhibitors.

The costs for anti-HIV combination therapy using the protease inhibitors is expected to be about $12,000/year for life. **Who will be able to afford the therapy? (Class Discussion).**

PEDIATRIC ANTI-HIV THERAPY

Recommendations for the optimal anti-HIV therapy for children with HIV infection are confused at best. Results of AIDS Clinical Trials Group protocols 152, 240, 245, 300, 327, and others which address the use of nucleoside analog monotherapy and combination therapy, through the end of 1997, have created

many questions, some of which are: At what point during the course of HIV infection should therapy be initiated? How does one determine the need for a change in treatment regimen? What is the best way to monitor responses to anti-HIV therapy and detect HIV disease progression? Further, the use of protease inhibitors available to adults is, in 1997, just becoming an option for children. The development of protease inhibitors for pediatric use was seriously impeded by the poor oral bioavailability and unpalatable nature of the liquid formulations. In March of 1997, ritonavir and nelfinavir became FDA approved for use in children.

PROTEASE INHIBITORS AND PREGNANCY

The use of zidovudine (often referred to as AZT) during pregnancy has cut the transmission rate of HIV into children to 8%. In mid-

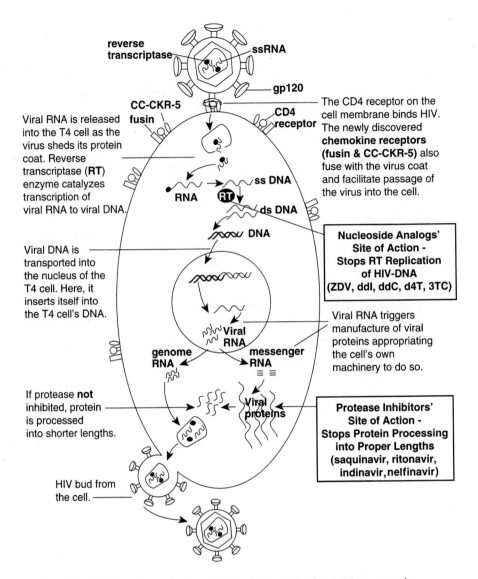

reverse transcriptase

ssRNA

gp120

CC-CKR-5 fusin

CD4 receptor

Viral RNA is released into the T4 cell as the virus sheds its protein coat. Reverse transcriptase (**RT**) enzyme catalyzes transcription of viral RNA to viral DNA.

RNA **RT** **ss DNA**

ds DNA

DNA

The CD4 receptor on the cell membrane binds HIV. The newly discovered **chemokine receptors (fusin & CC-CKR-5)** also fuse with the virus coat and facilitate passage of the virus into the cell.

Viral DNA is transported into the nucleus of the T4 cell. Here, it inserts itself into the T4 cell's DNA.

Nucleoside Analogs' Site of Action - Stops RT Replication of HIV-DNA (ZDV, ddI, ddC, d4T, 3TC)

Viral RNA

genome RNA **messenger RNA**

Viral RNA triggers manufacture of viral proteins appropriating the cell's own machinery to do so.

If protease **not** inhibited, protein is processed into shorter lengths.

Viral proteins

Protease Inhibitors' Site of Action - Stops Protein Processing into Proper Lengths (saquinavir, ritonavir, indinavir, nelfinavir)

HIV bud from the cell.

FIGURE 4-13 Diagram of Anti-HIV Therapy. The five FDA-approved nucleoside analogs and four protease inhibitors represented with respect to their anti-HIV activity. The nucleoside analogs act early after infection, while the protease inhibitors act later in the HIV life cycle, after viral proteins have been synthesized into long strands. Those strands of amino acids contain the individual HIV proteins that become functional after they are cut into their appropriate amino acid sequence lengths. **NOTE: The enzyme integrase is required for HIV DNA to enter human DNA. Drugs called INTEGRASE INHIBITORS are in development.**

THE COST OF STAYING ALIVE INCREASES WITH EACH NEW THERAPY

Even if protease inhibitors live up to their potential, it is not clear who will be able to afford them. By some estimates, the new drugs will cost $500 to $600 a month for the rest of a patient's life. And that is in addition to the cost of the nucleoside analogs that cost about $400 a month. Hospitalization and other medical care in the final stages of the disease can add $150,000. Future treatments could dwarf even that. Where is this going to stop?

Where will all this money come from? In an era of managed care, insurers do not wish to take on additional liability. And, funds are beginning to dry up. The **AIDS Drug Assistant Programs** (ADAPs) were set up in 1987 as a safety net to help provide low-income uninsured and underinsured persons with HIV access to treatment. In 1996, about 80,000 clients were served by these programs but experts estimate that anywhere from 140,000 to 280,000 persons may be eligible. This number does not include those persons who may not know their HIV status and who are not in a system of care.

All 50 states have **ADAP**s which are partly funded by Washington. But 20 states do not cover protease inhibitors. The rest face a funding crisis as requests for the protease inhibitors and AIDS cocktails flood in. Some states have waiting lists. Others, including Indiana and Missouri, have organized lotteries to determine which patients will get the treatments.

In mid-1996 budget cuts from New York State's ADAP forced it to drop 130 reimbursable medications used by AIDS patients. ADAPs are in trouble mainly because protease inhibitors and AIDS cocktails are so expensive.

Beginning 1997, 30 state ADAPs offered at least one protease inhibitor drug to those with HIV disease. For fiscal year 1998, ADAPs will spend $195 million buying drugs for 95,000 Americans who are **not covered** by Medicaid or private insurance. This money, many states say, is all that is keeping them afloat. State after state is running low on money to buy the newest, most potent AIDS drugs for thousands of low-income Americans, leaving many patients without access to these medicines or with a possible rationing of their medicines.

Washington became the latest state, following Illinois, Kansas, Florida, Mississippi, and South Dakota, to dramatically cut its ADAPs as it tried to avert almost certain bankruptcy. Eleven other states reported drug assistance shortfalls in 1997.

More cutbacks are pending as states scramble to cover unexpected bills for today's patients, not counting the thousands suddenly demanding protease inhibitor drugs because of headlines promising unprecedented new hope. Illinois now offers one protease, but cut 82 of the 112 other drugs that patients had been able to take, including almost every antibiotic. Kansans can no longer enroll in ADAP unless other patients leave the program. In the state of Washington, the AIDS Director had to temporarily shut down their AIDS drug program after a 76% jump in AIDS patients between January and June (1996) pushed the bills from $53,000 a month to $144,000. It may well be that the more sophisticated and effective HIV treatments become in the developed nations, the fewer people will have access to them. What chance does someone with AIDS have to new therapies if they live in an undeveloped nation? Moving into 1998, **less than 3%** of over 30 million people with HIV infections in developing nations have access to drugs presented in this chapter. People in underdeveloped countries have neither the money to buy the drugs, sufficient people to dispense them if they had them, nor the means by which to keep patients in dosing compliance! And these are just a few of the problems with making medicines available in these nations.

Based just on access to affordable HIV/AIDS treatment, it appears that **AIDS is a two-world disease, the wealthy versus the indigent.** (**Class Discussion**)

1997, researchers will begin putting HIV-infected mothers on combination therapy with protease inhibitors to see if they can cut the rate to lower levels. But protease inhibitors are more powerful and potentially more toxic than zidovudine and no one knows what harm it might do to the developing fetus.

For additional considerations for antiretroviral therapy in the HIV-infected pregnant woman, see pages 13–18 of the "Guidelines for

the Use of Antiretroviral Agents in HIV-Infected Adults and Adolescents" (1997).

DISCLAIMER

This chapter is designed to present information about certain aspects of HIV/AIDS therapy. This chapter does **NOT** provide medical advice or replace the advice or care of a medical professional. **ALWAYS** consult a trained health care provider for medical advice and treatment options.

SUMMARY

New results in the field of HIV therapy have given HIV-infected persons new hope in their battle against HIV disease and AIDS. First, combinations of nucleoside analogs compared to zidovudine alone were shown to have a clinical benefit (prolonged survival and fewer AIDS-defining events) when given to asymptomatic individuals with relatively early-stage disease. This was the first demonstration that an intervention regimen used in patients with early-stage HIV disease could actually be clinically beneficial. Next came the demonstration of nucleoside combination therapy, then the extraordinary capability of protease inhibitors. The introduction of the protease inhibitors is the most powerful intervention against HIV to date. Marked reductions in viral load, striking clinical improvement, and reduction in mortality have been observed among patients able to take these medications **properly**. Whether to initiate protease inhibitor therapy in the very early stages of HIV disease is controversial.

Protease inhibitors do not work for all HIV-infected persons; the reasons for this lack of efficacy are not completely understood. Long-term adverse effects of protease inhibitors are not known at this time. It is hoped that cumulative toxicities from years of protease inhibitor therapy will not offset the benefits. Drug resistance to protease inhibitor therapy can occur during regular use and especially when the drugs are not taken as scheduled. Resistance to one protease inhibitor can also confer cross-resistance to other protease in-

hibitors, although cross-resistance has not yet been established for the new protease inhibitors currently under investigation. These factors will need to be considered when discussing antiretroviral strategies with patients and their families.

The use of protease inhibitors in combination with nucleoside and non-nucleoside reverse transcriptase inhibitors holds great promise for a level of control of established HIV disease that has, until now, eluded patients and physicians. Furthermore, the use of these drugs in primary HIV infection holds promise for interfering with the establishment of chronic persistent infection and dramatically altering the subsequent course of HIV disease.

In less than a year, the prospects for treatment of HIV-infected patients, at least those socioeconomically privileged, have improved dramatically. Important new questions about HIV pathogenesis can now be asked and investigated. Nevertheless, the prospects of drug resistance, the toxicities of current drugs, and the need for even greater antiretroviral activity will require the discovery and development of still more and better drugs.

SOME AIDS THERAPY INFORMATION HOTLINES

For HIV/AIDS treatment information, call:

The American Foundation for AIDS Research: 800-39AMFAR (392-6237)

AIDS Treatment Data Network: 212-268-4196

AIDS Treatment News: 800-TREAT 1-2 (873-2812)

For information about AIDS/HIV clinical trials conducted by National Institutes of Health and Food and Drug Administration-approved efficacy trials, call:

AIDS Clinical Trials Information Service (ACTIS): 800-TRIALS-A (874-2572)

For more information about HIV infection, call:

Drug Abuse Hotline: 800-662-HELP (4357)

Pediatric and Pregnancy AIDS Hotline: 212-430-3333

National Hemophilia Foundation: 212-219-8180

Hemophilia and AIDS/HIV Network for Dissemination of Information (HANDI): 800-42-HANDI (424-2634)

National Pediatric HIV Resource Center: 800-362-0071

National Association of People with AIDS: 202-898-0414

Teens Teaching AIDS Prevention Program (TTAPP) National Hotline: 800-234-TEEN (8336)

General information:

English: 800-342-AIDS (2437)

Spanish: 800-344-7432

TDD Service for the Deaf: 800-243-7889

General information for health care providers:

HIV Telephone Consultation Service: 800-933-3413

To locate a physician, call your local or state Medical Society.

Note: This is not an all-inclusive list. For other sources of information, contact your state HIV hotline. State HIV hotline numbers are located at the end of the "Introduction."

REVIEW QUESTIONS

(Answers to the Review Questions are on page 576.)

1. Can HIV infection be cured?

2. What is a surrogate marker?

3. From ___ of 1987 through ___ of 1997 ___ anti-HIV drugs were FDA approved.

4. How many FDA-approved anti-HIV drugs are nucleoside analogs?

5. What is the proper drug name for the following drug acronyms: ZDV, ddI, ddC, d4T, and 3TC?

6. How do nucleoside analogs inhibit HIV replication?

7. What are the two major problems in the use of nucleoside and non-nucleoside analogs in HIV therapy?

8. What is HIV viral load? What can its quantitative measurement reveal?

9. Name the four protease inhibitors that have FDA approval for use in the United States.

10. Which of the four FDA-approved protease inhibitors appears to be the most effective and why?

11. How do non-nucleoside drugs inhibit HIV replication?

12. Briefly describe the focus of HIV combination drug therapy.

13. After starting antiretroviral therapy, what is an acceptable target for viral load that indicates the therapy is effective?
    A. 5,000 copies/mL
    B. 5,000–10,000 copies/mL
    C. 10,000–15,000 copies/mL
    D. No acceptable target level has been set.

14. Which of the following statements is correct regarding HIV pathogenesis?
    A. HIV contains two copies of the viral DNA genome.
    B. Viral polyproteins are cleaved by protease.
    C. The RNA copy is integrated in the host-cell chromosome.
    D. gp120 envelope glycoprotein facilitates entry of HIV core particle into the cell's cytoplasm.

REFERENCES

AUTRAN, BRIGITTE, et al. (1997). Positive effects of combined antiretroviral therapy on CD4+ T cell homeostasis and function in advanced HIV disease. *Science*, 277:112–116.

British Guidelines Coordinating Committee. (1997). British HIV Association guidelines for antiretroviral treatment of HIV seropositive individuals. *Lancet*, 349:1086–1091.

CARPENTER, CHARLES, et al. (1997). Antiviral therapy for HIV infection in 1997. *JAMA*, 277:1962–1969.

CHUN, TAE-WOOK, et al. (1997). Quantification of latent tissue reservoirs and total body viral load in HIV infection. *Nature*, 387:183–188.

CLUMECK, NATHAN. (1995). Summary to the use of saquinavir for HIV therapy. *AIDS*, 9(Suppl. 2):S33–S34.

COFFIN, JOHN. (1995). HIV population dynamics *in vivo*: Implications for genetic variation, pathogenesis and therapy. *Science*, 267:483–489.

DANNER, SVEN, et al. (1995). Short term study of the safety, pharmacokinetics and efficacy of ritonavir. *N. Engl. J. Med.*, 333:1528–1533.

DEEKS, STEVEN, et al. (1997). HIV protease inhibitors. *JAMA*, 277:145–153.

DE MARTINO, MAURIZIO. (1995). Redox potential status in children with perinatal HIV-1 infection treated with zidovudine. *AIDS*, 9:1381–1383.

DICKOVER, RUTH, et al. (1996). Identification of levels of maternal HIV-RNA associated with risk of perinatal transmission. *JAMA*, 275:599–605.

ERICKSON, JOHN, et al. (1990). Design, activity, and 2.8 angstrom crystal structure of a C_2 symmetric inhibitor complexed to HIV protease. *Science*, 249:527–533.

FLEXNER, CHARLES. (1996). Pharmacokinetics and pharmacodynamics of HIV protease inhibitors. *Infect. Med.*, 13:16–23.

GERBER, JOHN. (1996). Drug interactions with HIV protease inhibitors. *Improv. Manage. HIV Dis.*, 4:20–23.

GOLDSCHMIDT, RONALD, et al. (1995). Antiretroviral strategies revisited. *J. Am. Board Fam. Pract.*, 8:62–69.

GUATELLI, JOHN. (1997). Basic science research. *Improv. Manage. HIV Dis.*, 4:51–52.

Guidelines for the Use of Antiretroviral Agents in HIV-Infected Adults and Adolescents. (1997). *Federal Register* 62;118:33417–33418 (pp. 1–37).

HAASE, ASHLEY, et al. (1997). Kinetics of response in lymphoid tissues to antiretroviral therapy of HIV infection. *Science*, 276:960–964.

HAMMER, SCOTT. (1996). Advances in retroviral therapy and viral load monitoring. *AIDS*, 10(Suppl 3):S1–S11.

HENRARD, DENIS, et al. (1995). Natural history of HIV cell-free viremia. *JAMA*, 274:554–558.

HO, DAVID, et al. (1995). Rapid turnover of plasma virions and CD4 lymphocytes in HIV-1 infection. *Nature*, 373:123–126.

HU, DALE, et al. (1996). The emerging genetic diversity of HIV. *JAMA*, 275:210–216.

JACOBSEN, HELMUT, et al. (1995). Reduced sensitivity to saquinavir: an update from genotyping from phase I/II trials. 4th International Workshop on HIV Drug Resistance, Sardinia.

JOHN, PATRICIA, et al. (1996). Predictive value of viral load measurements in asymptomatic untreated HIV infection: A mathematical model. *AIDS*, 10:255–262.

JURRIAANS, SUZANNE, et al. (1994). The natural history of HIV infection: Virus load and virus phenotype independent determinants of viral course? *Virology*, 204:223–233.

LAURENCE, JEFFREY. (1996). The clinical promise of HIV protease inhibitors. *AIDS Reader*, 6:39–41, 71.

MARKOWITZ, MARTIN, et al. (1995). A preliminary study of ritonavir, an inhibitor of HIV protease. *N. Engl. J. Med.*, 333:1534–1539.

MAYERS, DOUGLAS. (1996). Rational approaches to resistance: Nucleoside analogues. *AIDS*, 10(Suppl. 1):S9–S13.

MELLORS, JOHN, et al. (1995). Quantitation of HIV-1 RNA in plasma predict outcome after seroconversion. *Ann. Intern. Med.*, 122:573–579.

MELLORS, JOHN. (1996). Clinical implications of resistance and cross-resistance to HIV protease inhibitors. *Infect. Med.*, 13:32–38.

MERRICK, SAMUEL. (1997). Managing antiretrovirals in HIV-infected patients. *AIDS Reader* 7:16–27.

MERRY, CONCEPTA, et al. (1997). Saquinavir pharmacokinetics alone and in combination with ritonavir in HIV-infected patients. *AIDS*, 11:F29–F33.

Morbidity and Mortality Weekly Report. (1994). Zidovudine for the prevention of HIV transmission from mother to infant. 43:285–287.

MOYLE, GRAEME. (1995). Resistance to antiretroviral compounds: Implications for the clinical management of HIV infection. *Immunol. Infect. Dis.*, 5:170–182.

NIGHTINGALE, STUART. (1996). From the Food and Drug Administration: First protease inhibitor approved. *JAMA*, 275:273.

NOWAK, MARTIN. (1995). How HIV defeats the immune system. *Sci. Am.*, 273:58–64.

PIATAK, MICHAEL, et al. (1993). High levels of HIV-1 in plasma during all stages of infection determined by competitive PCR. *Science*, 259:1749–1754.

ROBERTS, JOHN, et al. (1988). The accuracy of reverse transcriptase from HIV-1. *Science*, 242:1171–1173.

RUIZ, LIDIA, et al. (1996). Efficacy of triple combination therapy with zidovudine plus zalcitabine plus lamivudine versus double combination therapy in patients previously treated with zidovudine plus zalcitabine. *AIDS*, 10:F61–F66.

SAAG, MICHAEL, et al. (1996). Strategies for continuing antiretroviral therapy. *Improv. Manage. HIV Dis.*, 4:16–19.

SAKSELA, KALLE, et al. (1994). Human immunodeficiency virus type 1 mRNA expression in peripheral blood cells predicts disease progression independently of the number of CF4+ lymphocytes. *Proc. Natl. Acad. Sci. USA*, 91:1104–1108.

SCHMIT, JEAN-CLAUDE, et al. (1996). Resistance-related mutations in the HIV protease gene of patients treated for 1-year with protease inhibitor ritonavir. *AIDS*, 10:995–999.

SIMBERKOFF, MICHAEL. (1996). Long-term follow-up of symptomatic HIV-infected patients originally randomized to early vs. later zidovudine treatment: Report of a Veterans Affairs cooperative study. *AIDS*, 11:142–150.

STASZEWSKI, SCHLOMO, et al. (1996). Safety and efficacy of lamivudine/zidovudine combination therapy. *JAMA*, 276:111–124.

STEPHENSON, JOAN. (1996). New anti-HIV drugs and treatment strategies buoy AIDS researchers. *JAMA*, 275:579–580.

VELLA, STEFANO. (1995). Clinical experience with saquinavir. *AIDS*, 9(Suppl 2):S21–S25.

VELLA, STEFANO. (1997). Clinical implications of resistance to antiretroviral drugs. *AIDS Clin. Care*, 9:45–47, 49.

VELLA, STEFANO, et al. (1996). HIV resistance to antiretroviral drugs. *Improv. Manage. HIV Dis.*, 4:15–18.

VOLBERDING, PAUL. (1996). Initiation of antiretroviral therapy. *Improv. Manage. HIV Dis.*, 4:4–6.

WAIN-HOBSON, SIMON. (1995). Virologies mayhem [editorial]. *Nature*, 373:102.

WEI, XIPING, et al. (1995). Viral dynamics in human immunodeficiency virus type 1 infection. *Nature*, 373:117–122.

The Nature of the Human Immune System and Its Function During HIV Disease/AIDS

CHAPTER CONCEPTS

♦ HIV attaches to the CD4 receptor sites on T4 lymphocyte, monocyte, and macrophages cells.

♦ CXCR4(FUSIN) and CC-CKR-5 are receptors that allow HIV to enter cells.

♦ Monocytes and macrophages serve as HIV reservoirs in the body.

♦ Basic immune system terminology is defined.

♦ T4, T8, and B cell function is related to HIV disease.

♦ Apoptosis is a normal mechanism of cell death.

♦ Cofactors may enhance HIV infection.

♦ Impact of T4 cell depletion is immune suppression.

♦ Latency refers to inactive proviral HIV DNA, but true latency may not exist for HIV.

♦ Clinical latency refers to infection with low-level HIV production over time.

Several cell types in the human body can become infected by HIV. The more important of these cells belong to the body's **immune system.** The immune system filters out foreign substances, removes damaged and dead cells and acts as a security system to destroy mutant and cancer cells. It is composed of a number of specialized cells, several organs, and a group of biologically active chemicals. The human immune system is like a jigsaw puzzle—many parts come together to form an overall defense against disease-causing agents. If parts of the immune system are missing or damaged, illness may occur due to an immune deficiency.

Over most of the body, the skin prevents disease-causing agents from entering the body. But they can enter through body openings, cuts, or wounds. Once they enter the body, they trigger an **immune response**. All body cells have special molecules, called **class I proteins**, on their membranes that are like flags with the word **"self"** on them. The cells of the immune system try to destroy anything present in the body that is not carrying the self molecules, anything that is **"nonself."** Nonself is any substance or object that triggers the creation of antibodies. Such substances are called **antigens**. Antigens may be whole virus or organisms or parts of virus, organisms, or their products.

————— BOX 5.1 —————

HOW LARGE IS A TRILLION?

The human body is made up of many trillions of cells. For example, the human immune system contains at least a trillion lymphocytes dedicated to destroying foreign substances that endanger health. But, a trillion of anything is a very large number. Can we **really appreciate just how large a trillion of something is?**? Perhaps the following will help.

1. A stack of 1 trillion dollar bills would reach a height of 69,000 miles.

2. It would take a person 11.5 days to count to 1 million and 31,688 years to count to 1 trillion—1, 2, 3, 4, 5. . . . !

3. A stack of 1 trillion HIV (Figure 5-1) would be **over** 62 miles high (diameter of HIV = 1,000 angstroms: (1×10^{12}) $(1,000)$ $(1 \times 10^{-10}) = 1 \times 10^5$ meters = 62.15 miles)

FIGURE 5-1 Dimensions of HIV in Angstroms. HIV has a diameter of 1,000 angstroms (Å). It would take 254,000 HIV laid side by side to equal 1 inch in length.

In general, most organisms that damage cells do so from the outside by producing toxic chemicals or in some way externally interfering with the cell's metabolism. But viruses generally invade or **enter** different cell types forcing them to produce viral replicas at the expense of the cells' own essential metabolic functions. Gradually, like a machine wearing out, host cells start to malfunction and die. The best thing a virus can do is find a host cell that does not die and that can produce replicas indefinitely. In a biological time frame, new disease-causing viruses are often very deadly to new hosts. If a new virus strain is too deadly, it kills its host before other hosts are infected, and the ensuing epidemic dies out. For example, the **Ebola virus**, which makes its victims very weak shortly after infection and kills them in 7 to 14 days, has had seven brief outbreaks since its first appearance in 1976, the latest in November 1996. This virus kills quickly and vanishes. Its origin is still unknown. Over biological time, successful viruses and their new hosts learn to accommodate each other. This will most likely happen with human-HIV associations, but how many people over how many years will have to die before human cells learn to accommodate HIV is unknown. Perhaps it will never happen. Smallpox virus has been infecting humans for thousands of years and has never been accommodated by humans.

HUMAN LYMPHOCYTES: T CELLS AND B CELLS

The hallmark of the human immune system is its ability to mount a highly specific response against virtually any foreign entity, even those never seen before in the course of evolution. It is able to do this because of the number of different kinds of cells called lymphocytes. The human immune system contains about 1 trillion (1×10^{12}) lymphocytes, a relatively small number when compared to the trillions upon trillions of other types of cells in the body (see Box 5.1, Figure 5-1). Most mature lymphocytes recirculate continuously, going from blood to tissue and back to blood again as often as one to two times per day. They travel among most other cells and are present in large numbers in the thymus, bone marrow, lymph nodes, spleen, and appendix (Figure 5-2). By 1968, lymphocytes had been divided into two classes: lymphocytes called **B cells** that are derived from and mature in bone marrow, and lymphocytes called **T cells** that are derived from bone marrow but travel to and mature in the thymus gland (Figure 5-3). T cells make up 70% to 80% of the lymphocytes circulating in the body. Circulating T cells are a heterogeneous group of cells with a wide range of different functions. Each individual T cell expresses a receptor (**T cell antigen receptor, TCR**) which recognizes a ligand (a compound that fits a particular receptor) composed of an antigenic peptide,

8–15-amino-acid-long, bound to a **self-major-histocompatibility-complex (MHC) molecule** (also referred to as HLA-human leukocyte antigen). Thus, a T cell does not directly recognize a soluble antigen, but rather recognizes an antigen displayed on the surface of an **antigen-presenting cell (APC)** like a B cell or macrophage (Table 5-1). Three major kinds of T cells are **cytotoxic or killer** T cells, **suppressor** T cells and helper T cells. Both killer and suppressor T cells carry the **CD8 antigen**. T suppressor cells are referred to as **T8 cells.** Helper T cells carry the **CD4 antigen** and are called **T4 cells** (for an explanation of CD8 and CD4 antigens, see Box 5.2, T lymphocytes). Killer T cells bind to cells carrying a foreign antigen and destroy them. T4 cells do not kill cells; they interact with B cells and killer T cells and **help** them respond to foreign antigens.

It is believed that T4 cells recognize only those antigens of viruses, fungi, and other parasites; and trigger only those parts of the immune system necessary to act against these agents. Indeed, it is the viruses, fungi, and other parasites that produce the majority of opportunistic infections when the T4 cells have been depleted by the AIDS virus.

The Microbial World Responds to the Human Immune System

Large DNA viruses such as adenovirus, herpes simplex viruses 1 and 2, Epstein-Barr virus, and cytomegalovirus have evolved sophisticated mechanisms to avoid detection by the human immune system. Most of these mechanisms are geared toward preventing the expression of antigenic viral peptides that are bound to major histocompatibility complex (MHC) class I molecules, on the surface of the infected cells (antigen presentation). In this way, the viruses turn off the signal that would alert the immune system to the presence of an intracellular pathogen and, undetected by antigen-specific T lymphocytes, the infected cells continue to provide a safe haven for the viruses.

T4 Cell Function and HIV Disease

In general, individuals with partial or absolute defects in T cell function have infections or

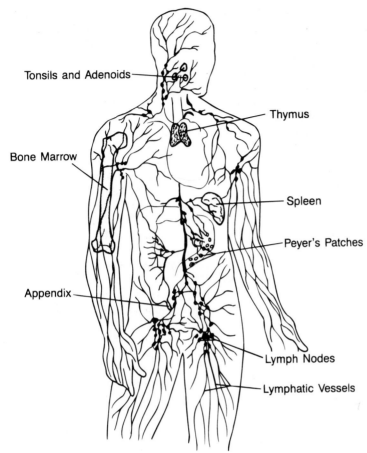

FIGURE 5-2 Organs of the Human Immune System. The organs of the immune system are positioned throughout the body. They are generally referred to as lymphoid organs because they are concerned with the development, growth, and dissemination of lymphocytes, or white cells, that populate the immune system. Lymphoid organs include the bone marrow, thymus, lymph nodes, spleen, tonsils, adenoids, appendix, and the clumps of lymphoid tissue in the small intestine called Peyer's patches. The blood and lymphatic fluids transport lymphocytes to and from all of the immune system organs.

clinical problems for which there is no effective treatment. The T cell disorders are more severe than the B cell disorders.

The discovery of the relationship between T4 lymphocyte count and HIV disease progression is based on the observation that losses in T4 counts leads to the development of opportunistic diseases, the diagnoses of AIDS, and death. T4 cell counts reliably track the natural history of HIV infection, particularly after an AIDS-defining illness is diagnosed. T4 cells are selectively deleted as a result of a series of events initiated by the binding of HIV to the CD4 molecule (located on the T4 cell membrane) by means of the viral envelope protein gp120. Once HIV enters a T4 cell, it begins to lose normal function. This change, however, is not immediately apparent. HIV's takeover is a quiet event. The virus joins the host cell's DNA, then, instead of functioning normally, the T4 cell manufactures new HIV and dies. The loss of T4 cells severely reduces cell-mediated immunity, eliminates the T4 cell dependent production of antibodies by B cells, and eventually makes HIV-infected people susceptible to opportunistic infection and subsequent death. **AIDS is diagnosed when the T4 cell count drops to less than 200/mL of blood.** (T4 counts from 800 to 1,200 are considered normal in adults.) T4 cell counts of less than 100 are associated with **profound** immunodefi-

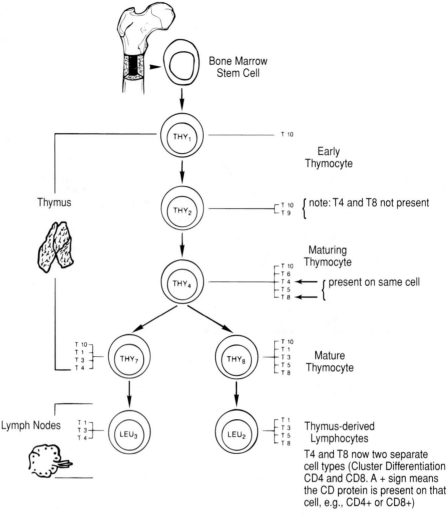

FIGURE 5-3 T lymphocyte Cluster Differentiation (CD) Antigens in Humans. Stages of thymic differentiation (i.e., the presence of the different antigens on their membrane surfaces) are defined on the basis of reactivity to monoclonal antibodies. Schematic pictures of cells represent thymocytes within specific stages of a defined phenotype: T1–T10 and membrane glycoproteins of T cells.

ciency and multiple or disseminated opportunistic infections (Crowe et al., 1991). (See Chapters 6 and 7.)

One of the most interesting findings has been the discovery of a subset of healthy, **long-term survivors** who have lived for years with T4 counts of less than 200 (see Chapter 7, Box 7.4). For the most part, they do not develop the secondary infections that are associated

with AIDS, or if they do, they tend to recover. This means that there is a lot about the immune system that immunologists still do not understand. Some researchers believe these men and women managed to press other white blood cells into service to make up for the T4 deficiency. It is also possible that persons with low T4 cell counts actually have more T4 cells than those detectable in peripheral blood

TABLE 5-1   Cells of the Human Immune System

Cell Type	Function
Stem cells	Self perpetuating cells that give rise to lymphocytes, macrophages, and other hematological cells
T helper cells (T$_H$), also called T4 or CD4 cells	Cells that interact with an antigen before the B cell interacts with the antigen
Cytotoxic cells (Tc)	Recruited by T helper cells to destroy antigens
Suppressor T cells (Ts), also called T8 or CD8 cells	Cells that dampen the activity of T and B cells; they somehow inhibit the immune response
B cells	Bone marrow stem cells that differentiate into plasma cells that secrete antibodies
Plasma cells	Cells devoted to the production of antibody directed against a particular foreign antigen
Monocytes	Precursors of macrophages
Macrophages	Differentiated monocytes that serve as antigen-presenting cells to T cells; they can also engulf a variety of antigens and antibody-covered cells
Killer cells (K)	Lymphocytes that recognize and kill any cell that is coated with antibody
Natural killer cells (NK or null cells)	Lymphocyte cells that detect and kill tumor cells and a broad range of foreign cells

--------- BOX 5.2 ---------

TO UNDERSTAND THE DIFFERENCE BETWEEN HEALTH AND DISEASE, IMMUNOLOGISTS NEED TO UNDERSTAND THE IMMUNE SYSTEM!

Basic Immune System Terminology

Of the many mysteries of modern science, the mechanism of **self** versus **nonself recognition** in the immune system must rank near the top. The immune system is designed to recognize foreign invaders. To do so it generates on the order of 10^{12} or one trillion different kinds of immunological receptors so that no matter what the shape or form of the foreign invader there will be some complementary receptor to recognize it and effect its elimination. Understanding how the immune system responds to any foreign substance is puzzle enough, but the added mystery is that the immune system can distinguish foreign carbohydrates, nucleic acids, and proteins from those that exist within us, often in shapes barely distinguishable from the invaders. When the immune system is working well it never gets activated by self substances, but unerringly responds to the nonself substances. When the system is not working well this distinction gets blurred and **diseases of autoimmunity occur—our immune cells attack our own tissue!**

To understand the human immune system certain basic terminology is reviewed:

Antibody—an immunoglobulin (a protein) which is produced and secreted by B lymphocytes in response to an antigen. Antibodies are able to bind to and destroy specific antigens. Antibodies contribute to the destruction of antigen by their interaction with other components of the immune system.

Antigen—a substance that is recognized as foreign by the immune system when introduced into the body. An antigen can be a whole microorganism (such as a bacterium or whole virus) or a portion or a product of an organism or virus.

Leukocytes—all white blood cells (WBCs) including neutrophils, lymphocytes, and monocytes (phagocytes).

Lymphocytes—mononuclear WBCs which are critical in immune defense because they provide the specificity and memory needed for immune function and long-term or even life-long immunity. The two major classes of lymphocytes are B cells and T cells; both recognize specific antigens. (For an excellent review of lymphocyte life span and memory, see Sprent et al., 1994.)

———— **BOX 5.2** (*continued*) ————

Lymphocyte Surface Receptors—Proteins are located on cell surfaces to serve a physiologic function. Some are enzymes, some are transport proteins, and many are **receptors**. All cells use specific receptors to communicate with their environment or with other cells. The receptors found on lymphocytes may be loosely classified according to their function. Thus lymphocytes require receptors that recognize antigen. They need receptors for antigen-presenting cells and receptors for the many factors that regulate lymphocyte responses.

Chemokines—are chemotactic cytokines that activate and **DIRECT** the migration of leukocytes. There are 28 known chemokines separated into two subfamilies, those whose protein amino acid structure begins with cytosine–amino acid–cytosine, called the CXC chemokines, and those whose protein amino acid structure begins with cytosine–cytosine, called the CC chemokines.

Cytokines—soluble factors secreted by T cells, B cells, and monocytes which mediate complex immune interactions by acting as messengers. Subcategories of cytokines include: (1) lymphokines (secreted by lymphocytes), and (2) monokines (secreted by monocytes and macrophages). Specific cytokines include interleukin-1 (IL-1), interleukin-2 (IL-2), gamma interferons (γINF), B cell stimulating factor (BCSF), and B cell differentiating factor (BCDF).

The two branches of the human immune system are: Cellular Immunity and Humoral Immunity. Basic terms for each are provided, but as the terms will show, the two branches overlap to provide our immunity. (Adapted from *Mountain-Plains Regional HIV/AIDS Curriculum*, 1992.)

I. ***Cellular Immunity***—immune protection resulting from direct action of cells of the immune system. Key cell types offering Cellular Immunity are:

A. ***Phagocytes***
   1. Phagocytes are leukocytes which are specialized for ingesting particles and molecules.
   2. The most active phagocytic cells are monocytes and macrophages. Monocytes circulate in the blood but eventually move into body tissues (brain, muscle, etc.) where they mature into macrophages.
   3. Phagocytes initiate the cellular immune response. When an invader (e.g., a virus

or bacteria) enters the body, it will be trapped and digested by a phagocyte. This attack against invaders occurs in various places in the body: the lining of the gut, throat, skin, bloodstream, or in organized lymphoid tissue such as the tonsils, other lymph nodes, or the spleen.
   4. The phagocyte ingests the foreign invader and partially digests it. Pieces of the invader (antigens) can then be displayed on the phagocyte's surface, making the phagocyte an **antigen-presenting cell**. This process alerts other cells in the immune system that a foreign substance is present.

B. ***Lymphocytes***
   1. Ninety-eight percent of lymphocytes reside in lymphoid tissue (Pantaleo et al., 1993). Lymphocytes are uniquely specialized. Each lymphocyte has receptors on its surface for one, and only one, of the many millions of possible antigens that can invade the body. When the receptors lock with their matched antigen, the process of neutralizing, inactivating, or destroying the foreign particle begins.
   2. This requires that the body have an immense variety of receptors for an immense number of antigens. Humans usually have about trillion lymphocytes.
   3. There are several types of lymphocytes that play major roles in the immune response.

   a. ***T Lymphocytes*** mature in the thymus and play a central role in the immune response by destroying infected cells, controlling inflammatory responses, and helping B cells make antibodies. There are several subsets of T lymphocytes **(*Subsets of T cells display different proteins in groups (antigens) on their cell membranes. For this reason they are referred to as cluster differentiation (CD) antigens. At least 95 different cluster differentiating antigens are known to reside on different human cell types. The different CD antigens located on T lymphocyte subsets allow investigators to distinguish between the different T cell lines. For example, in physical appearance it is nearly impossible to distinguish T cells from B*** cells. But each carries a different CD antigen. T lymphocytes attached by HIV carry type 4 antigen and are referred to as CD4 + T lymphocytes or T4 cells, likewise for T8 cells. B lymphocytes do not carry the T4 or T8 antigen.)

1) **Helper T cells** (T_H) alert the immune system to the presence of an antigen and activate other cells in the system. Helper T cells carry about 10,000 copies of the CD4 protein molecule on the surface of each helper T cell so these **CD4+** cells are most often referred to as **T4** cells.

   a) T4 cells have receptors on their surface which are specialized for the recognition of antigens found on the surface of antigen-presenting cells.

   b) When the T4 cell randomly contacts the surface of a phagocyte, its receptor binds to antigen on the phagocyte and the T4 cell becomes activated.

   c) The T4 cell then begins to secrete a variety of stimulatory factors (*lymphokines*) *into the space around it.*

   d) The T4 cell will eventually divide into two cells of exactly the same specificity. If the foreign substance persists, the two daughter cells will divide, and so on. Thus, the number of cells specific for that foreign antigen is greatly expanded.

   e) The T4 cell probably does little to repel the intruding substance on its own, but it is vital for activating the other main classes of lymphocytes (e.g., B cells, natural killer cells and phagocytes). It does this by means of the lymphokines it secretes when activated. The most familiar of these are interleukin-2 (IL-2) and gamma interferon (γIFN).

   f) As a result of activation by T4 cells, B lymphocytes multiply and produce specific antibodies. The antibodies attach to the antigens on free organisms and infected cells, leading to inactivation and destruction of organisms and cells.

2) **Inducer T cells** (T_i) were previously known as the delayed sensitivity T cells. Inducer T cells also carry the CD4 molecule.

   a) When an inducer T cell recognizes antigen on the surface of a phagocyte and is helped by factors from a T4 cell, it also becomes activated and secretes its own family of lymphokines. IL4, IL5, and IL10. These factors attract many more phagocytes from around the body which accumulate in the area where antigen is being recognized.

   b) Phagocytes are specialized for ingesting and destroying the foreign invader.

3) **Cytotoxic T cells** are lymphocytes also known as killer T cells. Cytotoxic T cells express the CD8 molecule and are most often referred to as **T8** cells. They are crucial for the immune response to viral infections. Although they cannot neutralize free virus, by eliminating virus infected-cells they are largely responsible for recovery from a viral infection.

   a) When a cytotoxic T8 cell recognizes antigen and is assisted by an activated T4 cell, it becomes *activated*. An activated cytotoxic T8 cell has the ability to "look inside" other cells and detect abnormalities within and destroy the infected cells.

   b) As the infected cell breaks apart, infectious particles can be released from the cell. The released infectious particles may be phagocytized, neutralized by antibody, or may infect new cells.

   c) Cytotoxic T8 cells have antigen specificity; this specificity is determined when the cytotoxic T8 cell is exposed to the antigen.

b. **B Lymphocytes** or **B cells** arise principally in the bone marrow and are responsible for making antibodies. The B cell response is referred to as humoral immunity.

   1) B lymphocytes have receptors for antigen and also require help from T4 cells to become activated.

   2) When activated, they release large amounts of immunoglobulins, called *antibodies*, into the bloodstream and mucosal surfaces.

———— **BOX 5.2** (*continued*) ————

3) Antibodies circulate in body fluids. When they encounter the specific antigen with which they can interact, they bind to it.

4) Antigen–antibody interactions block the antigen's harmful potential in a variety of ways. For example, if the antigen is a toxin it may be neutralized or if it is a virus, it may lose its ability to bind to its target tissue.

5) In addition, the complex of antigen and antibody activates a group of proteins in the blood called *complement,* which then facilitates the removal of the antigen by calling in a large number of phagocytes.

c. *Memory cells*
   1) Two groups of T and B lymphocytes become separate T and B memory cells for when the same antigen invades the body again.
   2) Memory cells initiate immune response upon re-exposure to an antigen.
   3) Memory cells remember, recognize, and induce a more rapid immune response against the antigen.
   4) Memory cells are responsible for disease resistance after immunization and

are also responsible for natural immunity.

d. *Suppressor T cells* also carry the CD8 molecule.
   1) The function of suppressor T8 lymphocytes in the immune system is not well understood.
   2) Suppressor T8 cells turn off antibody production and other immune responses after an invader has been destroyed or eliminated from the body. This provides a balance in the immune system and allows it to rest when its functions are not required.

e. *Natural killer (NK) cells*
   1) NK cells are antigen nonspecific lymphocytes which recognize foreign cells of many different antigenic types. That is, one NK cell can recognize many different types of invaders. Therefore, NK cells can attack without first having to recognize specific antigens.
   2) NK cells are important in fighting viral infections.

II. *Humoral Immunity*—immune protection by the circulating antibodies which are produced by B cells. (See preceding section on **B Lymphocytes**.)

measurements. In fact it is now known that most T4 cells are sequestered in lymphoid tissue. Thus the true number of T4 cells in the body can only be established by measuring their presence in tissues other than blood. Thus long-term survivors may have less damage to their lymphoid tissues than do those with less survival time.

B Cell Function and HIV Disease

The ultimate product of the B cells is **immunoglobulin.** Any abnormalities in the transition of the B lymphocyte from the stem cell level to the plasma cell may affect imunoglo-

bulin synthesis. The earlier the rupture in the developmental pathway, the more extensive the loss in antibody-forming capacity.

The B lymphocytes can produce and secrete soluble antibodies in response to direct contact with an antigen (T cell-independent B cell response), or the **B cell with the help of T4 cells can produce antibodies specific for a given antigen** (T4 cell-dependent B cell response). The antibodies enter the circulatory system and are carried throughout the body.

HIV does not normally infect B cells. However, in laboratory experiments, HIV is able to infect B cells, if the B cells are first in-

CLASS I AND CLASS II PROTEINS

There is a series of genes located on human chromosome 6 that is referred to as the **major histocompatibility** (tissue type) **complex (MHC)**. The genes in this region produce a series of proteins that are **almost** unique to the individual. Because these proteins belong to the individual, they would be recognized as foreign or as an **antigen** when placed in another human, for example, as in a transplanted heart (**transplantation antigens**). **Almost** all cells in an individual have a sample of their own MHC proteins or transplantation antigens located on the surface of each cell's membrane. Thus, a person's transplantation antigens are recognized as **self-proteins** by their immune system. Such MHC proteins are referred to as **class I** (type 1) tissue compatibility proteins. So, every individual will have their own set of class I proteins on their cell membranes. It is these proteins that cause **transplant graft rejections**. So, with minor exceptions, there is not much of your body tissue that would not be rejected if placed in another human body because your class I proteins would be recognized as foreign by the recipient body's immune system. **But how does the recipient's immune system recognize these class I proteins as foreign? ANSWER:** By using a second class of MHC proteins, **class II**, that are **immune response** gene products. Relatively few human cell types carry this **protein on their cell membranes**. All such cells carrying the class II protein are derived from a monocyte-macrophage cell series which includes macrophages located in the lung, liver and spleen, dendritic cells of the gut, skin, spleen and lymph nodes, Langerhans' cells of the skin, and microglial cells of the nervous system.

This class II protein, located on the membrane of these cell types, allows these cell types to act as the body's police force. These cells **digest** foreign protein into smaller products. Some of these products, a small series of amino acids or **peptides**, are then escorted to the cell surface alongside a molecule of the class II protein. In this way, the cells carrying a class II protein **serve up** or **present** the foreign substance or antigen alongside or adjacent to the class II protein or "self molecule" so that immune system cells, **notably** the T4 cells and B cells, can sense the presence of the foreign protein and initiate an immune response against it—the activation of a variety of immune system attack cells (cytotoxic T cells, killer T cells) and the production of very specific antibodies.

In medically important viral infections, neutralizing antibodies are generated within 6 to 14 days. In contrast, such protective antibodies generally appear 50 to 150 days after infection with HIV and the hepatitis B virus (HBV) in humans (Pianz et al., 1996).

JEFFREY GETTY'S HIV-RESISTANT BABOON CELL TRANSPLANT FAILS

In December of 1995 Jeff Getty received a transfusion of prepared HIV-resistant baboon bone marrow immune stem cells. After 2 months there were no signs of remaining immune baboon cells. Investigators believe the experiment failed because the low doses of radiation and chemotherapy failed to suppress his immune system. His immune system, sensing the foreign protein, rejected (destroyed) the baboon stem cells.

fected by the Epstein-Barr virus, which is the cause of infectious mononucleosis. The Epstein-Barr virus appears to change B cells in some way, allowing subsequent HIV infection. HIV can grow and replicate within B cells transformed by the Epstein-Barr virus, without destroying the host cell. Whether similar events occur within humans is not known. B cell function is almost normal in most HIV-infected persons. Small defects in B cell function exist, seemingly resulting from the disrupted communication with other cells, not from some internal B cell defect.

THE BIG QUESTIONS:

- How does HIV, which at first glance does not appear to be a highly formidable foe, persist in the body for such long periods of time and continue multiplying and progressively causing more and more damage until a fatal outcome is reached?

- Why does the immensely powerful immune system of the body, an organ system which has evolved over millenia of challenges from a wide variety of infectious and noninfectious invaders to become an exceedingly effective defender of the body against agents far more virulent than HIV, now appear to be powerless against it?

THE ANSWER:

Because HIV, unlike other agents that enter the human body, (virus, bacteria, fungus, and protozoa) infects immune system cells, in particular **the T4 cell which governs the response of the entire immune system!** Without T4 cells the immune system cannot function—like a car without gas, all the parts are there but nothing happens when called on to operate.

T8 Cell Function and HIV Disease

Together, T4 cells and T8 cells regulate the body's immune response to invaders. Also, T8 cells help the immune system recognize (and not attack) the cells of its own body. But some T8 cells are lost in HIV-infected persons. Depending on how many are lost, the immune system may not be properly suppressed when necessary and an autoimmune response (the immune system attacks self) may occur.

Summary: Immune Dysfunction Caused by HIV/AIDS

HIV enters the body via infected body fluids: blood, semen, and vaginal secretions. Once inside, HIV specifically infects a type of white blood cell called the T4 cell. These cells direct the body's immune response against infection. As HIV takes over the T4 cells, it alters their growth and reproduction through a complicated process that leads to the T4 cells' destruction. The ratio of T4 to other cells called T8 then

changes. In healthy people, the number of T4 cells is greater than the number of T8 cells. In HIV-infected individuals, a decline in the T4 count signals the progress of immune system deterioration. The results are debilitating: the T4 cells are not as responsive to antigen identification, macrophages become less responsive, and B cells produce fewer specific antibodies and lose their normal responsiveness. At this point, the immune system becomes dysfunctional and the host becomes vulnerable to attack from opportunistic infections that would normally be held in check by a healthy immune system. (A normal T cell count ranges from 800 to 1,200.)

ANTIBODIES AND VIRUSES

Twenty-four hours a day, 365 days a year, the body's lymphocytes must be on the lookout for harmful bacteria, viruses, and other pathogens. And these agents of disease don't look very different, biochemically, from most of the regular molecules lymphocytes normally encounter in the blood. Yet a mistake by these immune cells can leave the body open to infection.

But, the immune system has evolved antibodies for distinguishing the body's own molecular debris from potentially harmful material.

The Antibody

Antibodies are Y-shaped molecules that bind to specific foreign proteins, or pieces of protein, called antigens. If the immune system mistakenly identifies the body's own proteins as foreign, an autoimmune disorder can result.

When antibodies on the surface of a B cell snag an undesirable or foreign protein, **both disappear inside the cell**. Eventually, a bit of the foreign protein may reemerge, attached to a "self" recognizable protein molecule called a **class II protein** (Figure 5-4). The pair, the small piece of foreign protein attached to a "self" **class II protein**, acts as a red flag to T4 cells, which set off an aggressive immune response.

The self or class II protein molecules play a critical part in the immune defensive response because they determine which viral peptides will be displayed on certain cells, antigen-presenting cells (APC), and how effectively they are showcased. Any two individuals are

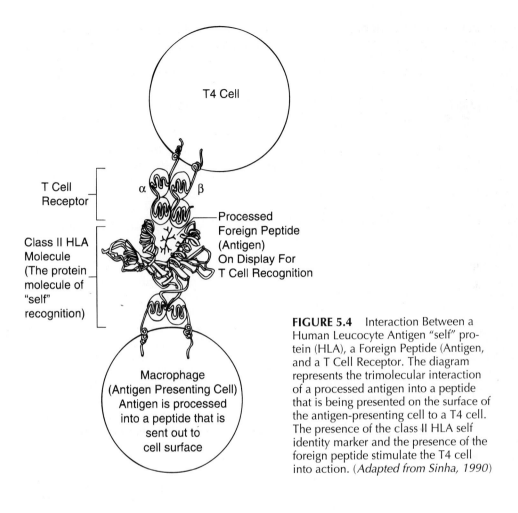

T4 Cell

T Cell
Receiver

α   β

Processed
Foreign Peptide
(Antigen)
On Display For
T Cell Recognition

Class II HLA
Molecule
(The protein
molecule of
"self"
recognition)

Macrophage
(Antigen Presenting Cell)
Antigen is processed
into a peptide that is
sent out to
cell surface

FIGURE 5.4 Interaction Between a Human Leucocyte Antigen "self" protein (HLA), a Foreign Peptide (Antigen, and a T Cell Receptor. The diagram represents the trimolecular interaction of a processed antigen into a peptide that is being presented on the surface of the antigen-presenting cell to a T4 cell. The presence of the class II HLA self identity marker and the presence of the foreign peptide stimulate the T4 cell into action. (*Adapted from Sinha, 1990*)

likely to differ in the precise structure of these class II molecules they possess. Thus, they will also differ in the peptides their cells exhibit and in the ability of the class II-peptide units to attract the attention of the immune system. Most people infected with HIV seem to recognize just a few of the many potential small peptide units generated from the virus's proteins, usually between one and 10.

Until now, scientists did not know where the cell degraded this undesirable protein and attached it to a "self" recognizable protein.

In mid-1994, four research teams announced the discovery of a special compartment, or organelle, inside cells where this processing occurs. Using sophisticated biochemical and immunological techniques, they independently determined that both the "self" recognizable protein and the antibody-antigen complex wind up in this new compartment called an endosome (Amigorena et al., 1994; Pennisi, 1994; Schmid et al., 1994; Tulp et al., 1994).

The characterization of a specialized vesicle is an important step. It permits an understanding of the trafficking events and defines the intracellular event of antigen processing. (For an excellent review of the concept of antigen processing and presentation, see Unanue, 1995; for class I and class II proteins, Strominger et al., 1995; for the concept of self, Zinkernagel, 1995; for cell-mediated immunity, Doherty, 1995).

B Cells Make Antibodies and Release Them into the Bloodstream

After an antibody and virus join, they are digested by macrophages or cleared from the blood by the liver and spleen. Some B cells and T cells become **memory cells** which are stored by the immune system. Memory cells can remember the antigen they have previously encountered. If the same virus ever gets into the bloodstream again, these cells rapidly begin antibody production. However, if the virus has mutated (changed), as the flu virus does yearly, previous antibodies will not affect it. New antibodies must be created to neutralize the new mutant virus. While this antibody production is taking place, the viral invader has time to multiply and infect new cells, and the infected person suffers the symptoms of the flu.

ANTIBODIES AND HIV DISEASE

Resistance to HIV does not seem to be the same as more common examples of immunity. The body's protective countermeasures against measles and mumps are absolute. Years after exposure, there is no hint within the body of the foreign agents that cause those diseases. After children become immune to mumps, they can no longer infect other people.

The human body makes apparently effective antibodies against HIV, but over time, the ratio of antibody production to new virus production becomes disproportionate, that is, more virus than antibody is made and at this time the level of T4 cells begin to drop. T4 cells drop because antibodies to HIV reduce circulating HIV in the plasma (viral load) without affecting HIV replication or cell-to-cell spread of HIV. This means that the production of mutant HIV to existing antibody nevers ceases, resulting in continued T4 cell infection and loss. Eventually there are too few T4 cells to ward off opportunistic infections (see Chapter 7 for additional information on T4 cell replacement and HIV production).

The rapid production of HIV mutants without the same rapid production of neutralizing antibody against each mutant means that

sometime after infection, many if not most of the antibody in some people may be nothing more than useless antibody copy (antibody to the initial strain or strains of HIV). In these people, HIV disease would most likely progress more swiftly than in persons whose immune system can keep up with the production of new antibody to match the formation of HIV mutants. This may be one important reason why some people progress to AIDS and death so rapidly when compared to other HIV-infected people.

HIV Protected from Human Antibodies

Humans create antibodies against a number of HIV proteins, namely the envelope proteins (gp120), the transmembrane protein (gp41), and the proteins of HIV's core (gp24). **But, antibodies cannot enter cells.** The antibody can only attack HIV in the plasma. Plasma is the fluid part of the blood and does not include the blood cells. **Once inside a host cell, HIV is protected from antibody.** Cells can generate antiviral chemicals within themselves, but these too seem ineffective against the hidden HIV.

Once HIV gets inside T4 or other cell types as a provirus, it is likely to remain there for the rest of the cells life (person's life?) unless some other antiviral mechanism within the body or some chemical agent is able to destroy the provirus. To date, no such drug has been found to be effective against the HIV provirus.

How HIV ATTACHES to the T4 Cell

The envelope of HIV is studded with proteins made by the virus. The major envelope protein is called gp120:

1. gp120 proteins protrude from the viral envelope. The gp120 region contains a conserved or **constant region** (in this region the sequence of amino acids remains constant from virus to virus) and a **variable region** (among HIV, the amino acid sequence is often different in this region). With respect to building a vaccine, the variable or **V** region, made up of five domains, each containing a separate sequence of amino acids, is the more important region of the envelope proteins. The region of the five domains is referred to as the hypervariable region of gp120 because of the ex-

tensive number of amino acid substitutions (new amino acids) that occur within the five areas. Each of the five domains, because of its amino acid arrangement, contains a loop-like structure. These are referred to as the V1 through V5 loops. The V3 loop is the most hypervariable (changeable). The V3 loop is located near the midportion of gp120 and appears to be involved in helping HIV lock into the CD4 receptor of a lymphocyte. A number of investigators are currently attempting to produce V3 loop antibody, believing that if the V3 loop is neutralized, HIV could not attach to the cell. **In summary**, each V-loop undergoes antigen change as its amino acids are replaced by different amino acids as genetic mutations occur in sections of HIV-RNA that code for the amino acid arrangement in the loop regions. Each loop acts as a separate antigen in that each stimulates the production of a loop-specific antibody. The V3 loop, the area that binds to the T4 lymphocyte (CD4 binding domain) is the principal site in the viral envelope for antibody neutralization (antibodies that inactivate HIV) and is believed to be the most important site responsible for HIV's-cell attachment (Belshe et al., 1994; Cohen, 1994; Ghiara et al., 1994). The V3 loop also contains the determinants responsible for the formation of T4 cell syncytium (fusion of uninfected T4 cells with HIV-infected T4 cells) (Bobkov et al., 1994). A more complete knowledge of the V3 loop should facilitate the design of new drugs and vaccines to inhibit HIV infection.

2. When HIV enters the body, it circulates in the blood until by chance it bumps into a cell with the CD4 receptor on its surface.

3. The viral protein gp120 then binds specifically and tightly to a CD4 receptor site, as well as to other receptors described below.

How HIV ENTERS CD4+ Cells: T4 Cells and Macrophage

HIV researchers have known since 1984 that human CD4 cell membrane receptors alone are sufficient for **binding** HIV to the T4 lymphocyte membrane but CD4 receptors are not sufficient for **HIV envelope fusion** with the T4 cell membrane or for **HIV penetration** or entry into the cell's interior. This knowledge has enticed many groups of AIDS researchers to search for additional receptors, coreceptors to CD4, that HIV uses to enter a cell after binding to it. Various candidate receptor molecules were put forward, sometimes with more fan-

fare than fact, but have not stood the test of critical examination.

In May of 1996, Ed Berger and colleagues reported on finding a receptor that allowed syncytium-inducing (SI) strains of HIV (HIV that causes T4 cells to form clusters—they attach to each other) to enter T4 cells. Strains of HIV that do not induce T4 cell syncytium formation (NSI) could not enter T4 cells. Berger and colleagues named this T4 cell receptor **FUSIN** (Figure 5-5). In August of 1996 Conrad Bleul and colleagues identified a chemokine, **CXC stromal cell-derived factor-1 (SDF-1)** that binds to the FUSIN receptor and blocks HIV entry. They named this chemokine **CXCR-4**. So FUSIN and CXCR-4 are one, a receptor which HIV can use to enter T cells (HIV T-tropic).

After the FUSIN receptor data was reported, **five separate research teams** reported on an additional coreceptor called **CC-CKR-5** (CKR-5). CKR-5 is the fifth of seven known human chemokine receptors that respond to β-Chemokines. β-Chemokines are chemicals released by T cells and other cells to attract macrophages and other immune cells to sites of inflammation. CKR-5 is known to be a receptor for three β-chemokine proteins called RANTES, MIP-1α, and MIP-1β. The β-chemokine RANTES (<u>r</u>egulated-upon-<u>a</u>ctivation <u>n</u>ormal <u>T</u> <u>e</u>xpressed and <u>s</u>ecreted), chomokine MIP-1α and 1β (macrophage inflammatory proteins) are all produced by T8 cells and are known to inhibit HIV replication, particularly in macrophage-tropic HIV strains (HIV strains that infect macrophage over T4 cells) (Deng et al., 1996; Dragic et al., 1996) **and are powerful suppressors of HIV infection, especially HIV infection of macrophage!** That is, these three chemokine proteins suppress HIV entry into macrophage by somehow blocking the coreceptor CKR-5. CKR-5 serves as a membrane receptor for all three chemokines. Members of the research teams who have contributed to the discovery of the CKR-5 receptor believe that **macrophage-tropic or M-tropic HIV strains occur in greatest number early on after HIV infection and then, sometime later during HIV disease the predominant HIV strain shifts to HIV strains that use the FUSIN receptor (CXCR-4) on T4 cells.** HIV, by shifting receptors, may be avoiding the suppressive activity of the chemokines that block the CKR-5 receptor. Figure 5-5 shows a diagram of this suggested **receptor swap** that occurs sometime during HIV disease progression.

GENETIC RESISTANCE TO HIV INFECTION

At this point in the HIV/AIDS pandemic it is believed that about 95% of HIV-exposed people are susceptible to HIV infection and HIV disease progression. This statement is made because it has long been known that persons who have deliberately avoided safer sex practice and who have had unprotected sex with HIV-infected persons failed to become HIV-infected! The question that has continued to puzzle HIV investigators is, how can multiple HIV-exposed persons remain uninfected. Pieces of that puzzle, why some frequently

HIV-exposed people remain uninfected, began to fall into place when two gay males who, despite repeated unprotected sex with companions who died from the disease, remain HIV-negative. Neither quite understood why he was spared but they were public-spirited enough to press scientists to come up with the answer. HIV investigators Rong Liu and co-workers (1996) and Michel Samson and co-workers (1996) reported that repeated HIV-exposed but uninfected people have a **32-nucleotide deletion in the gene that produces the CKR-5 receptors on macrophage**. The protein produced by this gene is severely damaged and does **not** reach the cell surface to act as a chemokine receptor. Without these receptors, the envelope of HIV cannot fuse with the envelope of macrophage to gain entrance into the cell. Thus, people who carry both defective CKR-5 genes' **homozygotes** (they received one defective gene from each parent) are resistant to HIV infection. If one

FIGURE 5-5 Coreceptors Required for HIV to Enter Human Cells. HIV can broadly be divided into two classes: those more suitable (tropic) to infecting macrophage and those which infect T4 cells in the lymph nodes or other tissues. Macrophage-tropic nonsyncytium-inducing (NSI) HIV isolates infect macrophages but fail to infect HIV T cells lines, while T4 HIV syncytium-inducing (SI) strains fail to infect macrophage. But HIV of both classes efficiently infect T4 cells isolated from peripheral blood mononuclear cells (PBMC). **Macrophage-tropic NSI HIV appear to be preferentially transmitted by sexual contact and constitute the vast majority of HIV present in newly infected individuals (Zhu, 1993). The T-tropic SI viruses generally appear late in the course of infection during the so-called "phenotypic switch" that often precedes the onset of AIDS symptoms (Conner, et al., 1994).** The molecular basis of HIV-1 tropism appears to lie in the ability of envelopes of macrophage-tropic and T-tropic viruses to interact with different coreceptors located on macrophage or T4 cells. Macrophage-tropic viruses primarily use CKR-5 (for CC-CKR-5), and less often CKR-3, a newly described seven-transmembrane domain chemokine receptors while T-tropic HIV tend to use FUSIN (CXCKR-4), a previously identified seven-transmembrane protein (Hill et al., 1996; Moore, 1997).

is **heterozygous** (that is, one carries one defective gene and one normal gene), one will produce the CKR-5 receptor that HIV needs to penetrate macrophage, but they may be fewer in number, thus, chemokines (the chemicals that the receptors were made for) would have fewer receptors to fill so there is a greater chance that fewer CKR-5 receptors are open or available for HIV attachment. As a result, heterozygous people may be **less** resistant to HIV infection than the homozygous mutant (receptorless) people, but may be **more** resistant then people who have two normal genes (homozygous normal) who are the most susceptable to HIV infection.

Michael Dean and colleagues (1996) present evidence that the frequency of CKR-5 deletion heterozygotes (those with one copy of the gene) was significantly elevated in groups of individuals who had survived HIV infection for more than 10 years, and, in some risk groups, twice as frequent as their occurrence in **rapid progressors to AIDS**. Survival analysis clearly shows that disease progression s slower in CKR-5 deletion heterozygotes than in individuals with the normal CKR-5 gene. Jesper Eugene-Olsen and colleagues (1997) reported that individuals who are heterozygous for the 32-base-pair deletion in the CKR-5 gene have a slower decrease in their T4-cell count and a longer AIDS-free survival than individuals with the wild-type gene for up to 11 years of follow-up.

Will the Mutant CKR-5 Gene Protect People from All Subtypes of HIV?

This genetic defect, the 32-nucleotide deletion, prevents infection only with the strain of HIV (Subtype B) that is transmitted sexually and is prevalent in the United States and Europe. It does not necessarily protect against other strains of HIV transmitted through intravenous drug use or blood transfusions, or strains prevalent in Africa.

Should I Be Tested for the Presence of the CKR-5 Gene?

Researchers agreed that getting tested for the gene would not be difficult, but it would not be of great value because the tested person could still be infected by other stains of HIV.

Besides, it must be assumed that most people do not carry a pair of defective CKR-5 genes because 95% or more of HIV-exposed people become HIV-infected!

Who Carries the Defective CKR-5 Gene?

Perhaps most surprising, HIV investigators found that the homozygous genetic defect is common: **It is present in 1% of whites of European descent.** But it appears to be absent in people from Japan and Central Africa; about 20% of whites are heterozygous for this gene.

Why Does This Gene Exist?

Scientists speculate that the mutant form of CKR-5 protected against some disease that afflicted Europeans but not Africans. The obvious candidate would be the Black Death of 1346, the plague. If the mutant CKR-5 blocked plague bacteria, the survivors would be more likely to carry the trait and pass it to the next generations.

T4 CELL DEPLETION AND IMMUNE SUPPRESSION

An understanding of the mechanisms by which HIV reduces the number of CD4 cells is important. However, we do not yet understand just how the T4 helper cell is killed or impaired by HIV infection. Recent research using the **polymerase chain reaction** (a method of amplifying present but unmeasurable quantities of HIV DNA in T4 cells into measurable quantities) has revealed that about *one in every 10 to 100* T4 cells is HIV-infected in an AIDS patient. Thus T4 cells serve as reservoirs of HIV in the body (Schnittman et al., 1989; Cohen, 1993). Collectively, T4 cell depletion leads to cumulative and devastating effects on the cell-mediated and humoral parts of the immune system.

Means by Which T4 Cells May Be Lost

1. Filling CD4 Receptor Sites—There is evidence from in vitro studies that HIV can attack CD4 receptor sites in at least two ways. First, HIV can attach, via its gp160 "spikes," to CD4

———— BOX 5.3 ————

MUTANT CKR-5 HIV RESISTANCE MAY JUST BE AN INDICATOR OF THE MORE COMPLEX BIOLOGY INVOLVED IN LONG-TERM SURVIVAL

A red flag has been raised by AIDS investigators as to just how important the CKR-5 mutation is in preventing HIV infection. It would appear, based on available data, that CKR-5 is not a major mechanism of HIV resistance.

First, too few people worldwide carry the mutant gene and some of those who do, have become HIV-infected and are progressing to AIDS (Biti et al., 1977; O'Brien et al., 1997; Theodorou et al., 1997).

Second, scientists at the University of California–San Francisco studied a group of uninfected individuals at high risk for contracting HIV. All were known to be engaging in unprotected sex and/or sharing needles with HIV-infected individuals. Among these apparently resistant people, one third were found to be heterozygous (they carried one copy) for the mutant

CKR-5 gene, but NONE were reported to be homozygous (carry both mutant copies of the gene). Thus among this substantial group of high-risk individuals, the underlying cause of their resistance was NOT defective CKR-5 receptors preventing the entry of HIV into the cells. If both mutant CKR-5 were required for resistance to HIV, then some of these people should have carried two copies of the mutant CKR-5 gene—but NONE did.

Third, there is ample evidence that black, Hispanic, and Japanese people multiply exposed to HIV have NOT become HIV-infected. And, since mutant CKR-5 genes have not yet been found in these people, clearly some other biological mechanism for conferring HIV resistance must exist (Fauci, 1996).

---

receptor sites. Second, HIV is capable of releasing or freeing its exterior gp120 envelope glycoprotein, thereby generating a molecule that can actively bind to CD4-bearing cells (Gelderblom et al., 1985). As a result of filling the receptor sites on the T4 cells, the T4 cells lose their immune functions; that is, the T4 cell does not have to be infected with HIV to lose immune function. In addition, CD4-bearing cells that attach the free gp120 molecule then become targets for immune attack by antibody-mediated antibody-dependent cell cytotoxicity (ADCC) and nonantibody-mediated cytotoxic T cells. Both events can result in the destruction of uninfected CD4 bearing cells. The extent to which this occurs in vivo depends on the level of gp120 synthesis, secretion, and shedding. Free gp120 has not yet been measured in the circulation, but this is not surprising given its powerful affinity for CD4 (Bolognesi, 1989).

2. Syncytia Formation—The formation of syncytia involves fusion of the cell membrane of an infected cell with the cell membranes of uninfected CD4 cells, which results in giant multinucleated cells. A direct relation between

the presence of syncytia and the degree of the cytopathic effect of the virus in individual cells has been demonstrated in vitro, and HIV isolated during the accelerated phase of infection in vivo has a greater capacity to induce syncytia in vitro. Syncytia have rarely been seen in vivo.

In the asymptomatic phase of HIV infection, predominantly nonsyncytium inducing (NSI), HIV variants can be detected. In about 50% of the cases SI HIV variants emerge in the course of infection, preceding rapid T4 cell depletion and progression to AIDS (Groenink et al., 1993).

3. Superantigens—Superantigens are bacterial or viral antigens that are capable of interacting with a very large number of T4 cells. Unlike a conventional antigen, which usually evokes a response from less than one in a million (0.01%) T4 cells, a superantigen can interact with 5% to 30% of T4 cells. They directly bind to the exposed surfaces of MHC class II molecules on antigen-presenting cells (APCs) and to the variable region of the T cell receptors (TCR) β chain (V_β) on the responding T cells. Therefore, superantigens can interact with a large fraction of T cells, resulting in cellular activation, proliferation, anergy (absence of reaction to an antigen), or deletion of specific T cell subsets. Bacterial superantigens include staphylococcal enterotoxins and the toxic shock syndrome toxin-1, which are the causative agents for several human diseases such as food poisoning and toxic shock syndrome (Phillips et al., 1995). The superantigen hypothesis regarding HIV infection stems from the observations that endogenous or exogenous retroviral-encoded super-antigens stimulate murine T4 cells in vivo, leading to the anergy or deletion of a substantial percentage of T4 cells that have the specific variable β regions (Pantaleo et al., 1993).

4. Apoptosis—Programmed cell death, or apoptosis (a-po-toe-sis), is a normal mechanism of cell death that was originally described in the context of the response of immature thymocytes to cellular activation. It is a mechanism whereby the body eliminates autoreactive clones of T cells. It has recently been suggested that both qualitative and quantitative defects in T4 cells in patients with HIV infection may be the result of activation-induced cell death or apoptosis. Since apoptosis can be induced in mature murine T4 cells after cross-linking CD4 molecules to one another and triggering the T4 cell antigen receptor, there has been speculation that cross-linking of the CD4 molecule by HIV gp120 or gp120-anti-gp120 immune complexes prepares the cell for the programmed death that occurs when a MHC class II molecule in complex with an antigen binds to the T4 cell antigen receptor. Thus activation of a prepared cell by a specific antigen or superantigen could lead to the death of the cell, without direct infection by HIV (Pantaleo et al., 1993). For an excellent review of Apoptosis and its role in human disease, see Barr et al., 1994, and Hengartner, 1995.

5. Cellular Transfer of HIV—Infected macrophages, or antigen-presenting cells, which normally interact with the T4 cells to stimulate the immune function, can transfer HIV into uninfected T4 lymphocytes. **In any case, immediate viral or proviral replication, kills the T4 cell**.

——————— BOX 5.4 ———————

COFACTORS EXPEDITE HIV INFECTION

(An excerpt from Michael Callen's article, "Everything Must Be Doubted," *Newsline*, July/August 1988, pp. 44–5.)
(Michael Callen died in 1993.)

By the age of 27 (when I was diagnosed with crypto [cryptococcus infection] and AIDS) I had had over 3,000 different sex partners. Not coincidentally, I'd also had: hepatitis A, hepatitis B, hepatitis non-A, non-B; herpes simplex types I & II; syphilis; gonorrhea; non-specific urethritis; shigella; entamoeba histolitica; chlamydia; fungal infections; venereal warts; cytomegalovirus infections; EBV [Epstein-Barr virus] reactivations; cryptosporidium and therefore, finally, AIDS. For me, the question wasn't why I got AIDS, but how I had been able to remain standing on two feet for so long . . . If you blanked out my name and my age on my pre-AIDS medical chart and showed it to a doctor and asked her to guess who I was, she might reasonably have guessed, based on my disease history, that I was a 65-year-old malnourished equatorial African living in squalor . . . I believe that a small subset of urban gay men unwittingly managed to recreate disease settings equivalent to those of poor Third World nations and junkies.

This excerpt details many of the cofactors which play a role in the development of immune dysfunctions; while any one infection might not cause a problem for a healthy individual, repeated infection and exposure to foreign body fluids takes a cumulative toll. And certain infections and unquestionably more immune-suppressive than others—in particular, the sexually transmitted diseases.

6. Autoimmune Mechanisms—One of the older theories, namely that HIV tricks the immune system into attacking itself is back because of the recent work of Tracy Kion and Geoffrey Hoffmann (1991). Their work showed that mice immunized with lymphocytes from another mouse strain make antibodies to the HIV envelope protein gp120, as do autoimmune strains of mice, even though **none of the animals had ever been exposed to the AIDS virus**. One implication of these results is that some component on the lymphocytes resembles gp120 closely enough so that antibodies directed against it can recognize gp120 as well. The converse is that antibodies to gp120 should also recognize the lymphocyte component so that an immune response directed against HIV might also interfere with normal lymphocyte function. The autoimmune theory is consistent with results that show there is a selective loss of particular subsets of T cells in AIDS patients.

7. Cofactors May Help Deplete T4 Cells— HIV-infected people who are asymptomatic show a wide variation in HIV disease time and progression to AIDS. It is believed that cofactors may be responsible for some of the time variation with regard to disease progression.

Many agents may act as cofactors to activate or increase HIV production. Although, in general, it is not believed that any cofactor is necessary for HIV infection, cofactors such as nutrition, stress, and infectious organisms have been considered as agents that might accelerate HIV expression after infection. Three new human herpes virus (HHV-6, 7, and 8) may be cofactors and play a role in causing immune deficiency. They have been shown to infect HIV-infected T4 cells and activate the HIV provirus to increase HIV replication (Laurence, 1996). Cytomegalovirus and the Epstein-Barr virus have also been associated with increased HIV expression. Over time, investigators expect to find other sexually transmitted diseases that behave as cofactors associated with HIV infection and expression.

Shyh-Ching Lo and colleagues at the Armed Forces Institute of Pathology suggested in 1989 that a mycoplasma infection was a cofactor in HIV infection. Mycoplasma lack a cell wall, are simpler than bacteria, and are more complex than viruses. They are the smallest known organisms that can live outside a host cell. Lo identified the mycoplasma as *M. incognitus* (Lo et al., 1989, 1991).

Drugs may also be cofactors in infection. Used by injection drug users (IDUs), heroin and other morphine-based derivatives are known to reduce human resistance to infection and produce immunological suppression.

Pneumocystis carinii pneumonia is about twice as frequent in heroin users as in homosexuals. It is believed that the heroin has an immunosuppressive effect within the lungs (Brown, 1987).

Blood and blood products may also act as cofactors in infection because they are immunosuppressive. Because blood transfusions save lives, their long-range effects are generally overlooked. Transfusions in hemophiliacs, for example, result in lowered resistance to viruses such as cytomegalovirus (CMV), Epstein-Barr (Berkman, 1984; Blumberg et al., 1985; Foster et al., 1985), and perhaps HIV. Seminal fluid (fluid bathing the sperm) may also act as a cofactor in infection because it also causes immunosuppression. One of its physiological functions is to immunosuppress the female genital tract so that the sperm is not immunologically rejected (Witkin et al., 1983; Baxena et al., 1985).

Epidemiologically, homosexuals at greatest risk of AIDS are those who practice passive anal sex, that is, anal recipients (Kingsley et al., 1987). It is generally considered that this sexual behavior is a cofactor that enables the AIDS virus to enter the bloodstream by means of traumatic lacerations of the rectal mucosa.

Last but not least of the agents that can suppress the immune system and thereby act as a cofactor in HIV infection is **stress**. Stress can be mental or physical; but it is easier to measure the effects of physical stress.

Although moderate exercise appears to stimulate the immune system, there is good evidence that intensive exercise can suppress the immune system. We still do not really know why (Fitzgerald, 1988; LaPierre et al., 1992). The effect of stress on the immune system is one of the reasons why physicians did not want Earvin "Magic" Johnson to play basketball (see Box 8.6 in Chapter 8).

IMPACT OF T4 CELL DEPLETION

The overall impact of T4 cell depletion is multifaceted. HIV-induced T4 cell abnormalities alter the T4 cells' ability to produce a variety of inducer chemical stimulants such as the **interleukins** that are necessary for the proper maturation of B cells into plasma cells and the maturation of a subset of T cells into cytotoxic cells (Figure 5-6). Thus the critical basis for the immunopathogenesis of HIV infection is the depletion of the *T4 lymphocytes* which results in profound immunosuppression.

Presumably, with time, the number of HIV-infected T4 cells increases to a point where, in terminal AIDS patients, *few normal T4 cells exist.*

ROLE OF MONOCYTES AND MACROPHAGES IN HIV INFECTION

Some scientists now believe that T4 cell infection alone does not cause AIDS because not enough T4 cells are destroyed. They believe that equally important to T4 cell infection is **monocyte** and **macrophage** infection (Bakker et. al., 1992). Monocytes change into various types of macrophages (given different names) in order to search and destroy foreign agents within tissues of the lungs, brain, and interstitial tissues, tissues that connect organs. Despite the name changes, all forms of macrophages basically work the same way: they ingest things. Some macrophages travel around within the body, others become attached to one spot, ingesting.

Macrophages are often the first cells of the immune system to encounter invaders, particularly in the area of a cut or wound. After engulfing the invader, the macrophage makes copies of the invader's antigens and **displays** them on its own cell membrane. These **copies of the invader antigens sit right**

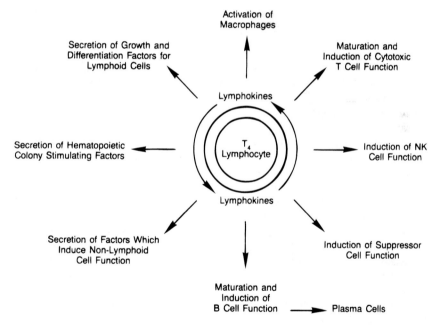

FIGURE 5-6 The T4 Cell Role in the Immune Response. T4 lymphocytes are responsible directly or indirectly for inducing a wide array of functions in cells that produce the immune response. They also induce nonlymphoid cell functions. T cell involvement is effected for the most part by the secretion of soluble factors or **lymphokines** that have trophic or inductive effects on the cells presented in the figure. Lymphokines serve to transfer control of the immune response from the external environmental proteins to the internal regulatory system consisting of ligands and receptors. (*Adapted from Fauci, 1991*)

next to the self molecules. **In effect, the macrophage makes a "wanted poster" of this new invader.** The macrophage then travels about showing the wanted poster to T4 cells, which triggers the T4 cells into action. Macrophages also release chemicals which stimulate both T4 cell and macrophage production and draw macrophages and lymphocytes to the site of infection.

Macrophages may play an important role in spreading HIV infection in the body, both to other cells and to HIV's target organs. **First,** HIV enters macrophase and spreads from macrophage to macrophage before the immune system is alerted. **Second,** macrophages, in their different forms, travel to the brain, the lungs, the bone marrow, and to various immune organs, carrying HIV to these organs.

HIV's ability to infect brain tissue is particularly important. The brain and cerebral spinal fluid (CSF) are specially protected sites. CSF cushions the brain and the spinal cord from sudden and jarring movements. The brain–blood barrier, a chemical phenomenon, normally stops foreign substances from entering the brain and the CSF. But HIV-infected monocytes can pass through this barrier. For HIV, monocyte-macrophages are Trojan horses, enabling HIV to enter the immune-protected domain of the central nervous system—the brain, the spine, the rest of the nervous system.

HIV isolates taken from macrophages appear to grow better in macrophages than in lymphocytes. In human cell culture experiments, HIV isolates taken from lymphocytes appear to grow better in lymphocytes than in macrophages. These peculiarities of replication rates may be evidence of separate tissue-oriented HIV strains.

HIV-infected macrophages have proven to be a major problem in efforts to control and stop HIV infection.

Clinical Latency: Where Have All the Viruses Been Hiding?

The immunodeficiency syndrome caused by HIV is characterized by **profound T4 cell depletion**. Prior to the progressive decline of T4 cells and the development of AIDS, there is a symptom-free period which may last for 10 or more years, during which the infection is thought to be clinically latent. Scientists thought little if any viral replication occurred during this period. In recent years, a number of studies have offered an alternative view. Some investigations suggest that there is no real latency period in HIV infection. Instead, **starting from the moment of infection, there appears to be a continuous struggle between HIV and the immune system, the balance of which slowly shifts in favor of the virus.** Cecil H. Fox of the Yale School of Medicine reported in December 1991 that HIV is not lying dormant at all but is continually infecting immune cells in the lymph nodes (Figure 5-7).

The **lymph nodes**, which are pea-sized capsules that trap foreign invaders and produce immune cells, are all over the body and are connected by vessels much like those that transport blood. Deep within the lymph nodes of 18 HIV-infected patients, researchers found millions of viruses. Based on those data, Fox suggested that HIV uses the lymph nodes as places to meet up with most immune cells. Fox believes that HIV begins replication in T4 cells in the lymph nodes soon after it enters the body. Infected T4 cells leave the lymph nodes and new uninfected cells arrive to become infected. Years later, when enough immune cells have been killed, the patient's defenses become so impaired that he or she is vulnerable to any one of a wide array of opportunistic infections—AIDS has arrived.

Anthony Fauci (Figure 5-8), the head of the National Institute of Allergy and Infectious Diseases (NIAID), and Sonya Heath and colleagues (1995) agrees that there are many more HIVs in the lymph nodes than in the blood. Studies in his laboratory have shown there are many millions of HIV particles stuck to what are known as follicular dendritic cells in the lymph nodes of an infected individual.

The follicular dendritic cells, which have thousands of feathery processes emanating from them and whose normal function is to filter and trap antigens for presentation to antibody-producing B lymphocytes, serve as highly effective trapping centers for extracellular HIV particles. Virtually every lymphocyte in a lymph node is enmeshed in the processes of

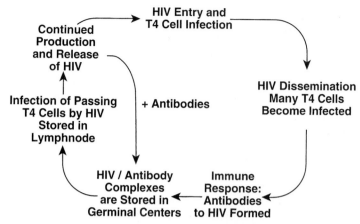

```
                          HIV Entry and
   Continued        →     T4 Cell Infection
   Production   ↗
   and Release  ─┐
     of HIV      │                              ↓

                                          HIV Dissemination
 Infection of Passing                      Many T4 Cells
  T4 Cells by HIV      + Antibodies        Become Infected
     Stored in
    Lymphnode

                                                │
       ↓                                        │
   HIV / Antibody        Immune                 │
    Complexes           Response:    ←──────────┘
   are Stored in   ←    Antibodies
  Germinal Centers   to HIV Formed
```

FIGURE 5-7   The Role of HIV Antibody in HIV Seeding of the Lymph Glands and Infection of New T4 Cells. To rid the body of HIV requires a way to cleanse the lymph nodes of HIV. (*Adapted from Fox, 1996*)

these cells. Although the follicular dendritic cells themselves do not seem to be susceptible to HIV infection, they appear to place huge numbers of virus particles into intimate contact with cells that are susceptible to HIV infection (Haase et al.,1996; Knight,1996).

During the clinically latent phase, the lymph nodes of an infected individual are slowly destroyed.

In the final phase of an infection, the follicular dentritic network completely dissolves and the architecture of the lymph node collapses to produce what Fauci called a "**burnt-out lymph node.**" With this collapse, large amounts of HIV are released into the circulatory system and an ever increasing number of peripheral cells are infected with HIV (Baum, 1992; Edgington, 1993).

In 1995, David Ho and colleagues, Xiping Wei and colleagues, and Martin Nowak and colleagues published separate reports on the rapid production of HIV which began soon after initial HIV infection. These studies, collectively demonstrated that, using early, frequent blood samples of HIV-infected persons taking the drug nevirapine, a non-nucleoside reverse transcriptase inhibitor and protease inhibitors ABT-538 and L-735.524 (protease is essential for HIV reproduction), it was possible to calculate how rapidly newly produced HIV turned over within HIV-infected persons by measuring the balance between HIV-RNA pro-

duction in and HIV RNA clearance from the blood plasma. The drugs worked well, dropping the amount of HIV-RNA in blood plasma to 1% of pretreatment level. In each case the treated person's T4 cell counts significantly in-

FIGURE 5-8   Anthony S. Fauci, M.D. (1989). Director, National Institute of Allergy and Infectious Diseases, National Institutes of Health; Associate Director of NIH for AIDS Research.

creased, in some by as much as 10-fold. By determining how quickly T4 cells increased once HIV RNA levels dropped, Ho and colleagues calculated that before treatment their patients had been producing over a billion T4 cells each day. That's an incredibly accelerated rate—between 25 and 75 times the rate seen in patients with less-advanced infections. But it still wasn't enough to stay ahead of the rapidly replicating virus, which was infecting and killing each new cell in less than 2 days. The patients' immune systems were functioning at full capacity but slowly losing the battle!

Such rapid viral replication countered by a strong immune response is not unknown; on the contrary, it is characteristic of acute, short-lived viral infections, such as measles or the flu. But in those infections, the immune system most often wins: it rids the body of the virus and builds resistance to future infection. The question is why can't the immune system do the same against HIV. Perhaps it's the length and intensity of the struggle that ultimately does in the immune system by encouraging the emergence of mutant viruses that outstrip the immune system's ability to continue making new types of antibody. During the time when the immune system is functioning well and producing new antibody against each new HIV variant, the struggle between HIV production and immune suppression of the viral load must move repeatedly from the virus to the immune system and back until the immune system is just overwhelmed with the number of different types of antibody it must rapidly produce in large quantity.

The viral load or quantitative amount of HIV RNA present in the HIV-infected persons studied by these investigators showed that about 30% of HIV and HIV-infected T4 cells in their blood plasma was turning over (produced and cleared from plasma) each day! Clearly HIV and T4 cells are being produced at about the same rate which is why the progression of HIV disease is so gradual.

T4 Cell Generation and Destruction

Ho and colleagues calculated that about 5% of the T4 cells are being regenerated per day, indicating a destruction rate of approximately 5% per day during steady state. The 5% figure is equivalent to a daily turnover of approximately 35 million cells in the bloodstream. Since the bloodstream accounts for approximately 2% of the total lymphoid population, it can be estimated that the total population minimum production and destruction rate is approximately 1.8 billion T4 cells per day. When Ho plotted the individual rates of T4 cell repopulation against initial T4 cell counts for his 20 patients studied, an inverse correlation was found, with those subjects with the lowest T4 cell counts exhibiting the greatest production rates.

This finding was a surprise, given the expectation based on prior literature that patients with more advanced illness would have the lowest T4 cell regenerative capacity. The implication is that the immune system continues trying even in late-stage HIV disease to counter the greater T4 cell destruction rates associated with the greater quantity of actively replicating virus.

Using the analogy of a faucet and basin, Ho equated the water level in the basin to the T4 cell count, the faucet to T4 cell replenishment, and the drain to HIV destruction of T4 cells. In the analogy, the basin drains just slightly faster than replenishment occurs, with the faucet turned full on in late-stage disease. Ho maintained that the major objective of treatment should be to plug the drain rather than solely attempt to increase the amount of water going into the basin—i.e., through immune-based therapies designed to boost T4 cell production. He suggested that it is difficult to imagine how T4 cell production rate could be augmented beyond that observed in late-stage HIV disease. Ho believes that the functional capacity of regenerating T4 lymphocytes may be limited; thus, efforts to restore immune function (saving or restoring T4 cells) is essential (Ho, 1995).

Another point established by Ho and colleagues investigations is that the rate of HIV clearance from the plasma is not affected by the stage of HIV progression or disease status. Ho concluded that viral load is **not** a function of viral clearance. HIV clearance efficiency varies little among individuals yet individuals can differ in viral load by several logs.

Therefore viral load is primarily a function of viral production.

Implications of a High HIV Replication Rate

Based on Ho and colleagues kinetic studies of viral replication, it can be estimated that the population of HIV undergoes between 3,000 and 5,000 replication cycles (**generations**) over the course of 10 years, producing a **minimum of 10^{12} (1 trillion) HIV** in an HIV-infected person. According to Ho, given the assumptions in the kinetics analysis that render the figures minimum estimates, the number of HIV produced is probably closer to 10^{13} (10 trillion) during the infected person's lifetime. This vast number of HIV replications over 3,000 to 5,000 generations creates a lot of opportunity for HIV RNA evolution, because genetic mutations occur most commonly during replication. Some mutations will weaken HIV in such a way as to expose it to attack by the immune system. But other mutations will aid the virus, speeding its replication and increasing the chances it can evade the immune system. Because HIV gets so many chances to replicate, it evolves and mutates, and those strains with the greatest replication efficiency gradually win out. **This is Darwinian evolution going on in one patient.**

HIV has been shown to have a random (any base has an equal chance of changing) mutation rate of approximately 1 mutation per 10,000 nucleotides **AND** one mutation caused by reverse transcriptase copy error (**transcription error**) per round of replication. The **combination** of events results in too many variants in the immune system to handle. For example, a single HIV-infected person, by the time he or she is diagnosed with AIDS, may have 1 billion to 10 billion or more HIV variants in his or her body. With so many variants present, some will be resistant to most if not all drugs currently used in therapy and to drugs that have **not yet been created**!. Thus it is the constant production of variant HIVs that produce the drug resistant mutants and not action of the drug.

In summary, the large number and excessive genetic diversity created by thousands of generations of HIV in one person allows HIV to surpass or exceed the ability of the immune system to recognize and respond to virus thus permitting resistant mutants to emerge and gain predominance. Ho and colleagues believe that because of the early rapid replication of HIV and production of such vast number of HIV variants, monotherapy (single drug) is not a rational strategy if a dramatic impact on the course of infection is to be achieved. They stated that a reasonable strategy is to use multiple potent agents simultaneously (e.g., three or four in combination), **requiring** HIV to simultaneously develop multiple mutations in order to escape the drugs. They also stated that given the dynamics of HIV in vivo, it makes sense to begin treatment as soon as infection is diagnosed, on the rationale that the more replicative cycles that are permitted, the more variants there will be when treatment is begun, stacking the deck in favor of the virus' ability to avoid both immune responses and effects of drug treatment.

Thus, through early 1995, scientists had vastly **underestimated** the extent of virus activity in an HIV-infected person, particularly during the asymptomatic or clinically latent phase. These and other recent studies should satisfy the major unanswered question concerning HIV disease/AIDS, which was, "**Where is the virus**?" During the 1980s, it was difficult to find medium to high levels of HIV in persons with HIV disease or even in those persons in the later stages of AIDS. We now know that there are large amounts of the HIV present early on in the lymph nodes of HIV-diseased people. Now, however, perhaps the most troubled group of researchers may be those currently developing AIDS vaccines. (See Chapter 9 for a discussion about possible HIV vaccines.) At present, vaccine strategies propose to introduce HIV antigen repeatedly during the long asymptomatic period to bolster B cell immunity. Vaccinated antigens, however, could wind up trapped in the lymph nodes, stimulating B cells to produce the cytokines that stimulate T4 cell infection and speed lymph node architecture destruction. Thus the vaccine's effect could backfire, compressing the clinically latent period and causing a more rapid onset of AIDS.

SUMMARY

After a healthy person is HIV-infected, he or she makes antibodies against those viruses that are in the bloodstream, but not against those that have become integrated as HIV proviruses in the host immune cell DNA. Over time the immune system cells that are involved in antibody production are destroyed. Evidence is accumulating that cofactors such as nutrition, stress, and previous exposure to other sexually transmitted diseases that increase HIV expression are associated with HIV infection and HIV disease. Agents that suppress the immune system may also play a significant role in establishing HIV infection. In short, HIV infection is permanent. It attaches to CD4-bearing cells and enters those cells using, at least, two separate coreceptors—FUSIN and CC-CRK-5. These coreceptors allow HIV to fuse with the cell membrane, and enter the cell, after HIV attachment to the CD4+-bearing cell. And, as seen in Chapter 3, HIV undergoes rapid genetic change, and, as far as is known, **attacks only human cells—mostly of the human immune system**. It has recently become quite clear that large amounts of the virus are produced within weeks after HIV infection. The virus remains, for the most part, in the lymph nodes until very late in the disease process.

REVIEW QUESTIONS

(Answers to the Review Questions are on page 576.)

1. Which cell type is believed to be the main target for HIV infection? Explain the biological impact of this particular infection.

2. What is CD4, where is it found, and what is its role in the HIV infection process?

3. Is there a period of latency after HIV infection—a time when few or no new HIV are being produced?

4. True or False: HIV is the cause of AIDS.

5. True or False: HIV primarily affects red blood cells.

6. True or False: Lymphocytes have a major role in the immune response to antigens.

7. True or False: All T and B lymphocytes inhibit or destroy foreign antigens.

8. True or False: CD4 and CD8 molecules are antibodies.

9. True or False: HIV belongs to the family of retroviruses.

10. True or False: Cytotoxic and suppressor T lymphocytes are the main targets of HIV.

11. True or False: The latent period is that time between initial infection with HIV and the onset of AIDS.

12. True or False: HIV can spread to infect new cells after it buds out of infected cells.

13. True or False: HIV causes the gradual destruction of cells bearing the CD4 molecule.

REFERENCES

AMEISEN, JEAN CLAUDE. (1994). Programmed cell death capoptosis and cell survival regulation: relavance to cancer. *AIDS*, 8:1197–1213.

AMIGORENA, SEBASTIAN, et al., (1994). Transient accumulation of new class II MHC molecules in a novel endocytic compartment in B lymphocytes. *Nature*, 369:113–120.

BAKKER, LEENDERT J., et al. (1992). Antibodies and complement enhance binding and uptake of HIV-1 by human monocytes. *AIDS*, 6:35–41.

BARR, PHILIP, et al. (1994). Apoptosis and its role in human disease. *BioTechnology*, 12:487–494.

BAXENA, S., et al. (1985). Immunosuppression by human seminal plasma. *Immunol. Invest.*, 14:255–269.

BELSHE, R. B., et al. (1994). Neutralizing antibodies to HIV in seronegative volunteers immunized with recombinant gp120 from the MN strain of HIV. *JAMA*, 272:475–480.

BERKMAN, S. (1984). Infectious complications of blood transfusions. *Sem. Oncol.*, 11:68–75.

BITI, ROBYN, et al. (1997). HIV infection in an individual homozygous for the CCR5 deletion allele. *Nature Med.*, 3:252.

BLEUL, CONRAD, et al. (1996). The lymphocyte chemoattractant SDF-1 is a ligand for LESTR/fusin and blocks HIV entry. *Nature*, 382: 829–833.

BLUMBERG, N., et al. (1985). A retrospective study of transfusions. *Br. Med. J.*, 290:1037–1039.

BOBKOV, ALEKSEI, et al. (1994). Molecular epidemiology of HIV in the former Soviet Union: analysis of ENV V3 sequences and their correlation with epidemiologic data. *AIDS*, 8:619–624.

BOLOGNESI, DANI P. (1989). Prospects for prevention of and early intervention against HIV. *JAMA*, 261:3007–3013.

CALLEBAUT, CHRISTIAN, et al. (1993). T cell activation antigen, CD26 as a cofactor for entry of HIV in CD4+ cells. *Science*, 262:2045–2050.

COHEN, JOEL. (1994). The HIV vaccine paradox. *Science*, 264:1072–1074.

COHEN, JON. (1993). Keystone's blunt message: "It's the virus stupid." *Science*, 260:292–293.

COHEN, JON. (1993). HIV cofactor comes in far more heavy fire. *Science*, 262:1971–1972.

COHEN, JON. (1997). Exploiting the HIV-chemokine nexus. *Science*, 275:1261–1264.

CONNER, RUTH, et al. (1994). Human immunodeficiency virus type 1 variants with increased replicative capacity develop during the asymptomatic stage before disease progression. *J. Virol.*, 68: 4400–4408.

CROWE, S.M., et al. (1991). Predictive value of CD4 lymphocyte numbers for the development of opportunistic infections and malignancies in HIV-infected persons. *AIDS*, 48:770–776.

DEAN, MICHAEL, et al. (1996). Genetic restriction of HIV infection and progression to AIDS by a deletion allele of the CKR5 structural gene. *Science*, 273:1856–1861.

DENG, HONGKUI, et al. (1996). Identification of a major co-receptor for primary isolates of HIV-1. *Nature*, 381:661–666.

DOHERTY, PETER. (1995). The keys to cell-mediated immunity. *JAMA*, 274:1067–1068.

DRAGIC, TATJANA, et al. (1996). HIV-1 entry into CD4+ cells is mediated by the chemokine receptor CC-CKR-5. *Nature*, 381:667–673.

EDGINGTON, STEPHEN M. (1993). HIV no longer latent, says NIAID's Fauci. *BioTechnology*, 11:16–17.

EMBRETSON, JANET, et al. (1993). Massive covert infection of helper T lymphocytes and macrophages by HIV during the incubation period of AIDS. *Nature*, 362:359–362.

Eugen-Olsen, Jesper, et al. (1997). Heterozygosity for a deletion in the CKR5 gene leads to prolonged AIDS-free survival and slower CD4 T-cell decline. *AIDS*, 11:305–310.

FAUCI, ANTHONY. (1996). Host Factors and the pathogenesis of HIV–induced disease. *Nature*, 384:529–534.

FAUCI, ANTHONY, et al. (1995). Trapped but still dangerous. *Nature*, 337:680–681.

FITZGERALD, LYNN. (1988). Exercise and the immune system. *Trends Genet.*, 2:1–12.

FOSTER, R,. et al. (1985). Adverse effects of blood transfusions in lung cancer. *Cancer*, 55:11951–12202.

FOX, CECIL H., et al. (1991). Lymphoid germinal centers for reservoirs of HIV type I RNA. *J. Infect. Dis.*, 164:1051–1057.

FOX, CECIL, (1996) How HIV causes disease. *Carolina Tips*, 59:9–11.

GELDERBLOM, H.R., et al. (1985). Loss of envelope antigens of HTLV III/LAV, a factor in AIDS pathogenesis. *Lancet*, 2:1016–1017.

GHIARA, JAYANT, et al. (1994). Crystal structure of the principal neutralization site of HIV. *Science*, 264:82–85.

GROENINK, MARTIJIN, et al. (1993). Relation of phenotype evolution of HIV to envelope V2 configuration. *Science*, 260:1513–1516.

HAASE, ASHLEY, ey al. (1996). Quantitative image analysis of Hiv infection in lymphoid tissue. *Science*, 274:985–990.

HEATH, SONYA, et al. (1995). Follicular dentritic cells and HIV infectivity. *Nature*, 377:740–744.

HENGARTNER, MICHAEL. (1995). Life and death decisions: Ced-9 programmed cell death in *C. elegans*. *Science*, 270: 931.

HILL, MARK, et al. (1996). Natural resistance to HIV. *Nature*, 382:668–669.

HO, DAVID. (1995). Pathogenesis of HIV infection. *International AIDS Society–USA*, 3:9–12.

HO, DAVID, et al. (1995). Rapid turnover of plasma virons and CD4 lymphocytes in HIV infection. *Nature*, 373:123–126.

KINGSLEY, L., et al. (1987). Risk factors for seroconversion to HIV among male homosexuals. *Lancet*, 8529:345–348.

KION, TRACY, et al. (1991). Anti-HIV and Anti-Anti-MHC antibodies in alloimmune and autoimmune mice. *Science*, 253:1138–1140.

KNIGHT, STELLA. (1996). Bone-marrow-derived dendritic cells and the pathogenesis of AIDS. *AIDS*, 10:807–817.

LaPIERRE, A., et al. (1992). Exercise and health maintenance in AIDS. In Galantino, M.L. (ed.), *Clinical Assessment and Treatment in HIV: Rehabilitation of a Chronic Illness*, Chap. 7. Thorofare NJ: Slack, Inc.

LAURENCE, JEFFREY. (1996). Where do we go from here? *AIDS Reader*, 6:3–4, 36.

LIU, RONG, et al. (1996). Homozygous defect in HIV-1 coreceptor accounts for resistance of some multiple-exposed individuals to HIV-1 infection. *Cell*, 86:367–377.

LO, SHYH-CHING, et al. (1989). A novel virus-like infectious agent in patients with AIDS. *Am. J. Trop. Med. Hyg.*, 40:213.

LO, SHYH-CHING, et al. (1991). Enhancement of HIV-1 cytocidal effects in CD4+ lymphocytes by the AIDS-associated mycoplasma. *Science*, 251:1074–1076.

Moore, John, (1997).Coreceptors: Implications for HIV pathogenesis and therapy. *Science*, 276:51–52.

Mountain-Plains Regional HIV/AIDS Curriculum, 4th ed. (1992). Mountain-Plains Regional AIDS Office, University of Colorado Health Sciences Center, Denver, CO 80262.

NOWAK, MARTIN, et al. (1995). HIV results in the frame: results confirmed. *Nature*, 375:193.

O'Brien, Thomas, et al. (1997). HIV-1 infection in a man homozygous for CCR5 Δ 32. *Lancet*, 349:1219.

PANTALEO, G., et al. (1993). HIV infection is active and progressive in lymphoid tissue during the clinically latent stage of disease. *Nature*, 362:355–358.

PENNISI, ELIZABETH. (1994). A room of their own. *Science News*, 145:335.

PIANZ, OLIVER, et al. (1996). Specific cytotoxic T Cells eliminate cells producing neutralizing antibodies. *Nature*, 382:726–729.

SAMSON, MICHEL, et al. (1996). Resistance to HIV-1 infection in Caucasion individuals bearing mutant alleles of the CCR-5 chemokine gene. *Nature*, 382:722–725.

SCHMID, SANDRA, et al. (1994). Making class II presentable. *Nature*, 369:103–104.

SCHNITTMAN, STEVEN M., et al. (1989). The reservoir for HIV-1 in human peripheral blood is a T cell that maintains expression of CD4. *Science*, 245:305–308.

SINHA, ANIMESH, et al. (1990). Autoimmune diseases: the failure of self-tolerance. *Science*, 248:1380–1387.

SPRENT, JONATHAN, et al. (1994). Lymphocyte life-span and memory. *Science*, 265:1395–1400.

STROMINGER, JACK, et al. (1995). The Class I and Class II proteins of the Human major histocompatibility complex. *JAMA*, 274:1074–1076.

THEODOROU, IOANNIS, et al, (1997). HIV-1 infection in an individual homozygous for CCR5 Δ 32. *Lancet*, 349:1219–1220.

TULP, ABRAHAM, et al. (1994). Isolation and characterization of the intracellular MHC class II compartment. *Nature*, 369:120–126.

UNANUE, EMIL. (1995). The concept of antigen processing and presentation. *JAMA*, 274:1071–1073.

WEI, XIPING, et al. (1995). Viral dynamics in HIV type I infection. *Nature*, 373:117–122.

WEISS, ROBIN, et al. (1996). Hot fusion of HIV. *Nature*, 381: 647–648.

WITKIN, S., and SONNABEND, J. (1983). Immune responses to spermatozoa in homosexual men. *Fertil. Steril.*, 39:337–341.

ZHU, TOUFU. (1993). Gentypic and phenotypic characterization of HIV-1 patients with primary infection. *Science*, 261:1179–1181.

ZINKERNAGEL, ROLF. (1995). MHC-restricted T-cell recognition: The basis of immune surveillance. *JAMA*, 274:1069–1071.

Profile of Opportunistic Infections, Their Treatments, and Cancers Associated with HIV Disease/AIDS

CHAPTER CONCEPTS

♦ Suppression of the immune system allows harmless agents to become harmful opportunistic infections (OIs).

♦ OIs in AIDS patients are caused by viruses, bacteria, fungi, and protozoa.

♦ Cancer in AIDS patients is not caused by OIs.

♦ There are two types of Kaposi's sarcoma (KS): classic and AIDS-associated.

♦ KS is rarely found in hemophiliacs, intravenous drug users, and women with AIDS.

WHAT IS AN OPPORTUNISTIC DISEASE?

Humans evolved in the presence of a wide range of parasites—viruses, bacteria, fungi and protozoa that do not cause disease in people with an intact immune system. But these organisms can cause a disease in someone with a weakened immune system, such as an individual with HIV disease. The infections they cause are known as **opportunistic infections** (OIs). Thus, OIs occur after a disease-causing virus or microorganism, normally held in check by a functioning immune system, gets the chance to multiply and invade host tissue because the immune system has been compromised. For most of medical history, OIs were rare and almost always appeared in patients whose immunity was impaired by cancer or genetic disease.

With improved medical technology, a steadily growing number of patients are severely immunosuppressed because of medications and radiation used in bone marrow or organ transplantation and cancer chemotherapy. **HIV disease also suppresses the immune system.** And perhaps as a corollary to their increased prevalence, or because of heightened physician awareness, OIs seem to be occurring more frequently in the elderly, who may be rendered vulnerable by age-related declines in immunity. New OIs are now being diagnosed because the pool of people who can get them is so much larger, and, in addition, new techniques for identifying the causative organisms have been developed. However, most of the infections considered opportunistic are not reportable, which precludes any clear-cut count of their growing numbers.

Although OIs are still not commonplace, they are no longer considered rare—they occur in tens of thousands of patients each year. But despite this increase, physicians and their patients have reasons to be optimistic about their ability to contain these infections. The reasons are: (1) in a massive federal effort, driven by the HIV/AIDS epidemic, researchers are finding drugs that can prevent or treat many of the OIs; and (2) various therapies have shown promise for warding off OIs by boosting patients' immune systems.

THE PREVALENCE OF OPPORTUNISTIC DISEASES

The prevalence of OIs in the United States is staggering. There are some 250,000 HIV-seropositive individuals with T4-cell counts below 200/µL of blood. More than 100 microorganisms—bacteria, viruses, fungi, and protozoa—can cause disease in such individuals, even though only a fraction of these (17) are included in the current surveillance definition for clinical AIDS. OIs are associated, directly or indirectly with about 90% of deaths in AIDS patients. In a large survey from the Centers for Disease Control and Prevention (CDC), such OIs were diagnosed in 33% of individuals at 1 year and in 58% at 2 years after documentation of a T4-cell count below 200/µL. In 1995, the CDC has promulgated guidelines for chemoprophylaxis of only 3 OIs: *Pneumocystis carinii* pneumonia (PCP), *Mycobacterium tuberculosis* (MTb), and *Mycobacterium avium-intracellulare* complex (MAC). PCP and MTb prophylaxis has extended the survival of AIDS patients, but it has also opened new issues. With the growing proportion of long-term AIDS survivors, new OIs

have become prominent, together with concerns about cost, compliance, drug interactions, and quality of life (Laurence, 1995; *MMWR*, 1995). For 1996, the five most common AIDS-related OIs were PCP, candidal esophagitis, pulmonary/disseminated TB, mycobacterium avium complex disease and herpes simplex reinfection.

PROPHYLAXIS AGAINST OPPORTUNISTIC INFECTIONS

Drug prophylaxis against OIs has become a cornerstone of treatment for AIDS patients. For example, the prevalence of *Pneumocystis carinii* pneumonia (PCP) dropped from about 80% in 1987 to about 20% by mid-1994 because of the use of excellent drug therapy. The mortality of PCP without treatment is almost 100%. (Dobkin, 1995). According to Laurence (1996), researchers at the University of California, San Francisco, found that it costs, on average, $215,000 to extend by 1 year, the life of an HIV-infected patient with *Pneumocystis carinii* pneumonia (PCP) who is treated in an intensive care unit. That is more than twice the comparable care cost for 1988. Part of the reason given was that as people with AIDS survived longer, they were presenting with second and third episodes of PCP, superimposed on other chronic infections. The downside to OI prophylaxis is that it is difficult to find drugs that work without harmful side effects. In addition, viruses and organisms that cause OIs become resistant to the drugs over time. This is one of the primary reasons researchers are looking for ways in which to boost an immunosuppressed patient's immune system (Zoler, 1991).

OPPORTUNISTIC INFECTIONS IN HIV-INFECTED PEOPLE

AIDS is a devastating human tragedy. It appears to be killing about everyone who demonstrates the symptoms. One well-known American surgeon said, **"I would rather die of any form of cancer rather than die of AIDS."** This statement was not made because of the social stigma attached to AIDS, or because it is a

AVAILABLE THERAPY FOR OPPORTUNISTIC INFECTIONS

Only 10 years ago there was hardly any standardized use of protective agents to block the infectious complications or opportunistic infections (OIs) associated with HIV-induced immunodeficiency. Now there is an array of drugs that can be used in strategies to prevent or delay nearly all the major OIs. With this advancement has come the need to weigh the pros and cons of various strategies. Cost, antimicrobial resistance, drug interactions, and pill overload are all important considerations.

EFFECT OF ANTI-HIV THERAPY ON OPPORTUNISTIC INFECTIONS

As presented in Chapter 4, the use of anti-HIV combination drug therapy (AIDS drug cocktails) has produced a number of unexpected results in patient response to those drugs. Soon after combination therapy began, physicians witnessed a rather **confusing** or **unusual** presentation of OIs. In some cases certain OIs improved, in others the situation deteriorated! Such changes in OIs expression are occurring now, at a time when hundreds of thousands of HIV-infected people want **highly active antiretroviral therapy** (HAART).

TREATMENT IN THE HAART ERA

For some people with HIV disease/AIDS, the use of AIDS cocktails containing one protease in-

hibitor (**PI**) unmasked subclinical (unnoticeable) *Mycobacterium avium* complex (**MAC**) disease. In others, cytomegalovirus (**CMV**) infection and CMV retinitis (retinal eye infection) developed within 8 weeks of starting HAART. In contrast, HAART offered an **improvement** in HIV wasting, Kaposi's sarcoma, and progressive multifocal leukoencephalopathy (**PML**) (Currier et al., 1997). The clinical presentation of OIs has been impacted by HAART. Physicians treating AIDS persons have to decide on how and when treatment for OIs can or should be altered. The choices involved in treatment strategy are not easily made!

VIRAL LOAD RELATED TO OPPORTUNISTIC INFECTIONS

HIV-clinicians have recently looked at the predictive value of plasma HIV RNA for the development of three OIs: *Pneumocystis carinii* pneumonia (PCP), CMV, and MAC. Using a database of 813 patients participating in AIDS Clinical Trial Groups (ACTG), for every 1-log increment increase in plasma HIV RNA level, the risk of developing one of these OIs was increased 2- to 3-fold. Plasma HIV RNA level was predictive of an increased risk of an OI independent of T4 cell count, which also predicted OI risk. This information confirms that maintaining control of viral replication may be a critical component of preventing OIs in HIV-infected patients.

---

lethal condition. It was made in recognition of the slow, demoralizing, debilitating, painful, disfiguring, helpless, and unending struggle to stay alive.

Because of a suppressed and weakened immune system, viruses, bacteria, fungi, and protozoa that commonly and harmlessly inhabit the body become pathogenic (Figure 6-1). In addition, organisms and viruses from old infections that have lingered in the body reactivate. The suppression of the immune system presents an **opportunity** for the harmless to become harmful. About 90% of deaths related to HIV infection and AIDS are caused by OIs, compared with 7% due to cancer and 3% due to other causes.

What makes HIV disease particularly horrible is that it leaves patients open to an endless series of infections that would not occur in people with healthy immune responses. *Pneumocystis carinii* pneumonia, toxoplasmosis, Kaposi's sarcoma, candidiasis, cytomegalovirus retinitis, cryptococcal meningitis, mycobacterium avium complex, herpes simplex, and herpes zoster are infections that sicken and disfigure, and some eventually kill most people with AIDS.

FIGURE 6-1 General Progression of Opportunistic Infections after HIV Infection. Normal T4 cell count in adolescent/adults is, on average, about 1,000/μL of blood. There is a relationship between the drop in T4 lymphocytes and the onset of opportunistic infections (OIs). The first sign of an OI begins under 500 T4 cells/μL. As the T4 cell count continues to drop, the chance of OI infection increases. Note the variety of OIs found in AIDS patients with 200 or less T4 cells/μL.

HIV-Related Opportunistic Infections Vary Worldwide

The course of HIV infection tends to be similar for most patients: infection with the virus is followed by seroconversion and progressive destruction of T4 cells. Yet the opportunistic infections and malignancies that largely define the symptomatic or clinical history of HIV disease vary geographically. People with HIV and their physicians in different regions confront distinct problems, mainly because of differences in exposure, in access to diagnosis and care, and in general health.

Comparisons between the data about opportunistic infections in different countries must be made with care. But, most developing nations lack the facilities and trained personnel to identify opportunistic infections correctly; consequently, their prevalence may be underreported. Clinicians in developed countries can order sophisticated laboratory analyses to identify pathogens. Those in developing countries must rely on signs and symptoms to make their diagnoses. Oral candidiasis and herpes zoster are easy to diagnose without laboratory backup because the lesions are visible. While some pneumonias and types of diarrhea can be specified, others, (such as extrapulmonary tuberculosis, cytomegalovirus infections, cryptococcal meningitis, and systemic infections, such as histoplasmosis, toxoplasmosis, microsporidiosis, and nocardiosis) go underreported due to the lack of laboratory facilities.

Socioeconomic Factors

Geography explains much about the varying patterns of opportunistic infections, but a decisive factor is often financial capacity. On the most fundamental level, money is needed to create an infrastructure that limits exposure to pathogens. Thus, while few people with HIV in wealthy countries develop certain bacterial or protozoal infections, they are a major cause of death in poor areas that cannot provide clean water and adequate food storage facilities.

Financial resources also affect clinicians' abilities to diagnose AIDS and, when appropriate, to provide the proper medicine. AIDS patients in Africa often die of severe bacterial infections because they don't have the antibiotics or the clinical care they need. They don't survive long enough to develop diseases such as PCP.

United States, Europe, and Africa—The United States and Europe on one end, and Africa on the other, represent the global extremes of financial resources for health care. The most common opportunistic infections each region faces reflect the overall quality of health care, sanitation, and diet. For example, Thailand and Mexico belong to the large group of nations that have intermediate incomes and correspondingly intermediate patterns of HIV complications (Harvard AIDS Institute, 1994).

AIDS patients rarely have just one infection (Table 6-1). The mix of OIs may depend on life

---

——— BOX 6.1 ———

THE DECISION

Speaking of things we don't talk about, a friend of mine was recently diagnosed with CMV. I asked her if she'd gotten a catheter and started gancyclovir. She said, "No, I haven't decided what I'm going to do. But everytime I bring up the idea of choosing not to treat this, my friends get really freaked out, even hostile. So I'm not telling anyone anymore except you." I told her that my roommate had been diagnosed with CMV and got a catheter and infused gancyclovir for four hours a day, and eventually failed on it and started foscarnet which gave him stomach problems, and started taking a new drug for his stomach. I used to watch him and wonder if I could ever do what he was able to do. I don't know if I could and I sympathize with my friend who has practiced walking around her apartment with a blindfold to experience what it would be like to be blind. I'm sure many of us wrestle with decisions about treatments and the choice not to treat at all, but this sort of consideration runs contrary to our limited notion of empowerment and our mandate to live with AIDS.

TABLE 6-1 Some Common Opportunistic Diseases Associated with HIV Infection and Possible Therapy

Organism/Virus	Clinical Manifestation	Possible Treatments
Protozoa		
Cryptosporidium muris	Gastroenteritis (inflammation of stomach-intestine membranes)	Investigational only
Isospora belli	Gastroenteritis	Trimethoprim-sulfamethoxazole (Bactrim)
Toxoplasma gondii	Encephalitis (brain abscess), retinitis, disseminated	Pyrimethamine and leucovorin, plus sulfadiazine, or Clindamycin, Bactrim
Fungi		
Candida sp.	Stomatitis (thrush), proctitis, vaginitis, esophagitis	Nystatin, clotrimazole, ketoconazole
Coccidioides immitis	Meningitis, dissemination	Amphotericin B, fluconazole, ketoconazole
Cryptococcus neoformans	Meningitis (membrane inflammation of spinal cord and brain), pneumonia, encephalitis, dissemination (widespread)	Amphotericin B, fluconazole, itraconazole
Histoplasma capsulatum	Pneumonia, dissemination	Amphotericin B, fluconazole, itraconazole
Pneumocystis carinii	Pneumonia	Trimethoprim-sulfamethoxazole (Bactrim, Septra), pentamidine, dapsone, clindamycin, trimetrexate
Bacteria		
Mycobacterium avium complex (MAC)	Dissemination, pneumonia, diarrhea, weight loss, lymphadenopathy, severe gastrointestinal disease	Rifampin + ethambutol + clofazimine + ciprofloxacin +/- amikacin; rifabutin, clarithromycin & azithromycin
Mycobacterium tuberculosis (TB)	Pneumonia (tuberculosis), meningitis, dissemination	Isoniazid (INH) + rifampin + ethambutol +/- pyrazinamide
Viruses		
Cytomegalovirus (CMV)	Fever, hepatitis, encephalitis, retinitis, pneumonia, colitis, esophagitis	Ganciclovir, Foscarnet
Epstein-Barr	Oral hairy leukoplakia, B cell lymphoma	Acyclovir
Herpes simplex	Mucocutaneous (mouth, genital, rectal) blisters and/or ulcers, pneumonia, esophagitis, encephalitis	Acyclovir
Papovavirus J-C	Progressive multifocal leukoencephalopathy	none
Varicella-zoster	Dermatomal skin lesions (shingles), encephalitis	Acyclovir, Foscarnet
Cancers		
Kaposi's sarcoma	Disseminated mucocutaneous lesions often involving skin, lymph nodes, visceral organs (especially lungs & GI tract)	Local injection, surgical excision or radiation to small, localized lesions; Chemotherapy with vincristine & Bleomycin
Primary lymphoma of the brain	Headache, palsies, seizures, hemiparesis, mental status, or personality changes	Radiation and/or chemotherapy
Systemic lymphomas	Fever, night sweats, weight loss, enlarged lymph nodes	Chemotherapy

Patients with compromised immune systems are at increased risk for all known cancers and infections (including bacterial, viral, and protozoal). Most infectious diseases in HIV-infected patients are the result of proliferation of organisms already present in the patient's body. Most of these opportunistic infections are not contagious to others. The notable exception to this is tuberculosis.

(**Disclaimer**: This table was developed to provide general information only. It is not meant to be diagnostic nor to direct treatment.)

(Adapted from Mountain-Plains Regional Education and Training Center *HIV/AIDS Curriculum*, 4th Ed., 1992 updated, 1996)

style and where the HIV/AIDS patient lives or has lived. Thus a knowledge of the person's origins and travels may be diagnostically helpful. (Note: a number of the symptoms listed in the CDC definition of HIV/AIDS can be found associated with certain of the OIs presented.)

Fungal Diseases

In general, healthy people have a high degree of innate resistance to fungi. But a different situation prevails with opportunistic fungal infections, which often present themselves as acute, life-threatening diseases in a compromised host (Medoff et al., 1991).

Because treatment seldom results in the eradication of fungal infections in AIDS patients, there is a high probability of recurrence after treatment (DeWit et al., 1991).

Fungal diseases are among the more devastating of the OIs and are most often regional in association. AIDS patients from the Ohio River basin, the Midwest, or Puerto Rico have a higher than normal risk of histoplasmosis (*his-to-plaz-mo-sis*) infection. In the Southwest, there is increased risk for coccidioidomycosis (*kok-sid-e-o-do-mi-ko-sis*). In the southern Gulf states, the risk is for blastomycosis. Other important OI fungi such as *Pneumocystis carinii (nu-mo-sis-tis car-in-e-i), Candida albicans (kan-di-dah al-be-cans),* and *Cryptococcus neoformans (krip-to-kok-us knee-o-for-mans)* are found everywhere in equal numbers. Because of their importance as OIs in AIDS patients, a brief description of **histoplasmosis, candidiasis,** *Pneumocystis carinii* **pneumonia (PCP), and cryptococcosis are presented** (Table 6-1).

Histoplasmosis (Histoplasma capsulatum)— Spores are inhaled and germinate in or on the body (Figure 6-2, A and B). This fungal pathogen is endemic in the Mississippi and Ohio river valleys. Signs of histoplasmosis include prolonged influenza-like symptoms, shortness of breath, and possible complaints of night sweats and shaking chills. In AIDS patients there is a multisystem involvement: the liver, central nervous system, lymph nodes, and gastrointestinal tract are affected, while mucosal ulcers and enlarged spleen may also occur. Histoplasmosis in an HIV-positive person is considered diagnostic

of AIDS. In about two-thirds of AIDS patients with histoplasmosis, it is the initial OI. Over 90% of cases have occurred in patients with T4 cell counts below 100/µL (Wheat, 1992).

In non-HIV-infected patients, amphotericin B is almost always successful in treating histoplasmosis (Table 6-1). Only 50% to 80% of AIDS patients respond, however, and relapse is common during maintenance therapy. Nonetheless, amphotericin B followed by weekly maintenance therapy remains the recommended strategy. Amphotericin B is a toxic drug, increases one's temperature, and may also cause uncontrollable shaking; it is sometimes referred to as the "shake and bake" treatment. Earlier reports suggested ketoconazole as a potential alternative for initial or maintenance therapy, but it had an even higher failure rate than amphotericin B and is no longer recommended in HIV-infected patients.

Itraconazole (Sporanox) has recently been approved for treating histoplasmosis and some now consider it the drug of choice for HIV-related histoplasmosis (Daar et al., 1993; *Guidelines, U.S. Publich Health Service,* 1995).

Candidiasis (Candida albicans)— This fungus is usually associated with yeast infections of the vagina. It is a fungus quite common to the body and in particular inhabits the alimentary tract. It is normally kept in check by the presence of bacteria that live on the linings of the alimentary tract. However, in immunocompromised patients, especially those who have received broad spectrum antibiotics, candida multiplies rapidly. Because of its location in the upper reaches of the alimentary tract, if unchecked, it may cause mucocutaneous candidiasis or thrush, an overgrowth of candida in the esophagus and in the oral cavity (Figure 6-3, A and B). Mucosal candidiasis was associated with AIDS patients from the very beginning of the AIDS pandemic (Powderly et al., 1992). In women, overgrowths of candidiasis also occur in the vaginal area.

Gynecological conditions in women with HIV disease have been found to be more aggressive and to occur with a greater frequency than in noninfected women. Vaginal candidiasis (VC) is generally caused by *C. albicans*. VC is seen at all stages of HIV disease, with increasing

FIGURE 6-2 A, Anal Histoplasmosis. Histoplasmosis is caused by
Histoplasmosis capsulatum and causes infection in immunocompromised
patients. (*Courtesy CDC, Atlanta*) **B**, AIDS patient's tongue showing multiple
shiny, firm Histoplasma erythematous nodules (see arrow A) and Thrush (see
arrow B). (Courtesy Marc E. Grossman and Celeste Cole, New York)

FIGURE 6-3 Thrush. **A,** An overgrowth of *Candida albicans* on the soft palate in the oral cavity of an AIDS patient. **B,** Creamy patches of candida that can be **scraped off** leaving a red and sometimes bleeding mucosa. (**A,** *Courtesy CDC, Atlanta;* **B,** *Courtesy of Drs. M. Schiodt, D. Greenspan, J.S. Greenspan, Oral AIDS Center, University of California, San Francisco, and* Journal of Respiratory Diseases, *1989, 10:91-109)*

frequency in conjunction with PCP and genital herpes in patients with <200 T4 cells per μL of blood. It is sometimes associated with the use of birth control pills, chemotherapeutic regimens, corticosteroids, and immune suppression related to pregnancy. Common symptoms include a thick, whitish discharge; severe itching; localized, sometimes severe pain; and infrequently, the development of lesions. Vaginal manifestations of the disease are thought to precede esophageal and/or oral thrush. HIV-related vaginal candidiasis may be characterized by resistance to standard therapy. Candida infections should be monitored for frequency and response to antifungal treatments (Table 6-1). If candidiasis is limited to the mouth and oropharynx and the patient is not debilitated, treatment with topical nystatin (Mycostatin Pastilles) or clotrimazole (Mycelex Troches) is often sufficient. If the patient does not respond adequately, or esophageal involvement is possible, a systemic agent such as ketoconazole (Nizoral) or fluconazole (Diflucan) is appropriate (Daar et al., 1993; *Guidelines, U.S. Public Health Service,* 1995). Difficult to treat cases may require IV amphotericin B (Fungizone). Acidopholis supplementation appears to be beneficial, especially in women receiving PCP

prophylaxis with TMP/SMX (Bactrim or Dapsone). Persons often self-administer alternative treatments, either alone or in conjunction with approved therapies. These include changes in diet, with the avoidance of foods containing yeast, sugar, and dairy products. Vitamin C supplementation and herbal products are often used (Willoughby, 1989).

Some people with oropharyngeal candidiasis may experience a sore mouth. This is particularly painful when acidic foods and juices are taken. In addition, the taste of food is often altered. Treatment is aimed at relieving the symptoms, as therapy is rarely successful at eliminating the fungus (Hay, 1991).

Impaired cell-mediated immunity, as occurs in people with HIV disease, may allow for a disseminated infection (distributed to other areas of the body). Oral or **esophageal candidiasis** causes thick white patches on the mucosal surface and may be the first manifestation of AIDS. Because other diseases can cause similar symptoms, candidiasis by itself is not sufficient for a diagnosis of AIDS.

***Pneumocystis carinii*—** This fungus, until recent reclassification, was considered a protozoan (Edman et al., 1988). The life cycle and reproductive characteristics of *P. carinii* are not completely understood because the organism is difficult to culture for laboratory study. However, the molecular biology and molecular taxonomy are now being rapidly constructed (Walzer, 1993; Stringer et al., 1996). Virtually everyone in the United States by age 30 to 40 has been exposed to *P. carinii*. It lies dormant in the lungs, held in check by the immune system. Prior to the AIDS epidemic, *P. carinii* pneumonia was seen in children and adults who had a suppressed immune system as in leukemia or Hodgkin's disease and were receiving chemotherapy. In the AIDS patient, the onset of *P. carinii* pneumonia is insidious—patients may notice some shortness of breath and they cannot run as far. It causes extensive damage within the alveoli of the lung.

The *P. carinii* fungus develops from a small unicellular trophozoite into a cyst containing eight sporozoites (Figure 6-4A). These sporozoites are disseminated throughout the body, but they show a greater affinity for the lungs, where they multiply in the spaces between the lung sacs and cause pneumonia (Figure 6-4B). Prior to 1981, fewer than 100 cases of *P. carinii* infection were reported annually in the United States; yet 80% of AIDS patients develop *P. carinii* pneumonia at some time during their illness. This is one of the few AIDS-related conditions for which there is a choice of relatively effective drugs. The first of these to be made available was the intravenous and aerosolized versions of pentamidine. There are frequent recurrences of this infection. With treatment, there is a 10% to 30% mortality with each PCP episode. (Montgomery, 1992). PCP accounted for a diagnosis of AIDS in over 65% of AIDS cases in 1990. In 1994 it had fallen to 20% due to available therapy (Ernst, 1990; Murphy, 1994). The triad of symptoms that almost always indicates the onset of PCP during HIV disease is fever, dry cough, and shortness of breath (Grossman et al., 1989). *P. carinii* pneumonia is unlikely to develop in people with HIV disease unless their T4 cell count drops below 200 (Phair et al., 1990).

The antifolate (blocking action to folic acid) drugs pentamidine and trimethoprim/sulfamethoxazole are currently treatments of choice for *P. carinii* pneumonia (Zackrison et al., 1991; Dobkin, 1995).

A

B

FIGURE 6-4 **A,** A concentration of *Pneumocystis carinii* cysts. (See text for details.) **B,** Scanning electron microscope image of *P. carinii* attached to lung tissue. Note the tubular extensions through which it extracts nutrients from host lung tissue. (*Courtesy of Linda L. Pifer, St. Jude Children's Research Hospital, Memphis and* Pediatric Research, *1977, 11:305-306*)

PNEUMOCYSTIS CARINII PNEUMONIA IN CHILDREN. PCP is the most common opportunistic infection in children who have AIDS. Despite the publication of guidelines for prophylaxis against PCP for children infected with HIV in 1991, ongoing AIDS surveillance has detected no substantial decrease in PCP incidence among HIV-infected infants. This continued incidence is associated with failure to identify HIV-infected children before PCP occurs and with limitations in the ability of T4 measurements to identify children at risk for PCP. In March 1994, the National Pediatric & Family HIV Resource

Center, in collaboration with CDC, convened a working group to review additional data about the occurrence of PCP among HIV-infected children. This report summarizes these new data and presents revised PCP prevention guidelines that recommend : 1) promptly identifying children born to HIV-infected women and initiating regular diagnostic and immunologic monitoring of such children; 2) beginning PCP prophylaxis at 4–6 weeks of age for all children who have been perinatally exposed to HIV; 3) continuing prophylaxis through 12 months of age for HIV-infected children; and 4) making decisions regarding prophylaxis for HIV-infected children ≥12 months of age based on T4 measurements and whether PCP previously has occurred (*MMWR*, 1995).

Cryptococcosis (Cryptococcus neoformans)— Since its discovery in 1894, *C. neoformans* has been recognized as a major cause of deep-seated fungal infection in the human host. The infection can affect many sites, including skin, lung, kidney, prostate, and bone. However, symptomatic disease most often represents infection of the central nervous system. Cryptococcal

meningitis is the most common form of fungal meningitis in the United States (Ennis et al., 1993). This fungus is shed in pigeon feces, the spores of which enter the lung. If the lung does not eliminate it, it gets into the bloodstream, travels to the brain, and can cause cryptococcal meningitis.

In a healthy person, *C. neoformans* may cause pulmonary problems or meningeal infection (infection of the membranes that envelop the brain and spinal cord). It is more commonly seen in people with immunosuppression, especially in HIV/AIDS cases. *C. neoformans* is a fatal OI that occurs in about 13% of AIDS patients (Brooke et al., 1990). It is acquired through the respiratory tract and most commonly causes cryptococcal meningitis. Disseminated *C. neoformans* (Figure 6-5A) infection may involve bone marrow, the central nervous system (CNS), and the lungs, causing cryptococcal pneumonia. In AIDS patients, *C. neoformans* also causes infection of the skin (Figure 6-5B), lymph nodes, and kidneys. *Cryptococcus* cannot be cured and it does recur. What drugs should be used is a subject of controversy. Eric Darr and colleagues (1993) report that fluconazole and itraconazole

FIGURE 6-5 *Cryptococcus neoformans.* **A,** Large, budding, and encapsulated *C. neoformans* shows white against an India ink stain. Isolated from the cerebral spinal fluid of a patient with meningitis. **B,** Skin lesions caused by *C. neoformans* may be single or multiple. The "ulcer" is usually painless but is an early sign of infection. (**A,** *Courtesy CDC, Atlanta.* **B,** *Courtesy of Ronald P. Rappini, University of Texas Medical School and reprinted with permission from* Cutis, *1988, Vol. 42:125-128)*

A

B

are effective in treating cryptococcal meningitis (Table 6-1). Since then, flucytosine and amphotericin B have been used (Dobkin, 1995; *Guidelines, U.S. Public Health Service*, 1995).

Viral Diseases

Because of a depleted T4 cellular component of the immune system, AIDS patients are at particularly high risk for the herpes family of viral infections: cytomegalovirus, herpes simplex virus types 1 and 2, varicella-zoster virus, and Epstein-Barr virus.

Cytomegalovirus (CMV)— This virus is a member of the human herpesvirus group of viruses. CMV is the consummate parasite. It infects most people asymptomatically. When illness does occur, it is mild and nonspecific. There have been no epidemics to call attention to the virus. Yet CMV is now considered the most common infectious cause of mental retardation and congenital deafness in the United States. It is also the most common viral pathogen found in immunocompromised people (Balfour, 1995).

A **latent state** follows initial infection, with CMV probably located in the white blood cells and involving many organs and organ systems. Later it is reactivated, usually by some form of immunosuppression such as organ or bone marrow transplantation, cancer chemotherapy, or HIV disease (Jacobson et al., 1992; Hardy, 1996).

FIGURE 6-6 Cytomegalovirus. This is an electron micrograph magnified 49,200 times. (*Courtesy CDC, Atlanta*)

The virus is very labile and survives only a few hours outside a human host. It can be found in saliva, tears, blood, stool, cervical secretions, and in especially high levels in urine and semen. Transmission occurs primarily by intimate or close contact with infected secretions. The incidence of CMV infection varies from between 30% and 80% depending on the geographical community tested. However, over 90% of homosexual males have tested positive for CMV (Jacobson et al., 1988). CMV causes the more important viral infections in AIDS patients (Figure 6-6). This virus causes a broad spectrum of diseases in HIV-infected people, ranging from mild or severe gastrointestinal problems to infections of the brain, the liver (hepatitis), and the onset of fulminant (sudden and severe) pneumonia. Gastrointestinal infection may result in severe ulceration of the esophagus, stomach, small intestines, and colon. CMV pneumonia occurs in 10% to 20% of AIDS patients and can be lethal because therapy is unsuccessful.

CMV infection of AIDS patients usually results in prolonged fever, anemia (too few red blood cells), leukopenia (too few white blood cells), and abnormal liver function. CMV also causes severe diarrhea and HIV-associated retinitis resulting in eventual blindness (*Emergency Medicine*, 1989; Lynch, 1989; Dobkin, 1995).

Perhaps 75% of AIDS patients have an eye disease, with the retina the most common site (Russell, 1990). The retina, which is a light-sensitive membrane lining the inside of the back of the eye, is also part of the brain and is nourished by blood vessels. AIDS-related damage to these vessels produces tiny retinal hemorrhages and small **cotton wool spots**—early indicators of disease that are often detected during a routine eye examination (Figure 6-7).

Symptoms of CMV retinitis may be subtle, such as blurred vision, haze or floaters, or small dim spots in side vision. In unusual circumstances, the virus can produce dramatic symptoms, such as loss of vision within 72 hours. Without treatment, CMV can destroy the entire retina in 3 to 6 months after infection.

In August 1991, the United States Food and Drug Administration (FDA) approved the use of **foscarnet** (Foscavir) and **ganciclovir** (Cytovene) for the treatment of CMV retinitis

———— BOX 6.2 ————

A PHYSICIAN'S AGONIZING DILEMMA

Opportunistic infections are the primary threat to patients with AIDS; they are the main causes of illness and death. The cruel irony is that although there are 26 or more FDA approved drugs to treat these infections, most cannot be used in patients receiving zidovudine (ZDV) *because the combination drug therapy is devastatingly toxic to bone marrow.*

EXAMPLE:

Cytomegalovirus (CMV) Retinitis

CMV retinitis is one of the *worst* of the opportunistic infections and it develops in 90% of AIDS patients (Gottlieb et al., 1987). Both the patient who contracts CMV retinitis and the treating physician confront an almost impossible dilemma: whether to continue the zidovudine and risk blindness or to treat the retinitis and risk death from another infection. A physician recently said, "In my experience, I have never yet been able to combine zidovudine with the experimental drug ganciclovir (DHPG), which is the only recognized treatment for CMV retinitis, because the combination destroys the bone marrow. I therefore face the virtually impossible task of asking a 25-year-old person: 'Which of these options do you prefer: to take zidovudine and keep on living but go blind, or to preserve your sight by having retinitis treatment but risk dying?' That is a truly terrible question to ask of any patient, especially a young one." He continued, "Recently, I treated just such a young patient. He had been taking zidovudine for AIDS when he contracted CMV retinitis. When I presented him with this agonizing choice, he told me, `I definitely don't want to go blind. I want to be treated for this retinitis.' So he stopped taking zidovudine and was started on DHPG treatment. He started to have seizures, which were a consequence of the toxoplasmosis brain abscess that eventually ended his life. Just before he died, he told me that the worst decision he ever made was to stop taking zidovudine. 'I should have stayed on it,' he said, 'and gone blind.'" (Robert J. Awe, M.D., 1988)

Cryptococcal Meningitis

The situation for AIDS patients with cryptococcal meningitis is similarly depressing. Because of the severe bone marrow toxicity, it is virtually impossible to use amphotericin B, the effective treatment for this meningitis, at the same time as zidovudine. Besides, the use of amphotericin B has its own side effects as can be noted from this excerpt from Paul Monette's *Borrowed Time: An AIDS Memoir:*

> Amphotericin B is administered with Benadryl in order to avoid convulsions, the most serious possible side effect. It was about nine or ten when they started the drug in his veins, and I sat by the bed as nurses streamed in and out. A half hour into the slow drip, the nurse monitoring the IV walked out, saying she'd be right back, and a couple of minutes later Roger began to shake. I gripped him by the shoulders as he was jolted by what felt like waves of electric shock, staring at me horror-struck. Though Cope [the physician] would tell me later, trying to ease the torture of my memory, that "mentation" [mental activity] is all blurred during convulsions, I saw that Roger knew the horror. (Page 336)
>
> When the nurse returned she looked at him in dismay: "How long has this been going on?" Then she ordered an emergency shot of morphine to counteract the horror. When at last he fell into a deep sleep they all told me to go home, saying they would try another dose of the ampho in a few hours. I was so ragged I could barely walk. So I left him there with no way of knowing how near it was [Roger's death], or maybe not brave enough to know.

Whichever option is chosen, the patient is bound to suffer, and perhaps die, either of cryptococcal meningitis or of some other infection.

(Table 6-1). The drugs slow the progression of CMV retinitis (Danner, 1995; Hermans, 1996). Recently (1996) eye implants of ganciclovir have shown to be a more effective way to delay CMV retinitis.

Herpes Viruses Types 1 & 2 (HSV 1 & 2)— Both viruses cause *severe* and progressive eruptions of the mucous membranes. HSV 1 affects the membranes of the nose and mouth. Also, when herpetic lesions involve the lips or throat,

FIGURE 6-7 Cytomegalovirus retinitis. The disease, as seen in this photograph, involves the posterior pole of the right eye. Fluffy white infiltrate (cotton wool spots) with a small amount of retinal hemorrhage can be seen in the distribution of the superior vascular arcade. (*Courtesy of Scott M. Whitcup, M. D., National Eye Institute, National Institutes of Health, Bethesda, MD*)

─────── **POINT OF INFORMATION 6.2** ───────

NEW THERAPIES, LONGER LIFE, HIGHER INCIDENCE OF CYTOMEGALOVIRUS (CMV)

The incidence of CMV disease is increasing as patients with HIV live longer with more profound degrees of immunosuppression. They are living longer due to the use of AIDS drug combination cocktails which include protease inhibitors. However, once CMV disease has been diagnosed (using clinical findings for CMV retinitis and histology and virology for gastrointestinal and central nervous system disease), the prognosis for the patient is poor. Initial treatment usually consists of 3 to 6 weeks of therapy, depending on the end organ involved, followed by lifelong maintenance therapy for retinal and neurological disease. Regardless, despite good initial responses to licensed anti-CMV therapies, management is limited to controlling rather than eradicating CMV and eventually the disease progresses or recurs and the cycle of treatment has to be restarted.

80% to 90% of the time they either precede or occur simultaneously with **herpes-caused pneumonia** (Gottlieb et al., 1987). Bacterial or fungal superinfections occur in more than 50% of herpes-caused pneumonia cases and are a major contributory cause of death in AIDS patients.

Mortality from HSV pneumonia exceeds 80% (Lynch, 1989). Herpes may also cause blindness in AIDS patients. The following is from Paul Monette's *Borrowed Time*:

I woke up shortly thereafter, and Roger told me—without a sense of panic, almost puzzled—that his vision seemed to be losing light and detail. I called Dell Steadman and made an emergency appointment, and I remember driving down the freeway, grilling Roger about what he could see. It seemed to be less and less by the minute. He could barely see the cars going by in the adjacent lanes. Twenty minutes later we were in Dell's office, and with all the urgent haste to get there we didn't really reconnoiter till we were sitting in the examining room. I asked the same question—

A **B**

FIGURE 6-8 Perirectal Ulcer in an AIDS Patient. **A,** This ulcer was caused by the herpes type II virus. Herpes infections out of control in AIDS and other immunocompromised patients are a serious threat. **B,** The chronic expression of herpes type II virus on the scrotum of an AIDS patient. (*Courtesy of Ronald P. Rappini, University of Texas Medical School and reprinted with permission from* Cutis, *1988, 42:125-128*)

what could he see?—and now Roger was getting more and more upset the more his vision darkened. I picked up the phone to call Jamiee, and by the time she answered the phone in Chicago he was blind. *Total blackness, in just two hours!*

The retina had detached. (An operation on retinal attachment was successful and sight was restored. The cause of the retinal detachment was a herpes infection of the eyes.)

HSV 2 also affects the membranes of the anus, causing severe perianal and rectal ulcers primarily in homosexual men with AIDS (Figure 6-8, A and B). Herpes of the skin can generally be managed with oral **acyclovir** (Zovirax) or Foscavir (Table 6-1).

Herpes Zoster Virus (HZV)— Like herpes simplex, this virus has the potential to cause fulmi-nant pneumonia in AIDS patients. Untreated HZV pneumonia has a mortality rate of 15% to 35%. HZV is now monitored as an early indicator that HIV-positive people are progressing toward AIDS.

Protozoal Diseases

An increasing number of infections *which have not been observed in immunocompromised* patients are being found in AIDS patients. Three such infections are caused by the protozoans *Toxoplasma gondii, Isospora belli,* and *Cryptosporidium muris.*

Toxoplasma gondii— *T. gondii* is a small intracellular protozoan parasite that lives in vacuoles inside host macrophages and other nucleated cells. It appears that during and after entry, *T. gondii* produces secretory products that modify vacuole membranes so that the normal *fusion* of cell vacuoles with lysosomes containing digestive enzymes is blocked. Having blocked vacuole-lysosome fusion, *T. gondii* can successfully reproduce and cause a disease called **toxoplasmosis** (Joiner et al., 1990). It can infect any warm-blooded animal, invading and multiplying within the cytoplasm of host cells. As host immunity develops, multiplication slows and tissue cysts are formed. Sexual multiplication occurs in the intestinal cells of cats (and apparently only cats); oocysts form and are shed in the stool (Sibley, 1992). Transmission may occur transplacentally, by ingestion of raw or undercooked meat and eggs containing tissue cysts or by exposure to oocysts in cat feces (Wallace et al., 1993).

In the United States, 10% to 40% of adults are chronically infected but most are asymptomatic. *T. gondii* can enter and infect the human brain causing **encephalitis** (inflammation of the brain). Toxoplasmic encephalitis develops in over 30% of AIDS patients at some point in their illness (Figure 6-9). The signs and symptoms of cerebral toxoplasmosis in AIDS patients have been presented in detail by Rossitch and colleagues (1990). They may include fever, headache, confusion, sleepiness, weakness or numbness in one part of the body, seizure activity, and changes in vision. These symptoms can get worse and progress to coma and death unless toxoplasmosis is promptly diagnosed

FIGURE 6-9 *Toxoplasma gondii* Lesions in the Brain. Radiographic imaging shows a deep ring-enhancing lesion located in the basal ganglia. (*By permission of Carmelita U. Tuazon, George Washington University*)

and treated. Toxoplasma infection affecting other parts of the body is rare, and symptoms vary depending on which organs the disease affects. Based on the projected incidence of AIDS cases in the United States in 1992, 40,000 to 70,000 cases of toxoplasmic encephalitis were expected to occur (Dannemann et al., 1989). Similar to a variety of other OIs manifested in HIV-infected people, toxoplasmosis appears to represent a reactivation of an earlier infection. In the United States, 30% of the population between the ages of 10 and 19 demonstrate serological evidence (antibody) to *T. gondii* exposure. *T. gondii* lies dormant in the reticuloendothelial system until it becomes reactivated within the immunocompromised host. Thus, for most AIDS patients, it is believed that *T. gondii* is latent within their bodies and is reactivated by the loss of immune competence. Once activated, symptoms can be as mild as chills, headaches that do not respond to common pain killers, low fevers, and delusions; or as severe as hard seizures, coma, and death. Arthur Ashe, tennis champion who died in February of 1993, was being treated for *T. gondii* infection.

Current treatment (Table 6-1) is with pyrimethamine combined with sulfadiazine or clindamycin and with trimethoprim/sulfamethoxazole (Bactrim) or dapsone (Daar et al., 1993; Hunt, 1996). Treatment keeps toxoplasma under control but it does not kill it. Therapy must be continued indefinitely.

Cryptosporidium— *Cryptosporidium* is the cause of cryptosporidiosis, and is a member of the family of organisms that includes *Toxoplasma gondii* and *Isospora*. Its life cycle is similar to that of other organisms in the class Sporozoa. Oocysts are shed in the feces of infected animals and are immediately infectious to others. In humans, the organisms can be found throughout the GI tract, including the pharynx, esophagus, stomach, duodenum, jejenum, ileum, appendix, colon, and rectum. Various case reports of patients with AIDS describe infection in the gallbladder and pulmonary dissemination which clinically resembles *Pneumocystis carinii* pneumonia. *Cryptosporidium* causes profuse watery diarrhea of six to 26 bowel movements per day with a loss of 1 to 17 liters of fluid (a liter is about 1 quart). It is an infrequent infection in AIDS patients, usually occurring late in the course of disease as immunological deterioration progresses.

Studies of transmission patterns have shown infection within families, nursery schools, and from person to person, probably by the fecal-oral route. The infection is particularly common in homosexual men, perhaps as a consequence of anilingus (oral-anal sex). Cryptosporidiosis made headlines in March and April 1993 when an outbreak of the infection in Milwaukee resulted in diarrheal illness in more than 400,000 people. Following that outbreak, testing for *Cryptosporidium* in people with diarrhea increased substantially in some areas of Wisconsin. As a result of the investigations, *Cryptosporidum* contamination was found in several public swimming pools. At this time, there are no effective prophylaxes against cryptosporidiosis (Church, 1992; MMWR, 1995). The prevention of transmission rests on good hygiene, hand washing, and awareness of the risks of direct fecal-oral exposure (Wofsy, 1991).

Isospora belli— *Isospora belli* enters the body via feces-contaminated food and drink or is sexually transmitted (DeHovitz, 1988). This organism infects the bowels. Isosporiasis is characterized by an acute onset of profuse watery diarrhea (eight to 10 stools per day), fever, malaise, cramping, abdominal pain, and in some cases significant weight loss and anorexia. According to the 1987 revised definition for AIDS, isosporiasis persisting for longer than 1 month and a positive test for HIV is indicative of AIDS.

Treatment (Table 6-1) calls for high doses of trimethoprim-sulfamethoxazole, furazolidone, and pyrimethamine-sulfadiazine (Wofsy, 1991).

Bacterial Diseases

There is a long list of bacteria that cause infections in AIDS patients. These are the bacteria that normally cause infection or illness after the ingestion of contaminated food, such as species of *Salmonella*. Others, such as *Streptococci, Haemophilus,* and *Staphylococci* are common in advanced HIV disease. A number of other bacterial caused sexually transmitted diseases such as syphilis, chancroid, gonor-

rhea, and chlamydial diseases are also associated with HIV disease.

One difference between AIDS and non-AIDS individuals is that bacterial diseases in AIDS patients are of greater severity and more difficult to treat. In fact, drug treatments for HIV/AIDS patients have been associated with an increase in the incidence of bacterial infections (Rolston, 1992). Two bacterial species, *Mycobacterium avium intracellulare* and *Mycobacterium tuberculosis* are of particular importance as agents of infection in AIDS patients (Table 6-2).

***Mycobacterium avium intracellulare (MAI)*—** Over the past 40 years, MAI has gone from a rare, reportable infection to something that is common in most large American communities. Unlike tuberculosis, which is almost exclusively spread person-to-person, MAI is, in most instances, environmentally acquired. MAI exists in food, animals, water supplies, soil and enters people's lungs as an aerosol when they take showers.

When an elderly person develops MAI infection, it is invariably confined to his or her lungs. In contrast, MAI infections in AIDS patients run rampant and are clearly systemic (Zoler, 1991).

The fact that MAI produced disseminated disease in AIDS cases was recognized in 1982. The epidemiology of MAI continues to evolve. MAI occurs in 18% to 43% of people with HIV disease and has been implicated as the cause of a nonspecific **wasting syndrome**. AIDS patients demonstrate anorexia (inability to eat), weight loss, weakness, night sweats, diarrhea, and fever. Some patients also experience abdominal pain, enlarged liver or spleen, and malabsorption. In contrast to viral infections, this bacterium rarely causes pulmonary or lung problems in AIDS patients. Among persons with AIDS, the risk of developing disseminated MAI increases progressively with time. AIDS patients surviving for 30 months had a 50% risk of developing disseminated MAI. It appears most HIV-infected persons will develop disseminated MAI if they do not first die from other OIs (Chin, 1992). Some new drugs in use are clofazimine, ciprofloxacin, ethambutol, amikacin, azithromycin (Zithromax), clarithromycin (Biaxin), and rifabutin, but their

TABLE 6-2 Categories of Organism and Viral Involvement in Opportunistic Diseases

Symptoms	Causative Agent
Generally Present	
Fever, weight loss, fatigue, malaise	*Pneumocystis carinii*
	Cytomegalovirus
	Epstein-Barr virus
	Mycobacterium avium intracellulare
	Candida albicans
Diffuse Pneumonia	
Dyspnea, chest pain, hypoxemia, abnormal chest X-ray	*Pneumocystis carinii*
	Cytomegalovirus
	Mycobacterium tuberculosis
	Mycobacterium avium intracellulare
	Candida albicans
	Cryptococcus neoformans
	Toxoplasma gondii
Gastrointestinal Involvement	
Esophagitis (sore throat, dysphagia)	*Candida albicans*
	Herpes simplex
	Cytomegalovirus (suspected)
Enteritis (diarrhea, abdominal pain, weight loss)	*Giardia lamblia*
	Entamoeba histolytica
	Isospora belli
	Cryptosporidium
	Strongyloides stercoralis
	Mycobacterium avium intracellulare
Proctocolitis[a] (diarrhea, abdominal pain, rectal pain)	*Entamoeba histolytica*
	Campylobacter
	Shigella
	Salmonella
	Chlamydia trachomatis
	Cytomegalovirus
Proctitis[a] (pain during defecation, diarrhea, itching and perianal ulcerations)	*Neisseria gonorrhoeae*
	Herpes simplex
	Chlamydia trachomatis
	Treponema pallidum
Neurological Involvement	
Meningitis, encephalitis, headaches, seizures, dementia	Cytomegalovirus
	Herpes simplex
	Toxoplasma gondii
	Cryptococcus neoformans
	Papovavirus
	Mycobacterium tuberculosis
Retinitis (diminished vision)	Cytomegalovirus
	Toxoplasma gondii
	Candida albicans

[a]Especially in those persons practicing anal sex.

Adapted from Amin, 1987

For Sexual Exposures—People should use male latex condoms during every act of sexual intercourse to reduce the risk of exposure to cytomegalovirus, herpes simplex virus, and human papillomavirus, as well as to all other sexually transmitted pathogens. Use of latex condoms will also prevent the transmission of HIV to others. People should avoid sexual practices that may result in oral exposure to feces (e.g., oral-anal contact) to reduce the risk of intestinal infections such as cryptosporidiosis, shigellosis, campylobacteriosis, amebiasis, giardiasis, and hepatitis A and B (*MMWR*, 1995).

effectiveness is limited—resistance to these drugs develops quickly (Table 6-1) (Kaplan et al., 1995).

Mycobacterium tuberculosis—Tuberculosis (TB) is an infectious disease caused by the bacterium *Mycobacterium tuberculosis*, which is spread almost exclusively by airborne transmission. TB has been observed in elephants, cattle, mice, and other animal species. In 1993, TB was transmitted from an infected seal to its trainer in Australia. In the United States, monkeys are the primary source of animal-to-human transmission.

The disease can affect any site in the body, but it most often affects the lungs. When persons with pulmonary TB cough, they produce tiny droplet nuclei that contain TB bacteria, which can remain suspended in the air for prolonged periods of time. (With respect to transmission, the cough to TB is similar to sex to HIV.) Anyone who breathes air that contains these droplet nuclei can become infected with TB. It has been suggested that there is a minimal chance of inhaling HIV in blood-tinged TB sputum (Harris, 1993).

A person who becomes infected with the TB bacillus remains infected for years. Usually a person with a healthy immune system does not become ill, but is usually not able to eliminate the infection without taking an antituberculosis drug. This condition is referred to as a latent tuberculosis infection.

About 10% of otherwise healthy persons who have latent tuberculosis infection will become ill with active TB at some time during their lives (*MMWR*, 1992). With HIV disease the risk is 10% per year (Daar et al., 1993).

Tuberculosis is not generally considered to be an OI because people with healthy immune systems contract TB. After infection with *M. tuberculosis* about 5% of immunocompetent individuals will develop TB (Daley, 1992). But, people with a depressed immune system are much more likely to develop the disease (Zoler, 1991). Tuberculosis in people with AIDS does not look like ordinary tuberculosis. In the usual presentation of the disease, TB is usually restricted to a given area in the chest. People with AIDS may have tuberculosis throughout the chest cavity.

WASTING SYNDROME

Wasting syndrome is defined as weight loss in excess of 10% from baseline that is associated with chronic diarrhea, fever, or weakness. Between 1987 and 1991, wasting was the second most common AIDS-associated condition reported to the CDC and the only AIDS-associated illness noted in 7% of reported cases. Unpublished data from the CDC's Adult-Adolescent Spectrum of Disease Program, which studied AIDS deaths in 10 cities, found that between 1990 and 1994, wasting occurred in 21.6% of cases. This was the fourth most common AIDS-associated condition, after PCP, MAC, and esophageal candidiasis. CDC statistics from 1995 documented wasting as the third most common AIDS-indicator condition, after severe immunosuppression and PCP. Wasting is more prevalent in people of low socioeconomic status and women.

Although weight loss is not always an accurate measure of wasting, it can cause or be a sign of other problems associated with HIV disease. In addition to the weight loss associated with wasting, for example, people with HIV lose weight when they are fighting opportunistic infections. Once an opportunistic infection has been treated effectively, people often stop losing weight. While there are periods of weight stability, people usually do not return to baseline—they progress in a downward, stepwise fashion.

People with HIV typically sustain a 5% loss of body weight with each new infection. Because weight loss is correlated with mortality, oral supplements or artificial diets by vein or feeding tube may be needed. This means that although supplemental nutrition may not restore body composition, it may be useful in counteracting weight loss due to an opportunistic infection and in maintaining overall nutrition.

Weight loss may be caused by antiretrovirals and medications used to treat opportunistic infections. They frequently cause anorexia, as do infections themselves. Also, people experiencing nausea, diarrhea, difficulty swallowing, or infection with any pathogen that affects the digestive tract may not feel like eating. Similarly, people with HIV may not have the energy or resources to maintain a nutritious diet. Two appetite stimulants have been approved for use by people with HIV—Megestrol acetate and Dronabinol. Megestrol acetate has been shown to increase body fat rather than lean body mass, however, and the type of weight gain with Dronabinol use is unclear.

There is a strong association between HIV disease and TB: HIV infection is the highest risk factor for progression from latent *M. tuberculosis* infection to TB (Bermejo et al., 1992).

HIV infection is now considered to be the single most important risk factor in the expression of TB. HIV disease is associated with the reactivation of a dormant or inactive TB infection (Stanford et al., 1993).

M. tuberculosis infection occurs in about 35% of HIV-infected individuals, usually as the result of *M. tuberculosis* reactivation from a latent prior infection (Brooke et al., 1990). The CDC defines extrapulmonary TB combined with an HIV-positive test as diagnostic of AIDS.

According to the World Health Organization (1995) TB is, worldwide, the leading cause of death in HIV-infected people and among adults from a single, infectious organism.

Drugs used to treat TB are isoniazid, rifampin, pyrazinamide, streptomycin, and ethambutol. Ethambutol is used in combination with the other four drugs when the infecting organism is suspected to be drug-resistant (Bernardo, 1991; Dannenberg, 1993). However, health officials state that between 40% and 60% of those developing multidrug resistant TB will die (Ezzell, 1993).

Other Opportunistic Infections

Other opportunistic infectious organisms and viruses and the diseases they cause and possible therapies are listed in Table 6-1. Table 6-2 separates OIs into the body parts most affected by a particular organism or virus.

From diagnosis until death, the AIDS battle is *not just against its cause*, HIV, but against those

TUBERCULOSIS (TB), A MAJOR KILLER

About **2 billion** people carry the bacterium that causes tuberculosis worldwide. Tuberculosis is a killer with impressive credentials. Over the past two centuries, it has killed over a billion people. Currently it is the leading cause of mortality from a single infectious agent—accounting for 26% of preventable adult deaths in the developing world. In the coming decade, it is slated to kill at least 30 million people.

RELATIONSHIP OF TB TO HIV

The synergy between the epidemics of TB and HIV constitutes a global public health crisis of staggering dimensions. In persons infected with HIV, infection with *Mycobacterium tuberculosis* is much more likely to progress rapidly to active disease, which is increasingly difficult to diagnose and more complicated to treat. Globally, TB is now the leading cause of death among persons with AIDS,

killing 1 of every 3 people who die with AIDS. In addition, there are about 6 to 10 million people globally infected with both TB and HIV! Each year, worldwide, there are 8 million new TB cases and 3 million deaths from TB. About 9% of global TB cases are attributed to HIV infection. And projected to the year 2000, 14% of TB cases will be attributed to HIV disease (DeCock et al., 1996). In the United States, about 10% of those HIV-infected are also infected with TB! To date, the dual scourge of TB and HIV has affected predominantly the African continent, but the rapid spread of HIV in Asia, home to the majority of the world's TB-infected persons, is a time bomb. While industrialized nations rejoice in the increased survival associated with the use of combination antiretroviral therapy for HIV-infected patients, it is important to remember that for most people in developing nations access to relatively inexpensive anti-TB therapy is the most significant life-prolonging medical intervention (Small, 1996).

organisms and viruses that cause OIs. Opportunistic infections are severe, tend to be disseminated (spread throughout the body), and are characterized by multiplicity. Fungal, viral, protozoal, and bacterial infections may be controlled for some time but are rarely curable.

CANCER IN AIDS PATIENTS

Because of the severe and progressive impairment of the immune system, host defense mechanisms that normally protect against certain types of cancer are lost. Cancers develop in approximately 40% of AIDS patients. Four kinds of cancer that occur with increased frequency are: **progressive multifocal leukoencephalopathy**, **squamous cell carcinoma** (oral and anal), **non-Hodgkin's lymphoma**, and **HIV/AIDS-associated Kaposi's sarcoma (KS)**. None of these cancers, except for KS, is considered to be an opportunistic infection because they are not infections. They are cancers arising from cells that have lost control of their division processes. Of the eight types of AIDS-associated cancers, KS occurs

with the greatest frequency and is discussed in some detail. Lymphomas are briefly described (Table 6-3).

Kaposi's Sarcoma (cap-o-seas sar-comb-a)

HIV-1 infection represents an overwhelming risk factor for the development of KS, which was a rare tumor in the United States (incidence less than 1/100,000/year) before the HIV-1 epidemic. Today, KS remains the most frequent **neoplasm** affecting HIV-infected individuals. Approximately 25% to 30% of homosexual males with HIV infection develop clinically significant KS, and autopsy studies indicate an even higher prevalence of the disease up to approximately 40%. It is an aggressive disease, with involvement of the gut, lung, pleura, lymph nodes and the hard and soft palates.

KS, as it occurs in HIV/AIDS patients, may not be an opportunistic infection. Its cause is still unknown. It is uncertain whether KS is really a cancer because unlike cancer, which arises from one cell type, KS arises from several cell types. KS lesions are made up of an overgrowth of blood vessels.

——— BOX 6.3 ———

LIFE GOES ON!

by Wendi Alexis Modeste

What this epidemic has cost me is the complete faith I had in the medical profession. I was raised believing that doctors were second only to priests and God. They were never to be questioned. Whatever the doctor said was law. If a person didn't get well after seeing the doctor, somehow they (the patient) had done something wrong. This was pretty much standard thinking for middle-class African-Americans. For a variety of reasons (mainly no self-esteem) I became a drug addict, prostitute, convict, battered, homeless woman, in that order! With the exception of emergency room admissions (which are a joke and a whole `nother story) I had no access to health care.

Now, as a PWA (person with AIDS) fortunately/unfortunately on SSI, Medicaid pays for my nine different AIDS medications, clinic visits, treatment, tests, etc. When I received the "exciting news" that I was eligible for "all" Medicaid benefits, I was still under the impression doctors were those super-intelligent, gifted, Christian, saint-like people. Girlfriend, I am here to tell you, AIDS has totally shot that Marcus Welby theory straight to hell!

Early in my diagnosis, I went to my physician because my tongue was almost completely covered with what looked like cottage cheese. There was also a horrible pink lesion dead center. The first time I showed it to my doctor he said, "Ugh," and made a face. He told me to wait a month. If nothing changed or got worse when I returned he'd have someone look at it. Being ignorant about the disease at that time, and still blindly believing in the medical profession, I waited a month, then returned. Again I showed the doctor my tongue. He asked me if I wanted him to write me a prescription for codeine and Valium. I totally freaked! By this time, I'd done some reading and realized I probably had thrush and some sort of herpes. This physician was aware of my serostatus. He also knew that I was a person with a 20-year history of drug abuse. I'd been in recovery less than a year and this jerk wanted to prescribe for me two of the most addictive and abused prescription drugs. I'd never mentioned being in pain or that I was experiencing any type of anxiety. I contacted the Executive Director of this health facility and asked to have a different doctor assigned to me. In an attempt to make me feel guilty about requesting a change, I was told about the problems doctors have in getting Medicaid reimbursement. I was neither intimidated nor impressed. A new doctor was assigned. My new physician was very nice. After I told *him* what I thought my diagnosis was, he prescribed the appropriate medications. He was not trained in AIDS/HIV. I could have dealt with his ignorance because I knew he was trying. His nurse, however, was a different story. Every time she came to do my vitals she'd say the same thing: "I always get nervous when taking the temperature of you guys." She'd then force a little chuckle and go on to say, "Oh, well, I figure we all have to die of something." (I assume this was to show me what a courageous Florence Nightingale she was.)

Let me tell you, when you are burning up with a 103 degree temp. and your bowels haven't stopped running for a week, causing your butt to feel like it's on fire, it's real hard to be the patient, understanding AIDS educator. I really get crazy when the person I'm forced to educate is someone whose been privileged to more information than myself.

But life goes on!

One day I had a toothache. I go to the dentist. After waiting half the day, I'm brought into the treatment room for an X-ray. At first I thought the dental assistant had made a mistake. Surely this room had been prepared for a paint job. Everything was draped in white towels. The entire dental unit, including where my head, arms and feet went, was completely covered. The seat of the unit was securely wrapped up, as was the metal extension arm that holds the overhead dental lamp. All surfaces of the walls were also draped. When I asked the reason for this "painter preparation," I was informed it was done because I have AIDS, and they had to protect their other patients from coming into contact with my contaminated blood. Needless to say, I saw red! I knew I had to protect myself. I mean, what kind of dentistry were they practicing if they were concerned about my blood splattering that far and wide? What was even more frightening was that they'd done all this unnecessary draping and I was only having an X-ray. I filed a complaint with the Human Rights Dept.

I became a patient at the AIDS Care Center in Syracuse. My physician, a woman (need I say more?), is a caring person and well-educated about AIDS/HIV. My nurse/social worker is ex-

———— **BOX 6.3** *(continued)* ————

cellent, but as all of us living with AIDS know, shit happens. One day I awaken with enough yeast in my body to make all the baked goods in Central New York rise. My doctor isn't in. I wait a couple of days but can no longer stand the discomfort. I beg to see a doctor in the AIDS Care Unit. I'm assigned the doctor who sees the HIV-infected prisoners. (My heart and soul truly go out to those guys.) First he talks with me over the phone to find out if I can possibly wait another week when my doctor is due to return. I tell him my tongue is unrecognizable, the yeast in my esophagus is burning like a heart attack, and the Roto-Rooter service couldn't satisfy the itch caused by the yeast in my vagina. HELL NO, I can't wait another week! I go in to see him. I show him my tongue. I can't believe it, but like the first doctor, he uses that medical term, "Ugh," then says, "That does look nasty." At this point I'm ready to French kiss this idiot. But it gets worse. He won't touch me, let alone examine anything. He asks me what I think will work. I feel too badly to curse, so I tell him Mycelex, Myastatin suspension, Monistat 7. He writes the prescriptions and for good measure increases my acyclovir. For this he gets paid? He did nothing!

I'm now as educated as a lay person can be about HIV disease/AIDS. In addition to my doctor at the AIDS Care Center, I have a private primary care physician. Sometimes it's easier to get in to see this doctor. I call his office one day because there is swelling and burning on the sides of my tongue. I cannot eat. My regular doctor isn't in, but one of his associates assures me if I come in to the office he'll see me right away and give me something to ease the pain so I can at least eat. As a fat person who proudly admits a genuine fondness for food, I can tell you not being able to eat registers serious panic in my soul. Nothing stops me from eating. I was probably the only overweight homeless dope addict living on the streets of NYC. Being scared is putting it mildly. I scrape up the carfare and go to the office. After waiting an unreasonably long time, Doogie Howser's twin comes in to see me and announces he's Dr. Jones, whom I spoke to on the phone. OK, I know not to judge a book by its cover. I mean, Doogie is pretty good on TV. Dr. Jones looks at my tongue and proceeds to ask a zillion questions, all of which are answered in my chart. Finally he says he's never seen an HIV-infected person or a person with AIDS, and frankly he doesn't know what to do. He then sug-

gests I eat popsicles for a few days because the cold will soothe the pain and the sugar should help give me energy. I kid you not, this actually happened. This jerk prescribed me popsicles. I truly wished I could transmit the virus by biting at this point. He used me so he could write in his journal or resume (or somewhere) that he'd treated a person with AIDS. He could also charge Medicaid for nothing.

But this type of quackery must stop.

The last gripe I'm going to list is this patient statement I hear all the time when I get an unexplained fever or infection and no one can determine its origin. I'm told, "there hasn't been enough studies done on the paths this disease takes in women. Even less has been done on the effects of different AIDS medications on people of color." This is said to me as if it's my fault they don't know. This disease has been documented for ten years in both men and women. I know African-Americans were dying of AIDS long before the gay white community mobilized and, thank God, refused to lay down and die quietly. There is no excuse for the fact that there's no studies done on these populations.

I am thankful to Dr. Sallie Klemmens and nurse/clinician/social worker Judith Swartout at University Hospital's designated AIDS Care Center here in Syracuse. I am thankful for Dr. Barbara J. Justice who with God's help kept me alive when I lived on the streets of NYC. They are all examples of what the medical profession should be about. Dr. Justice made me feel that I counted and should be assertive about my health care. Though no longer my surgeon, she continues to be a source of inspiration and a fountain of information for me. These three are gems in a field I think is greatly overrated, overpaid, and run by capitalist male chauvinist pigs.

Though medical people wear white, that absence of color symbolizing purity and goodness, I beg you all, "Don't believe the hype!" We need a national health care system for everyone. As PWAs we must be assertive about our health care. Good health care is a right not a privilege.

As a child I cried when I learned there was no Santa Claus. When my illusion about the medical profession was shattered I got angry. I decided to fight with the only ammunition I had, education! Knowledge gives one power. A close friend of mine told me I shouldn't submit this article because I might offend some members of the medical profession. He also felt because I'm on Medicaid I'm not supposed to complain, I should be grateful. To his comments I respond, raised with two college-educated parents, never wanting or needing anything, I wasn't supposed to be a drug addict. Unfortunately I was. After 20 years of addiction, I wasn't supposed to be able to stop. I've been in recovery almost two years now. I'm not supposed to be living with AIDS, but with God's help I'm happy and living large (as the kids say now).

The best things I do have always been what I'm not supposed to do!

Power to all PWAs!

Wendi Alexis Modeste, a PWA who was diagnosed in 1990, died August 25, 1994.

Source: MODESTE, W.A., August 1991, Issue 68, *PWA Coalition Newsline.* Reprinted with permission.

In the United States, Kaposi's sarcoma is at least 20,000 times more common in people with HIV/AIDS than in the general population, and 300 times more common than in other immunosuppressed groups (Beral et al., 1990).

KS was first described by Moritz Kaposi in 1877 as a cancer of the muscle and skin. Characteristic signs of early KS were bruises and birthmark-like lesions on the skin, especially on the lower extremities. KS was described as a slow growing tumor found primarily in elderly Mediterranean men, Ashkenazi Jews, and equatorial Africans.

Kaposi's sarcoma as described by Moritz Kaposi is called classic KS and it differs markedly from the KS that occurs in AIDS patients (Figure 6-10, A and B). Classic KS has a variable prognosis (forecast), is usually slow to develop, and causes little pain (**indolent**). Patient survival in the United States ranges from 8 to 13 years with some reported cases of survival for up to 50 years (Gross et al., 1989). Symptoms

of classic KS are ulcerative skin lesions, swelling (**edema**) of the legs, and secondary infection of the skin lesions.

The AIDS epidemic has brought a more virulent and progressive form of KS marked by painless, flat to raised, pink to purplish plaques on the skin and mucosal surfaces which may spread to the lungs, liver, spleen, lymph nodes, digestive tract, and other internal organs. In its advanced stages it may affect any area from the skull to the feet (Figure 6-11, A–C). In the mouth, the hard palate is the most common site of KS (Figure 6-12) but it may also occur on the gum line, tongue, or tonsils.

KS in AIDS patients is fulminant; it comes on swiftly and spreads aggressively. However, there have been *no reported* AIDS deaths due to KS. Most AIDS deaths are due to opportunistic infections.

The prevalence of KS among gay men in 1981 was 77%; by 1987, it had fallen to 26% and by 1995 to less than 20%. This drop in KS among gay men was paralleled by a fall in CMV cases. However, as reasons for these drop-offs remain unknown, KS continues to decline in frequency.

Two questions provide differing views of the basic nature of the KS lesion: **Is KS merely a polyclonal proliferation of blood vessel cells? Or is it a true neoplastic process?** Whatever the answer, there must be additional host factors modulating the expression of KS to ex-

---

——— **BOX 6.4** ———

AUTOPSY DIAGNOSES OF DISEASES IN AIDS PATIENTS

Between 1984 and 1991, autopsy diagnoses of AIDS-defining diseases were determined in 250 AIDS patients. Forty-seven percent of diseases found at autopsy had not been diagnosed during life. Examples of diseases found at autopsy but not in life were CMV visceral infection, mycoses, HIV-specific brain lesions, cerebral lymphomas, and progressive multifocal leukoencephalopathy. Another important finding was that only a small number of AIDS-diagnostic diseases present at some point during life were *not* observed at autopsy. This indicates that AIDS-related diseases are seldom cured (Monforte et al., 1992).

TABLE 6-3 Malignancies Associated with HIV/AIDS

Kaposi's sarcoma (epidemic form)
Burkitt's lymphoma
Non-Hodgkin's lymphomas
Hodgkin's disease
Chronic lymphocytic leukemia
Carcinoma of the oropharaynx
Hepatocellular carcinoma
Adenosquamous carcinoma of the lung

A.

Early oral involvement

Early lymph node involvement

KS moves upward to arms

Visceral involvement in late stages of disease

Develops dark blue macules

B.

Lesions first appear red and turn dark

Early visceral involvement

Classic Kaposi's Sarcoma

Upper body usually free of KS macules

AIDS Associated Kaposi's Sarcoma

KS macules appear first in upper body

FIGURE 6-10   Classic and AIDS-Associated Kaposi's Sarcoma. **A,** Patients with classic KS (non-AIDS-related) demonstrate violet to dark blue bruises, spots, or macules on their lower legs. Gradually, the lesions enlarge into tumors and begin to form ulcers. KS lesions may, with time, spread upward to the trunk and arms. The movement of KS appears to follow the veins and involves the lymph system. In the late stages of the disease, visceral organs may become involved. **B,** For AIDS patients, initial lesions appear in greater number and are smaller than in classic KS. They first appear on the upper body (head and neck) and arms. The lesions first appear as pink or red oval bruises or macules that, with time, become dark blue and spread to the oral cavity and lower body, the legs, and feet. Visceral organs may be involved early on and the disease is aggressive. However, death is usually caused by opportunistic infection.

plain its **male predominance** both in mice and in humans and, among AIDS patients, its preferential occurrence among gays, greater than 15:1 male: female overall, approximately 4:1 male:female in AIDS patients when homosexual males are excluded (Looney, 1996). It has a low rate of incidence in hemophiliacs, intravenous drug users, women with AIDS(Cooley et al., 1996), and in pediatric AIDS cases. In summary, KS does *not* appear to be caused by HIV, but the immunosuppression which is caused by HIV infection may be an essential element in the evolution of this disease.

***Proposed Kaposi's Virus*—** Some researchers suspect that the AIDS virus is not the primary pathological agent for Kaposi's sarcoma. Beral and colleagues (1990) at the Centers for Disease

FIGURE 6-11 Kaposi's Sarcoma in AIDS Patients. **A,** KS on the right thigh. **B,** On heel and foot. **C,** On lower leg. (**A** *and* **C,** *courtesy of Nicholas J. Fiumara, M.D., Boston;* **B,** *courtesy of CDC, Atlanta*)

Control and Prevention concluded that the epidemiological data on Kaposi's distribution suggest that it is caused by a sexually transmitted pathogen other than HIV. They found, for example, that KS was more common in people infected with HIV by sexual contact (gay males)

than those infected by contaminated needles or blood (Palca, 1992).

Friedman-Kien and colleagues believe that human papillomavirus-16 (HGPV-16) is a major cofactor, if not the direct cause of KS. They have detected HPV-16 DNA in 95% of KS cells tested

FIGURE 6-12 Oral Kaposi's Sarcoma. KS can be seen on the hard palate and down the sides of the oral cavity. (*Courtesy of Nicholas J. Fiumara, M.D., Boston*)

(Palca, 1992). Other scientists believe the cause of KS is another retrovirus. In December of 1994, Yuan Chang and colleagues reported that they found DNA sequences that appear to represent a **new** human herpes virus (HHV-8) in KS tissue. Preliminary data showed that this unique DNA sequence occurred in KS tissue of 25 out of 27 gay men who had died of AIDS, but was found in only 6 of 39 non-KS tissues from AIDS patients. Investigations are in progress (Schulz et al., 1995; Moore et al., 1996). In addition, Chang and colleague Patrick Moore reported that they have transmitted the suspect "herpes virus" to a cell line and identified two dozen of its genes. They also know that its DNA includes 270 kilobases (270,000 nucleotide base pairs), making it the largest known herpesvirus, (Cohen, 1995). Gianluca Gaidano and colleagues (1996) report that their data confirm that HHV-8 DNA sequences are found, at high frequency, with selected types of AIDS-related KS. However, there are a number of nationally recognized oncologists and virologists who do not agree with current findings that associate a herpes virus with KS (Cohen, 1995; Gallo, 1995). Philip-Browning offers evidence that HHV-8 may be widespread in populations that don't develop KS (Cohen, 1996; Gaidano, 1996). And the disagreement continues. Beginning 1998, the exact role of HHV-8 in the biology of KS remains unknown (Kedes et al., 1997).

KS is rare in Caucasian women, but those who acquired HIV through *heterosexual contact* were more likely to have it if their partners were bisexual men than if their partners were injection drug users (3% vs. 0.7%) (Gorin et al., 1991; Serrano et al., 1995; Cooley et al., 1996; Warren et al., 1996). For men and women who acquired HIV through heterosexual contact, Kaposi's sarcoma was more frequent among those born in the Caribbean, Mexico, Central America, or Africa than those born in the United States (6% vs. 2%).

Risk of Kaposi's sarcoma within each HIV transmission group was not consistently related to age or race and varied across the United States. Kaposi's sarcoma in AIDS patients decreased 50% between 1983 and 1988, a trend that could be due to changes in reporting, the short incubation period for Kaposi's sarcoma, and a declining exposure to the causal agent (Beral et al., 1990).

The theoretical "Kaposi's virus" may have entered the same population in which the AIDS virus is endemic, which would explain why the two are often transmitted together. HIV may produce the right conditions for Kaposi's development by causing growth factor production, and possibly by suppressing the body's immune defenses against cancer.

Lymphoma (lim-fo-mah)

Lymphoma is the second most common cancer in HIV and is now the seventh most common cause of death for people with AIDS. A lymphoma is a neoplastic disorder (cancer) of the lymphoid tissue (Figure 6-13). *B cell* lymphoma occurs in about 1% of HIV-infected people, but makes up about 90% to 95% of all lymphomas found in people with HIV disease (Herndier et al., 1994). Although it occurs most often in those demonstrating persistent generalized lymphadenopathy (swollen lymph glands), the usual site of lymphoma growth is in the brain, the heart, or the anorectal area (Brooke et al., 1990). The most common signs and symptoms are confusion, lethargy, and memory loss. Lymphomas are increasing in incidence primarily due to the extension of the life span of AIDS patients, by medical therapy (Table 6-1).

There were approximately 36,000 cases of non-Hodgkin's lymphoma (NHL) diagnosed in 1992, between 8% and 27% occurred in individuals infected with HIV. A recent large prospective observational study indicated an incidence of approximately 1.6% per year in a population with advanced HIV infection treated with zidovudine. It is clear that as HIV infection increases in the population and as individuals infected with HIV survive for longer periods because of more successful treatment, NHL cases will continue to rise (Kaplan, 1992).

Progressive Multifocal Leukencephalopathy

Progressive multifocal leucoencephalopathy (PML) is an opportunistic infection caused by a papovavirus [Jamestown Canyon virus (JCV)] affecting 4% of AIDS patients. It is usually fatal within an average of 3.5 months and there is no treatment. In a few patients spontaneous improvement and prolonged survival have been reported. Some observations have indicated that cytosine arabinoside (ARA-C), a potent antiviral, may reverse the symptoms of PML. Symptoms of PML include altered mental status, speech and visual disturbances, gait difficulty and limb incoordination (Guarino et al., 1995).

FIGURE 6-13 HIV/AIDS Patient Demonstrating a Lymphoma of the Neck. (*Courtesy CDC, Atlanta*)

HIV Provirus: A Cancer Connection

In early 1994 AIDS investigators reported that HIV, on entering lymph cell DNA, activated nearby cancer-causing genes (oncogenes). The evidence suggests that HIV itself can trigger cancer in an otherwise normal cell (Figure 6-14).

These findings may mean that a variety of retroviruses that infect humans may also cause cancer (McGrath et al., 1994). Such findings raise concerns for developing an HIV vaccine. Using a weakened strain of HIV to make the vaccine may, when used, increase the incidence of lymphoma and other cancers.

NEUROPATHIES IN HIV DISEASE/AIDS PATIENTS

Neuropathies are functional changes in the peripheral nervous system, therefore, any part of the body may be affected. Although neuropathies are not OIs, they may result from the presence of certain OIs. Peripheral neuropathy is caused by nerve damage and is usually characterized by a sensation of pins and needles, burning, stiffness, or numbness in the feet and toes. It is a common, sometimes painful, condition in HIV-positive patients, affecting up to 30% of people with AIDS. At autopsy, two-thirds of AIDS patients have neuropathies (Newton, 1995). Neuropathy has been a continuous problem for patients throughout the HIV/AIDS epidemic. It is most common in people with a history of multiple opportunistic infections and low T4 cell counts. There is a wide range of expression among patients with neuropathy, from a minor nuisance to a disabling weakness. The kinds of neuropathies occurring in people with HIV/AIDS are numerous and must be identified before appropriate treatment can be prescribed. The underlying cause of the most common type of peripheral neuropathy remains elusive. What was a common complaint early in HIV infection of severe neuropathy—usually, burning feet, causing patients to walk on their heels—has diminished. The decrease in such complaints may be attributable to the antiviral effects of the drug ZDV. On the other hand, new varieties of drug-induced nerve damage (neuropathies) have been recognized in the

Cancer: The HIV Connection

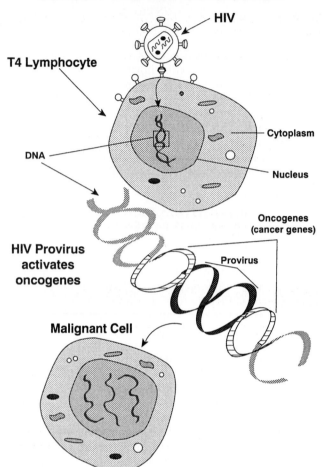

FIGURE 6-14 An HIV-AIDS cancer connection. HIV invades the lymph or other cell types. Its RNA-produced DNA enters cell DNA, becoming an HIV provirus. Sometime during or after integration into host cell DNA, dormant oncogenes, located nearby, become activated and a cancer results. In lymph cells the cancer becomes a lymphoma.

use of antivirals like dideoxyinosine (didanosine) (ddI) and dideoxycytosine (zalcitabine) (ddC). Researchers have also identified cytomegalovirus as a contributing factor in some different kinds of neuropathies in HIV disease.

HIV/AIDS SURVEILLANCE CHECKLIST/REPORT

A few of the most prevalent OIs found in HIV/AIDS patients have been discussed. Figure 6-15 lists those OIs and cancers that are used in the CDC criteria for defining AIDS. The report form presented in Figure 6-15 is in use at a public health HIV/AIDS clinic in Florida.

DISCLAIMER

This chapter is designed to present information on opportunistic infections in HIV/AIDS patients. It is not intended to provide medical advice. Consult proper health care providers for medical advice before undertaking any treatment discussed herein.

SUMMARY

One of the gravest consequences of HIV infection is the immunosuppression caused by the depletion of the T4 helper cell population; suppressed immune systems allow for the ex-

HIV/AIDS SURVEILLANCE CHECK LIST/REPORT FORM

A person will have CDC defined AIDS (MMWR Vol. 36, No. 1S, Aug. 14, 1987) if they have a positive test result for Human Immunodeficiency Virus (HIV) and at least one of the following:

(If HIV test is not performed or inconclusive, please refer to the MMWR for additional criteria)

Disease   Disease

(Please indicate definitive diagnosis (D) with laboratory data or presumptive diagnosis (P) where option exists)

____ Candidiasis, bronchi, trachea, or lungs   ____ Candidiasis, esophageal (D or P)
____ Cervical cancer   ____ Cryptococcosis, extrapulmonary
____ Coccidiodomycosis, dissem. or extrapul.   ____ Cytomegalovirus, other than liver, spleen, nodes
____ Cryptosporidiosis, chronic intestinal   ____ HIV Encephalopathy (AIDS Dementia Complex)
____ Cytomegalovirus retinitis with vision loss (D or P)   ____ Histoplasmosis, dissem. or extrapul.
____ Herpes Simplex, chronic ulcers   ____ Kaposi's Sarcoma (D or P)
       >1 month duration, or bronchitis, pneumonitis, or esophagitis
____ Isosporiasis, chronic intest.   ____ Lymphoma, immunoblastic or equivalent
       >1 month duration
____ Lymphoma, Burkitt's or equivalent   ____ Mycobacterium avium, M. kansasii, dissem. or extrapul. (D or P)
____ Lymphoma, primary in brain   ____ Mycobacterium tuberculosis, any site (pulmonary or extrapul.)
____ M.Tuberculosis, dissem. or extrapul. (D or P)   ____ Mycobacterium, other, dissem. or extrapul. (D or P)
____ Pneumocystis carinii pneumonia (PCP)(D or P)   ____ Pneumonia, recurrent
____ Salmonella septicemia, recurrent   ____ Progressive multifocal leukoencephalopathy
____ Wasting (>10% baseline body weight + diarr or fatigue)   ____ Toxoplasmosis of brain

Pediatrics (<13 years of age) include:

____ Bacterial infections, multiple, recurrent   ____ Lymphoid interstitial pneumonia and/or
                                                pulmonary lymphoid hyperplasia

HIV+ Test/Laboratory Date ____/____/____ Current CD4 cell count _____ Diagnosed as Inpatient _____ or Outpatient _____?

Risk Factor: male/male sex _____ IVDU _____ Transfusion/Hemophilia _____ male/female sex with HIV infected person _____

Mom to Baby _____ none of the above _____ other _____

Patient Name: _____ Date of Birth: ____/____/____ Male/Female: _____ Race: _____

Address: _____ Zip: _____ Country of Birth: _____

Clinic/Hospital Name: _____ Med. Record #: _____ SS Number #: ____/____/____

Physican Name: _____

Name of person notifying Surveillance Office: _____ Date sent/called: ____/____/____

Instructions: Place form in chart of each HIV+ patient. When at least one of the opportunistic infections listed is diagnosed, complete the form and either call the Surveillance Office, or mail a copy of this form in an envelope marked "CONFIDENTIAL" to:

AIDS Surveillance Office

Keep the original in each medical record for documentation of having reported to the Surveillance Office.
Thank you!

* THIS FORM WAS ALTERED TO REFLECT THE JANUARY, 1993 CDC AIDS DEFINITION. THE MAJOR CHANGE IS THAT ALL PERSONS WITH A T4 CELL COUNT OF LESS THAN 200/mm^3 HAS AIDS. THREE MORE DISEASES WERE ADDED TO THE LIST (See Table 1-3.)

FIGURE 6-15 HIV/AIDS Surveillance Report Form. The form is completed and sent to an AIDS Surveillance Office. The information is then sent on to the CDC in Atlanta.

pression of opportunistic diseases and cancers. It is the OI that kills AIDS patients, not HIV per se. The major OIs are listed in Table 6-1. It is the cumulative effect of several OIs that creates the chills, night sweats, fever, weight loss, anorexia, pain, and neurological problems.

One tragic disease that does not result from an OI is Kaposi's sarcoma (KS), a cancer (?) that can spread to all parts of an AIDS patient's body. About 20% of AIDS patients, mostly gay men, have KS. It is not usually found in hemophiliacs, intravenous drug users, or female AIDS patients.

REVIEW QUESTIONS

(Answers to the Review Questions are on page 576.)

1. Define opportunistic infection (OI).

2. Which OI organism expresses itself in 80% of AIDS patients? Where is it located and what does it cause?

3. Which of the protozoal OI organisms causes weight loss, watery diarrhea, and severe abdominal pain?

4. Which of the bacterial OIs causes "wasting syndrome," night sweats, anorexia, and fever?

5. True or False: Kaposi's sarcoma (KS) is caused by HIV. Explain.

6. Name the two kinds of KS.

7. True or False: KS affects all AIDS patients equally. Explain.

8. True or False: Candidiasis and ulceration may be present in patients with HIV infection.

9. True or False: Oral candidiasis occurs frequently with HIV infection.

REFERENCES

AMIN, NAVIN M. (1987). Acquired immunodeficiency syndrome, Part 2: The spectrum of disease. *Fam. Pract. Recert.,* 9:84–118.

AWE, ROBERT J. (1988). Benefits, promises and limitations of zidovudine (AZT). *Consultant,* 28: 57–72.

BALFOUR, HENRY (1995). Cytomegolovirus retinitis in persons with AIDS. *Postgrad. Med.,* 97: 109–118.

BERAL, VALERIE, et al. (1990). Kaposi's sarcoma among persons with AIDS: A sexually transmitted infection? *Lancet,* 335:123–138.

BERMEJO, ALVERO, et al. (1992). Tuberculosis incidence in developing countries with high prevalence of HIV infection. *AIDS,* 6:1203–1206.

BERNARDO, JOHN. (1991). Tuberculosis: A disease of the 1990s. *Hosp. Pract.,* 26:195–220.

BROOKE, GRACE LEE, et al. (1990). HIV disease: A review for the family physician Part II. Secondary infections, malignancy and experimental therapy. *Am. Fam. Pract.,* 42:1299–1308.

CHANG, YUAN, et al. (1994). Identification of Herpes virus-like DNA sequences in AIDS-Associated Kaposis Sarcoma. *Science,* 266:1865–1869.

CHIN, DANIEL. (1992). Mycobacterium avium complex infection. *AIDS File: Clin. Notes,* 6:7–8.

CHURCH, DEIRDRE L. (1992). Fatal diarrhea in an AIDS patient. *Patient Care,* 26:280–283.

Coalition News. (1993). Pet guidelines for people with HIV. 2:4–5.

COHEN, JON. (1995). AIDS mood upbeat for a change. *Science,* 267:959.

COHEN JON. (1995). Controversy: Is KS really caused by new herpesvirus? *Science,* 268:1847–1848.

COHEN, JON, (1996). Reports bolster viral cause of KS. *Science,* 273:573.

COOLEY, TIMOTHY, et al. 1996). Kaposi's sarcoma in women with AIDS. *AIDS,* 10:122–125.

CURRIER, JUDITH, et al. (1997). Pathogenesis, prevention and treatment of opportunistic complications. *Improv. Manage. HIV Dis.,* 4:S17-S18.

DAAR, ERIC S., et al. (1993). The spectrum of HIV infection. *Patient Care,* 27:99–128.

DALEY, CHARLES L. (1992). Epidemiology of tuberculosis in the AIDS era. *AIDS File: Clin. Notes,* 6:1–2.

DANNEMANN, BRIAN R., et al. (1989). Toxoplasmic encephalitis in AIDS. *Hosp. Pract.,* 24:139–154.

DANNENBERG, ARTHUR M. (1993). Immunopathogenesis of pulmonary tuberculosis. *Hosp. Pract.,* 28:51–58.

DANNER, SVEN, (1995). Management of CMV disease. *AIDS,* 9:53–58.

DE COCK, KEVIN, et al.(1996).Research issues involving HIV-associated TB in research-poor countries. *JAMA,* 276:1502–1508.

DEHOVITZ, JACK A. (1988). Management of *Isospora belli* infections in AIDS patients. *Infect. Med.,* 5:437–440.

DEWIT, STEPHANE, et al. (1991). Fungal infections in AIDS patients. *Clin. Adv. Treatment Fungal Infect.,* 2:1–11.

DOBKIN, JAY, (1995). Opportunistic infections and AIDS. *Infect. Med.,* 125:58–70.

EDMAN, JEFFREY C., et al. (1988). Ribosomal RNA sequence shows *Pneumocystis carinii* to be a member of the fungi. *Nature,* 334:519–522.

ENNIS, DAVID M., et al. (1993). Cryptococcal meningitis in AIDS. *Hosp. Pract.,* 28:99–112.

Emergency Medicine. (1989). Fighting opportunistic infections in AIDS. 21:24–38.

ERNST, JEROME. (1990). Recognize the early symptoms of PCP. *Med. Asp. Hum. Sexuality,* 24:45–47.

EZZELL, CAROL. (1993). Captain of the men of death. *Science News,* 143:90–92.

GAIDANO, GIANLUCA, et al. (1996). Distribution of human herpesvirus–8 sequences throughout the spectrum of AIDS-related neoplasia. *AIDS,* 10:941–949.

GALLO, ROBERT, (1995). Human retroviruses in the second decade: a personal perspective. *Nature Med.,* 1:753–759.

GANEM, DONALD. (1996) Kaposi's sarcoma-associated herpesvirus. *Improv. Manage. HIV Dis.,* 4(3):8–10.

GORIN, ISABELLE, et al. (1991). AIDS-associated Kaposi's sarcoma in female patients. *AIDS,* 5:877–880.

GOTTLIEB, MICHAEL S., et al. (1987). Opportunistic viruses in AIDS. *Patient Care,* 23:139–154.

GROSS, DAVID J., et al. (1989). Update on AIDS. *Hosp. Pract.,* 25:19–47.

GROSSMAN, RONALD J., et al. (1989). PCP and other protozoal infections. *Patient Care,* 23:89–116.

GUARINO, M., et al. (1995). Progressive multifocal leucoencephalopathy in AIDS: treatment with cytosine arabinoside. *AIDS,* 9:819–820.

Guidelines, U.S. Public Health Service, (1995). Preventing OIs in persons with HIV disease. *AIDS Reader,* 5:172–179.

HARDEN, C.L., et al. (1994). Diagnosis of central nervous system toxoplasmosis in AIDS patients confirmed by autopsy. *AIDS,* 8:1188–1189.

HARDY, DAVID. (1996). Lessons learned from HIV pathogenesis and therapy: Implications for better management of cytomegalovirus disease. *AIDS,* 10(Suppl, 1):S31–S35.

HARRIS, CHARLES. (1993). TB and HIV: The boundaries collide. *Medical World News,* 34:63.

Harvard AIDS, Institute, (1994). *Special Report—Opportunistic Infections.* Fall issue:1–14.

HAY, R.J. (1991). Oropharyngeal candidiasis in the AIDS patient. *Clin. Adv. Treatment Fungal Infect.,* 2:10–12.

HERMANS, PHILIPPE, (1995), Haematopoietic growth factors as supportive therapy in HIV-infected patients. *AIDS,* 9:59–514.

HERNDIER, BRIAN, et al. (1994). Pathogenesis of AIDS lymphomas, *AIDS,* 8:1025–1049.

HUGHES, WALTER. (1994). Opportunistic infections in AIDS patients. *Postgrad. Med.,* 95:81-86.

HUNT, SUSAN, (1996). Office management of HIV: OIs. I. *Resp. Dis.,* 17:235–238.

JACOBSON, MARK A., et al. (1988). Serious cytomegalovirus disease in the acquired immunodeficiency syndrome (AIDS): Clinical findings, diagnosis, and treatment. *Ann. Intern. Med.,* 108:585-594.

JACOBSON, MARK A., et al. (1992). CMV disease in patients with AIDS: Introduction. *Clin. Notes,* 6(2):1–11.

JOINER, K.A., et al. (1990). Toxoplasma gondii: Fusion competence of parasitophorous vacuoles in Fe receptor-transfected fibroblasts. *J. Cell Biol.,* 109:2771.

KAPLAN, LAWRENCE. (1992). HIV-associated lymphoma. *Clin. Notes,* 6(1):1–11.

KAPLAN, JONATHAN, (1995). USPHS/IDSA guidelines for the prevention of opportunistic infections in persons infected with human immunodeficiency virus an overview *Clin. Infect. Dis.,* 21 (suppl 1):S12–S31.

KEDES, DEAN, et al. (1997). The prevalence of serum antibody to human herpesvirus 8 among HIV-seropositive and high-risk HIV-seronegative women. *JAMA,* 277:478–481.

LAURENCE, JEFFREY, (1995). Evolving management of OIs. *AIDS Reader,* 5:187–188, 208.

LAURENCE, JEFFREY, (1996). Where do we go from here? *AIDS Reader,* 6:3–4, 36.

LOONEY, DAVID, (1996). Kaposi's sarcoma. *Improv. Manage. HIV Dis.,* 4:21–24.

LYNCH, JOSEPH P. (1989). When opportunistic viruses infiltrate the lung. *J. Resp. Dis.,* 10:25–30.

MCGRATH, MICHAEL, et al. (1994). Identification of a common clonal human immunodeficiency virus integration site in human immunodeficiency virus-associated lymphomas. *Cancer Res.,* 54:2069.

MEDOFF, GERALD, et al. (1991). Systemic fungal infections: An overview. *Hosp. Pract.,* 26:41–52.

MONETTE, PAUL. (1988). *Borrowed Time: An AIDS Memoir.* New York: Avon Books.

MONFORTE, ANTONELLA D'ARMINIO, et al. (1992). AIDS-defining diseases in 250 HIV-infected patients; A comparative study of clinical and autopsy diagnoses. *AIDS,* 6:1159–1164.

MONTGOMERY, BRUCE A. (1992). *Pneumocystis carinii* pneumonia prophylaxis: Past, present and future. *AIDS,* 6:227–228.

MOORE, PATRICK, et al. (1996). Kaposi's sarcoma—Associated herpesvirus infection prior to onset of Kaposi's sarcoma. *AIDS,* 10:175–180.

Morbidity and Mortality Weekly Report. (1993). Estimates of future global TB morbidity and mortality. 4:961–964.

Morbidity and Mortality Weekly Report. (1995). USPHS/IDSA guidelines for the prevention of opportunistic infections in persons infected with HIV: a summary. 44:1–34.

Morbidity and Mortality Weekly Report. (1995). 1995 Revised guidelines for prophylaxis against PCP for children infected with or perinatally exposed to HIV. 44:1–10.

MURPHY, ROBERT. (1994). Opportunistic infection prophylaxis. *Int. AIDS Soc.–USA,* 2:7–8.

NEWTON, HERBERT. (1995). Common neurologic complications of HIV infection and AIDS. *Am. Fam. Phys.*, 51:387–398.

PALCA, JOSEPH. (1992). Kaposi's sarcoma gives on key fronts. *Science*, 255:1352–1354.

PHAIR, JOHN, et al. (1990). The risk of *Pneumocystis carinii* among men infected with HIV-1. *N Engl. J Med.*, 322:161–165.

POWDERLY, WILLIAM G., et al. (1992). Molecular typing of Candida albicans isolated from oral lesions of HIV-infected individuals. *AIDS*, 6:81–84.

ROLSTON, KENNETH. (1992). Changing pattern of bacterial and fungal infections in patients with AIDS. *Primary Care and Cancer*, 12:11–15.

ROSSITCH, EUGENE, et al. (1990). Cerebral toxoplasmosis in patients with AIDS. *Am. Fam. Pract.*, 41:867–873.

RUSSELL, JAMES. (1990). Study focuses on eyes and AIDS. *Baylor Med.*, 21:3.

SCHULZ, THOMAS, et al. (1995). Karposi's Sarcoma; A finger on the culprit. *Nature*, 373:17.

SERRAINO, DEIGO, et al. (1995). HIV transmission and Kaposi's sarcoma among European women. *AIDS*, 9:971–973.

SIBLEY, L. DAVID. (1992). Virulent strains of *Toxoplasma gondii* comprise single clonal linage. *Nature*, 359:82–85.

SMALL, PETER. (1996). Tuberculosis research: Balancing the portfolio. *JAMA*, 276:1512–1513.

STANFORD, J.L., et al. (1993). Old plague, new plague, and a treatment for both? *AIDS*, 7:1275–1276.

STRINGER, JAMES, et al. (1996). Molecular biology and epidemiology of pneumocystis carinii infections in AIDS. *AIDS*, 10:561–571.

TUAZON, CARMELITA, et al. (1991). Diagnosing and treating opportunistic CNS infections in patients with AIDS. *Drug Therapy*, 21:43–53.

WALLACE, MARK R., et al. (1993). Cats and toxoplasmosis risk in HIV-infected adults. *JAMA*, 269:76–77.

WALZER, PETER D. (1993). *Pneumocystis carinii:* Recent advances in basic biology and their clinical application. *AIDS*, 7:1293–1305.

WHEAT, L. JOSEPH. (1992). Histoplasmosis in AIDS. *AIDS Clin. Care*, 4:1–4.

WILLOUGHBY, A. (1989). AIDS in women: Epidemiology. *Clin. Obstet. Gynecol.*, 32:15–27.

WOFSY, CONSTANCE. (1991). Cryptosporidiosis and isosporiasis. *AIDS Clin. Care*, 3:25–27.

ZACKRISON, LEILA H., et al. (1991). *Pneumocystis carinii:* A deadly opportunist. *Am. Fam. Pract.*, 44:528–541.

ZOLER, MITCHELL L. (1991). OI's widening realm. *Medical World News*, 32:38–44.

Stages of HIV Disease and Biological Indicators for Progression to AIDS

CHAPTER CONCEPTS

♦ The terms **incubation** and **latency** are defined.
♦ Clinical signs and symptoms of HIV infection and AIDS are presented.
♦ Stages of HIV disease vary substantially.
♦ From infection, HIV replication is rapid and continuous.
♦ AIDS Dementia Complex presents as mental impairment.
♦ Clues to adult AIDS diagnosis are listed.
♦ Clues to long-term survival are presented.
♦ Serological changes after HIV infection are presented.
♦ The evolution of HIV during HIV disease progression is discussed.
♦ The development of AIDS over time is discussed.
♦ Classification of HIV/AIDS progression is presented.
♦ Clinical indicators to track HIV disease progression are listed.
♦ Diarrhea is the most common gastrointestinal sign and symptom of HIV/AIDS infection.
♦ Clues to pediatric AIDS diagnosis are presented.

HIV DISEASE DEFINED

The CDC feels that enough has now been learned about HIV infection to call it a disease. This makes sense, as the vast majority of those who become infected become ill. HIV infection leads to the loss of T4 cells, which in turn produces a variety of signs and symptoms of a **non-specific disease** with initial acute febrile illness or mononucleosis-like symptoms which may last up to 4 weeks or longer. After the initial symptoms most individuals enter a clinically asymptomatic phase. (see Case in Point 7.1) This means the infected person feels well while his or her immune system is slowly compromised. It has been shown that long-lasting symptomatic primary HIV infection predicts an increased risk of rapid development of HIV-related symptoms and AIDS, but it is not known whether the different responses to HIV infection are caused by viral or host factors. Virulent strains of HIV have been characterized by their rapid replication, **syncytium-inducing (SI)** capacity, and tropism (attraction) for various types of T cells. It is

161

VARIATION OF INITIAL SYMPTOMS AFTER HIV INFECTION

Case I: Male, Age 35, Los Angeles, California

One evening, for no apparent reason, John began sweating profusely. Soon after a red rash began on his arms, face, and legs and then covered his body. Simultaneously, breathing became difficult and he was rushed to an emergency room. By then he was shaking violently. After medication and a battery of tests his problem could not be defined. This brief illness passed, he felt fine but some years later, during a blood screen for insurance purposes he came up HIV-positive. He immediately reflected back on his earlier illness and its cause.

Case II: Male, Age 29, Los Angeles, California

This case is in marked contrast to case I. Feeling the pinch of a sore throat, this male went to his physician for an antibiotic. On examination, he had a yeast infection which appeared far back in his throat. This raised suspicion and he agreed to an HIV test. It came back positive. He had no other illness, he was treated, the sore throat vanished, and he is thriving in a long asymptomatic period.

ONE MISTAKE COST HIM HIS LIFE

I held my son today while he died from AIDS. There is no pain like the pain in a mother's heart. He was 28 years old, and now, he is dead.

This wonderful young man will never have a family. He will never again have a chance to do the things he enjoyed so much — water ski, snow ski, travel. He loved *Star Trek* and music. He loved working for the airlines and traveling all over the world. He was delightful and smart — a computer whiz — could take one apart and put it back together.

He wasted away from a handsome young man to a skeleton — nothing more than skin and bones. His weight dropped from 160 pounds to 80 pounds. His hair fell out. His beautiful teeth fell out. Sores broke out all over his body. He couldn't hold down any food, and eventually, he starved to death.

No, young people, he was not gay, nor was he a drug user. He just went to bed with a girl he didn't know.

His Mom

(Source: Ann Landers, Syndicated Columnist, 1994)

known that the biological properties of HIV strains in asymptomatic HIV-infected individuals with normal T4 cell counts may predict the subsequent development of HIV-related disease, and that patients who harbor SI isolates develop immune deficiency more rapidly. It is not clear whether the appearance of more virulent strains during the chronic phase of the infection is a cause or an effect of progressive immune deficiency (Nielson et al., 1993). Several studies have demonstrated that a long period of fever around the time of **seroconversion** (the presence of detectable HIV antibody in the serum) is associated with more rapid development of immune deficiency (Pedersen et al., 1989).

Spectrum of HIV Disease

Because the immune system slowly falters, HIV disease is really a spectrum of disease. At one end of the spectrum are those infected with HIV who look and feel perfectly healthy. At the opposite end are those with advanced HIV disease

(symptomatic AIDS) who are visibly sick and require significant medical and psychosocial support (Figure 7-1). Between these two extremes, HIV-infected people may develop illnesses that range from mild to serious. Symptoms can include persistent fevers, chronic fatigue, diarrhea, swollen lymph nodes, night sweats, skin rashes, significant weight loss, visual problems, chest pain, and fungal infections of the mouth, throat, and vagina. Illness from these conditions can be **severe** and **disabling**, and some people may die without ever being diagnosed with AIDS. Also, people with HIV disease may develop **neurologic disorders**, which can cause **forgetfulness, memory loss, loss of coordination and balance, partial paralysis, leg weakness, mood changes and dementia**. These symptoms may occur in the absence of any other symptoms. The interval between initial HIV infection and the presence of signs and symptoms that characterize AIDS is variable and may range from several months to a median duration of about 11 years (Figure 7-2).

FIGURE 7-1 (**a**) The HIV/AIDS Pyramid for the United States. This figure demonstrates that current AIDS cases are coming from an existing pool of HIV-infected persons living in the United States. Most of those infected (about 80%) do not yet know they are HIV positive. Although both the asymptomatic and symptomatic periods may last for years, once diagnosed with AIDS the average life expectancy **without AIDS drug cocktails is 2 to 3 years**. Average life expectancy for those now on combination drug cocktails has not yet been determined. (**b**) Clinical outcomes 10 to 16 years after HIV infection in a population tracked by the San Francisco City Clinic from the beginning of the AIDS outbreak.

Defining Incubation and Latency

Because of the long delay in determining what happened after HIV infection and progression to AIDS, the terms **incubation** and **latency** are used, in many cases interchangeably, causing some confusion. In this text, these two terms are used with respect to **clinical** observations as follows: **clinical incubation** is that period after infection through the window period or when anti-HIV-antibody production is measurable. **Clinical latency** is the time period from detectable anti-HIV-antibody production (seroconversion—the person now tests HIV-antibody-positive) through the asympto-

matic period—a time prior to the expression of opportunistic diseases. The beginning and end of these periods will vary from person to person and their susceptibility and expression of HIV disease.

STAGES OF HIV DISEASE

The course of the disease in the infected individual varies substantially. At the extremes are individuals who show either little evidence of progression (loss in T4 cells) 10 to 20 years following infection (1% to 3%) or extremely rapid progression and death within less than 2

Adult/Adolescent HIV Disease Continuum to AIDS

1. Some studies described neurologic problems in otherwise asymptomatic HIV-infected persons, such problems are seen mostly in advanced HIV disease.
2. With advancing immune suppression, the HIV antibody titer is sometimes low or indeterminate.
3. Antibody may appear 1 week after infection but the most common finding is antibody appears 6 to 18 weeks post infection; in one study, gay men did not produce antibody for at least 3 years.
4. Groups 1, 2, 3, and 4 are positioned from HIV infection through progression to diagnosed AIDS according to CDC classification (see Table 6-2).
5. The spectrum of HIV disease to AIDS will vary with individual cases.
6. Recent studies suggest that KS is a separate sexually transmitted disease. However, when it ocurs in HIV/AIDS patients, it occurs during this time frame.

FIGURE 7-2 Spectrum of HIV Infection, Disease, and the Expression of AIDS. Seroconversion means that HIV antibodies are measurably present in the person's serum. With continued depletion of T4 cells, signs and symptoms appear announcing the progression of HIV disease to AIDS. Although HIV antibodies have been found as early as 1 week after exposure, most often seroconversion occurs between weeks 6 and 18; 95% within 3 months, 99% within 6 months (see Figure 7-4). The early stage of HIV infection can be separated from the symptomatic stage by years of **clinical latency**. Early infection is characterized by a high number of infected cells and a high level of viral expression. AIDS is characterized by increased levels of viremia and p24 antigenemia, activation of HIV expression in infected cells, an increased number of infected cells, and progressive immune dysfunction. Stages of HIV disease blend into a continuum ranging

(continued on next page)

to 3 years. In general, HIV-infected adults experience a variety of conditions, categorized into four stages: acute infection, asymptomatic, chronic symptomatic, and AIDS.

Acute or Primary HIV Disease Stage

The acute stage usually develops in 2 to 8 weeks after initial infection or exposure to the virus. Up to 70% of infected individuals develop a self-limited (brief) illness similar to influenza or mononucleosis: fever, sore throat, headaches, and swollen lymph nodes. Some may develop a rash, vomiting, diarrhea, and thrush (yeast infection in the mouth).This is referred to as the acute retroviral syndrome. The symptoms last about 2 to 4 weeks and resolve spontaneously (Table 7-1). The acute stage can be even quickly and easily missed. The acute phase is marked by high levels of HIV production. During this phase, large numbers of HIV spread throughout the body, seeding themselves in various organs, particularly lymphoid tissues such as the lymph nodes, spleen, tonsils, and adenoids (Figure 7-3).

During acute primary infection, patients have extremely high levels of viral replication **but no notable immune response**. Plasma HIV RNA levels increase to 10^5 to 10^8 copies/mL. This period of high viral replication in the absence of detectable antibody is called the **Window of infectivity before seroconversion**. During this period, patients may be highly infectious because their viral levals are at the highest—over 10^6 RNA copies/mL of blood. The viral burden in genital secretion is particularly high during this time. Mathematical models suggest that 56% to 92% of all HIV infections may be transmitted during this period of acute infection (Quinn, 1997).

TABLE 7-1 Clinical and Laboratory Analyses of Acute HIV Infection

Signs

Erythematous truncal maculopapular rash
Generalized urticaria, roseola-like exantham, palm and sole desquamation
Generalized lymphadenopathy, splenomegaly
Acute meningo-encephalitis
Myelopathy, Guillain-Barre syndrome
Radiculopathy (brachial or sacral plexopathy)
Peripheral neuropathy
Myopathy
Pharyngitis
Hepatitis
Mental changes
Oral or esophageal ulcerations
Weight loss

Symptoms

Fever, night sweats, chills, malaise, fatigue
Arthralgias, myalgias
Anorexia, nausea and vomiting, abdominal cramps, diarrhea
Headache, retro-orbital pain, photophobia, lethargy
Sore throat, dry cough

Laboratory Analysis

Mild-moderate neutropenia, relative monocytosis
Lymphopenia to lymphocytosis/atypical lymphocytes
Elevated erythrocyte sedimentation rate
Appearance of HIV antibodies
HIV in serum and/or CSF
Abnormal liver function tests
Raised levels of beta-2 microglobulin

A true state of **biological latency**, according to the work of Xiping Wei and co-workers (1995) and David Ho and co-workers (1995), does not exist in the lymph nodes at any time during the course of HIV infection. The investigations of Wei and Ho show that from the time of infection HIV replication is rapid and continuous, and within 2 to 4 weeks the infecting HIV strain is replaced by drug-resistant mutants. Each day

(continued)

from the asymptomatic with apparent good health, to increasingly impaired health, to the diagnosis of AIDS. Thus the spectrum of HIV disease ranges from the silent infection to unequivocal AIDS. Clinical expression moves from one condition to another, often without a clear-cut distinction. The level of an individual's infectiousness is believed to be greatest within the first months after infection and again when the T4 cell count drops below 200 (see Figure 7-3). However, people who are HIV-infected can transmit HIV at any time.

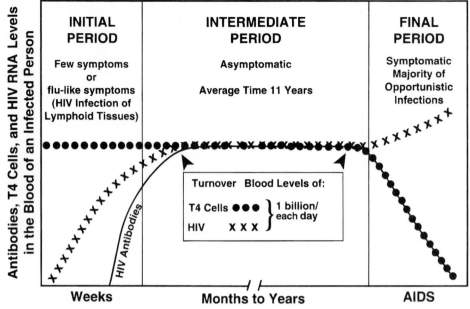

FIGURE 7-3 Relationship of T4 cells, HIV antibodies, and HIV RNA Levels (Viral Load) Beginning with HIV Infection through AIDS. Within a week to weeks after HIV infection, HIV becomes seeded throughout the body's blood and lymph system. HIV reproduction (infection of T4 cells) begins almost immediately in the lymph system. The T4 cell population also begins rapid reproduction to replace T4 cell loss. This is why the T4 graph line stays at the same level through the **asymptomatic** period. The immune system begins to turn out HIV antibodies, in general 6 to 18 weeks later (window period, see Figure 7-4). Note that during the asymptomatic period T4 cell and HIV replication and antibody production keep pace. With time, however, T4 cells fail to replace losses, HIV continues to replicate, antibody levels drop due to loss of T4 signals to B cells to produce antibodies and opportunistic infections begin—the **symptomatic** period. **Without** therapy this period lasts on average about 2 to 3 years. When a person is able to use the AIDS drug cocktails containing a protease inhibitor, the average number of years this period lasts has yet to be determined.

1 billion to 10 billion HIV are produced and mostly destroyed and a billion T4 cells or more are infected, dying, and replaced. Over time the immune system fails to destroy HIV and replace its T4 cell losses and HIV disease progresses. Also, over time, many T4 cells in the lymphoid organs probably are **activated** by the increased secretion of certain cytokines such as tumor necrosis factor-alpha and interleukin-6. **Activation** allows uninfected cells to be more easily infected and causes increased replication of HIV in infected cells. Other components of the immune system also are chronically activated, with negative consequences that may include the suicide of cells by a process known as programmed cell death or apoptosis (pronounced a-po-toe-sis) and an inability of the immune system to respond to other invaders.

Asymptomatic HIV Disease Stage

Following acute illness, an infected adult can remain free of symptoms from 6 months to a median time of about 11 years. During the

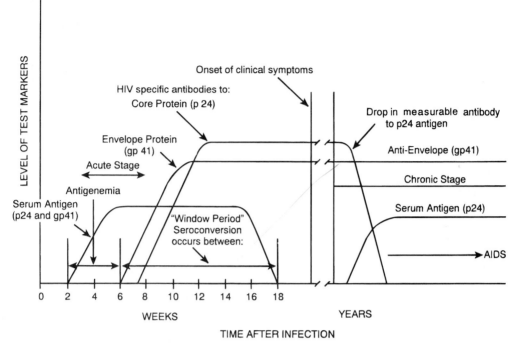

FIGURE 7-4   Profile of Serological Changes after HIV Infection. The dynamics of antibody response to HIV infection was determined by enzyme immunoassays (EIA). Note that during antigenemia, specific HIV proteins (antigens) can be detected before seroconversion occurs. Perhaps other HIV proteins will allow even earlier detection of HIV infection. Once antibodies appear, some antigens like p24 and gp41 disappear only to show up again later on. Note also that although antibody production is a sign that the immune system is working, in HIV-infected people, it is not working well enough. Although envelope and core protein antibodies are being produced as clinical illness begins, as the p24 antibody drops, the illness becomes more serious. *(Adapted from Coulis et al., 1987)*

asymptomatic period, measurable HIV in the blood drops to a low level but it continues to replicate and continues to destroy T4 cells within the lymph nodes while the body continues to produce new T4 cells and antibodies to the virus (Figure 7-4). An asymptomatic individual appears to be healthy and can assume normal activities of daily living.

Chronic Symptomatic HIV Disease Stage

The chronic phase can last for months or years before a diagnosis of AIDS occurs. During this phase, as viral replication continues, T4 cells become depleted. As the number of immune system cells decline, the individual develops a variety of symptoms such as fever, weight loss, malaise, pain, fatigue, loss of appetite, abdominal discomfort, diarrhea, night sweats, headaches, and swollen lymph glands. Ultimately, HIV overwhelms the lymphoid organs. The follicular dentritic cell networks break down in late-chronic stage disease and virus trapping is impaired, allowing spillover of large quantities of virus into the bloodstream. The destruction of the lymph node structure seen late in HIV disease may stop a successful immune response against not only HIV but other pathogens as well, and heralds the onset of the opportunistic infections and cancers

AIDS: Advanced HIV Disease Stage

DESCRIPTION OF AN AIDS PATIENT

Cecilia Worth is a registered nurse and author. In a recent edition of The New York Times Magazine she wrote:

Clustered near the bed, framed photos show a burly athlete who placed in the triathlon, a handsome man who grins disarmingly, an arm slung around his wife's shoulders. Now, transformed into a skin and bones caricature of himself, he is ruled by fatigue. After an interminable struggle to reach the bathroom, knees buckling, leg muscles barely able to hoist his feet forward over the floor, a heroic effort of will, he collapses back in bed, exhausted, motionless, glaring from huge, haunted eyes when I speak to him.

Only in his wife's presence is he calm, though no less armored. She is angry, too, and afraid of him. She cooks for him but will not touch him. His children, parents, brother visit often, struggle for words, and leave without embracing.

He rejects kindness in any form. To my cordial first greeting, he responds with silence, slamming shut his eyes. To suggestions of television, music, back rubs, his response is emphatic, curt: "No!"

Worth vividly describes some of the agony of this terrible disease. She also describes the mental and emotional strain that tears at family life.

There is a point at which sickness and dying cease to offer insights into the human condition and become instead an unbearable, unredeemable absurdity. This is most often how AIDS appears to those who know it.

The diagnosis of AIDS is a marker, not an end in itself. Currently most people recover from their first, second, and third AIDS-defining illnessess. People with AIDS are a very heterogeneous group—some feel well and continue working for several years, others are chronically ill, and some die rather quickly.

Patients with AIDS became an even more diverse group after the 1993 expansion of the Centers for Disease Control and Prevention's (CDC's) definition of AIDS. People, in excellent health, are diagnosed with AIDS because their T4 cell count is less than $200/\mu l$ of blood.

The final stage of HIV infection is called AIDS. During this time there is continued rapid viral replication which finally upsets the delicate balance of HIV production/T4 cell infection to T4 cell replacement and the virus largely depletes the cells of the immune system. It has been suggested that during the AIDS stage, serious immunodeficiency occurs when HIV diversity exceeds some threshold beyond which the immune system is unable to control HIV replication (Nowak et al., 1990; Wei et al., 1995; Cohen, 1995).

In addition to the symptoms and conditions caused by HIV, opportunistic infections, and malignancies, HIV-infected patients often experience side effects from various drugs they are taking for primary conditions. In many instances, the toxic side effects of the drugs are life-threatening.

In the symptomatic stages of HIV disease, an individual's ability to carry on the activities of daily living is impaired. The degree of impairment varies considerably from day to day and week to week. Many individuals are debilitated by the symptoms of the disease to the point where it becomes difficult to hold steady employment, shop for food, or do household chores. However, it is also quite common for people with AIDS to experience phases of intense life-threatening illness, followed by phases of seemingly normal functioning, all in a matter of weeks. For a good review on the mechanisms of HIV disease, read "The Immunopathogenesis of HIV Infection" by Giuseppe Pantaleo et al. (1993).

that characterize AIDS. Individuals at this stage, with a T4 cell count of 200 or less/μL of blood often develop thrush, oral lesions, and other fungal, bacterial, and/or viral infections. The duration of these symptoms varies, but it is common for HIV-infected individuals to have them for months at a time. Of those persons in the chronic stage, and not using HIV drug therapy, about 30% developed AIDS-associated infections within 5 years.

——— BOX 7.2 ———

EVOLUTION OF HIV DURING HIV DISEASE PROGRESSION

HIV is a unique retrovirus. For example, mitosis, a form of cell division, is a requirement for the nuclear entry of most retroviral nucleic acids. In contrast, mitosis does not appear to be required for nuclear entry of HIV nucleic acids, particularly in terminally differentiated cells (e.g., macrophages and dendritic cells) (Freed et al., 1994). And second, HIV lacks any mechanism to correct errors that occur as its genetic material is being duplicated. This means that every time the virus makes a copy of itself there will be, on average, at least one genetic "mistake" incorporated in the new virus. So a few days or weeks after initial infection, there may be a large population of closely related, but not identical, viruses replicating in an infected individual. In the **quasi**—steady-state condition, there are successive generations of viral progeny, with each generation following the next by about 2.6 days. Approximately 140 generations of virus are produced over the course of a year and 1,400 generations over the course of 10 years, allowing production of an extraordinary number of genetic variants. Some variants can provide pre-existing drug-resistant forms or enable rapid development of resistance under drug pressure, and some enable the viral population to escape immune activity.

VIRAL POOL

The viral pool is estimated to be a minimum of 10^{10} particles. It is known from experimental data that only 1 in 1,000 particles is infectious, so the infectious viral pool may be on the order of 10^7 particles. At the reverse transcription stage, errors are made at the rate of 3×10^5 per nucleotide per cycle. With a genome of approximately 10^4 nucleotides, there is potential for generation of at least 10 million variants daily, ensuring that mutations can occur at every nucleotide position on a daily basis (Ho, 1996). This creates an enormous potential for genetic mutations and viral evolution. On average, the HIV that is transmitted to another individual will be over 1,000 generations removed from the initial HIV infection. This extent of replication per transmitted infection (transmission cycle) is probably without equal among viral and perhaps bacterial infections (Coffin, 1995). Regardless of the underlying mechanism of immunodeficiency, it is becoming apparent that **the force that is driving the disease is the constant repeated cycles of HIV replication**. Simon Wain-Hobson (1995) suggests that because of 24-hour-a-day HIV replication, as shown by Wei and co-workers (1995), an HIV-infected asymptomatic person can harbor at least 1 million distinct HIV variants and an AIDS patient more than 100 million HIV variants. With so many genetic variants, some are going to be resistant to *any* given drug. (This would include drugs not yet used in therapy). During the investigations of Ho and co-workers (1995) and Wei and co-workers (1995), variants of HIV, resistant to the drugs, ABT-538, **now called Ritonavir**, (a protease inhibitor), and nevirapine (a non-nucleoside agent that inhibits reverse transcriptase function), occurred within days or weeks! Alan Perelson and colleagues (1996) reported data collected from five HIV-infected people after administering Ritonavir through 7 days. Each person responded with a similar pattern of decline in plasma HIV-RNA. Their results: Infected T4 cells had an average life span of 2.2 days. Plasma HIV-RNA had an average life span of 0.3 days. The estimated average total HIV production was over 10 billion HIV per day, which is substantially greater than previous minimum estimates. The results also suggest that the minimum duration of the HIV life cycle in humans is 1.2 days on average and that the average HIV generation time—defined as the time from release of a virus until it infects another cell and causes the release of a new generation of HIV—is 2.6 days.

Number	1 to 10 billion plus HIV produced each day.	About 2 billion T4 cells infected each day.
After two days	Half of HIV are destroyed and are replaced by about an equal amount of new HIV.	About half of the infected T4 cells die and are replaced by new T4 cells. (4% of total body T4 cell count).
After 14 days	After mutations, almost all of new HIV are drug resistant.	The healthy T4 cell count decreases and new T4 cells are infected with the drug-resistant viruses.

Effect of anti-HIV drugs	Initially, over 99% percent of HIV are destroyed using combination drugs like proteases and nucleoside and non-nucleoside reverse transcriptive inhibitions.	The healthy T4 cell count increases.

HIV CLEARANCE

Douglas Richman (1995) states that HIV clearance rate can be calculated based on the rate of reduction in viral RNA load. In cases in which viral RNA load attains a constant level, it can be assumed that there is a dynamic equilibrium resulting in a steady-state level, with production rates matching clearance rates. When viral resistance emerges, as in cases of drug resistance, the production of resistant virus may double every 2 days. The proportion of virus with resistance mutations can also be calculated. According to Richman, in the case of the nonnucleoside reverse transcriptase inhibitors, this has been found to be approximately 1 to 2 per 1,000 RNA copies circulating in the plasma; that is, a patient with 60,000 copies/mL plasma has approximately 100 copies/mL of resistant mutants prior to the **beginning of treatment**. A similar scenario probably holds for all drug-resistance mutations. Thus it is reasonable to expect the HIV-resistant mutants will emerge to almost any antiretroviral compound.

IMPLICATIONS OF HIV DYNAMICS

The rapid turnover of HIV RNA populations has several implications for pathogenesis and treatment of HIV disease. High levels of replication persist throughout HIV disease, with the rate of replication appearing to be fairly constant. Clearance of HIV RNA is also rapid and remains fairly constant throughout the disease. It is only the steady-state levels of HIV RNA that appear to change, which is affected by the production rate of HIV-RNA. Treatment can affect HIV steady-state levels by inhibiting its production. What is

not clear, however, is whether the rate of HIV RNA clearance can be increased.

The implications of the presence of high levels of HIV RNA and high HIV RNA turnover for the assessment of antiretroviral drug activity are clear. With new techniques for quantitating plasma HIV RNA, nearly every HIV-infected individual can be evaluated for response to antiretroviral therapy. While the immune system will recognize most members of a population of viruses, some mutants will evade the immune response for a time. Until they are brought under immune control, these so-called escape mutants will attack T4 cells. It is these cells that are key to orchestrating the overall immune response, and once they are gone the immune system collapses.

OVERWHELMING THE IMMUNE SYSTEM

As HIV multiplies and mutant forms are produced, the immune system responds to these new forms. But ultimately the sheer number of **different** viruses to which the immune system must respond becomes overwhelming. It's a bit like the juggler who tries to keep too many balls in the air: The result is disastrous. Once the immune system is overwhelmed, the latest escape mutant—which may not necessarily be the most pathogenic one to come along—will predominate and immune deficiency will progress. If, as investigators now believe, immunodeficiency or HIV disease is due to accumulated damage over the course of the clinically latent phase, then drug treatment at almost any time during this period, or even after the onset of symptoms, could have a virtually identical effect with regard to prolonging the time of progression to more serious disease or death. That is, it will make no difference when the drug is administered because the drug, whenever present, selects for HIV-resistant mutants which then replicate to increase their numbers and continue to infect T4 cells. As the number of drug-resistant mutants increase, the drug becomes less and less effective while the disease progresses (Japour, 1995).

HIV Can Be Transmitted During All Four Stages

A person who is HIV-infected, even while feeling healthy, may unknowingly infect others. Thus the term HIV disease, rather than

AIDS, more appropriately describes the entire scope of this public health problem. **The greatest risk of HIV transmission occurs within the first several months after infection and again when the T4 cell count drops below 200.**

HIV DISEASE WITHOUT SYMPTOMS, WITH SYMPTOMS, AND AIDS

A person may have no symptoms (asymptomatic) but test HIV-positive. This means that the virus is present in the body. Although he or she has not developed any of the illnesses associated with HIV disease, it is possible to pass the virus on to other people.

Persons may develop some symptoms early on in HIV disease such as swollen lymph glands, night sweats, diarrhea, or fatigue. (This stage used to be called ARC for AIDS-Related Complex; the term is no longer used by the Centers for Disease Control and Prevention.)

In time, most, people with HIV disease progress to AIDS. (This is sometimes referred to as full-blown AIDS. This term is not used in this text; one either is or is not diagnosed with AIDS.) A person has HIV/AIDS when the defect in his or her immune system caused by HIV disease has progressed to such a degree that an unusual infection or tumor is present or when the T4 cell count has fallen below 200/µl of blood. In AIDS patients, a number of diseases are known to take advantage of the damaged immune system. These include opportunistic infections usually caused by viruses, bacteria, fungi, or protozoa; or tumors such as Kaposi's sarcoma, a form of skin cancer (?), or lymphoma, a malignancy of the lymph glands. It is the presence of one of the opportunistic diseases, or a T4 cell count of less than 200, along with a positive HIV test that establishes the medical diagnosis of AIDS. Thus the disease we call AIDS is actually the end stage of HIV disease. It is important to remember that AIDS itself is not transmitted—the virus is. AIDS is the most severe clinical form of HIV disease.

INCREASES IN THE NUMBER OF HIV/AIDS CASES

Prior to 1988, there were between 5 and 10 million HIV-infected people worldwide, an estimated 1.5 million of them living in the United States. Relatively few of these people were actually sick. The majority of these people were infected by HIV in the early 1980s. But from 1988 on (there is an average clinical latency period of about 11 years), the number of new HIV infections, new AIDS cases, and AIDS-related deaths began to rise rapidly; and by the beginning of 1998, over 400,000 AIDS patients in the United States out of an accumulated 648,000 AIDS cases died. (AIDS cases are still being underreported by 10% to 15% in the United States.) The point is that the number of AIDS cases and deaths will continue to rise in the 1990s because those who became infected by HIV in the 1980s will progress to AIDS. In addition, the CDC estimated that there will be at least 40,000 new HIV infections in the United States for each year from 1991 through at least the year 2000.

ASPECTS OF HIV INFECTION

HIV infection depends on a variety of events, for example, the amount and strain of HIV that enters the body (some strains of HIV are known to be more pathogenic than others), perhaps where it enters the body, the number of exposures, the time interval between exposures, the immunological status of the exposed person, and the presence of other active infections. These are referred to as cofactors that contribute to successful HIV infection.

Post Infection

Estimating the date of initial HIV infection helps predict the likely timing of disease progression. The task is easiest when there has been a known blood exposure, but even in other cases, the patient may have experienced a limited number of high-risk sexual or drug-use exposures—or perhaps only one such exposure.

The virus may be present in the bloodstream or within cells for various lengths of time prior to antibody formation. (Normally it takes 7 to 10 days after antigen exposure for the first antibody to appear.) When the antibody appears it is called **seroconversion** (sero = serum of the

———— BOX 7.3 ————

DEVELOPMENT OF AIDS OVER TIME

A spectrum of clinical expression of disease can occur after HIV infection. Approximately 10% of HIV-infected subjects progress to AIDS within the first 2 to 3 years of HIV infection (**rapid progressors**). People with greater than 50,000 HIV RNA copies/mL at 6 months after infection are the most likely to be rapid progressors. About 60% of adults/adolescents will progress to AIDS within 12 to 13 years after HIV infection (**slow progressors**). Approximately 5% to 10% of HIV-infected subjects are clinically asymptomatic after 8 to 15 years and have stable peripheral blood T4 cell levels (**nonprogressors**). Data from the Multicenter AIDS Cohort Study suggest that 20 years after infection, 10% to 17% of HIV-infected individuals will still be AIDS-free (Haynes et al., 1996).

In summary, true **nonprogressors**—people who have had HIV for up to 15 years or more with no symptoms and with continually normal and stable T4 cell counts—are rare. The majority of nonprogressors are, in fact, **slow progressors**—people who have had HIV for 12 years or more and who are healthy but whose T4 cell counts, although not falling below 500, have gradually declined. These people have about 10,000 or fewer HIV RNA copies/mL of plasma.

People with AIDS and a very low T4 cell count who have survived for exceptionally long periods of time (5 years or more) are usually described as long-term survivors. Thus, if one has lived with AIDS for 5 or more years, he or she is a long-term survivor. Some 6% of persons diagnosed with clinical AIDS are long-term survivors (Laurence, 1996).

Current and contained use of AIDS drug cocktails containing at least one protease inhibitor will increase the number of long-term survivors! It will take at least another 1 or 2 years to determine the actual percentage increase in long-term survivors using the drug cocktails. Survival after the onset of AIDS has been increasing in industrialized countries from an average of less than 1 year to over 3 years at present. Survival time with AIDS in developing countries remains short and is estimated to be less than 1 year. Longer survival appears to be directly related to routine treatment with antiretroviral drugs, the use of drugs for opportunistic infections, and a better overall quality of health care.

The majority of AIDS cases occur before age 35, and over 90% of all AIDS deaths occur in people under the age of 50 worldwide.

Philip Rosenberg and colleagues (1994) reported that the length of incubation, progression from HIV infection to AIDS, varied according to the age at the time of infection. Younger ages were associated with a slower progression to AIDS. The estimated median treatment-free clinical incubation period was 12 years for those infected at age 20, 9.9 years for infection at age 30, and 8.1 years for infection at age 40.

THE CLINICAL COURSE OF AIDS AMONG MEN AND WOMEN

Andrew Phillips and colleagues (1994) compared the development of AIDS-defining diseases between 566 women and 1988 men with AIDS who were HIV-infected via similar routes, mainly by sharing IDU equipment and by heterosexual sexual contact. **They concluded that there was little if any difference between men and women in the clinical course of AIDS.**

---

blood; conversion from antibody negative to antibody present or positive). Seroconversion for HIV may occur as early as 1 week, but most often is detected between 6 and 18 weeks after infection (Figure 7-4).

Immunosilent HIV Infection: Time Before Seroconversion

The period after HIV infection necessary to induce production of specific antibodies,

immunological defect, and AIDS is variable and probably depends on the characteristics of both the virus and the host. It has been estimated that between 95% and 99% of infected individuals seroconvert (produce HIV antibodies) within 6 months of infection (Horsburg et al., 1989). However, according to some investigators, antibodies may not appear for up to 36 months or more (Ranki et al., 1987; Imagawa et al., 1989; Ensoli et al., 1990, 1991).

Incubation and Window Period

The time from HIV infection to the first signs and symptoms of HIV disease is called the clinical incubation period. Evidence suggests that the route or manner of HIV infection may influence the **incubation period**. For example, exposure through sexual intercourse has a mean incubation time of 6 months. Infection by transfusion has a mean incubation time of 2.5 years. It appears that for unknown reasons, **free viruses** (those not inside cells) present at the time of infection do not stimulate the immune system. Infected cells in the transfused blood have a **latent** (inactive) proviral state and antibody will not be made until new viruses are produced which then engender HIV disease symptoms. Infected newborns have a mean incubation period of 10 months. (Newborns in general begin making their own antibody about 3 to 6 months after birth, but may not make antibody against HIV for several years.)

The time between infection and the presence of first HIV antibody or seroconversion is called the **window period**. Because it can be quite lengthy, HIV antibody tests performed during the window period that are negative may be falsely negative (Figure 7-4).

PRODUCTION OF HIV-SPECIFIC ANTIBODIES

During the 15 years (1983–1998) since the discovery of HIV, scientists have constructed a serological or antibody graph of HIV infection and HIV disease. The graph reveals how soon the body produces HIV-specific antibodies after infection and about when the virus begins its reproduction. Different parts of the graph (Figure 7-4) have been filled in by Paul Coulis and colleagues (1987), Dani Bolognesi (1989), and Susan Stramer and colleagues (1989). **The history of the HIV antibody is not yet complete, but the order of appearance and disappearance of antibodies specific for the serologically important antigens over the course of HIV disease has been described.**

The time period from seroconversion to the presentation of clinical symptoms is quite variable and may last for 10 or more years in adults and adolescents, but occurs earlier in children and older persons with HIV disease. The time period for moving from clinical symptoms of HIV disease to AIDS is also quite variable (Figure 7-2). Much depends on the individual's genetic susceptibility and his or her response to medical intervention. The **average** time from HIV infection to AIDS from 1990 through 1997 was 11 years. Note that Figure 7-4 shows that HIV plasma viremia (the presence of virus in blood plasma) and antigenemia (an-ti-je-ne-mi-ah—the persistence of antigen in the blood) can be detected as early as 2 weeks after infection. This demonstrates that viremia and antigenemia occur prior to seroconversion. Using HIV proteins produced by recombinant DNA methods (making synthetic copies of the viral proteins), antibodies specific for gp41 (a subunit of glycoprotein 160) are detectable prior to those specific for p24 (a core protein) and persist throughout the course of infection. Levels of antibody specific for p24 rise to detectable levels between 6 and 8 weeks after HIV infection but may disappear abruptly. The drop in p24 antibody has been shown to occur at the same time when there is a rise in p24 antigen in the serum. This strange phenomenon is thought to be due to the loss of available p24 antibody in immune complexes—too little p24 antibody is being made to handle the new virus being produced. It is believed that this imbalance is one of the important factors that moves the patient towards AIDS. Thus a sudden decrease in anti-p24 is considered by many scientists to be a prognostic indicator that people with HIV disease are moving towards AIDS.

It is now believed by some AIDS researchers and health care professionals that 90% to 95% of those persons infected with HIV will eventually develop AIDS. It has been estimated that approximately 50% of people with HIV disease will progress to AIDS within 8 years after infection. At 10 years 70% will have developed AIDS. After that, an additional 25% to 45% of the remainder will develop AIDS. It is **most improbable** that 100% of those infected will develop AIDS.

HIV EXPOSURE: FAILURE TO SEROCONVERT

A recent study has shown that 10% of 260 female prostitutes who work in Nairobi **have not developed antibodies to HIV**. They have remained seronegative for 3 years despite ongoing unprotected sexual exposure to HIV-infected men (Matheson et al., 1996).

During the past few years it has become clear that apparently harmless, and possibly protective, encounters with HIV can occur. Some individuals who have been exposed to the virus and are therefore at high risk for HIV infection remain apparently uninfected; they do not have antibodies to HIV in their blood, and neither HIV nor its nucleic acids can be detected in blood samples. In one study of 97 HIV exposed individuals who were seronegative for HIV, 49% exhibit cell-mediated immunity to HIV (their T cells respond to HIV peptides in vitro), whereas only 2% of 163 individuals not known to be exposed to HIV exhibit responses to these peptides. Such HIV-specific, cell-mediated responses have been seen in gay men with known sexual exposure, injection drug users, health care workers exposed by accidental needlestick, and newborn infants of HIV-positive mothers. HIV-specific lymphoproliferation or cytotoxic T lymphocyte activity, hallmarks of cell-mediated responses, have also been observed by other investigators in some exposed, but apparently uninfected subjects (Salk et al., 1993). Mario Clerici and colleagues (1994) have also reported on HIV-specific T-helper cell activity in six of eight HIV-negative health care workers with exposure to HIV-positive body fluids. High HIV specific T-helper cell activity was detectable 4 to 8 weeks after the exposure and was lost in individuals followed up for 8 to 64 weeks. Exposure to HIV without evidence of subsequent infection appears to result in activation of cellular immunity without activation of antibody production.

Through 1997, separate cases of HIV-positive, seronegative (do not make HIV antibody) gay men have been reported on (*MMWR*, 1996). In each case the men were confirmed HIV-positive, demonstrated OIs consistent with HIV disease, e.g., PCP and low T4 cell counts, but never produced HIV antibody. To date such cases are rare—**but they do happen!** (See **Genetic Resistance to HIV Infection** in Chapter 5.)

AIDS Survival Time Has Nearly Doubled

A National Institute of Allergy and Infectious Diseases study followed more than 5,000 homosexual and bisexual men with HIV infection or who were at risk of infection from 1984 through 1991. For men diagnosed with AIDS during the years 1984 and 1985, 50% had a survival time of less than 11.6 months. For men diagnosed with AIDS in 1990 or 1991, a large percentage had survived for nearly 2 years. The greatest gain in survival time occurred among those whose AIDS-defining illness was *Pneumocystis carinii* pneumonia (PCP). Survival time following the diagnosis of AIDS among the participants who developed *P. carinii* increased from a median of 12.8 months in 1984 and 1985 to a median of 26.3 months in 1990 and 1991. The increase in survival time is related to effective PCP therapy. The survival estimate of persons classified with AIDS using the 1993 definition will be considerably longer than for those diagnosed with AIDS using the 1987 definition. Using the 1987 definition, the median survival for patients enrolled in the registry was 24 months; using the new definition, 53% were still alive after 57 months. Jeffrey Laurence (1995, 1996) reports that 5% to 6% of clinically defined AIDS patients now live beyond 5 years. With many thousands of AIDS-diagnosed people now using the drug cocktails which include at least one protease inhibitor, the number of people with AIDS living past 5 years will greatly increase! These findings have important implications for health planners as well as for those involved in providing care and counseling for patients with AIDS.

Classification of HIV/AIDS Progression

There are several classifications that spell out the progression of signs and symptoms from HIV infection to the diagnosis of AIDS. The classifications were developed to provide a framework for the medical management of pa-

————— BOX 7.4 —————

ARE THERE LONG-TERM ADULT NONPROGRESSORS OF HIV DISEASE—YES!—WHY?

Long-term nonprogressors of HIV disease are defined as those persons who are still alive 10 or more years after they tested HIV-positive, with seroconversion documented by history or stored serum samples, absence of symptoms, and normal and stable T4 cell counts (at least 600 T4 cells/microliter of blood). The long-term nonprogressors who are of particular interest to AIDS investigators, are those who after 8 years, in the absence of antiviral therapy, continue to maintain T4 cell counts of 500 or more. Studies through 1997 suggest that 12% to 15% of HIV-infected people remain asymptomatic with about normal T4 cell counts for at least 8 to 12 years (Conant, 1995; Levy, 1995). At least one person is known to be asymptomatic 21 years after HIV infection! (Shernoff, 1997). **The question is: How does their immune system differ from those who do not live as long?**

In 1983, at age 71, a man became HIV-positive. He received a contaminated blood transfusion while undergoing colon surgery. Unlike most long-term HIV survivors, he has suffered no symptoms and no loss of immune function. He is celebrating his 81st birthday. He is one of five patients who came to the attention of an AIDS researcher as he was preparing a routine update on transfusion-related HIV infections. All five people were infected by the same donor. And 7 to 10 years later, no one has suffered any effects.

The blood donor was a gay male who had contracted the virus during the late 1970s or early 1980s and gave blood at least 26 times before learning he was infected. After locating the donor it was found that the man was just as healthy as the people who got his blood.

A 39-year-old San Francisco artist has beaten the odds by living with the virus that causes AIDS for 15 years. He has only routine medical complaints: the stuffiness of an occasional head cold or the aches and pains of a flu. He has never taken an anti-HIV drug. His own immune system seems to have held the virus at bay.

Susan Buchbinder and colleagues (1992, 1994) reviewed 588 HIV-infected gay men. Thirty-one percent were still AIDS-free 14 years after infection. They attempted to determine why these men lived while others died of HIV/AIDS. Some long-term survivors have low T4 cell counts, some have never taken antiviral therapy, and some have high T4 cell counts. The question is, what is keeping them healthy? If it can be determined why or how their bodies have delayed the progression of HIV disease, then perhaps new approaches to treating all HIV-infected persons will follow. Understanding their defense may help in preventing HIV infection per se.

Buchbinder and colleagues have found that three aspects of the healthy survivors' immune system appear to delay HIV disease progression: Survivors have strong cytotoxic lymphocyte activity, strong suppressor or T8 cell activity, and have higher levels of antibodies against certain HIV proteins.

It is also possible that long-term nonprogressors carry a less pathogenic virus or that these men have not been reexposed to the virus through unprotected sexual activities. Nicholas Deacon and colleagues (1995) have sequenced HIV DNA from a blood donor and a group of six recipients who have not shown HIV disease symptoms despite being infected for 10 to 14 years. Deletions were found in the *nef* gene and in the U3 region of the long terminal repeat. Because the lack of disease progression appears to depend on the virus instead of the host immune system, these results suggest a possible use of such HIV strains in live vaccines. One thing found in the studies that leads to confusion is that, in general, the healthy long-term positives in the study are living very healthy **lifestyles**, but so are many of the other men who are not doing as well. In addition, physicians who treat HIV/AIDS persons do not notice any trends that would lead one to recognize the type of patient or factors that would lead to long-term survival. It was concluded that, at the moment, there is a dire lack of advice for longer life for persons who have become HIV-infected. AIDS investigators at the National Institute of Allergy and Infectious Diseases are studying the immune systems of 14 people who have been HIV positive for 12 or more years.

Current evidence suggests that between 5% and 10% of HIV-infected people will live 10 to 20 or more years. The second longest documented case of long-term nonprogressor to date is that of a gay male who tested HIV-positive 18 years ago. His T4 count remains at 1,000 or normal. It should be mentioned that if the average time from infection to AIDS is 11 years, statistically speaking, survivors at 20+ years, are expected to occur. Time will tell! For other accounts of long-term survivors, see the articles by Cayo (1995), Pantaleo (1995), Kirchhoff (1995), and Baltimore (1995).

UPDATE 1996

John Mellors studied how viral load (amount or numbers of copies of HIV RNA per milliliter of blood) regardless of treatment, affected a person's survival or nonprogression to AIDS. He found that the baseline viral load accurately predicted survival, while the person's T4 cell count did not. Mellors and his colleagues divided HIV-infected men into two groups, one including those with more than 10,190 HIV RNA copies per milliliter of blood and the other including men with fewer copies. After 10 years, he found that 70% of the people in the low viral-load group had survived compared to only 30% survival of the group with an initial high load—even though the two groups had nearly identical baseline T4 counts (Cohen, 1996). These data should transform the way physicians make decisions on when to treat and what drug(s) to use. The data strongly suggest that viral loads be determined for each HIV-infected person. (Refer to Chapter 4 for further explanation of Viral Load.)

LONG-TERM AIDS SURVIVORS

Parade Magazine, January 31, 1993, carried a review of 16 long-term AIDS survivors who date back to 1982. On April 16, 1995, the same magazine reported that 12 of the 16 had since died. Of the four survivors, all have refused zidovudine (ZDU) therapy (Figure 7-5).

On April 6, 1997, *Parade Magazine* continued its follow-up on the four survivors seen in Figure 7-5. All four remain alive and productive. They are Cristofer Shihar, 46, a Hollywood hair-stylist; Michael Leonard Marshall, 51, a floral designer in Culver City; George Melton, 44, an author in San Francisco; and Niro Asistent, 51, a therapist now living in France. Of the four, only Marshall said he was taking an AIDS cocktail: Viramune, Crixivan, and 3TC. Niro Asistent remarried in 1996. She said HIV **cannot** be detected in her body!

FIGURE 7-5   Long-Term AIDS Survivors. In 1988, *Parade Magazine* began tracking 16 long-term AIDS survivors. The longest living of these survivors was diagnosed with AIDS in 1982. Only one of the 16, a woman, was HIV-infected through a heterosexual relationship. Her sexual partner was bisexual. In June 1990, 13 were alive. By January 1993, six of the original 16 were alive. In April 1995 and April 1997, *Parade Magazine* updated interviews with the four remaining survivors.

tients from the time of infection through the expression of AIDS. All classification systems are fundamentally the same—they group patients according to their stage of infection, based on signs that indicate a failing immune system (Royce et al., 1991).

The Walter Reed Army Medical Center System (WRS) classifies HIV infection through six stages. The stages are based on signs and symptoms associated with immune dysfunction. Although individual parts of the immune system appear to function independently of one another, all parts appear to depend on the function of T4 cells (see Chapter 5).

A second classification, the most widely accepted because of its greater clinical applicability, comes from the CDC (Table 7-2). The CDC classification uses four mutually exclusive groupings (Figure 7-6). The groupings are based on the **presence** or **absence** of signs and symptoms of disease, and clinical and/or laboratory findings and the chronology of their occurrence. Group 1, acute infection, means the person is **viremic** (i.e., many virus particles are present in his or her blood or serum). There are **no measurable antibodies;** one is HIV-positive but lacks HIV antibodies and signs and symptoms of HIV disease.

The majority of people in Group 1 remain asymptomatic. Some may experience flu- or mononucleosis-like symptoms that generally disappear in a few weeks. In relatively few cases the patient moves rapidly from mild symptoms into severe opportunistic infections and is diagnosed with AIDS.

In Group 2, antibodies are present but most patients remain free of HIV disease symptoms. Regardless of the lack of outward clinical symptoms, 90% of those who are asymptomatic experience some form of immunological deterioration within 5 years (Fauci, 1988).

In Group 3, asymptomatic people from Groups 1 and 2 become symptomatic and demonstrate lymphadenopathy in the neck, armpit, and groin areas. Although a number of other diseases may cause the lymph nodes to swell, most swelling declines as the other symptoms of illness fade. However, with HIV infection, the lymph nodes remain swollen for months, with no other signs of a related infectious disease. Consequently, lymphadenopathy is sometimes called **persistent generalized lymphadenopathy** (PGL). People with PGL may experience night sweats, weight loss, fever, on and off diarrhea, fatigue, and the onset of oral candidiasis or thrush (a fungus or yeast infection of the oral cavity) (see Figure 6-3). Such signs and symptoms are prodromal (symptoms leading to) for AIDS. Studies have shown that people in group 3 appear to become more infectious as the disease progresses.

People in Group 4 have been diagnosed with AIDS. They fit the 1987 CDC criteria for AIDS diagnosis (The CDC AIDS diagnostic criteria are listed in Tables 7-2 and 1-1). Hairy leukoplakia (Figure 7-7, Table 7-2, Category C-2) is virtually diagnostic of AIDS in group 4 patients. Statistics show that about 30% of all the newly HIV-infected will progress to group 4 (AIDS) every 5 years, so that about 90% will have been diagnosed with AIDS within 15 years. Not all of the opportunistic diseases (OIs) or cancers will appear in any one AIDS patient. But some OIs, like *Pneumocystis carinii* pneumonia occur in some 80% of AIDS patients prior to their deaths.

PROGNOSTIC BIOLOGICAL MARKERS RELATED TO AIDS PROGRESSION

The **ideal marker** would be able to predict HIV disease progression, be responsive to antiretroviral therapy, and explain the variance in clinical outcome due to therapy. It is, however, unlikely that any one marker will be able to fulfill all these criteria in HIV infection completely. Therefore, individual markers used to track HIV infection to AIDS are presented.

p24 Antigen Levels

p24 is a specific protein located in the core or inner layer of HIV. Because the immune system produces antibody against foreign protein, antibody is made against p24. A positive test for p24 antigen in the blood means that HIV production is so rapid that it overcomes the available antibody (Figure 7-4). That is, there is more HIV antigen than antibody to neutralize it. During this state of HIV-antibody imbalance, HIV is believed to spread into uninfected cells. This raised p24 antigen level condition occurs at least twice; once shortly after infection and again during the AIDS period when the immune system is rapidly deteriorating and unable to produce sufficient antibody to deal with newly produced HIV.

Those who, during the early stage of HIV infection, test p24 antigen positive are likely to progress to AIDS earlier than those who test p24 negative. Thus, a positive p24 test is an early and serious warning sign for HIV-infected people (Escaich et al., 1991; Phillips et al., 1991a).

p24 Antibody Levels

High levels of p24 antibody indicate that the immune system is functioning well and clearing the body of free HIVs. High antibody levels appear to slow the progression toward AIDS. Typically, p24 antibody levels are high

SEROREVERSION: CHANGING FROM HIV-POSITIVE TO HIV-NEGATIVE!

INFANTS AND ADULTS WHO CLEAR HIV FROM THEIR BODIES

Infants

An infant's mother tested HIV-positive during her 4th month of pregnancy. She was asymptomatic then and continues to be so at the time of the report by Yvonne Bryson and colleagues (1995). The child was born by vaginal delivery. No blood products were received and the child was not breast-fed. HIV tests of the baby's blood at 19 days and 51 days after birth were positive, but tests done 3 months after birth were negative. The boy is now 5 years old and in kindergarten and by all measures, including DNA tests, remains free of the virus.

A case such as this one only heightens the mystery of why 70% of babies born to HIV-positive mothers escape HIV infection.

Since the report of Bryson, Pierre Roques and colleagues (1995) reported on the clearance of HIV from 12 infants with perinatal exposure to HIV. And, a series of investigations from the European Collaborative Study adds more data to the growing literature on this phenomenon. From a series of 264 children born to HIV-infected mothers in Padua, Genoa, Brussels and Stockholm, nine infants were positive by viral culture or PCR and subsequently reverted to negative during follow-up ranging from 16 months to almost 9 years.

All the infants lost HIV antibody by the age of 18 months. Six of them were positive on one or more viral culture or PCR assays during early infancy, then reverted to consistently negative tests for the remainder of the study period. The other three had sporadically positive tests well into childhood. None had HIV-related symptoms or received anti-HIV treatments (Newell et al., 1996).

Adults

David Schwartz of the Johns Hopkins School of Public Health reported in January 1995, a 43-year-old woman who became HIV-infected from a blood transfusion after the birth of her second child in 1981. Despite over 40 attempts, investi-gators have not been able to culture HIV from her blood. Although she is a nonprogressor, the donor died of AIDS and two other people who received the same virus through blood transfusions developed AIDS. Prior to learning that she received HIV-positive blood she had two children. Each was breast-fed for a year. In 1985 she read about blood transfusion HIV cases, was tested and turned up HIV-positive. At this time the mother, the children, and the husband are HIV-negative.

Schwartz's team is studying four other cases that are similar with the hope of learning what might be unusual about the virus in those people or in their immune system.

Australian researchers have been studying a group of six people who each received HIV contaminated blood products infected by a single common donor and tested positive. Both the donor and the people infected have now been under scrutiny for up to 11 years, and after this length of time both the donor and five of the recipients have remained symptom free, with no decline of T4 cells and no sign of the P24 antigen, a specific marker that identifies the presence of HIV in the blood, which is considered a sign of worsening AIDS conditions. In only one of the six has it been possible to isolate HIV. In the others, the researchers were unable to find evidence of the presence of HIV, despite repetitive testing of body fluids.

The researchers have no clear-cut answer for their findings, stating that it is not clear whether the benign course of HIV infection was due to host, viral, or other unknown factors.

UPDATE 1997/1998

Through the use of combinations of AIDS drugs now available in the United States, thousands of persons with HIV disease and those with AIDS have essentially become HIV-negative. HIV has been reduced to unmeasurable levels in their blood plasma. The AIDS drug cocktails have now suppressed HIV replication in some persons for about 3 years (1995–beginning 1998).

TABLE 7-2 CDC Classification of HIV-Related Diseases

HIV Disease
Group 1: Acute infection—HIV antibodies absent; asymptomatic or if symptomatic mononucleosis-like symptoms which subside in most cases

Group 2: Asymptomatic infection—HIV antibodies present; eventually moves on to

Group 3: Persistent generalized lymphadenopathy; eventually moves on to group 4

AIDS
Group 4:
Subgroup A: Constitutional symptoms (previously called ARC, aids-related complex) and <200 T4 cells/μl of blood.

Subgroup B: Neurologic, symptoms (AIDS dementia complex, neuropathy)

Subgroup C
  Category C-1: Secondary infections listed in the CDC surveillance definition for AIDS: *Pneumocystis carinii* pneumonia, recurrent pneumonia, chronic cryptosporidiosis, CNS toxoplasmosis, extraintestinal strongyloidosis, isosporiasis, esophageal candidiasis, cryptococcosis, histoplasmosis, *Mycobacterium avium intracellulare* or *Mycobacterium kansasii*, cytomegalovirus, chronic or disseminated herpes simplex, progressive multifocal leukoencephalopathy
  Category C-2: Other specified secondary infections: oral hairy leukoplakia, multidermatomal herpes zoster, recurrent *Salmonella* bacterium, nocardiosis, pulmonary tuberculosis, oral candidiasis
Subgroup D: Secondary cancers: Kaposi's sarcoma, non-Hodgkin's lymphoma (small, noncleaved lymphoma; immunoblastic sarcoma), primary brain lymphoma
Subgroup E: Other conditions: lymphocytic interstitial pneumonitis, neoplasms, infections not previously listed

during a person's asymptomatic or latent stage (Figure 7-4). However, antibody levels begin to decrease over time. As measurable antibody falls, p24 antigen levels rise, indicating a loss of immune function. When both p24 antigen and antibody levels are high, the body may be expressing an autoimmune disorder—the immune system is attacking its own body cells. Why this occurs is not understood.

Other Markers

Beta-2 microglobulin (B-2M) is a low molecular weight protein that is present on the surface of almost all nucleated cells. As cells die, this compound is released into body fluids. Thus there is always some B-2M in the blood because of normal cell degeneration and replacement. However, in a chronic illness with increased cell destruction, as in HIV infection, B-2M increases beyond normal levels.

To date, a B-2M level of 5 mg/L or higher is the best available indicator of progression to AIDS within 3 years. Levels below 2.6 are considered normal. Similar to p24 antigen, B-2M protein increases dramatically shortly after infection occurs, then declines, and finally rises again with AIDS. B-2M can be used with T4 counts to foretell which HIV-positive individuals face the greatest immediate risk of progressing to AIDS.

Neopterin is a metabolite of guanosine triphosphate which is produced in stimulated monocytes and macrophages and is found in increased levels in HIV disease. In some studies, the presence of these two compounds have been better HIV disease progression indicators than T4 cell counts (Cohen, 1992).

Interferon is a protein that transfers chemical signals between subtypes of lymphocytes (white blood cells). Levels are generally increased in proportion to the stage of HIV disease.

Delayed type hypersensitivity (DTH) means that persons with HIV disease progressively lose their ability to respond to antigens. DTH is a gauge of functioning cell-mediated immunity rather than antibody response.

T4 and T8 Lymphocyte Levels

The most extensive use of data for AIDS progression risk identification involve the number of T4 and T8 cells circulating in the blood (Anderson et al., 1991; Burcham et al., 1991; Phillips et al., 1991b).

T4 cells and the ratio of T4 cells to T8 cells found in the blood have, beginning 1997, been widely used as prognostic indicators for AIDS progression. T4 cell counts, however, are not ironclad predictors of HIV disease progression. In some cases persons with HIV disease and very low (less than 50 or 100) T4 counts remain healthy; conversely some HIV-diseased persons

FIGURE 7-6 Clinical History of HIV Infection According to Center for Disease Control and Prevention Groupings. Seroconversion means that HIV antibodies are measurably present in the person's serum. With continued depletion of T4 cells, various signs and symptoms appear announcing the progression of HIV disease into AIDS. Although HIV antibodies have been found as early as 1 week after exposure, most often seroconversion occurs between weeks 6 and 18 but may not occur for up to 1 year or more.

have relatively high counts (over 400) and are quite ill. T4 counts are notoriously fickle, they can vary widely between labs or because of a person's age, the time of day a measurement is taken, and even whether the person smokes (Sax et al., 1995).

CDC Insists That Performing T4 Cell Counts in HIV-Infected People Continues to Be Essential

Accurate and reliable measures of CD4+ T lymphocytes (CD4+ T cells or T4 cells) are essential to the assessment of the immune system of

FIGURE 7-7 Oral Hairy Leukoplakia (lu-ko-pla-ki-ah) of the Tongue. An early manifestation, it is virtually diagnostic of AIDS. The white corrugated or "hairy" patches are caused by the Epstein-Barr virus (EBV).These white plaques cannot be removed. **A,** A milder form of the disease. **B,** A more severe manifestation of the disease. Note that the white plaques may cover the entire tongue. (*Courtesy of Drs. M. Schiodt, D. Greenspan, and J.S. Greenspan, Oral AIDS Center, University of California, San Francisco* and Journal of Respiratory Diseases, *1989, 10:91–109*).

A

B

HIV-infected persons. The progression to AIDS is largely attributable to the decrease in T4 lymphocytes. Progressive depletion of T4 lymphocytes is associated with an increased likelihood of clinical complications. Consequently, the Public Health Service (PHS) has recommended that T4 lymphocyte levels be monitored every 3 to 6 months in all HIV-infected persons. The measurement of T4 cell levels has been used to establish decision points for initiating *Pneumocystis carinii* pneumonia prophylaxis and antiviral therapy and to monitor the efficacy of treatment. T4 lymphocyte levels are also used as prognostic indicators in people who have HIV disease and recently have been included as one of the criteria for initiating prophylaxis for several opportunistic infections that indicate an HIV infection. Moreover, T4 lymphocyte levels are a **criterion** for categorizing HIV-related clinical conditions by CDC's classification system for HIV infection and surveillance case definition for AIDS among adults and adolescents (*MMWR*, 1997).

Levels of HIV RNA in the Blood: VIRAL LOAD

David Baltimore, the Nobel Prize-winning retrovirologist, and co-workers have found a useful clinical predictor of HIV disease progressors, levels of HIV RNA in the blood. More RNA means more HIV, and that makes patients get sicker sooner. HIV RNA is a more sensitive measure than other assays and may detect the virus earlier than it would be seen otherwise.

Since the reported work of Baltimore and others on the levels of HIV RNA in the blood, Dennis Henrard and co-workers (1995) have concluded that the stability of HIV RNA levels suggests that an equilibrium between HIV replication rate and efficacy of immunologic response is established shortly after infection and persists throughout the asymptomatic period of the disease (Figure 7-3). Thus, a defect in immunologic control of HIV infection may be as important as the viral replication rate for determining AIDS-free survival. Because individual steady-state levels of HIV RNA were established soon after infection, HIV RNA levels can, as

Baltimore suggests, be useful markers for predicting clinical outcome. In that regard, when researchers analyzed HIV RNA levels in HIV-positive men they found that HIV RNA—but not CD4 counts—tightly correlated with AIDS progression (Holden, 1994; Cohen, 1996) (see Chapter 4 for additional information on RNA-viral load). Data from many HIV RNA plasma load studies through 1996 suggest that viral load is superior to T4 cell count as a marker for HIV disease progression. However, the best monitor of disease progression is the use of both, the T4 cell count and viral load (Merigan et al., 1996; Katzenstein et al., 1996; Voelker, 1995).

No current viral or immunological markers adequately reflect drug toxicities caused by therapy.

HIV INFECTION OF THE CENTRAL NERVOUS SYSTEM

A wide variety of central nervous system (CNS) abnormalities occur during the course of HIV infection. They result not only from the opportunistic infections and malignancies in the immunodeficient individual, but also from direct HIV infection of the CNS. Certain brain cells have surface molecules similar to the CD4 antigen on T4 lymphocytes and are receptive to HIV infection. In other brain cells, an alternative receptor for HIV has recently been identified. It was shown that a glycolipid in these cells can mediate HIV infection. In addition, HIV-infected monocytes can migrate to the brain, become tissue macrophages, and release HIV to infect adjacent cells. HIV investigators believe that HIV may invade the brain within a few weeks to months after HIV infection (Ranki et al., 1995). Although the precise mechanisms by which HIV gains entry into the CNS and produces nerve cell dysfunction are still undetermined, infection of the brain is an integral component of the biology and natural history of HIV infection; the resulting clinical manifestations are summarized in Table 7-3.

AIDS Dementia Complex

In addition to cancers and opportunistic diseases, a progressive dementia (mental deterioration) due to HIV infection of the central

VIRAL LOAD AND T4 CELL COUNTS: THEIR USE IN CLINICAL PRACTICE

VIRAL LOAD

Viral load assays measure only viral RNA present in the plasma. They do not account for **intact virus** in the lymph system or other tissues. Individual measurements are a good surrogate (substitute) for virus replication. Although the relationships among viral replication, T4 cell count, and disease progression are not entirely clear, viral load correlates fairly well with all of them. Viral load measurements can be effectively used to monitor therapy.

HIT EARLY, HIT HARD

The level of plasma HIV RNA at 6 months after primary infection is called the **SET POINT**, but treatment should be considered regardless of **set point** RNA values. The idea is to stop HIV replication early rather than later.

T4 CELL COUNTS

T4 cell counts remain helpful in determining the stage of the disease. But, T4 counts are highly variable, even from hour to hour in some HIV-infected people. They are also significantly influenced by other current viral infections. Although T4 cell counts function well as reliable markers of disease progression and antiretroviral drug efficacy in large populations, they are less reliable for prescribing therapy for the individual. Viral load determinations present a better basis on which to present therapy. Until viral load determination costs fall and until physicians become more familiar with them and insurance companies pay for them, the T4 tests will remain the more practical determinant of disease stage and when to begin therapy. (Medicaid, Medicare, and some HMOs do cover HIV RNA determinations.)

It is suggested that HIV RNA levels be used as a means to prescribe medication. RNA levels should be determined, after exposure, at 6 weeks, 12 weeks, and at 6 months—the **set point**.

SUMMARY

The level of circulating RNA in plasma is a direct reflection of ongoing HIV replication in the host. The T4 lymphocyte, being a **target** of HIV replication, is an **indirect** marker of antiretroviral therapy. The T4 count itself is a measurement of the relative production and destruction of the T4 cell population. For example, if there is a production problem, either due to nutritional, toxicity, or other factors, the T4 count may not rise proportionately to the **decrease** in viral load. Thus, the change in viral load is more precisely measuring the effect of antiretroviral therapy and, therefore, is the best marker of how well drugs are working.

TABLE 7-3 Neurological Manifestations Associated with Direct HIV Infection of the Nervous System

AIDS dementia complex
Asymptomatic infection
Acute encephalitis
Aseptic meningitis
Vacuolar myelopathy
Inflammatory demyelinating polyneuropathy
Radiculopathy
Mononeuropathies
Distal sensory neuropathy

nervous system develops in 55% to 65% of AIDS patients. Pathological changes in the CNS are observed in up to 80% of those autopsied (McGuire, 1993). But the mystery remains as to why some HIV infected people develop dementia while others do not. Some people with high viral loads were not demented, while others with low viral loads had AIDS dementia. A study by Johnson and colleagues (1996) suggests that factors other than viral load lead to dementia. Investigators have found that this dementia is solely associated

ANTI-HIV DRUG THERAPY AND THE BLOOD–BRAIN BARRIER

Within the brain there are reservoirs of HIV within macrophage and microglia. However, the newer triple-drug combination therapies, which include protease inhibitors, are, in general, not capable of crossing the blood–brain barrier and eradicating infection in the central nervous system. Among these drugs, zidovudine alone may penetrate the brain to some degree, but its effects on the dramatic cognitive decline are manifest in about one-third of patients, who develop AIDS dementia, level off, or fail after about 3 months of treatment (Lipton, 1997).

with HIV infection and progression to AIDS. HIV-caused dementia has a unique set of clinical and pathological features. Some authorities estimate that 90% of AIDS patients in the terminal stages of the disease have AIDS Dementia Complex (ADC) (Hanley et al., 1988). Information presented by the National Institute of Allergy and Infectious Diseases in June 1989 indicated that **asymptomatic** HIV-infected persons **do not demonstrate mental impairment** (Figure 7-8). Therefore, the onset of mental impairment must begin sometime after the HIV-infected person becomes symptomatic (Update, 1989). Initially, investigators thought that OIs caused ADC, but it was later discovered that HIV is carried into the brain by HIV-infected macrophages.

Early Symptoms— Early symptoms of cognitive (quality of knowing or reasoning) dysfunction include forgetfulness, recent memory loss, loss of concentration and slowness of thought, social withdrawal, slurring of speech, loss of balance (inability to walk a straight line), deterioration of handwriting, and impaired motor function. An early diagnosis of ADC in AIDS patients is difficult because the early signs of neurological disease are very similar to those symptoms used to identify emotional depression. However, neurological symptoms may be the first sign of illness in about 10% of adult AIDS patients.

FIGURE 7-8 Central Nervous System Events after HIV Infection. Note that aseptic meningitis (an inflammation of the membrane of the brain and spinal cord in the absence of viral or bacterial infection), when it occurs, occurs early after HIV infection. Although usually apparent later, AIDS dementia complex may begin during the early–late phase. The late phase represents the period during which major AIDS-defining opportunistic infections occur. The headings acute, latent, early-late and late refer to periods after HIV infection. It appears that OI infection of the brain occurs after the onset of ADC. (*Adapted from Price et al., 1988*)

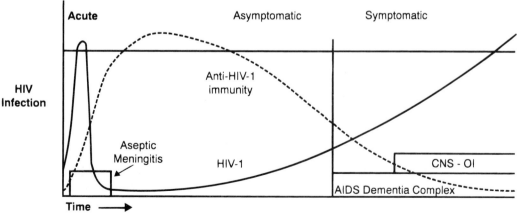

Late Symptoms— These symptoms are characterized by loss of speech, great fatigue, muscle weakness, bladder and bowel incontinence (loss of control), headache, seizures, coma, and finally death. About 95% of patients with ADC have HIV antibodies in their cerebral spinal fluid.

PEDIATRIC CLINICAL SIGNS AND SYMPTOMS

Currently over 90% of pediatric AIDS cases are newborns and infants who received HIV from mothers who were injection drug users or the sexual partners of IDUs. For those who become HIV-infected during gestation, clinical symptoms usually develop within 6 months after birth. Few children infected as fetuses live beyond 2 years and survival past 3 years used to be rare; but with better therapy for opportunistic diseases now available, some children born with HIV are still alive at 5, 10, and 12 years old.

The clinical course of rapid HIV disease progression in infants diagnosed with AIDS is marked by failure to thrive, persistent lymphadenopathy, chronic or recurrent oral candidiasis, persistent diarrhea, enlarged liver and spleen (hepatosplenomegaly), and chronic pneumonia (interstitial pneumonitis). Bacterial infections are common and can be life-threatening. Bacterial infection and **septicemia** (the presence of a variety of bacterial species in the bloodstream) was the leading cause of death in one group of affected infants in Florida. An excess of gamma globulin and depressed cell-mediated immunity and T cell function are frequently encountered.

Less than 25% of AIDS children express the kinds of OIs found in adult AIDS patients. Kaposi's sarcoma occurs in about 4% of them. Young AIDS children experience delayed development and poor motor function. Older AIDS children experience speech and perception problems.

SUMMARY

The clinical signs and symptoms of HIV infection and AIDS have been addressed in the previous chapters. However, there are two major classification systems used to diagnose patients as they progress from HIV infection to AIDS. The first is the Walter Reed System. It recog-

--------- BOX 7.5 ---------

LONG-TERM SURVIVORS AMONG HIV-INFECTED CHILDREN

Mark Kline (1995) reports that now, in the 1990s, many if not most HIV-infected children demonstrate relatively slow HIV disease progression. European studies suggest that 70% to 75% of children who truly were HIV-positive at birth survive to at least 5 years of age; 60% survive to age 10 or beyond (Italian Register for HIV Infection in Children, 1994; The European Collaborative Study, 1994). Investigators from the CDC Pediatric Spectrum of Disease Project recently reported an estimated mean survival time of 9.4 years for U.S. children born HIV-positive (Barnhart et al., 1995). The CDC study suggests that the average child is moderately or severely symptomatic for most of his or her expected life span. In a recently published study from New Jersey, 24 (57%) of 42 children over the age of 9 had a history of an AIDS-defining condition, and 33 (79%) children had moderate or severe immunologic compromise as reflected by T4 counts of 500/μL of blood or less (Grubman et al., 1995). Only 2 of 41 children over 5 years of age are asymptomatic and have no evidence of immunologic compromise. It is apparent that long-term survival with true nonprogression of disease is unusual among children born with HIV infection.

According to Susan Davis and co-workers (1995), from 1978 through 1993, approximately 14,920 children were born with vertically acquired HIV infection in the United States. Among these children, approximately 5,330 had developed AIDS and 2,680 had died. Thus, an estimated 12,240 children with vertically acquired HIV infection were alive at the beginning of 1994. More than half (56%) of these children had been born since 1988 and thus were younger than 5 years.

nizes six stages of signs and symptoms which a person passes through to AIDS. The CDC uses four groupings that identify the stage of illness from infection to AIDS. Both systems revolve around the recognition of a failing immune system, persistent swollen lymph nodes, and opportunistic infections. Mysteries still to be resolved are exactly why and how HIV attacks the body cells, and why some people stabilize after the initial symptoms of HIV infection while others move directly on to AIDS.

One disorder that was not immediately recognized in AIDS patients is AIDS dementia complex (ADC), a progressive mental deterioration due to HIV infection of the central nervous system. ADC develops in over 50% of adult AIDS patients prior to death. Research has shown that some of the symptoms of this dementia can be reversed with the use of the drug zidovudine.

REVIEW QUESTIONS

(*Answers to the Review Questions are on page 577.*)

1. Name the two major AIDS classification systems in use in the United States.

2. What percent of HIV-infected individuals will progress to AIDS in 5 years; in 15 years?

3. What is the neurological set of behavioral changes in AIDS patients called?

4. Name three body organs and their associated AIDS related diseases.

5. True or False: Currently the single most important laboratory parameter that is followed to monitor the progress of HIV- infection is the T4 cell count.

6. True or False: The average time from infection to seroconversion is 2 weeks. Explain.

7. True or False: Being infected with HIV and being diagnosed with AIDS are the same thing. Explain.

8. True or False: The average length of time from infection with HIV to an AIDS diagnosis is approximately 2 years.

REFERENCES

ABOULKER, JEAN-PIERRE, et al. (1993). Preliminary analysis of the concorde trial. *Lancet,* 341: 889–890.

ANDERSON, ROBERT E., et al. (1991). CD8 T lymphocytes and progression to AIDS in HIV-infected men: Some observations. *AIDS,* 5: 213–215.

BALTIMORE, DAVID. (1995). Lessons from people with non progressive HIV infection. *N. Engl. J. Med.,* 332:259–260.

BARNHART, HUIMAN, et al. (1995). *Abstracts of the 2nd National Conference on Human Retroviruses,* Washington, D.C., p. 161, abstr. 575.

BOLOGNESI, DANI P. (1989). Prospects for prevention of and early intervention against HIV. *JAMA,* 261:3007–3013.

BRYSON, YVONNE J., et al. (1995). Clearance of HIV infection in a prenatally infected infant. *N. Engl. J. Med.,* 332:833–838.

BUCHBINDER, SUSAN P., et al. (1992). Healthy long-term positives: Men infected with HIV for more than 10 years with CD4 counts of 500 cells. *Eighth International Conference on AIDS,* Amsterdam, July 1992, abstr. TUCO572.

BUCHBINDER, SUSAN P., et al. (1994). Long-term HIV infection without immunologic progression. *AIDS,* 8:1123–1128.

BURCHAM, JOYCE, et al. (1991). CD4 % is the best predictor of development of AIDS in a cohort of HIV-infected homosexual men. *AIDS,* 5:365–372.

CAO, YUNZHEN, et al. (1995). Virologic and immunologic characterization of long-term survivors of human immunodeficiency virus type 1 infection. *N. Engl. J. Med.,* 332:201–208.

CLERICI, MARIO, et al. (1994). HIV-specific T helper activity in seronegative health care workers exposed to contaminated Blood. *JAMA,* 271: 42–46.

COFFIN, JOHN M. (1995). HIV population dynamics in vivo: implications for genetic variation, pathogenesis and therapy. *Science,* 267: 483–489.

COHEN, JON. (1992). Searching for markers on the AIDS trail. *Science,* 258:387–390.

COHEN, JON. (1993). Keystone's blunt message: It's the virus stupid. *Science,* 260:292–293.

COHEN, JON. (1995). High turnover of HIV in blood revealed by new studies. *Science,* 267:179.

COHEN, JON. (1996). Results of new drugs bring cautious optimism. *Science,* 271: 755–756.

CONANT, MARCUS. (1995). The current face of the AIDS epidemic. *AIDS Newslink,* 6 (Fall):1–9.

COULIS, PAUL A., et al. (1987). Peptide-based immunodiagnosis of retrovirus infections. *Am. Clin. Prod. Rev.,* 6:34–43.

DAVIS, SUSAN, et al. (1995). Prevelance and incidence of vertically acquired HIV infection in the U.S.A. *JAMA,* 274:952–955.

DEACON, NICHOLAS, et al. (1995). Genomic structure of an attenuated quasi species of HIV from a blood transfusion donor and recipients. *Science,* 270:988–991.

ENSOLI, F., et al. (1990). Proviral sequences detection of human immunodeficiency virus in seronegative subjects by polymerase chain reaction. *Mol. Cell Probes,* 4:153–161.

ENSOLI, F., et al. (1991). Plasma viraemia in seronegative HIV-1 infected individuals. *AIDS,* 5:1195–1199.

ESCAICH, SONIA, et al. (1991). Plasma viraemia as a marker of viral replication in HIV-infected individuals. *AIDS,* 5:1189–1194.

FAUCI, ANTHONY S. (1988). The scientific agenda for AIDS. *Issues Sci. Technol.,* 4:33–42.

FREED, ERIC, et al. (1994). HIV infection of non-dividing cells. *Nature,* 369:107–108.

GRUBMAN, SAMUEL, et al. (1995). Older children and adolescents living with perinatally acquired HIV infection. *Pediatrics,* 95:657–663.

HANLEY, DANIEL F., et al. (1988). When to suspect viral encephalitis. *Patient Care,* 22:77–99.

HAYNES, BARTON, et al. (1996). Toward an understanding of the correlates of protective immunity to HIV infection. *Science,* 271:324–328.

HENRARD, DENIS, et al. (1995). Natural history of HIV cell-free viremia *JAMA,* 274:554–558.

HO, DAVID, et al. (1995). Rapid turnover of plasma virons and CD4 lymphocytes in HIV infection. *Nature,* 373:123–126.

HO, DAVID. (1996). HIV pathogenesis. *Improv. Manage. HIV Dis.,* 4:4–6.

HOLDEN, CONSTANCE. (1994). New tool for predicting AIDS onset. *Science,* 263:606.

HORSBURG, C.R., et al. (1989). Duration of HIV infection before detection of antibody. *Lancet,* ii:637–639.

IMAGAWA, D.T., et al. (1989). Human immunodeficiency virus type I infection in homosexual men who remain seronegative for prolonged periods. *N. Engl. J. Med.,* 320:1458–1462.

Italian Register for HIV Infection in Children. (1994). *Lancet,* 343:191–195.

JAPOUR, ANTHONY. (1995). Antiviral drug resistance: Clinical significance and implications for HIV pathogenesis. *AIDS Clin. Care,* 7:63–67.

JOHNSON, RICHARD, et al. (1996). Quantitation of human immunodeficiency virus in brains of demented and nondemented patients with acquired immunodeficiency syndrome. *Ann. Neurol.* 39:392–395.

KATZENSTEIN, TERESE, et al. (1996). Longitudinal Serum HIV RNA quantification: Correlation to viral phenotype at seroconversion and clinical outcome. *AIDS,* 10:167–173.

KELLY, MAUREEN, et al. (1991). Oral manifestations of human immunodeficiency virus infection. *Cutis,* 47:44–49.

KIRCHHOFF, FRANK, et al. (1995). Brief report: Absence of intact NEF sequences in a long-term survivor with nonprogressive HIV-1 infection. *N. Engl. J. Med.,* 332:228–232.

KLINE, MARK. (1995). Long-term survival in vertically acquired HIV infection. *AIDS Reader,* 5:153.

LAURENCE, JEFFREY. (1995). A primary care condition. *AIDS Reader,* 5:110–111.

LAURENCE, JEFFREY. (1996). Where do we go from here? *AIDS Reader,* 6:3–4; 36.

LEVY, JAY. (1995). HIV and long-term survival. *Int. AIDS Soc. USA,* 3:10–12.

LIPTON, STUART. (1997). Treating AIDS dementia. *Science,* 276:1629–1630.

MATHESON, PAMELA, et al. (1996). Heterosexual behavior during pregnancy and perinatal transmission of HIV. *AIDS,* 10:1249–1256.

McGUIRE, DAWN. (1993). Pathogenesis of brain injury in HIV disease. *Clin. Notes,* 7:1–11.

MERIGAN, THOMAS, et al. (1996). The prognostic significance of viral load, codon 215-reverse transcriptase mutation and CD4 + T cells on HIV Disease Progression. *AIDS,* 10:159–165.

Morbidity and Mortality Weekly Report. (1996). Persistent lack of detectable HIV-antibody in a person with HIV-infection—Utah, 1995. 45:181–185.

Morbidity and Mortality Weekly Report. (1997). Revised guidelines for performing CD4+ T-cell determinations in persons infected with HIV. 46:1–4.

NATIONAL INSTITUTE OF ALLEGY AND INFECTION DISEASES. (1989). Tests confirm lack of mental impairment in asymptomatic HIV-infected homosexual men. June:1–2.

NEWELL, MARIE, et al. (1996). Detection of virus in vertically exposed HIV-antibody-negative children. *Lancet,* 347:213–215.

NIELSON, CLAUS, et al. (1993). Biological properties of HIV isolates in primary HIV infection: Consequences for the subsequent course of infection. *AIDS,* 7:1035–1040.

NOWAK, M.A., et al. (1990). The evolutionary dynamics of HIV-1 quasispecies and the development of immunodeficiency disease. *AIDS,* 4:1095–1103.

PANTALEO, GUISEPPE, et al. (1993). The immunopathogenesis of HIV infection. *N. Engl. J. Med.,* 328:327–335.

PANTALEO, GUISEPPE, et al. (1995). Studies in subjects with long-term nonprogressive human immunodeficiency virus infection. *N. Engl. J. Med.,* 332:209–216.

PEDERSEN, C., et al. (1989). Clinical course of primary HIV infection: Consequences for subsequent course of infection. *Br. Med. J.,* 299:154–157.

PERELSON, ALAN, et al. (1996). HIV dynamics in vivo: Viron clearance rate, infected cell life-span and viral generation time. *Science*, 271: 1582–1586.

PHILLIPS, ANDREW N., et al. (1991a). p24 Antigenaemia, CD4 lymphocyte counts and the development of AIDS. *AIDS*, 5:1217–1222.

PHILLIPS, ANDREW N., et al. (1991b). Serial CD4 lymphocyte counts and development of AIDS. *Lancet*, 337:389–392.

PHILLIPS, ANDREW, et al. (1994). A sex comparison of rates of new AIDS-defining disease and death in 2554 AIDS cases. *AIDS* 8:831–835.

PRICE, RICHARD W. (1988). The brain in AIDS: Central nervous system HIV infection and AIDS dementia complex. *Science*, 239:586–593.

QUINN, THOMAS. (1997). Acute primary HIV infection. *JAMA*, 278:58–62.

RANKI, A., et al. (1987). Long latency precedes overt seroconversion in sexually transmitted human immunodeficiency virus infection. *Lancet*, ii:589–593.

RANKI, ANNAMARI, et al. (1995). Abundant expression of HIV NEF and Rev proteins in brain astrocytes *in vivo* is associated with dementia. *AIDS*, 9:1001–1008.

RICHMAN, DOUGLAS. (1995). Antiretroviral resistance and HIV dynamics. *Int. AIDS Soc.*, 3:15–16.

ROQUES, PIERRE, et al. (1995). Clearance of HIV infection in 12 perinatally infected children: Clinical, virological and immunological data. *AIDS*, 9:F19–F26.

ROSENBERG, PHILIP, et al. (1994). Declining age at HIV infection in the United States. *N. Engl. J. Med.*, 330:789–790.

ROYCE, RACHEL A., et al. (1991). The natural history of HIV-1 infection: Staging classifications of disease. *AIDS*, 5:355–364.

SALK, JONAS, et al. (1993). A strategy for prophylatic vaccination against HIV. *Science*, 260: 1270–1272.

SAX, PAUL, et al. (1995). Potential clinical implications of interlaboratory variability in CD4+ T-lymphocyte counts of patients infected with human immunodeficiency virus. *Clin. Infect. Dis.*, 21:1121–1125.

SHERNOFF, MICHAEL. (1997). A history of hope: the HIV roller coaster. *Focus*, 12: 5–7.

STRAMER, SUSAN L., et al. (1989). Markers of HIV infection prior to IgG antibody seropositivity. *JAMA*, 262:64–69.

THE EUROPEAN COLLABORATIVE STUDY. (1994). *Pediatrics*, 94:815–819.

VOELKER, REBECCA. (1995). New studies say viral burden tops CD4 as a marker of HIV-disease progression. *JAMA*, 275:421–422.

WAIN-HOBSON, SIMON. (1995). Virological mayhem. *Nature*, 373:102.

WEI, XIPING, et al. (1995). Viral dynamics in HIV type 1 infection. *Nature*, 373:117–122.

Transmission of HIV: High-, Moderate-, and Low-Risk Behaviors

CHAPTER CONCEPTS

♦ In 1985, HIV-2 was isolated in West Africa.

♦ Transmission of HIV into the United States may have been via Haiti.

♦ Lifestyle is associated with HIV transmission.

♦ HIV is not casually transmitted.

♦ HIV is not transmitted to humans by insects.

♦ HIV transmission is being reported from 194 countries and among all age and ethnic groups.

♦ The major route of HIV transmission involves an exchange of body fluids.

♦ The body fluids involved in HIV transmission are exchanged during sexual activities, injection drug use, blood transfusions, use of blood products and during pre- and postnatal events.

♦ First documented case of HIV transmission via deep kissing.

♦ Highest frequency of HIV transmission in the United States is among homosexual and bisexual males and among injection drug users.

♦ Bloodbanks in several countries knowingly allowed the distribution of HIV-contaminated blood.

♦ Should HIV infected athletes be allowed to compete?

♦ Death due to HIV infection is placed in perspective.

♦ Interactions between HIV and STDs are discussed.

♦ National AIDS Resources phone numbers are listed.

♦ Highest frequency of HIV transmission in Africa is among heterosexuals.

♦ Prenatal HIV transmission generally occurs after the 12th to 16th week of gestation, most often during childbirth.

♦ Zidovudine decreases perinatal HIV transmission.

When a population becomes infected with a contagious disease, an epidemic results. **Epidemic** is derived from Greek and means "in one place among the people." To understand how an infectious disease can spread or remain established in a population, investigators must consider the relationship between an infectious disease agent and its host population. The study of diseases in populations is an area of medicine known as **epidemiology**.

We learned from earlier epidemics, the danger of complacency. Complacency about HIV infection is especially dangerous because the infection can remain hidden for years. Because many infected people remain symptom-free for years, it is hard to be sure just who is infected with the virus. The more sexual partners you have, the greater your chances of encountering one who is infected and subsequently becoming infected yourself.

With regard to HIV infection, it is your behavior that counts. **The transmission of HIV can be prevented. HIV is relatively hard to contract and can be avoided.** HIV is a communicable disease in a limited sense. A communicable disease is one in which the causative agent passes from one person to another. The modes of transmission for communicable diseases include: direct contact with body fluids, contact with inanimate objects, and contact with vectors, including flies, mosquitoes, or other insects capable of spreading disease. HIV is communicable only in the first of the three modes, that is, through direct contact with certain body fluids. HIV is transmitted in human body fluids by **three** major routes: (**1**) sexual intercourse through vaginal, rectal, or penile tissues; (**2**) direct injection with HIV-contaminated drugs, needles, syringes, blood or blood products; and (**3**) from HIV-infected mother to fetus in utero, through intrapartum inoculation from mother to infant or during breast-feeding.

Epidemiological data suggest that **sexual transmission, in general, is relatively inefficient, in that exposure often does not produce infection.** HIV is transmitted more efficiently through intravenous than through sexual routes. However, worldwide the predominant mode of transmission of HIV is through exposure of mucosal surfaces to infected sexual fluids (semen, cervical/vaginal, rectal) and during birth.

HIV is not communicable through contact with inanimate objects or through vectors. Thus people do not "catch" HIV in the same way that they "catch" the cold or a flu virus. Unlike colds and flu viruses, HIV **is not**, according to the CDC, spread by tears, sweat, coughing or sneezing. The virus **is not** transmitted via an infected person's clothes, phone or toilet seat. HIV **is not** passed on by eating utensils, drinking glasses, or other objects that HIV-infected people have used that are free of blood.

HIV **is not** transmitted through daily contact with infected people, whether at work, home, or school. Insects do not transmit the virus. Kissing is also considered very low risk: There has never been a documented case to prove that HIV is transmitted by kissing. However, Paul Holmstrom and colleagues (1992) report that salivary HIV antibodies are detected regularly in HIV seropositive subjects. This suggests that these antibodies neutralize HIV producing the negative results of HIV cultivation or antigen detection in the saliva. The route of HIV into saliva is not fully understood. Both salivary glands and salivary leukocytes have been shown to harbor HIV. Gingival fluid, which is a transudate of serum, has been regarded as the main source of salivary HIV antibodies and infectious HIV.

In its 1990 supplemental guidelines for cardiopulmonary resuscitation (CPR) training and rescue, the Emergency Cardiac Care Committee of the American Heart Association (AHA) noted that there is an extremely small theoretical risk of HIV or hepatitis B virus (HBV) transmission via cardiopulmonary resuscitation (CPR). No known case of seroconversion for HIV or HBV has occurred in these circumstances.

WE MUST STOP HIV TRANSMISSION NOW!

We are standing at a moment in the AIDS epidemic when we have what may be our last opportunity to stem a major new wave of HIV infection of heterosexuals and in particular minorities in the urban areas, and of gay men and drug users in the smaller cities and suburban and rural areas where infection is currently of less intensity. Stephen Joseph, Commissioner of Health of New York City from 1986 to 1990, states that 10% to 15% of reproductive age men and women in poor minority neighborhoods will be infected. This of course will lead to the birth of a steady stream of HIV-infected infants and the orphaning of a steady stream

HIV/AIDS CAN BE STOPPED NOW!

Some HIV/AIDS experts now believe that the AIDS epidemic in America can be all but stamped out, without a vaccine or wonder drug. The strategy would involve concentrating on prevention of risky behavior that is particularly prevalent in 25 to 30 neighborhoods nationwide, in such cities as New York, Miami, Los Angeles, San Francisco, Houston, Newark, and Camden, New Jersey. Among the measures on which public health officials want to concentrate in those neighborhoods are some that many conservatives oppose, including free distribution of clean hypodermic needles, many more drug treatment programs, and explicit sex education adapted to the language and mores of affected neighborhoods. For example, a medical anthropologist at Montefiore Medical Center in the Bronx told of a recent examination that revealed that a patient had been engaging in anal sex. But when the doctor asked him if he had ever had sex with another man, he repeatedly said no. Finally, at the end of the interview, the doctor asked him, "Has another man's penis ever touched your anus?" The man replied, "Oh yeah, all the time." This man practiced anal sex as a trade, for a living; he was homeless. Sex, for him, he said, was something you did with a woman.

Once the controversial idea of stopping HIV/AIDS was proposed, persons of various disciplines immediately began voicing their support or opposition to the idea that the HIV/AIDS epidemic in the United States can be stopped NOW! The following are items of interest both pro and con. After reading both points of view, formulate your own.

PRO:

As Stephen Joseph writes in his book, *Dragon Within the Gates: The Once and Future AIDS Epidemic,* an epidemic requires not only a microbe but also an appropriate social context. HIV/AIDS has found both contexts in the United States: the artistic, cultural, and fashion enterprises and large numbers of gay men. In the late 1980s came the great epidemiological shift away from gay white males and toward minority heterosexuals and needle-sharing injection drug users and their sexual partners. AIDS, like lung cancer, coronary artery disease, and motor vehicle accidents, is a characteristic 20th century epidemic: It is closely related to current behavior—related, in

fact, to voluntary, conscious, and intimate behavior, involving sex and drugs. And much of the high-risk behavior is highly concentrated in a few small areas. Because AIDS in America has been associated with stigmatized and illegal behavior, and has been concentrated among marginalized groups—homosexuals and inner-city poor—that feel vulnerable to oppression, there has been a concerted effort to "democratize" the disease. The politically correct message is that everyone is vulnerable—"AIDS does not discriminate." And there has been resistance to targeting the risky behavior of particular groups, groups that tend to be concentrated in given geographical areas of the United States.

Gina Kolata (*New York Times,* March 7, 1993) quotes Don Des Jarlais (day-zhar-lay), a drug-abuse specialist and AIDS researcher at Beth Israel Medical Center in New York, "We could stamp AIDS out. I think that's a realistic goal."

Other experts from a variety of disciplines are also arguing that AIDS can be stopped. They cite two reasons: the pattern of AIDS's spread and the success of programs that have focused tightly on affected groups and neighborhoods.

Their view of the disease's pattern of spread has emerged from a recent analysis by a committee of the National Research Council that suggests AIDS is devastating a handful of neighborhoods while leaving most of the nation relatively unscathed.

In its report, "The Social Impact of AIDS," released in February 1993, the council said the epidemic was "settling into spatially and socially isolated groups and possibly becoming endemic in them." As a result, the committee wrote, "many geographic areas and strata of the population are virtually untouched by the epidemic and probably never will be," while "certain confined areas and populations have been devastated."

The second reason for a new approach is that data now emerging, mostly from abroad, show it is possible to reverse the course of an AIDS epidemic or even to prevent one if efforts are intense and narrowly focused. Such efforts have succeeded even among supposedly recalcitrant populations like injection drug users.

Australia, for example, has managed to control the rate of new infection in the last 5 years by targeting high-risk groups. And Tacoma, Washington, has kept its HIV infection rates among injection drug users negligible while rates in New York and other cities have soared to between 50% and 80%. To this end, Allan Brandt of Harvard University states, "If we want to really deal with the epidemic, we have to go where the epidemic is."

Until recently, health officials in Russia performed some 24 million HIV tests a year on pregnant women, hospital patients, soldiers, and just about anyone else. The result: Between 1990 and the end of 1993, 338 people tested positive. It's a similar story throughout much of the former eastern bloc. Out of almost 100,000 AIDS cases so far reported across Europe, only 3.4% are from the continent's eastern half, and some countries—including Azerbaijan, Kazakhstan, Tajikistan, and Albania—have yet to diagnose their first AIDS case. The AIDS virus was not rapidly spread under communism.

A big question facing these countries now is whether the virus can continue to be kept at bay in the wake of the social liberalization and increase in foreign travel that are following the collapse of the old, repressive regimes. The guarded answer from officials at the World Health Organization (WHO) is: Yes, at least in theory. They calculate that the epidemic in eastern Europe and the former Soviet Union is lagging 5 years behind that in the West—just enough time, they argue, to mount an effective anti-HIV effort. Eastern Europe is one of the few parts of the world where it may be possible to stop the virus in its tracks. "These countries have a good chance," says Johannes Hallauer, European coordinator for WHO's Global Program on AIDS, "because it is early enough to prevent a big spread of the virus" (Balter, 1993).

Albert Jonsen, an ethics professor at the University of Washington and the chairman of the National Research Council's Committee on AIDS believes that epidemics throughout history have behaved in a pattern similar to that of HIV/AIDS. "The thing that leaps out at you is the way that almost every historical epidemic was socially-culturally determined." People were not felled indiscriminately.

A second feature of epidemics is that they require a concentration of cases to sustain the disease. In the case of AIDS, if you are going to have sexual transmission outside of infected communities, you need a fairly high rate of contact. The disease can and does break out of the tight communities where it festers, but it cannot sustain itself there.

In concluding the PRO discussion, Jeff Stryker and Ronald Bayer (1933), both members of NRC, believe that if the people of the United States come to believe that AIDS no longer threatens every hamlet and every citizen, political support for AIDS prevention and research might be eroded. Those who agree with this idea believe that focusing on "the universality of risk among all people" helps meet the need of the truly vulnerable (Stryker et al., 1993). Stryker and Bayer believe the time is ripe for new leadership in the fight against AIDS.

The rethinking they propose involves asking some hard questions. Does current AIDS prevention policy in the United States suffer because of a scattershot approach divorced from epidemiological reality? Would a more targeted approach place those outside the current epicenters of HIV infection at risk? Would such an approach to prevention foster stigmatization, possibly weakening the delicate political alliance that currently supports HIV prevention and research?

CON: The Opposing Force

The contention that AIDS is sustained by a small number of epicenters is unrealistic. The opposing force counters that it is, in fact, very unwise to focus prevention efforts on a relatively small number of neighborhoods at the expense of those with fewer AIDS cases. They emphasize that everyone needs help and should be assured of receiving it. June Osborn, chairwoman of the National Commission of AIDS, states that, "AIDS sustains itself awfully well. As soon as the virus is present, as it now is everywhere, risk-taking behavior becomes significant."

Osborn takes issue with the very notion of targeting a few areas: "It is much too broad a brush to say, 'Focus your money in some areas, and everyone else can forget it.' Nobody can forget it. The AIDS epidemic is very rapidly spreading throughout smaller and smaller communities each year." Still others warn that the strategy of focusing on a few target areas could threaten and offend the very groups it is meant to help. There is a real concern among many people that public discussions of HIV and AIDS as a problem among minorities will further stigmatize them without necessarily leading to an allocation of resources to help correct the problem.

Osborn and colleague David Rogers (1993) state that the NRC report "subtly encouraged the virus spread through all segments of society" and feel it is a "cruel influence" and "painful setback [for] responsible public policy."

Another point of view is that if this idea had been tried early on it might have worked—if one could possibly have gotten around the charges of racial discrimination. But it is too late, the horse is out of the barn.

Class Discussion:

What do you think? Is it too late? Has the horse left the barn? Can the barn still be locked up?

Can charges of discrimination be justly filed if large sums of money and medical personnel were assigned to those areas with the largest concentration of AIDS cases while the lower incidence areas were left to a lower level of support?

of older uninfected children as mothers and fathers die of AIDS. To get a sense of the magnitude of the AIDS orphan problem, consider the following: New York City will have 10,000 to 20,000 of these children by the late 1990s (Josephs, 1993). World wide there will be 10 million orphans by the year 2000.

Education and advocacy for risk reduction remain important tools for preventing HIV infection, but, alone, they will never accomplish the objective of slowing the speed and extent of the virus's spread. This can only be achieved by combining educational and early intervention efforts with specific measures guiding those resources to the people who need them most: those who are already infected and to their sex and drug partners.

Beginning 1998, there were about 650,000 AIDS cases in the United States. Figure 8-1 breaks this number down according to means of HIV infection that is, sexual behavior, drug use, medical exigencies, and undetermined causes. Figure 8–2 gives a breakdown by transmission category for 61,300 AIDS cases reported for 1997. An estimated 57,500 AIDS cases will be reported for 1998. There were 69,151 AIDS cases for 1996 and 74,180 for 1995.

EPIDEMIOLOGY OF HIV INFECTION

The first scientific evidence of human HIV infection came from the detection of HIV antibodies in preserved serum samples collected in Central Africa in 1959. The first AIDS cases appeared there in the 1960s. By the mid-1970s

FIGURE 8-1 AIDS Cases by Route of Transmission. Beginning 1998, there were about 650,000 AIDS cases in the United States. By the end of 1998 there will be about 710,000 AIDS cases. This diagram gives the percentage of adults and adolescents in each group for 1997. Groupings are according to sexual preference, drug use, medical conditions, and others not associated with any of these. (*Courtesy of CDC,* Atlanta)

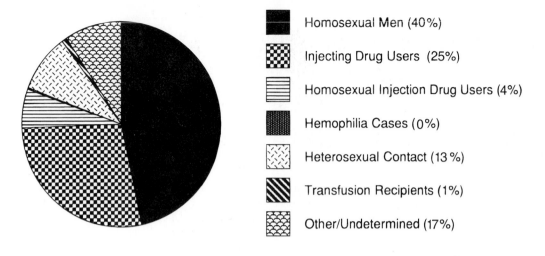

Homosexual Men (40%)

Injecting Drug Users (25%)

Homosexual Injection Drug Users (4%)

Hemophilia Cases (0%)

Heterosexual Contact (13%)

Transfusion Recipients (1%)

Other/Undetermined (17%)

Total Cases 69,151   (Courtesy CDC, Atlanta)

FIGURE 8-2   Adult/Adolescent AIDS Cases by Transmission Category Reported for 1996 , United States. Reported for 1995, 74,180. (Pediatric, for 1996, 678)

HIV was being spread throughout the rest of the world. The earliest places to experience the arrival of HIV were Central Europe and Haiti. Transmission into the United States may have been by tourists who had vacationed in the area of Port-au-Prince, Haiti (Swenson, 1988).

On entry into the United States the virus first spread among the homosexual populations of large cities such as New York and San Francisco. The first **recorded** AIDS cases in the United States occurred in 1979 in New York. The first CDC **reported** AIDS cases were in New York, Los Angeles, and San Francisco in 1981 (Figure 8-3). In both cases, the diagnosis of AIDS was based on clinical descriptions.

─────── **POINT OF INFORMATION 8.1** ───────

CONSEQUENCES OF IGNORING HIV

You may be offended by the description of how HIV is transmitted. You may feel invulnerable to HIV infection. You may think that given time, HIV infection and AIDS will go away. You may choose to ignore that it exists. **But ignoring HIV may kill you.** The cost of ignorance about any of the STDs is always high, but with AIDS the cost is a disfiguring, painful death.

According to the CDCs first clinical AIDS definition, at least one case of AIDS occurred in New York City in 1952 and another in 1959. Both males demonstrated opportunistic infections and *Pneumocystis carinii* pneumonia, today a hallmark of HIV infection. This early evidence of AIDS suggests that the virus might have been in the United States, Europe and Africa at about the same time (Katner et al., 1987). If HIV has been present for decades as suggested, its failure to spread may reflect a recent HIV mutation, a major change in social behaviors conducive to HIV transmission, or both. For example, the sexual revolution and the widespread use of birth control pills, which began in the 1960s, and the subsequent decrease in the use of condoms may be involved with the transmission of HIV.

TRANSMISSION OF TWO STRAINS OF HIV (HIV-1/HIV-2)

The spread of HIV-1 is global. The clinical presentation of AIDS caused by HIV-1 is similar regardless of geographical area.

HIV-2 is a genetically similar but distinct strain. HIV-2 was first discovered in 1985 in West Africa. It is believed to have been present

The Spread of AIDS

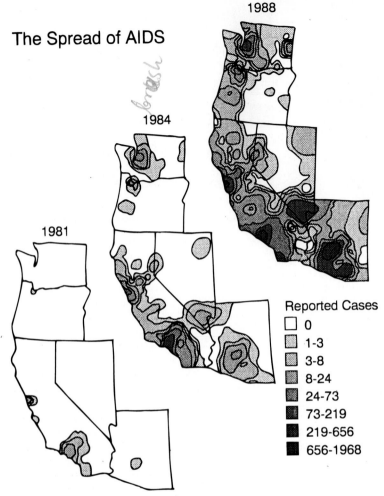

FIGURE 8-3 The Spread of HIV/AIDS on the West Coast. The three separate maps show the rapid spread of AIDS along the Pacific Coast from 1981 through 1988. The maps depict a movement from urban centers into the suburbs and surrounding rural areas. The AIDS epidemic in the West first appeared in Los Angeles and San Francisco, followed by Las Vegas and Phoenix. By 1983, Seattle and Portland encountered the epidemic. The number of AIDS cases continues to increase as HIV infection continues to spread. (*Courtesy of Peter Gould and colleagues, Pennsylvania State University*)

Reported Cases

- ☐ 0
- 1-3
- 3-8
- 8-24
- 24-73
- 73-219
- 219-656
- 656-1968

in West Africa as early as the 1960s. Clinical data demonstrate that HIV-2 has a reduced virulence compared to HIV-1 (Marlink et al., 1994).

What appears certain is that HIV-2, like HIV-1, will spread worldwide. HIV-2 has already spread from West Africa to other parts of Africa, Europe, and the Americas. Both HIV-1 and HIV-2 are transmitted or acquired through the same kinds of exposure.

(Because over 99% of global AIDS cases are caused by the transmission of HIV-1, only data that pertain to HIV-1 (HIV) will be presented unless otherwise stated.)

IS HIV TRANSMITTED BY INSECTS?

In spite of convincing evidence of the ways in which HIV can be transmitted, it remains difficult for the general public to believe that a virus that appears to spread as rapidly as HIV is not either highly contagious or transmitted by an environmental agent. After all, there are many viral and bacterial diseases that are either highly contagious or transmitted by insects. The question was asked: Is this virus being transmitted by insects?

Necessary data to resolve the question were

available. Epidemiological data from Africa and the United States suggested that AIDS was not transmitted by insect bites. If it were, many more cases would be expected among school-age children and elderly people, groups that are proportionally underrepresented among AIDS patients. In one study of the household contacts of AIDS patients in Kinshasa, Zaire, where insect bites are common, not a single child over the age of 1 year had been infected with the AIDS virus, while more than 60% of spouses had become infected.

In 1987, the Office of Technology Assessment (OTA) published a detailed paper on the question of whether blood-sucking insects such as biting flies, mosquitoes, and bedbugs transmit HIV (Miike, 1987). The conclusion was that the conditions necessary for successful transmission of HIV through insect bites and the probability of their occurring rule out the possibility of insect transmission as a significant factor in the spread of AIDS. Jerome Goddard reported (1997) that blood-sucking arthropods (e.g., **mosquitoes** and **bedbugs**) for good biological reasons, **can not** transmit HIV. The virus has to overcome many obstacles. It must avoid digestion in the gut of the insect, recognize receptors on the external surface of the gut, penetrate the gut, replicate in insect tissue, recognize and penetrate the insect salivary glands, and subsequently escape into the lumen of the salivary duct. Webb and colleagues (1989) inoculated bedbugs intraabdominally (belly) and mosquitoes intrathoracically (chest) with HIV to enable the virus to bypass gut barriers. The virus failed to replicate in either potential carrier.

EXPOSURE TO HIV AND SUBSEQUENT INFECTION

Early on, it was believed that certain aspects of one's lifestyle and medical status predetermined the risk of HIV infection upon HIV exposure. For example, if the HIV-exposed individual had some previous sexually transmitted disease or an open sore, used drugs, or had an already weakened immune system, he or she would be more susceptible to HIV infection. Such conditions are called **cofactors**. (See Chapter 5 for a discussion on cofactors.)

TRANSMISSION OF HIV

If most HIV-exposed people can become HIV-infected, can most infected people **transmit** HIV to others? This is a difficult question to answer. Infection with HIV appears to depend on a large number of variables that involve the donor, recipient, and portal of entry. The most important variables are mode of transmission, viral load, which subtype and variant of HIV is present, and the recipient's genetic resistance.

CASUAL TRANSMISSION

There is overwhelming evidence that **HIV is not transmitted casually**. Assurances that HIV is not spread through casual contact are based on observation of health care workers and family members of AIDS patients. These individuals have much closer contact with AIDS patients and their body fluids than the average person would in a social, educational, or occupational setting. Thus, if HIV could be transmitted through casual contact, it would be found in much larger numbers of health care workers.

Several studies of the family members of AIDS patients have failed to demonstrate the spread of the HIV through household contact. The only cases in which family members have become infected involved the sexual partners of AIDS patients or children born to mothers who were already infected with the virus. Even individuals who bathed, diapered, or slept in the same bed with AIDS patients have not become infected. In one study, 7% of the family members shared toothbrushes with the infected person and none became infected.

Perhaps the best evidence against casual HIV transmission comes from studies of household members living with blood-transfused AIDS patients (Peterman et al., 1988). Transfusion infection cases are unique because their dates of infection are known retrospectively. Prior to the onset of AIDS symptoms, the families were unaware that they were living with HIV-infected individuals. Family life was not altered in any way, yet family members remained uninfected. In some cases, the transfusion patients were hemophiliacs who received weekly or monthly injections of blood products and became HIV-infected. From the combined studies of these households, only the sexual partners of infected hemophiliacs became infected. In some cases, the sexual partners of hemophiliacs remained HIV free after 3 to 5 years of unprotected sexual intercourse.

HIV TRANSMISSION IN HOUSEHOLD SETTINGS

Although contact with blood and other body substances can occur in households, transmission of HIV is rare in this setting. Through 1997, at least eight reports have described household transmission of HIV not associated with sexual contact, injection drug use, or breast feeding (Table 8-1). Of these eight reports, five were associated with documented or probable blood contact. In one report, HIV infection was diagnosed in a boy after his younger brother had died as the result of AIDS; however, a specific mechanism of transmission was not determined.

Home Nursing Exposure

Three reports involved home nursing care of terminally ill persons with AIDS in which a blood exposure might have occurred but was not documented; in these reports, skin contact with body secretions and excretions occured.

In another reported case in the United States, a mother apparently became infected with HIV as a result of extensive, unprotected exposure to her infected child's blood, body secretions, and excretions. The child, who underwent numerous surgical procedures to correct a congenital intestinal abnormality, had become infected through multiple blood transfusions. The mother did not wear gloves when performing procedures such as drawing blood, removing intravenous lines, emptying ostomy bags, changing diapers, and changing surgical dressings. On numerous occasions her hands became contaminated with blood, feces, saliva, and nasal secretions. Although she reported no accidental needlesticks or open wounds on her hands, she often failed to wash her hands immediately after such exposures.

In a similar case, a woman in England developed AIDS after caring for a man who died of AIDS. Again, the care involved frequent contact with body secretions and excretions. The woman reported that she had some small cuts and eczema on her hands during the time that she cared for the man.

HOME CARE PREVENTION

Because of the social, economic, and medical benefits of home care, the number of persons with AIDS who receive health care outside of hospitals is increasing. Persons infected with HIV and persons providing home care for those who are HIV-infected should be fully educated and trained regarding appropriate infection control techniques. In addition, health care providers should be aware of the potential for HIV transmission in the home and should provide training and education in infection control for HIV-infected persons and those who live or provide care to them in the home. Such training should be an intergral and ongoing part of the health care plan for every person with HIV infection.

The findings of the investigations described in Table 8-1 indicate the transmission of HIV as the result of contact with blood or other body secretions or excretions from an HIV-infected person in the household.

Additional infection control recommendations are contained in a recently updated brochure published by CDC, *Caring for Someone with AIDS: Information for Friends, Relatives, Household Members, and Others Who Care for a Person with AIDS at Home.* This brochure is available free in English or Spanish from the CDC National AIDS Clearinghouse, P.O. Box 6003, Rockville, MD 20849–6003; Telephone (800) 458–5231 or (301) 217–0023. (*MMWR,* 1994)

Living in the Same Household

In December 1993, investigators found two cases in which HIV was transmitted from one child and one adolescent to others but not by the usual routes.

One case involved two New Jersey boys, whose ages were given only as between 2

Case-Patient	Source-Patient	Activity During Which Transmission May Have Occured	Type of Exposure	Body Substance Through Which Transmission May Have Occured	HIV DNA Sequence Match	Comment
Mother	Child	Home nursing	Cutaneous	Blood/stool	ND[a]	Mother provided extensive care without gloves (e.g., drawing blood, removing intravenous catheters, and emptying and changing ostomy bags).
Child	Child	Home intravenous therapy for hemophilia	Possible intravenous percutaneous[2]	Blood	Y	Mother administered intravenous therapy to both children in succession and placed used needles in bag within reach of case-patient.
Child	Child	Living in same household	Cutaneous[2]	Blood	Y	Source-patient had frequent bleeding; case-patient had excoriated rash.
Adolescent	Adolescent	living in same household	Cutaneous/percutaneous	Blood	Y	Case-patient and source-patient shared a razor; each cut himself while shaving with the razor and bled as a result. Both have hemophilia.
Child	Mother	Living in same household	Cutaneous	Blood/exudate	Y	Source-patient had drained skin lesions; source-patient picked at case-patient's scabs.
Child	Child	Living in same household	Bite[b]	Not specified	ND	Source-patient bit case-patient, skin was not broken, and there was no bleeding. Details of home care not reported.
Adult	Adult	Home nursing	Cutaneous	Body secretions and excretions, including urine and saliva	ND	Case-patient wore no gloves while caring for source-patient; case-patient had eczema and small cuts on her hands.
Mother	Adult son	Home nursing	Cutaneous	Body secretions and excretions, including urine and feces	ND	Case-patient usually wore gloves.

[a]Not done.
[b]No definite exposure documented.
(Source: *MMWR*,1994a-updated)

and 5. The other involved two teenage brothers who are hemophiliacs.

In the New Jersey case, the older, infected child had frequent nosebleeds, and the younger child had dermatitis, a condition that can break the surface of the skin.

The brothers with hemophilia shared a razor on one occasion. They told investigators that they did not know who used the razor first. Each had his own injection equipment to deliver the drug needed to prevent uncontrolled bleeding.

In August of 1994, There was a single report of HIV being transmitted during a bloody fight (Ippolito et al., 1994). Two brothers had a severe fight. Brother (1) had been diagnosed with AIDS. Brother (2) beat (1) until blood from (1) flowed freely from both sides of his face. Brother (2) reported that blood from (1) came into contact with his mucosal surfaces of his eyes and lips. Brother (2) developed mononucleosis symptoms and tested positive 30 days after the fight. Brother (2) denied contact with needles used by his brother, or sharing of razors, toothbrushes, manicure scissors, or a common sexual partner. Tests for other bloodborne and sexually transmitted diseases were negative. HIV isolated from both brothers showed the same pattern of mutations associated with resistance to zidovudine (ZDV) even though only brother (1) had taken the drug.

Since transmission in such a manner has rarely, if ever, been documented, these cases are of special interest to scientists. But these two cases are not cause for alarm and are not cause for changing CDC recommended guidelines for allowing HIV-infected children to attend schools.

The exposures in these nine cases are not typical of the household or social contact most people would have with an HIV-infected or AIDS patient. Nevertheless, they underline the need for observance of commonsense sanitary precautions when caring for an AIDS patient.

NONCASUAL TRANSMISSION

The routes of HIV transmission were established **before** the virus was identified. The appearance of AIDS in the United States occurred first in specific groups of people: homosexual men and injection drug users. The transmission of the disease within the two groups appeared to be closely associated with sexual behavior and the sharing of IV needles. By 1982, hemophiliacs receiving blood products, as well as the newborns of injection drug

users, began demonstrating AIDS. By 1983, heterosexual female partners of AIDS patients demonstrated AIDS. **Sixteen years** of continued surveillance of the general population has failed to reveal other categories of people contracting HIV/AIDS (Table 8-2). It became apparent that the infectious agent was being transmitted within specific groups of people, who by their behavior were at increased risk for acquiring and transmitting it (Table 8-3). Clearly, an exchange of body fluids was involved in the transmission of the disease.

With the announcement that a new virus had been discovered, further research showed that this virus was present in most body fluids. Thus, even before there was a test to detect this virus, the public was told that it was transmitted through body fluids exchanged during intimate sexual contact, contaminated hypodermic needles, contaminated blood or blood products, and from mother to fetus. In addition it was concluded that the widespread dissemination of the virus was most likely the result of multiple or repeated viral exposure because the data from transfusion-infected individuals indicated that they did not necessarily infect their sexual partners. In other words, it was con-

TABLE 8-2   HIV Transmission and Infection

TRANSMISSION ROUTES

Blood Inoculation

Transfusion of HIV-infected blood and blood products
Needle sharing among injection drug users
Needlesticks, open cuts, and mucous membrane exposure in health care workers
Use of HIV-contaminated skin-piercing instruments (ears, acupuncture, tattoos)
Injection with unsterilized syringe and needle (mostly in Africa)

Sexual Contact: Exchange of semen, vaginal fluids, or blood

Homosexual, between men
Lesbian, between women
Heterosexual, from men to women and women to men
Bisexual men

Perinatal

Intrauterine
Peripartum (during birth)
Breast feeding

(Adapted from Friedland et al., 1987)

TABLE 8-3 Adult/Adolescent AIDS Cases by Sex and Exposure Categories, through June 1997, United States[a]

Male Exposure Category (85%)	Total No.	(%)
1. Men who have sex with men	298,699	(58)
2. Injecting drug use	113,635	(22)
3. Men who have sex with men and inject drugs	38,932	(8)
4. Hemophilia/coagulation disorder	4,378	(1)
5. Heterosexual contact:	18,811	(4)
a. Sex with injecting drug user	6,906	
b. Sex with person with hemophilia	44	
c. Sex with transfusion recipient with HIV infection	342	
d. Sex with HIV-infected person, risk not specified	11,519	
6. Receipt of blood transfusion, blood components, or tissue	4,634	(1)
7. Other/undetermined	32,858	(6)
Total male AIDS cases	511,934	(100)

Female Exposure Category (15%)		
1. Injecting drug use	41,029	(44)
2. Hemophilia/coagulation disorder	189	(0)
3. Heterosexual contact:	35,760	(39)
a. Sex with injecting drug user	15,984	
b. Sex with bisexual male	2,768	
c. Sex with person with hemophilia	346	
d. Sex with transfusion recipient with HIV infection	525	
e. Sex with HIV-infected person, risk not specified	16,137	
4. Receipt of blood transfusion, blood components, or tissue	3,441	(4)
5. Other/undetermined	11,823	(13)
Total female AIDS cases	92,242	(100)
Total cases	**604,176**	

[a]Pediatric cases, 7,902.

TABLE 8-4 How HIV is Transmitted Worldwide, 1997

Exposure	Efficiency, %	% of Total
Blood transfusion/blood products	>90	3
Perinatal	20–40	9
Sexual intercourse[a]	0.1–1.0	80
Injection drug use	0.5–1.0	8

[a]Heterosexual intercourse 70%
(Source: WHO/Global Programme on AIDS and UNAIDS, 1997)

stage of the HIV/AIDS epidemic, for example, the route of the virus could be associated with mobility.

The first HIV-infected people in some Latin American and European countries reported a history of foreign travel. In some African countries, spread of the virus could be traced along international roads. Today, increasing numbers of HIV infection have been observed to be associated with the relaxation of travel restrictions in Central and Eastern Europe.

Few countries are **unaffected** by HIV/AIDS. This has made it clear that restrictive measures such as refusal of entry to people living with HIV/AIDS and compulsory testing of mobile populations are inappropriate and ineffective measures to stop spread of the virus. In times of increasing international interdependency, it is an illusion to think that the disease can be stopped at any border (see related information in Point of Information 8.2).

TABLE 8-5 An Approximation of How 612,078 Americans Become Infected with HIV, June 1997

55	health care workers got infected from the blood or body fluids of patients;
7,902	children infected through their mothers;
12,852	people got HIV from infected blood or blood products;
42,840	people did not know how they were infected, did not report their risk, or died before anyone could find out;
37,211	people were infected who had both unprotected sex and shared needles;
153,000	people were infected who shared needles;
358,218	people were infected through unprotected sex.

(Based on data from HIV/AIDS Surv. Rpt, CDC, Mid-Year Edition, 1997)

cluded early on and later confirmed that this viral infection did not occur as easily as other blood-borne viral diseases such as hepatitis B, or viral and bacterial sexually transmitted diseases. Table 8-4 lists the means of HIV transmission worldwide. Table 8-5 lists the means of HIV transmission in the United States.

Mobility and the Spread of HIV/AIDS

Mobility is an important epidemiological factor in the spread of communicable diseases. This becomes particularly obvious when a new disease enters the scene. In the early

AIDS AND IMMIGRATION

Time magazine reported (February 1993) the results of a telephone poll of 1,000 American adults. The question was: Should the United States allow foreigners who have the AIDS virus to enter [the USA]? Twenty-two percent said yes, 71% said no.

In 1992, the National Commission on AIDS urged the Clinton Administration to scrap the continued prohibition against HIV-infected foreigners. International visitors are questioned by the Immigration and Naturalization Service, and those who admit to testing HIV-positive can be denied visas. An exemption for travelers attending international conferences or business meetings was added in 1990.

Under current regulations, there is a list of communicable diseases—including AIDS, syphilis, gonorrhea, leprosy, and tuberculosis—that are grounds for barring entry into the United States. A Clinton proposal (1993) is to remove all of them except active tuberculosis, which unlike the others can spread through the air. The National Commission on AIDS estimates that as a result between 300 and 600 people with AIDS or infected with HIV might immigrate into the country every year.

Clinton's plan to lift the current ban is supported by most of the medical community, including officials at the Public Health Service, the Centers for Disease Control and Prevention, and the National Academy of Sciences. "AIDS is not transmitted by casual contact, so we don't have a public health concern with Clinton's proposal," says Dr. Charles Mahan, Florida's state health officer. "The argument has been that it's expensive to take care of these patients, but we let in chronic kidney and cancer patients, whose treatment can be even more costly."

Meanwhile, in an interim order in March of 1993, U.S. District Court Judge Sterling Johnson, Jr., ordered the government to immediately move all HIV-infected Haitian refugees in detention at the U.S. naval base at Guantanamo Bay in Cuba. This order moved 158 HIV-positive Haitian immigrants into South Florida and the New York area on humanitarian grounds—medical care at Guantanamo was inadequate to treat HIV-positive persons. By the end of 1993, the U.S. Senate voted 76 to 23 to bar HIV-infected foreigners from permanent immigration into the United States.

Class Discussion:

Is the case for barring HIV-positive persons from establishing permanent residence in the United States based on scientific fact, political fear, or both/neither?

HIV Patterns in Different Countries

HIV infection is a global pandemic. Within the global community, three general patterns of HIV transmission have been identified by the World Health Organization and the U.S. Communicable Disease Center: Patterns I, II, and III. The three pattern designations are of limited use now because of the global nature of the pandemic.

Pattern I transmission occurs in industrialized parts of the world such as the United States, Canada, Western Europe, Australia, and New Zealand, and some Latin American countries such as Brazil, Mexico, and Puerto Rico. HIV was introduced to these countries in the late 1970s. The principal modes of transmission are through homosexual sex, bisexual sex, prostitution, injection drug use, and sex with a drug user. The ratio of male to female AIDS cases is 10:1 to 15:1. However, if the number of gay AIDS cases is subtracted, the male-to-female ratio is about 3:1. Hetero-sexual transmission and perinatal infection account for a small but gradually increasing number of cases. IDUs account for a significant number of AIDS cases in Italy, Spain, and Puerto Rico. Transfusion-associated disease is steadily declining due to effective screening of donated blood.

Pattern II transmission occurs in developing countries in Africa, the Caribbean (Haiti and the Dominican Republic), and parts of South America. Here, HIV was introduced in the early to mid-1970s and has been predominantly spread by heterosexual intercourse. The male to female ratio is about 1:1. Homosexual transmission is believed to be rare. Transmission by IDUs is infrequent due to lack of money and drug availability. Transfusion-associated infection is still significant due to lack of resources required to screen donated blood.

Early in 1994, the World Health Organization stopped using the term "Pattern II" to describe regional differences in transmission because this is no longer a useful way to describe all countries where heterosexual contact is a major mode of HIV transmission. Adult/adolescent heterosexual contact cases formerly classified under "Born in Pattern II country" and "Sex with person born in Pattern II country" are now tabulated under the category "Risk not reported or identified." Pediatric perinatal transmission cases in which the child's mother was formerly classified under "Born in Pattern II country" and "Sex with person born in Pattern II country" are now tabulated under the exposure category "Mother with/at risk for HIV infection: Has HIV infection, risk not specified." This change in reporting heterosexual contact is reflected in the data presented in Table 8-3.

Pattern III transmission occurs in countries of Eastern Europe, the Middle East, North Africa, Asia, and the Pacific. In Thailand and India, HIV infection is rapidly increasing, and most cases have been associated with sexual or IDU contact with foreigners. Imported contaminated blood has also been a significant problem in some countries.

Number of HIVs Required for Infection

Robert Coombs and colleagues (1989) calculated the dose of HIV necessary to cause an HIV infection. They reported that **"one infective dose"** of 1,000 HIV particles is necessary to establish HIV infection in human tissue culture cells. To establish HIV infection in the body, it was reasoned that it would take **10 to 15 infective doses**. Their study indicated that a pint of blood from an AIDS patient contains 1.8 million infective doses, or about 2 billion HIV particles per pint of blood, or about 4.2 million HIV particles per milliliter.

Placing HIV Numbers in Perspective— In cases of hepatitis B there may be 100 million to

RELATIVE DOSE: THE SWIMMING POOL ANALOGY

An analogy on the number of viruses it would take to cause an infection can be made by diluting the number of viruses in 1 mL of blood in a swimming pool full of water.

Basically the analogy goes like this: If 1 mL of blood carrying the hepatitis B virus were dropped into 24,000 gallons of water and mixed well, and if 1 mL of that solution were injected into a susceptible individual, that individual would develop hepatitis B. He or she might not develop jaundice, gray stools, chocolate urine, or other clinical conditions, but would develop serological markers indicating hepatitis B infection.

In contrast, if 1 mL of blood from an AIDS patient were dropped into a quart of water and 1 mL of that solution were injected into a susceptible individual, there is only a 1 in 10 chance that the individual would develop HIV antibody indicating HIV infection (Cottone et al., 1990). The implication here is that HIV is not easy to acquire.

1 billion hepatitis viruses in *just 1 milliliter* of blood (25 to 250 times more virus/mL than for HIV). A pint of blood contains 473 mL. Yet only one in three people who stick themselves with a needle contaminated with blood from a hepatitis B patient becomes infected.

The epidemiology of HIV infection is similar to that of HBV infection, and much that has been learned over the last 15 years about the risk of acquiring hepatitis B in the health care workplace can be applied to understanding the risk of HIV transmission in similar settings. Both viruses are transmitted in the same manner.

Current evidence indicates that despite the epidemiological similarities of HBV and HIV infection, the risk of HBV transmission in health care settings far exceeds that of HIV transmission. The risk of HIV transmission from a needlestick (including probable cases) is less than 0.5% (1 in 200). By contrast, the risk of hepatitis B infection from a needlestick has been estimated at 6% to 30%, or anywhere from 12 to 60 times more likely than for HIV. Approximately 12,000 health care workers in the United States develop symptomatic hepatitis B annually. About 1,000 of them become carriers, and approximately 250 die of cirrhosis, fulminant hepatitis, or primary liver carcinoma. A health care worker's risk of dying of hepatitis B after 15 years on the job is about 27 in 10,000; the annual risk of dying in a car crash is 2.4 in 10,000 (Sadovsky, 1989).

Body Fluid Transmission

HIV has been isolated from blood, semen, saliva, serum, urine, tears, vitreous, breast milk, vaginal secretions, lung fluid, and cerebrospinal fluid (Friedland et al., 1987). HIV has not been found in sweat. Because HIV has been identified in these fluids does not mean they are important in HIV transmission. Jay Levy and colleagues (1989) isolated HIV from 10 cell-free body fluids and from the cells found in five of them (Table 8-6). The results indicated that except for cerebrospinal fluid, large

TABLE 8-6 HIV in Body Fluids and in Cells within Body Fluids

	Estimated Number of HIV[a]
Cell-free fluid	
Plasma	10–50
Serum	10–50
Tears	<1
Ear secretions	5–10
Saliva	<1
Urine	<1
Vaginal/cervical	<1
Semen	10–50
Sweat	0
Breast milk	<1
Cerebrospinal fluid	10–1,000
Infected cells (T4 and macrophages)	
PBMC	0.001–0.1
Saliva	<0.01
Bronchial fluid	not detected
Vaginal/cervical fluid	present but not quantitated
Semen[b]	0.01–5

[a]Cell-free fluid is expressed in infectious particles per milliliter; infected cells, in percentage of infected cells observed.
[b]HIV has been detected in cell-free seminal fluid and in nonspermatazoal mononuclear cells and in the DNA of sperm from some HIV-infected men (Meriman et al., 1991; Bagasra et al., 1994).
(Source: Adapted from Levy, 1989)

quantities of cell-free HIV are not present in any of the nine other body fluids tested.

The low levels of HIV in cell-free body fluids and within the cells of these fluids does not mean that HIV cannot be transmitted via these fluids or cells—it can, but the dose (number of viruses) is so small that the risk of infection is minimal, thus the reason for the low number of health care workers contracting HIV infection after touching, being splashed by, or needlesticking themselves with blood containing HIV. Particularly interesting is the finding that there is no detectable HIV in bronchial fluid or sweat.

HIV is found in greatest numbers (100 to 10,000 infectious units per mL) *within T4 cells, macrophage, and monocytes of blood, vaginal fluids, and semen;* yet these fluids carry relatively low levels of **cell-free** HIV. Laboratory findings, along with overwhelming empirical observations, support the scientific conclusion that the major route of HIV transmission is through human blood and sexual activities involving exchange of semen and vaginal fluids. Semen carries significantly larger numbers of HIV than vaginal fluid. It appears that of all body fluids, these three contain the largest number of infected lymphocytes (Figure 8-4), which provide the largest HIV concentration in a given area at a given time.

Cell-to-Cell Transmission

According to classic models of viral infection, which draw heavily from research on bacteriophage (viruses that attack bacteria), the process of infection starts with adherence of free virus to host cells. This view has dominated the thinking about mechanisms of infection by HIV. But now there is overwhelming evidence that HIV infection can be initiated by the direct transfer of HIV from one cell to another by syncytia (group) formation and by cell-to-cell transmission without this formation. Cell-to-cell HIV transfer may take place either between host and donor cells within the host or between a donor HIV-infected mononuclear cell and intact host epithelium of the genital, digestive or urinary tract, or the placenta. Different mechanisms of cell-mediated transmission are illustrated in Figure 8-5.

FIGURE 8-4　Electron Micrograph of an HIV-Infected T4 Lymphocyte. The T4 cell has produced a large number of HIVs that are located over the entire lymphocyte. Each HIV leaves a hole in the cell membrane. The photograph shows part of the convoluted surface of the lymphocyte magnified 20,000 times. (*Courtesy of The National Biological Standards Board, South Mimms, U.K. and David Hockley*)

Presence of HIV-Infected Cells in Body Fluids

Blood— Cell-to-cell transmission assumes that HIV-infected cells are present in the body fluid of the infected donor individual. Recent observations indicate that both latent and HIV-producing cells are present throughout the course of infection. Although virus is primarily confined to lymphatic organs, considerable numbers of HIV-infected cells can also be detected in the blood. Thus it is probable that HIV-infected people harbor substantial numbers of HIV-infected mononuclear cells from soon after the initial infection to the terminal stage of the disease.

Semen— Semen from healthy men typically contains many leukocytes, including T4 cells. But the number and type of all mononuclear cells in the semen of a healthy man differs considerably from day to day.

Reducing the numbers of T4 cells (lymphocytes and macrophages) in semen could decrease the chances of infection. Lymphocytes and macrophages can originate from the testes, epididymis, seminal vesicles, prostate and the inflammation of the genital tract also results in an increased number of these cells in semen. In one recent study on 94 semen samples from HIV-infected men, HIV DNA was found in 35% of the mononuclear cells (Bagasra, 1996). It has been suggested that vasectomy could reduce the infectivity of HIV-infected men because it would eliminate mononuclear cells or cell-free virus in semen originating from the testes and epididymis. Although vasectomy has been reported to reduce the number of these white blood cells in

FIGURE 8-5 Schemes of Four Possible Mechanisms of Cell-Mediated Transmission of HIV. (**1**) An HIV-secreting donor mononuclear cell (MC) releases virus that infects nearby host cells; (**2**) an HIV-infected donor MC fuses with a host cell; (**3**) and (**4**) adhesion-based cell-to-cell transmission without syncytia. Cell-to-cell transfer of virus could hypothetically take place either between cells within the body of the host (**3**) or between a donor HIV-secreting MC and a host epithelial cell at the portal of entry (**4**). (*Source:* Phillips, 1994)

semen, HIV-infected mononuclear cells have been detected in semen from seropositive vasectomized men. Further studies are necessary to determine the efficacy of vasectomy for AIDS prevention.

In summary, semen from HIV-infected men can contain both cell-free and cell-associated virus. From the available evidence, as in blood, it is not yet possible to determine to what extent cell-free and cell-associated virus mediate HIV infectivity (Phillips, 1994).

Sperm— Omar Bagasra (1996) reported that 33% of sperm samples, from 94 HIV-positive men, contained HIV RNA. Many investigators have now reported that the mitochondria of various tissue types are infected with HIV. The sperm midpiece contains large numbers of mitochondria.

Saliva— There has always been the fear that HIV could be transmitted by kissing, that is, by coming in contact with HIV-infected saliva. Several large-scale studies have failed to demonstrate HIV transmission to household members and health care workers by ca-

sual contact, suggesting that transmission by saliva is uncommon. Although saliva from healthy individuals may contain considerable numbers of leukocytes, very few of these are T4 mononuclear cells. Using the DNA polymerase chain reaction test (presented in Chapter 13), Goto and co-workers (1991) found that HIV provirus was present in saliva from all 20 AIDS patients they examined. Omar Bagasra (1996) found HIV DNA in nuclei of epithelial cells (cells scraped off the inner sides of the mouth oral scrapings) in 29 of 35 HIV-infected persons (83%). Saliva from the 29 people all contained HIV-positive mononuclear cells. It should also be noted that AIDS patients frequently have oral lesions that result in blood in the oral cavity. Thus, it is possible that both cell-free virus and HIV-infected mononuclear cells in saliva from AIDS patients could originate from blood (Phillips, 1994). A recent report suggests that a secretory protease inhibitor in saliva attaches to the surface of lymphocytes blocking HIV infection (see "Orogenital Sex," this chapter).

DANGER OF HIV INFECTION VIA ARTIFICIAL INSEMINATION

By early 1996, 13 women were reported to have been HIV-infected through the use of donor sperm to initiate pregnancy; four in Australia, two in Canada, and six in the United States. Thirty recipients of semen from HIV-infected donors refused to be HIV tested. (Guinan, 1995). About 80,000 women each year are artificially inseminated with donor sperm. But 16 years into the AIDS epidemic, the increasingly popular fertility business remains largely unregulated and unmonitored, even though it traffics in semen, long known to be one of the two main HIV transmission routes.

Only a few states (New York, California, Ohio, Illinois, and Michigan) require HIV testing of semen donors. **There are no federal regulations.**

Medical and public health experts agree that artificial insemination is an HIV risk that somehow fell through the cracks of public education and health regulations. They insist, however, that the risk is low.

In January of 1996 Washington State's top educator announced that she had AIDS. She received the virus trying to become pregnant through artificial insemination with donor sperm. HIV announcement has once again focused national attention on the problem, the lack of federal regulations for this industry.

Omar Bagasra and colleagues (1994, 1996) state unequivocally that there is a risk of HIV transmission during artificial insemination. To quote Bagasra, "As we have shown, the sperm easily penetrates other cells—and when this occurs, the midpiece also penetrates. A single ejaculation contains [millions of] sperm. We have data to show that the mitochondria in the midpieces of HIV-infected sperm are loaded with HIV. If 1 in 1,000 of these mitochondria contains HIV, that is a significant viral load. The viral load transmitted from a man to a woman in this manner is quite likely to be high."

Lack of federal and state regulations means you must protect yourself! (**1**) Stay away from private physicians unless you know the doctors are using only certified sperm banks to get their products. (**2**) Review a doctor's or clinic's testing and record-keeping procedures and demand to see donor medical records, which can be shared even if the donor's identity is protected. (**3**) Accept only frozen donor semen that has been HIV-tested twice at 3- to 6-month intervals.

There continues to be some concern over the presence of HIV in saliva because of the exchange of saliva during **deep kissing**, the saliva residue left on eating utensils, and saliva on instruments handled by health care workers, especially in dentistry. Results of studies on hundreds of dental workers, many of whom have cared for AIDS patients, have shown no evidence of HIV infection (Friedland et al., 1987). Also, in a recent CDC study, none of 48 health care workers became infected after parenteral (IV) or mucous membrane exposure to the saliva of HIV-infected patients (Curran et al., 1988). A recent study by Philip Fox (1991), National Institute of Dental Research, showed that saliva from three healthy men stopped HIV infection of lymphocytes in vitro. Additional studies by D.W. Archibald and colleagues (1990) and Pourtois and colleagues (1991) also showed that human saliva contains factors that inhibit HIV infectivity. Robert Woolley (1989) attempted to calculate the amount of hemo-globin that might be transferred during passionate kissing, and concluded that kissing **does not** pose a serious health threat. Further saliva inhibition tests are in progress. In July of 1997, the **first** documented case of HIV transmission via **deep kissing** was **reported** on by the CDC. In this **one** case, the man was HIV-positive, via IDU in 1988. Both he and his female partner had serious gum (periodontal) disease. His gums routinely bled with brushing or flossing. Investigators at the CDC believe that the HIV was transmitted via blood within the man's oral cavity due to oral lesions onto the mucus membrane of the woman (*MMWR*, 1997).

Spitzer and colleagues (1989) reported that a male became HIV-infected during unprotected fellatio with an HIV-infected prostitute. A second similar case has also been reported. The mechanism of transmission, saliva, in these cases may be suspected, but it is not conclusive!

The precise risk of oral sex is difficult to assess because most couples engage in other sexual practices. However, Rozenbaum and colleagues (1988) and Monzon and colleagues (1987) reported that this was a probable route of HIV transmission (see discussion under "Orogenital Sex" in this chapter). Regardless, special precautions for dentistry are recommended by the CDC. A small number of hepatitis B viral infections have been documented in dental workers (*MMWR*, 1988b, 1991a).

Mother's Milk— Several studies have shown that HIV can be transmitted by breast-feeding. Van de Perre and co-workers (1993) found that infection of babies via breast milk was most strongly correlated with the presence of HIV-infected cells in the milk, suggesting that infection might be cell-mediated. However, infection was also correlated with low levels of antibodies to HIV, suggesting that infection was initiated by cell-free virus. Thus this study does not present strong evidence in favor of infection by cell-associated versus cell-free virus.

Transmission by Cell-to-Cell Fusion: Syncytia Formation

The idea that a virus could spread from one cell to another was recognized in the mid-1950s. Induction of syncytium formation, a fused group of cells (Figure 3-8), is a characteristic effect produced when HIV-infected cells expressing surface gp120 come in contact with T4 cells.

Hironori Sato and co-workers (1992) have suggested how syncytium formation may mediate HIV infection and spread. These workers compared the infection of T4 cells following either the addition of HIV-infected H9 cells or cell-free virus obtained from H9-infected cell culture fluids. Examination of the cultures by light microscopy revealed that addition of HIV-infected cells, but not free virus, resulted in numerous small syncytia 1 hour after infection, large syncytia by 2 to 4 hours, and giant syncytia, containing hundreds of nuclei, by 8 hours. Although the amount of the virus produced by HIV-secreting T4 cells may not be comparable to that of free virus in culture medium because T4 cells are a continuous source of virus, Sato

and co-workers' conclusion that cell-mediated infection was much more efficient than infection by cell-free virus appears justified in view of the striking difference in virus production (Phillips, 1994).

Transmission by Cell-to-Cell Adhesion

Cell Transmission of HIV to Epithelial Cells— To examine the possibility that HIV could directly infect epithelia at the portal of entry, David Phillips and co-workers (1994) grew established cell lines derived from the gut, genital tract, and placenta, potential sites of HIV entry. Initially they attempted to infect these epithelial cell lines with culture fluid containing free HIV. They had limited success. However, when they added HIV-infected T4 cells or monocyte cell lines to the epithelia, they were able to detect infection.

HIV-infected cells were much more efficient in infecting epithelical cells than free virus because the mononuclear cells continued to adhere to the epithelia even after the cultures were washed vigorously. In the scanning electron microscope they observed many cells attached to the epithelium. These cells frequently display pear shapes and ruffles disposed away from the epithelium (Figure 8-6, A and B).

Dentist with AIDS Infects Patient During Tooth Extraction?

In July of 1990, the CDC reported on the possible transmission of HIV from a dentist with AIDS to a female patient (*MMWR*, 1990a). This case, like no other before it, sent chills through many. But why this case? Because the vast majority of people go to dentists! They don't inject drugs and are not gay. This case, however, is difficult to resolve. For example, 2 years had elapsed from the time of the dental work to when the patient, Kimberly Bergalis (Figure 8-7), was diagnosed with AIDS. Both patient and dentist, David J. Acer of Stuart, Florida, were uncertain of exactly what happened. Some of the pertinent factors in this case are (**1**) review of dental records and radiographs suggest that the two tooth extractions were uncomplicated; (**2**) interviews with Bergalis and the dentist did not identify other

A

B

FIGURE 8-6 HIV Tisue Adherence and Infectivity. **A**, Scanning electron micrograph of HIV-infected T cells(MOLT-4/HIV-1$_{IIIB}$) adhering to an epithelium derived from the human intestine (1407). Following adherence T cells tend to become pear-shaped.(Original magnification × 4,500.) **B**, HIV-infected cervix-derived epitheial cell. The epithelium has been cut perpendicular to the filter. Budding HIV (*arrows*) are observed on both the apical (*A*) and basal (*B*) surfaces. (Original magnification × 17,000.) (*Reprinted with permission of David M. Phillips, The Population Council*)

FIGURE 8-7 Kimberly Bergalis, Age 23. Bergalis is being comforted by her mother after their train trip from their home in Florida to Washington, D.C. She made the trip to testify before a congressional committee on September 26, 1991. Bergalis favored mandatory HIV testing for health care personnel. She died December 8, 1991. (*Photograph courtesy of AP/Wide World Photos*)

risk factors for HIV infection (Bergalis, age 22, stated over national TV in 1990 that she was still a virgin;) This point was disputed on June 19, 1994, during the TV program *60 Minutes* (with Mike Wallace) as well as the CDC's genetic match between Dr. Acer's HIV and his patient's strain of HIV. Yes, she did engage in sexual foreplay, but not intercourse. Yes, she was infected with the human papilloma virus, which can be sexually transmitted, but this is not at all uncommon in immune-suppressed AIDS patients with no history of sexual intercourse; (**3**) nucleotide sequence data indicated a high degree of similarity between the HIV strains infecting her and the dentist; and (**4**) the time between the dental procedure and the development of AIDS was short (24 months), and Bergalis developed oral candidiasis 17 months after infection. Only 1% of infected homosexual/ bisexual men and 5% of infected transfusion recipients develop AIDS within 2 years of infection.

David Acer, a bisexual, was diagnosed with symptomatic HIV infection in 1986 and with AIDS in 1987. He died on September 3, 1990. Since then, 1,100 of his 2,500 patients were contacted for HIV testing. In January of 1991, the test results of 591 of these patients revealed that five were HIV-positive: a 68-year-old retired school teacher, a middle-aged father of two, a 37-year-old carnival worker, an unemployed drifter, and a 19-year-old student. As with Bergalis, infection in these patients may have come from some other source. All six patients denied having sexual contact with the dentist or with one another (*MMWR*, 1991a). If an absolute case can be made that Acer transmitted the virus to Bergalis, this will be the *first documented case of a health care professional infecting a patient.* Bergalis is reported to have settled her first claim for $1 million from Acer's malpractice insurance company. She settled a second claim against his estate for an undisclosed sum.

Bergalis died of AIDS on December 8, 1991. She was 23 years old and weighed 48 pounds. In January 1993 a life-size bronze statue of Kimberly Bergalis was unveiled at the high school she attended. Her dying wish was that

DEADLY INNOCENCE: A MURDER MYSTERY?

Kimberly Bergalis had just graduated from the University of Florida. She would spend that summer, 1989, waiting tables. One day she **fainted**. This was just the beginning of her 28-month odyssey to her death from AIDS. It was the beginning of a search for her illness—an investigative medical journey into her illness proved very puzzling. It was an unending illness, chronic vaginal infections, a mouth full of yeast, dizzy spells, exhaustion, and loss of appetite. First diagnosis—could it be leukemia? (A weakened immune system allows the presentation of many look-alike symptoms.) Almost unable to breathe, she was diagnosed with Pneumocystis pneumonia. The doctor found the agent causing the pneumonia—*Pneumocystis carinii*. An HIV test was positive; **the diagnosis, AIDS!** Kim said she was a virgin, did not use drugs, had never had a blood transfusion, surgery, acupuncture, or tattoos—**but wait**, she had two teeth extracted by a dentist who was sickly but his illness was said to be cancer.

THE INVESTIGATION

The CDC and other investigators tried but failed to find evidence that Ms. Bergalis was anyone other than who she professed to be. They even asked her if she had sex with animals (Burkett, 1995). She was, after the news broke nationally, demonized by some and defended by others. Even after her funeral, her parents received hate mail—"Thank God the bitch is finally dead" or "She got what was coming to her." **Such remarks took their place among so many other even more hateful remarks that people with AIDS had to endure then and NOW.**

AUTHOR'S NOTE

The absolute truth of how Ms. Bergalis became infected will never be known—too much time has passed, the dentist is dead, and the chain of transmission was never clearly established! A recent TV documentary of this case implies that the dentist **intentionally infected** Ms. Bergalis and at least five others who were his dental patients.

what happened to her should never happen to anyone else. To this end, weak and near death, she traveled by train to testify before the United States Congress urging mandatory testing for all health care workers. The 'Bergalis Bill' never got out of committee, the CDC and Congress rejected the call for mandatory testing of health care workers. On April 6, 1991, Ms. Bergalis wrote a two-page unmailed letter to the Florida State Department of Health and Rehabilitative Services. She wrote "Whom do I blame? I blame Dr. Acer and every single one of you bastards. Anyone who knew Dr. Acer was infected and had AIDS and stood by not doing a damn thing about it. You are all just as guilty as he was."

In July 1991, a guest on the *Sally Jessy Raphael Show* stated in front of Mr. and Mrs. Bergalis, that their daughter Kimberly, knowing she was HIV-infected, went to another dentist and did not tell him that she was infected.

Acer's Dental Practice— Staff reported that by 1987 all surgical instruments were routinely autoclaved. Nonsurgical heat-tolerant instruments (e.g., dental mirrors) were autoclaved

when practice conditions, such as time and instrument supply, allowed, or were immersed in a liquid germicide for varying lengths of time. Tests of the autoclave in October 1990, demonstrated that it was functioning properly (*MMWR*, 1991a).

There is no shortage of ideas as to how Acer might have infected his patients. For example, he could have used the same dental instruments on himself or his sexual partners that he used on his patients without sterilizing them. Or he could have had HIV in his sweat which could have dropped into his patients' oral cavities. However, the polymerase chain reaction (the latest in DNA detection technology) was used to detect the presence of HIV in the natural sweat from 40 HIV-infected people. All 40 tested HIV-negative. It appears that by the available methodology of detection HIV is **not** present in the sweat of HIV-positive people.

The actual route of HIV transmission in the Acer–Bergalis case will most likely never be known. There have been suggestions that the dentist did not wish to die alone and chose certain people to infect. It was suggested that he

DISTRIBUTION OF HIV-CONTAMINATED BLOOD: FRANCE, GERMANY, THE UNITED STATES, AND OTHER COUNTRIES

Near the end he could not bring himself to visit his youngest brother, to see him dying of AIDS. He too was dying of AIDS. Their deaths would close out a family of four HIV-infected hemophiliac brothers, all diagnosed with AIDS. The first died at age 24, the second committed suicide at age 33, the last two brothers died in 1993. The four brothers became HIV-infected about 1985 from using HIV-contaminated blood-clotting factor.

FRANCE

The French National Center of Blood Transfusions (CNTS) knowingly distributed HIV-contaminated blood products to hemophiliacs in 1985. The scandal, which broke in 1991, prompted the center's director to resign and an official government investigation.

In the confidential minutes of a 1985 CNTS meeting, agency officials concluded that 100% of the concentrated blood-clotting factors used to treat French hemophiliacs were contaminated with HIV. The agency, which has a monopoly on blood for transfusions, kept its secret and ignored a 1984 recommendation from the U.S. Centers for Disease Control and Prevention that blood products be heated in order to kill the deadly virus (Dorfman, 1991).

In July 1985, the CNTS decided to heat all blood products and to institute national testing of donated blood. But for the next 3 months, the agency continued to sell the HIV-contaminated blood products to hemophiliacs without warning them of the risk. That policy, which was approved by the Ministry of Health and the French Association of Hemophiliacs, was reportedly intended to ward off a blood shortage.

Whatever the reasons, the secrecy and delay produced catastrophic results. Nearly half of France's 3,000 hemophiliacs were infected with HIV; subsequently 256 have died. Bowing to public and media pressure, the French government will provide compensation for some 7,000 French citizens who have been infected with HIV through blood products and transfusions (Aldhous, 1991).

French Ministers to Face Poisoning Charges

Formal charges of "collusion in poisoning" were made in October 1994 against Laurent Fabius, the former Socialist prime minister, and four of his colleagues—Edmond Hervé, then deputy health minister, and Georgina Dufoix, then minister of social affairs, Francois Gros, scientific advisor to Fabius, and Claude Weisselberg, physician and advisor to Fabius—over their role in France's HIV-contaminated blood scandal in the mid-1980s. In 1995, Gerard Jacquin, former director of bioindustry at CNTS, was charged with poisoning and Louis Schweitzer and Patrick Baudry, advisors to Fabius and Dufoix, respectively, were charged with delaying the screening of blood products (Reichhardt, 1995). The charge carries a maximum sentence of 30 years in prison. In addition to these three men, the charge of collusion to poison were also brought against Jean-Pierre Allain (just released from prison) and Michel Garretta (still in prison) (Butler, 1994a, 1994b).

Update 1996— The latest charges in France's contaminated blood case threaten to involve the Pasteur Institute in Paris. Jean Weber, a former chief executive of Pasteur Diagnostic (PD)—in which Pasteur's foundation holds shares—was charged by an examining judge with "complicity in poisoning" for his alleged role in the scandal (Kaiser, 1996).

GERMANY

The German blood scandal began with two questions. The first question was how to explain several unexpected cases of HIV infection. And the second question, associated with the first, was how could 7,000 units of blood have been screened for HIV using 2,500 HIV blood testing kits (it takes one kit/unit of blood screened). The search for the answers led investigators to a blood supply company called UB Plasma in the city of Koblenz. The investigators concluded that either the firm had failed to test thousands of units, or it had "pooled" units from multiple donors before conducting the test, an illegal practice that reduces the chances of detecting HIV contamination.

Investigators discovered that after UB Plasma began running into financial trouble in 1991, technicians were told to pool units to save money on the $2 test kits. After German kit manufacturers stopped deliveries (UB Plasma failed to pay its bills) technicians switched to an unauthorized and less reliable test. There was also evidence that the firm may have distributed blood that was not screened at all.

Because of the extent of blood banking violations, German authorities closed UB Plasma. They arrested the manager and three employees on charges of fraud and "negligent bodily harm." The current health minister disbanded the German Federal Health Bureau. And the Director of Pharmaceuticals was relieved of his duties relating to the control of blood and blood products. In stark contrast to the HIV blood scandals in France and the United States, German investigators attribute the distribution of HIV-contaminated blood and blood products to incompetence rather than company greed—UB Plasma did not attempt to distribute known HIV-positive blood until current stocks were used up!

The question for the reader is whether incompetence is a crime and, if so, what kind of crime and what should be the punishment?

Update 1995

German laws for testing blood products have been tightened following the 1994 allegations that the company UB Plasma pooled blood donations before testing for HIV. Three customers were infected with HIV, and one has died of AIDS. Five officials were charged with grievous bodily harm, which carries a maximum 5 year prison sentence.

In 1995 the director and the head of product testing of Haemoplas, a German blood products company, have been charged with murder on the grounds that they had been motivated by greed. They are alleged to have conspired in the early 1980s to economize by not testing blood samples, and to have persisted after testing was made compulsory in 1985.

Fourteen people became infected with HIV through Haemoplas products between 1986 and 1987, and three have since died.

Both men have also been charged with 5,837 counts of attempted murder — corresponding to the number of batches distributed — infringing legislation on the control of pharmaceutical products, and fraud (Abbott, 1995).

THE UNITED STATES

In late 1993, a class action suit was filed on behalf of 9,000 hemophiliacs who became infected with HIV after using HIV-contaminated blood products, called Blood Factor 8, which is essential for proper blood clot formation following an injury. In the case of severe hemophilia, many persons spontaneously bleed into their joints. Blood Factor 8 is sometimes referred to as Anti-Hemolytic Factor or AHF. Hemophiliacs are now dying of AIDS at the rate of one a day.

The suit charges that five manufacturers of AHF and the National Hemophilia Foundation continued to pursue aggressive advertising and marketing of AHF while downplaying the risk of viral infection. In 1995, the United States Supreme court disallowed the suit.

By the mid-1970's, the dangers of viral infection from blood products was well known and methods had been provided for blood viral inactivation. Such methods were patented and available by 1977. In 1981, Donald Francis, an epidemiologist then with the CDC, and Max Essex, a retrovirologist at Harvard Cancer Biology Laboratory, were convinced that AIDS, then referred to as Gay Related Immune Deficiency or GRID, was caused by an infectious agent, most likely a virus. But others thought GRID was related to the gay male lifestyle. The disease was spreading rapidly among gay males through sexual contact. But the evidence continued to mount that the disease, or agent causing the disease, was being transmitted by blood. And in that same year, the president of an AHF-producing company stated the agent was in the blood supply. He said he thought it was a 100% fatal retrovirus. At this time, a major part of blood stocks came from paid donors, mostly from poor neighborhoods. To offset taking in contaminated blood, this single company began questioning donors face-to-face: Are you homosexual? In the first 2 weeks of new guideline operations, 308 donors said yes and their blood was not taken. Another 500 refused to answer and left.

The American Association of Blood Banks (AABB) and the American Red Cross issued a joint statement that "Direct or indirect questions about a donor's sexual preferences are inappropriate." Clearly, they kept open the door to high behavioral risk blood donors. The FDA went along with the joint statement and against the CDC recommendations for screening blood donors.

According to Milton Musin, former medical research director of Cutter Laboratories, by the end of 1983 he knew that the hemophiliacs clotting factor could transmit AIDS. And virtually all lots of the concentrate were contaminated with the AIDS virus. "You'll never convince me that profit margins and fear of the product liability and fear of losing a very lucrative business did not drive the CEOs and leaders of these companies."

In 1985, the FDA announced a blood test. "This test adds a major dimension of protection to our present safeguards. Its use will keep our blood supply safe and indeed make them even safer."

The HIV antibody test, called the ELISA test, would help make the blood supply, in large part, safe. But it came at a cost to the blood banks. Technicians had to be hired and trained. Donors had to be checked and every new unit of blood tested and logged. **But, astonishingly, the blood banks were not required to go back to the inventories on their shelves.** In hindsight, the current head of the AABB says that was a mistake.

But perhaps the worst was yet to be learned. While the AABB was stalling testing, it convinced the FDA to reduce the number of blood bank inspections at the very time HIV was entering the blood system of the country.

It wasn't until 1988 that the blood banks began recalling HIV-positive blood. FDA reports were discovered that told of errors and accidents. Between 1985 and 1987 thousands of units of potentially contaminated blood had been released and officially recalled. But recalling blood that was released for transfusion is a bit misleading because, depending on when and how you are trying to recall it, the chances of being able to get it all back are almost zero. Once it is released, it is used. Potentially contaminated blood had been used, most of it quickly, in emergency rooms. The FDA now had no choice but to take action. In September 1988, the FDA and the Red Cross entered into what is known as a voluntary agreement to comply with all FDA regulations. From now on there would be yearly inspections! But that did not work. The Red Cross kept poor records at local blood banks and the FDA constantly had to threaten license revocations.

Finally, in 1993, FDA commissioner, Dr. David Kessler, went to federal court and obtained an injunction against the Red Cross for failure to fulfill its promise under the 1988 voluntary agreement.

It is now estimated that as many as 30,000 Americans were infected with AIDS through blood. It is a tragedy that has exposed critical weaknesses in the rules and practices in blood banking. It's also a story of missed opportunities, vested interests, and lax regulations stretching back more than a decade when a mysterious virus entered America's bloodstream. In November 1993, Donna Shalala, Secretary of Health and Human Services, asked for a high-level investigation of how thousands of American hemophiliacs became HIV-infected from contaminated blood products. As of late 1995 the investigation is still underway.

Update April 1996/1997—The four major producers of blood-clotting factors made a $640 million offer to hemophiliacs of the United States. In the summer of 1997 over 6,000 hemophiliacs or their families recieved $100,000. Some refused and will go to court to settle.

Question: Do you feel this saga of delayed and controlled misuse of blood in the United States is equal to or greater than the French and/or German scandals? Explain. (Class discussion)

USE OF HIV-CONTAMINATED BLOOD OR BLOOD PRODUCTS IN OTHER COUNTRIES

Canada and Nova Scotia

A flood of lawsuits is expected to follow the decision to award more than half a million Canadian dollars to the HIV-infected wife of a man who died of AIDS after receiving a transfusion of HIV-contaminated blood. The outcome of this case was announced on the eve of a deadline set by all except one of Canada's provinces and territories for acceptance of a compensation package by more than a thousand recipients of HIV-infected blood. To obtain the money, victims had to sign wavers promising not to sue Ottawa, the provinces or territories, hospitals, the Red Cross, and pharmaceutcal and insurance companies. Compensation was set at C$515,000 per case or per person plus interest and legal fees.

The Canadian compensation is less generous than the province of Nova Scotia, which, as well as making annual payments of C$30,000 to the HIV-infected, pays for expensive AIDS drugs, as well as funeral costs and post-secondary education for their children (Spurgeon, 1994, 1996).

Switzerland

In mid-1994, the former head of the Swiss Red Cross Central Laboratory in Bern was charged with causing "grievous bodily harm" by allowing HIV-tainted blood-clotting factors to be distributed to Swiss hemophiliacs in 1985 and 1986.

The Swiss case resembles the French scandal. In both cases, a national lab continued to distribute blood products that were known to be potentially infected with HIV. France stopped using such products in October 1985, but in Switzerland they were marketed until April 1986.

The suspect Swiss factors were made with blood collected some months before July, 1985, when HIV testing became routine. The trial is likely to center on his failure to stop production of the factors in July, 1985, when the New York Blood Center identified one HIV-positive sample among 3,375 units of donated Swiss blood. But the Swiss Red Cross insists that no alternative supplies were available: "If these products would not have gone out, the hemophiliacs would have bled to death." (Holden, 1994)

Japan

In July of 1993, 92 Japanese hemophiliacs filed suit against the Japanese government and blood product manufacturers. They are seeking compensation for failure to protect them from blood products contaminated with HIV. Blood product manufacturers continued to advertise untreated blood products in Japan without warning until late-1985; Japanese hemophiliacs used them into 1986. They are seeking one million dollars each in compensation.

During 1983–1985, Japan dramatically increased its imports of untreated U.S. blood products and, as a result, about 2,000 of Japan's 5,000 hemophiliacs were infected with HIV. Through 1996 over 400 have died. (Swinbank, 1993, 1994).

Update 1996— After a 7-year court battle, Japan's hemophiliacs and their families reached an out of court settlement. Each HIV-affected hemophiliac will receive about $430,000. And those with AIDS will receive an additional $1,400 a month for life (Abbott, 1996).

In September of 1996, the president and two former presidents of Green Cross Corporation (Midori Juji), Japan's leading blood product manufacturer, were arrested in connection with the infection of thousands of Japanese with HIV through the use of non-heat-treated blood products in the 1980s. They were being held on suspicion of negligence in promoting the continued sale of non-heat-treated blood coagulants in 1986, after safer heat-treated products, including those of the Midori Juji Company, were approved for sale by the government in 1985. Their trial is pending.

India

A blood bank in Bombay operated by the India Red Cross Society (IRCS) has been closed down following a government decision to conduct an inquiry into charges that the center had supplied blood infected with HIV to hospitals in the city between 1992 and 1994.

The medical officer in charge of the blood bank has already been removed from his post, and more officials are expected to lose their jobs.

The affair has caused concern throughout India, as the IRCS is intended to set national standards for blood safety.

The affair came to light when the chairman of the IRCS subcommittee on blood transfusion services, examined the records of the blood bank. These showed that HIV-positive blood had been supplied to at least 10 city hospitals, including one that specializes in transfusion services.

In addition, there have been suspicions that employees of the blood bank, rather than discarding infected blood, have been selling it on the black market created by an overall shortage of blood supplies (Jayaraman, 1995).

CHINA

In October of 1996, China's Ministry of Public Health ordered thousands of state-run medical institutions to stop using a certain brand of serum albumin, a common blood product produced by a military-run factory.

Now, 2 years after Chinese journalists in Hong Kong and the United States first published reports that the blood product was contaminated with HIV, China's Foreign Ministry acknowledged that tests of some samples of the blood product have indicated the presence of HIV. But, at the Department of Medicine Administration and Control, a Mr. Liu said: "No, no, it has never happened. Some people outside China and some foreign journalists just made their reports on the basis of rumors."

OTHER BLOOD SCANDALS IN BRIEF

In Columbia, a drug-addicted bisexual who knew he had AIDS sold his blood 12 times to a laboratory. Twelve patients received the blood between 1989 and 1990 and went on to infect an additional 200 people through sexual contact.

In Romania during the Communist era, HIV-contaminated blood infected 2,376 children.

Developing countries at the moment must rely on paid donors, who may include gay and bisexual men, prostitutes, and drug addicts needing money. Countries like India, Pakistan, and Russia have an open paid donor system.

Parts of Africa and Latin America use family replacement donors—a scheme that allows paid donors to pose as relatives of the patient. Paying unquestioned donors without HIV screening their blood is an invitation for the transmission of HIV. But developing countries do not have the capital nor sufficient trained personnel to do anything else at the moment.

EFFECTIVENESS OF SCREENING HEALTH CARE WORKERS FOR HIV IN THE UNITED STATES

There is considerable public concern regarding the potential transmission of the human immunodeficiency virus (HIV) from health care worker to patient. This risk is manifest in the results of a 1991 *Newsweek* poll, which found that 90% of Americans favor testing health care workers for HIV and revealing the results to patients. The same poll indicated that 49% of the public believed health care workers should be forbidden to practice if they are HIV-positive, and the majority indicated they would no longer seek treatment from an infected practitioner.

In contrast to this perceived risk, the CDC has estimated the theoretical probability of this type of transmission to be between 0.000024 and 0.0000024. Daniels (1992) points out that the risk of being infected by an HIV-positive surgeon is roughly 10% of the chance of being struck by lightning, 25% as probable as being killed by a bee, and half as likely as being hit by a falling aircraft. Part of the basis of the public's concern is that, in contrast to the other risks mentioned, transmission of HIV from a health care worker to a patient is potentially avoidable. Still, the CDC has recommended against mandatory screening because the low risk does not warrant the anticipated cost associated with testing.

William Chavey and co-workers (1994) examined a screening protocol that included a sequence of antibody tests (enzyme-linked immunoabsorbent assay and the Western blot) and culture for HIV. The incremental cost-effectiveness of applying this protocol as opposed to the status quo for the prevention of transmission of HIV from health care worker to patient was evaluated. The incremental cost-effectiveness ratio was then compared with that of other interventions. Their study showed that the expected annual cost of screening for a large hospital would be $244,382 to prevent 0.02663 transmission. The incremental cost-effectiveness ratio was $9,177,615 per transmission prevented. (*Question:* Is it worth over $9 million to prevent the transmission of HIV to one person? *Discussion.*) The conclusion reached was that screening health care workers for prevention of potential HIV transmission to patients is an expensive use of health care resources.

The results of another cost-effectiveness study of HIV testing of just physicians and dentists in the United States by Kathryn Phillips and co-workers (1994) showed that, although one-time mandatory testing of surgeons and dentists with mandatory restriction of those found to be HIV-positive is more cost-effective than other policies, the cost-effectiveness varies tremendously under different scenarios. Results were highly sensitive to several data inputs, especially HIV seroprevalence of surgeons and dentists and transmission risk. For example, under a medium seroprevalence and transmission risk scenario, mandatory testing of all surgeons might avert 25 infections at a total cost of $27.9 million or $1,115,000 per infection averted and an incremental cost of $291,000 compared with current testing; however, the incremental cost-effectiveness per patient infection averted ranges from $29,807,000 under a low-risk scenario to a savings of $81,000 under a high-risk scenario.

may have attempted to infect still others, but was unsuccessful. A friend of the dentist said that he believed that Acer intentionally infected his patients to call attention to the HIV/AIDS problem in the United States. Acer felt that mainstream America was ignoring the problem. In mid-1994, Continental Broad-casting Systems (CBS), during an interview with Lionel Resnick, chief of retrovirology research at Mt. Sinai Medical Center in Miami, said that, based on his research, David Acer was not the source of HIV infection for the six persons. He said the CDC "vastly overstated the reliability of the DNA tests." But, to the contrary, the CDC believes it has **understated** its case based on the evidence!

A recent CDC estimate put the theoretical risk of HIV transmission from an HIV-infected dentist to patient during a procedure with potential blood exposure at 1 chance in 263,158 to 1 chance in 2,631,579 (Friedland, 1991). **Point for Discussion: Is this last point, one of revenge against society, reasonable?**

(Read: Denis Breo (1993). The dental AIDS cases—murder or an unsolved mystery? *JAMA*, 270:2732–2734.)

Summary— The CDC states that based on the following considerations, their investigation strongly suggests that at least three patients of Acer's were infected with HIV during dental care: (**1**) the three patients had no other confirmed exposure to HIV; (**2**) they all had invasive procedures performed by an HIV-infected dentist; and (**3**) DNA sequence analyses of the HIV strains from these three patients indicated a high degree of similarity to each other and to the strain that had infected the dentist—a finding consistent with previous instances in which cases have been linked epidemiologically. In addition, these strains are distinct from the HIV strain from another of Acer's patients who had a known behavioral risk for HIV infection, and from the strains of the eight HIV-infected people residing in the same geographic area and from the 21 other North American HIV isolates.

Ending 1997, two of the six patients believed to have been infected by Acer have progressed to AIDS but are still alive: Kimberly Bergalis, Richard Driskill, John Yecs, and Barbara Webb have died. To date, the six people have received $10 million from Acer's insurance company.

See Point of Information 8.6.

Sexual Transmission

Sexual transmission of HIV occurs when infected blood, semen, or vaginal secretions from an infected person enter the bloodstream of a partner. This can happen during

---

SIDEBAR 8.1

HIV INFECTIVITY

HIV infectivity is the average probability of transmission to another person after that person is exposed to an infected host. Infectivity plus two other parameters—the duration of infectiousness and the average rate at which susceptible people change sexual partners— determines whether the epidemic grows or slows. On a population level, host-related factors (the social, cultural, and political milieu) and agent factors (HIV) determine HIV infectivity. Host-related and environmental factors can promote the pandemic because they can accelerate infectivity (Royce et al., 1997).

BOX 8.2

VASECTOMY LOWERS BUT DOES NOT ELIMINATE HIV TRANSMISSION RISK DURING UNSAFE SEX

Vasectomized men infected with HIV have less of the virus in their ejaculate than do men who have not had the sterilization procedure, according to a study released at the recent American Urological Association meeting.

But HIV-positive men who have had a vasectomy still can transmit the virus during unprotected sex. Thus men must still use a condom to prevent HIV transmission.

Unlike sperm, which is not transmitted by vasectomized men, small numbers of lymphocytes still are present in the ejaculate of men who have had the proceedure. Therefore, a vasectomy cannot be viewed as a way to prevent transmission of HIV (Pudney et al., 1991).

---

anal, vaginal, or oral penetration, in descending order of risk. Unprotected anal sex by a male or female appears to be the most dangerous, since the rectal wall is very thin. Masturbation or self sex is the safest. In general, a person's risk of acquiring HIV infection through sexual contact depends on (**1**) the number of different partners, (**2**) the likelihood (prevalence) of HIV infection in these partners, and (**3**) the probability of virus transmission during sexual contact with an infected partner. Virus transmission, in turn, may be affected by biological factors, such as concurrent STD infections in either partner. If there is a genital ulcer caused by syphilis or chancroid or herpes, the risk of getting HIV increases 10- to 20-fold. If there is gonorrhea or chlamydial infection, which are more common, the risk increases probably 3- to 4-fold. Behavioral factors, such as type of sex practice and use of condoms, or varying levels of infectivity in the source partner (for example viral load) related to clinical stage of disease also increase the risk of HIV transmission/ infection. Based on these factors, the risk for HIV infection is highest for an uninfected partner of an HIV-infected person practicing unsafe sex. Persons who have sex partners with risk factors for HIV infection or who themselves have multiple partners from urban settings with high rates of injection drug and "crack" cocaine use, prostitution, and other STDs are also at increased risk.

Personal Choice–Personal Risks

About 90% of the HIV infections that occur within the heterosexual non-injection drug use population occur through one or more sexual activities. Some 90% of the HIV infections that occur among gay males occur through anal intercourse (Kingsley et al., 1990). In any sexual activity, HIV is transmitted via a body fluid. Transmission may occur between men, from men to women, women to men or possibly from women to women (see Chapter 11).

Heterosexual HIV Transmission

Heterosexual HIV transmission means that the virus was transmitted during heterosexual sexual activities. As such, the **proportion** of HIV infection and AIDS cases among the heterosexual population in the United States is now increasing at a greater rate than the proportion of HIV infections and AIDS cases among homosexuals or IDUs (Friedland et al., 1987). Persons at highest risk for heterosexually transmitted HIV infection include adolescents and adults with multiple sex partners, those with sexually transmitted diseases (STDs), and heterosexually active persons residing in areas with a high prevalence of HIV infection among IDUs. In 1985, fewer than 2% of AIDS cases were from the heterosexual population; by 1989, 5% were from the heterosexual population. For the year 1993, 9% of cases were from the heterosexual population. The large increase is a reflection of the new AIDS definition of 1993. Now overall, the incidence of heterosexual AIDS cases is 9% of the total number of reported AIDS cases in the United States. Of the number of the **heterosexual AIDS cases** reported in the United States, about two-thirds (66%) of cases occur among women and one-third among men.

Heterosexual HIV Transmission Outside the United States—Studies in Africa, Haiti, and other Caribbean and Third World countries indicate that HIV transmission is most prevalent among

---

──────── BOX 8.3 ────────

HIV/AIDS ROULETTE

Case I: The Woman Executive

I am a successful executive woman. A year ago I applied for life insurance. I was required to take an HIV antibody test. It came back positive.

I am not a prostitute or promiscuous. I am not and have never been an injection drug user. I am not a member of a minority group, indigent nor homeless, and I have not slept with a bisexual male (?).

I don't fit any of the stereotypes that people have designated for those infected with HIV. I got HIV from a man I love and have been seeing for 5 years. He is not homosexual or bisexual. He has never used injection drugs. He had no idea he was carrying the virus. He believes he may have been infected about 6 years ago by a woman with whom he had a brief, meaningless relationship. For that one indiscretion we will both pay the ultimate price.

Case II: The HIV-Infected Male

In February of 1994, a 21-year-old man walked into a sexually transmitted disease clinic and told the doctor he had "the clap," or gonorrhea. But he carried HIV.

When a counselor inquired about his sex partners, he told them about several, including a 12-year-old girl. The girl had gone elsewhere to be treated for gonorrhea and tested positive for HIV.

The man admitted to sleeping with 27 women, including 13 teenagers. Ten of the partners couldn't be found. Of the 17 others, 12 tested positive for HIV.

The man has since died, and the clinic has not been able to track all of his sexual partners.

There is a message to be found in these two cases: People with HIV are much more dangerous to a community than someone with AIDS. Those with AIDS are symptomatic. They are losing weight. They are sick. They have little or no sexual appetite. Those with HIV are healthy and vigorous. That's where the sexual roulette begins.

---

the heterosexual population. The male-to-female ratio in Africa is 1:1. In late 1991, the World Health Organization stated that 75% of worldwide HIV transmission occurred heterosexually. By the year 2000, up to 90% will occur heterosexually. Homosexuality and injection drug use occurs in Africa but the incidence is reported to be very low. The high frequency of AIDS cases in Third World countries is thought to be due to poor hygiene, lack of medicine and medical facilities, a population that demonstrates a large variety of sexually transmitted diseases and other chronic infections, unsanitary disposal of contaminated materials, lack of refrigeration, and the reuse of hypodermic syringes and needles due to supply shortages.

Transmission from men to women in Nairobi has been shown to be facilitated by common genital ulcers, the use of oral contraceptives rather than condoms, and the presence of chlamydia, a type of bacterium. Chlamydia infection probably increases the inflammatory response in the vaginal walls and increases the likelihood of having lymphocytes there that can attach to the virus and allow transmission. The damage that sexually transmitted ulcerative diseases cause to genital skin and mucous membranes is believed to facilitate HIV transmission. Prevention and early treatment of STDs could slow HIV transmission in the United States and in other countries.

Vaginal and Anal Intercourse— Among routes of HIV transmission, there is overwhelming evidence that HIV can be transmitted via anal and vaginal intercourse. In vaginal intercourse, male-to-female transmission is much more efficient than the reverse. This is believed to be due to (**1**) a consistently higher concentration of HIV in semen than in vaginal secretions, and (**2**) abrasions in the vaginal mucosa. Such abrasions in the tissue allow HIV to enter the vascular system in larger numbers than would occur otherwise, and perhaps at a single entry point.

The same reasoning explains why the receptive rather than the insertive homosexual partner is more likely to become HIV-infected during anal intercourse. It appears that the membranous linings of the rectum, rich in blood vessels, are more easily torn than are those of the vagina. In addition, recent studies indicate the presence of receptors for HIV in rectal mucosal tissue. A recent report by Richard Naftalin (1992) states that human semen contains at least two components, collagenase and spermine, that cause the breakdown of the membrane that supports the colonic epithelial cell layer of the rectal and colon mucosa. This leads to the loss of mucosal barrier function allowing substances to penetrate the rectal and colon mucosa.

Homosexual Anal Intercourse— Today about 60% of homosexual men in San Francisco are infected, probably the highest density of infection anywhere in the developed world. "It colors everything we do out here," says a gay activist, "the gay community, to a large extent, is about addressing AIDS. It has to be, because it's literally a war: your entire community is under siege."

In a single year, 1982, 21% of the uninfected gay male population became infected, and for some reason not yet known, many of those infected early, died early. "Soon everyone, and I mean everyone, had a friend who was dying" (Science in California, 1993). During 1995, 1996 and into 1997, three gay men died of AIDS each day and three become HIV-positive (seroconvert). This rate of seroconversion is down from 20 a day in the early 1980s (Conant, 1995).

--------- BOX 8.4 ---------

RE-INFECTION AMONG HIV-POSITIVE GAY MEN

Four HIV-positive gay men were talking about sex. The conversation turned to unprotected sex. It turned out that all four had unprotected sex with their HIV-positive partners. On reflection about what they know of their other HIV-positive friends and their sexual behavior, they agreed that unprotected sex among HIV-positive partners appeared to be the norm. One of the four men said that he had unprotected sex with hundreds of men, some with and without HIV. He guessed he must have been re-infected many times. Another commented that re-infection is occurring in the gay community more times than anyone can believe—we just don't talk about it!

It appears that of all sexual activities, **anal intercourse** is the most efficient way to transmit HIV (DeVincenzi et al., 1989). Information collected from cross-sectional and longitudinal (cohort) studies has clearly implicated receptive anal intercourse as the major mode of acquiring HIV infection. The proportion of new HIV infections among gay males attributable to this single sexual practice is about 90%.

Major risk factors identified with regard to HIV transmission among gay males include anal intercourse (both receptive and insertive), active oral-anal contact, number of partners, and length of homosexual lifestyle (Kingsley et al., 1990).

Heterosexual Anal Intercourse— A number of sexuality oriented surveys of the heterosexual population indicate that between one in five and one in 10 heterosexual couples have tried or regularly practice anal intercourse. Bolling (1989) reported that 70% to 80% of women may have tried anal intercourse and that 10% to 25% of

─────── BOX 8.5 ───────

GAY MEN PUTTING THEMSELVES AT HIGH RISK FOR HIV INFECTION

At the 11th International Conference on AIDS (July 1996), AIDS researchers said that a generation of young gay men across the industrialized world, tragically ignoring the lessons of the AIDS pandemic, risk a new wave of HIV infection by engaging in unsafe sex. In some parts of the United States, **as many as one in 10 gay men under the age of 25 carries HIV**, and the risk appears to be especially high for nonwhite minorities. Such figures are high, very high, especially considering that these young men have become sexually active in an era in which massive effort was exerted to increase awareness of HIV risk behaviors and to promote safer sex.

A variety of surveys have found that about one-third of young gay men in their 20s engage in anal sex without condoms, the riskiest form of homosexual behavior.

Experts believe one reason risky behavior continues among the young is that they have not yet seen their friends die of the disease.

Another is simply the kind of risk-taking common among the young—the same impulse that prompts teenagers to drive fast or take up smoking.

THE HIGH RATE OF HIV INFECTION AMONG GAY MEN ON SOUTH BEACH, MIAMI, FLORIDA

Miami's South Beach—hot music, hot spots, hot sun, hot bodies. The once sagging tip of Miami Beach has been turned into the playground of the beautiful, the rich, and the chic. South Beach is also a growing mecca for young gay men. In a world where homosexuality is often confined to the closet, it is a place to be out and to be open. But behind the perfect tans, there is the dark reality! According to a new study one in every six gay men between the ages of 18 and 29 in South Beach has tested HIV-positive.

William Darrow, AIDS researcher who surveyed 87 gay men ages 18 to 29 and 70 gay men age 30 and older, said, "People seem to think they're on a holiday there from everything—including AIDS." Darrow's survey showed that about 75% of gay men in both age groups had **unprotected anal sex** in 1996.

Testimonial—One gay male living at South Beach said he fell victim to **love**. "I was in a relationship, and we both got tested together and we tested negative, so we started having unprotected sex. But during the relationship, my partner was cheating on me and he was infected and in turn infected me."

A majority of young gay men have grown up thinking they won't reach middle age; for those who aren't positive, the specter of AIDS haunts them. For many of those who have grown up with the safer sex message, the words of warning are often lost. In addition, the media covering the new anti-AIDS drugs, protease inhibitors, are generating **hype and new hope**, but there is a downside: young gay men may be letting their guards down because of the hype. Another contributing high-risk behavioral factor is the growing number of gay bathhouses and sex clubs cropping up across the country. People come to South Beach to have anonymous sex; they pay to use the facility and condoms are free. Safer sex posters are everywhere. But, some argue that bathhouses are centers for HIV infection; others argue that shutting down bathhouses will drive men in search of sex to public parks or other unmonitored settings.

these women enjoyed anal sex on a regular basis. He also reported that 58% of women with multiple sex partners participated in anal sex. James Segars (1989) reported that the highest rates of anal sex occur among teenagers who use drugs and older married couples who are broadening their sexual experiences.

Although it may increase the risk of HIV infection, it must be emphasized that anal intercourse is not necessary for HIV transmission among heterosexuals. In fact, most HIV-infected heterosexuals say that they have never practiced anal intercourse.

Risk of HIV Infection; Number of Sexual Encounters— The risk of HIV infection to a susceptible person after one or more sexual encounters is very difficult to determine. In some cases, people claim to have become infected after a single sexual encounter.

In some reported transfusion-associated HIV infections, the female partners of infected males remained HIV-negative after 5 or more years of unprotected sexual intercourse. Television star Paul Michael Glaser said that he had normal sexual relations with his wife Elizabeth for 5 years prior to her being diagnosed as HIV-infected (Figure 8-8). He was not HIV-infected. She received HIV during a blood transfusion, but was not diagnosed until after their first-born child was diagnosed with HIV. In other studies of heterosexual HIV transmission, many couples had unprotected sexual intercourse over prolonged periods of time with no more than 50% of the partners becoming HIV-infected. There are many instances of heterosexuals and homosexuals who remained HIV-negative after having repeated sexual intercourse with HIV-infected partners.

The fact that not all who are repeatedly exposed become infected suggests that biological factors may play as large a role in HIV infection as behavioral factors. For biological reasons, some people may be more efficient transmitters of HIV; while others are more susceptible to HIV infection, that is, require a smaller HIV infective dose. And, it is now known that some people carry genes that may make them resistant to HIV infection (see "Mutant CKR-5 Genes" in Chapter 5).

FIGURE 8-8 Paul Michael and Elizabeth Glaser. (*Photograph couresy of AP/Wide World Photos*)

Number of Sexual Partners and Types of Activity— One relatively large risk factor for HIV infection in both homosexuals and heterosexuals is believed to be the number of sexual partners. The greater the number of sexual partners, the greater the probability of HIV infection.

The scale of multiple-partnering during the late 20th century is unprecedented. With over $5^1/_2$ billion people on earth, an ever-increasing percentage of whom are urban residents; with air travel and mass transit available to allow people from all over the world to go to the cities of their choice; with mass youth movements advocating, among other things, sexual freedom; with a feminist spirit alive in much of the industrialized world, promoting female sexual freedom; and with 47% of the world's population made up of people between the ages of 15 and 44—there can be no doubt that the amount of worldwide urban sexual energy is unparelleled.

The amount of protection one actually obtains from limiting one's number of partners depends mainly on who those partners are. Having one partner who is in a high-risk group may be more

———— BOX 8.6 ————

SPORTS AND HIV/AIDS: EARVIN "MAGIC" JOHNSON AND OTHER ATHLETES

HIV-INFECTED ATHLETES AND COMPETITION

The question regarding whether HIV-infected athletes should be allowed to compete has two facets:

1. Should these athletes be banned from competition to avoid the risk of spreading HIV infection?

2. Does the exercise that is demanded in competition accelerate progression of HIV disease?

As yet, there is no hard, fast, scientifically supported answer to either question. However, beginning 1998, there has not been a single reported case of HIV transmission in any sporting event worldwide! (Drotman, 1996, updated).

Magic Johnson: Age 32; Professional Basketball Player, Los Angeles Lakers, HIV-Positive

On November 7, 1991, Magic Johnson (Figure 8-9) appeared at a nationally televised press conference and said, "Because of the HIV virus I have obtained, I will have to announce my retirement from the Lakers today." He admitted having been "naive" about AIDS and added, "Here I am saying **it can happen to anybody,** even me, Magic Johnson." He also assured the world that his wife, Cookie Kelly, 2 months pregnant, had tested negative for the virus. As he spoke, Johnson promised to battle the disease and "become a spokesman" for it. New York AIDS activist Rodger McFarlane said, "If you tried to come up with the perfect person to carry the message of AIDS awareness to the people it ought to reach, you couldn't do better than Magic Johnson."

In 1995, it was reported on the Mary Lou Fenner TV Show that Magic had an outbreak of Shingles prior to learning he was HIV-positive. (Shingles is an infection caused by the varicella-zoster virus, a herpes virus. It is characterized by skin eruptions on one side of the body following the course of a nerve inflammation. The virus may lay dormant for years before being activated by some outside agent.)

The National AIDS Hotline lit up with 40,000 phone calls on the day of Johnson's announcement, instead of the usual 3,800. At the Centers for Disease Control and Prevention in Atlanta,

AIDS-related calls, which usually average 200 per hour, jumped to 10,000 in a single hour. And shares of Carter-Wallace, Inc., the maker of Trojan condoms, were up $3 on Johnson's announcement that he would become a spokesperson for safer sex. Following Johnson's HIV infection announcement, STD/HIV sexual risk behaviors of persons of an STD clinic in a Maryland suburb of Washington, D.C. were studied. Information was gathered during the 14 weeks prior to his announcement and for 14 weeks after his announcement. The same 283 people were interviewed before and after Johnson's announcement. The mean age was 25 years, 85% had a high school diploma, 60% were males, and 73% of the males were black. Johnson's announcement appeared to lower the number of one-

FIGURE 8-9 Earvin "Magic" Johnson, National Basketball Association Basketball Star. The photograph was taken on November 7, 1991 as he announced that he is HIV-positive and that because of the infection, he retired from the Los Angeles Lakers team. He was 32 years old at this time and at the peak of his basketball career. His wish is to become a spokesperson for the struggle against HIV/AIDS. (*Photograph courtesy of AP/Wide World Photos*)

night stands for persons between ages 16 to 48, but it had no effect on the use of condoms. Persons between 25 and 48 reduced their number of sexual partners but those between the ages of 16 and 24 did not (Boekeloo et al., 1993). Prior to Magic's announcement, the black community lacked a focal point for action: no leader of national stature had claimed a prominent space from which to address HIV disease. Few black politicians, entertainers, civil rights leaders, or sports figures had tackled the issue of AIDS either through public service announcements, television talk shows, radio addresses, church pulpits, theaters, or school auditoriums. Magic's announcement—at least for a time—changed that.

Some Events Since Magic's Announced Retirement

June 4, 1992—Earvin the III is born *without* antibody to HIV. (As of August 14, 1998, Magic is age 39. His wife, age 39, and baby, age 7, are HIV-negative.)

Magic announced in April 1997 that his AIDS drug combination which included a protease inhibitor has reduced his viral load to unmeasurable blood levels!

OTHER SPORTS, OTHER ATHLETES

Basketball players are not the only athletes whose behavior may place them at risk for HIV infection. In 1996 there were 6,114 professional athletes in the United States involved in Boxing (3,500), National Football League (1,590), National Hockey League (676), and the National Basketball League (348). Of these professionals, the CDC estimated 30 to be HIV-positive.

John Elson (1991) wrote a revealing article for *Time* magazine just after Magic Johnson revealed his HIV status. Elson tells of groupies that follow athletes in all sports. They are usually college-age or older. Mainly they seek money, attention, and the glamor of associating with celebrated and highly visible "hard bodies." According to a 31-year-old who has had affairs with athletes in two sports, "For women, many of whom don't have meaningful work, the only way to identify themselves is to say whom they have slept with. A woman who sleeps around is called a whore. But a woman who has slept with Magic Johnson is a woman who has slept with Magic Johnson. It's almost as if it gives her legitimacy."

Baseball players call them "Annies." To riders on the rodeo circuit, they are "buckle bunnies."

To most other athletes, they are "wannabes" or just "the girls." They can be found hanging out anywhere they might catch an off-duty sports hero's eye and fancy, or in the lobbies of hotels where teams on the road check in. To the athletes who care to indulge them—and many do—these readily available groupies offer pro sport's ultimate perk: free and easy recreational sex, no questions asked. Recently, an HIV-infected female stated publicly that she had had sex with at least 50 Canadian ice hockey players. She could not recall their names. The sex may be free, but now there is a price for the lifestyle—HIV/AIDS.

Concerns over the transmission of HIV are shared throughout sports, particularly those sports that cause blood-letting injuries—football, hockey, and boxing. In football Jerry Smith, a former Washington Redskin, died of AIDS in 1986; no others are known at this time. In 1996, the National Football League officials estimated that there was the **possibility** of one HIV transmission from body fluid exchange in 85 million football games played. In boxing, Esteban DeJesus, WBC lightweight champion, died of AIDS in 1989. Three other boxers are known to be HIV-positive. In February of 1996 Tommy Morrison, age 27, a heavyweight boxing title contender (Figure 8-10) said, on announcing that he is HIV-positive, "I honestly believed I had a better chance of winning the lottery than contracting this disease. I've never been so wrong in my life. I'm here to tell you I thought that I was bulletproof, and I'm not." Morrison went on to describe his promiscuous sexual lifestyle and ignorance about AIDS. Former heavyweight champ Floyd Paterson, the current chairman of the New York State Athletic Commission, who was asked why his organization waited until the Tommy Morrison case to institute HIV testing for boxers, said "AIDS just came out, I go back to the '50s. I fought for 23 years. There was no AIDS. **I just heard of AIDS a few weeks ago.**" Just heard of AIDS? Since Morrison's announcement, 12 states have banned HIV-positive professional boxers from the ring. In November 1996, Morrison fought in Japan. He knocked his opponent out in 1:38 (1 minute, 38 seconds). The fight would have been stopped at the first sign of Morrison's blood.

Update July 1997 POZ Magazine Interview—Tommy Morrison now believes that HIV is not a disease-causing virus! **"AIDS has been here since creation, but is doesn't do anything"** and as for AIDS, he says, **"Acquired Immune Deficiency Syndrome is something that's easily**

—————— **BOX 8.6** (*continued*) ——————

cured." With regard to taking anti-HIV drugs, he "fired" his physician who prescribed them for him (Dr. David Ho, *Time Magazine* **Man of the Year 1996**). He points to an HIV-infected friend and says **"this kid was perfectly healthy until he started taking medication."** He says that he and his wife have **unprotected** sex because **"HIV can't hurt you. There is no way you can get HIV from sex. It's scientifically impossible."**

Morrison refers to himself as the most educated person he knows regarding HIV (he read Peter Duesberg's book, *Inventing the AIDS Virus* and Richard Wilner's *Deadly Deception*). "I don't know how I know the things I know, I just know

FIGURE 8-11 Greg Louganis. (*Photograph courtesy of Archive Photos*)

I'm right—I have not been sick in 5 years—if it ain't broke don't fix it."

There is a certain irony in all of this because as part of his probationary terms of a suspended sentence for weapons violation and assault charges, he gives speeches to high school and college students on HIV/AIDS!

In professional ice skating, the Calgary Herald reported that, by 1992, at least 40 top United States and Canadian male skaters and coaches have died from AIDS (among them, Rob McCall, Brian Pockar, Dennis Coi, and Shawn McGill). In February 1995, Greg Louganis, the greatest diver in Olympic history, announced that he has AIDS (Figure 8-11).

In 1996, Tim Richmond, race car driver, age 34, died of AIDS. He won 13 Winston Cup races on The NASCAR racing circuit. One report states that Richmond may have infected up to 30 women (Knight-Tribune Service, March 27, 1996, A-1). His physician estimated that he was HIV-positive for at least 8 years. During this time, according to accounts of friends and so on he was sexually promiscuous. (Richmond actually died in 1989 but his story was kept silent until 1996.)

Bill Goldsworthy, five-time NHL All-Star, age 51, dies of AIDS. He played 14 seasons in the NHL. He was diagnosed with AIDS in 1994. Goldworthy said his health problem was caused by drinking and sexual promiscuity.

FIGURE 8-10 Tommy Morrison. Las Vegas, NV, 7 June 1993—Tommy Morrison raises his right hand after being declared the new WBO heavyweight champion. Morrison won the 12-round bout against former heavyweight champion George Foreman at the Thomas & Mack Center. (*Photograph courtesy of Archive Photos*)

dangerous than having many partners who are not. An example of this is seen in prostitutes, who may be more likely to be infected by their regular injection drug using partners than by customers, who are not in a high-risk group. The risk status of a person who remains faithful to a single sexual partner depends on that partner's behavior: if the partner becomes infected, often without knowing it, the monogamous individual is likely to become infected (Cohen et al., 1989).

Sexual Activities— In addition to a high-risk partner or a number of sexual partners, the types of sexual activities that occur are also significant (Table 8-7). Any sexual activity that produces skin, anal, or vaginal membrane abrasions prior to or during intercourse increases the risk of infection.

OROGENITAL SEX. Orogenital sex may be a greater risk factor for becoming HIV-infected than previously thought. Of 82 HIV-infected gay men in three San Francisco area studies, 14 (17%) gave orogenital sex as their only high-risk behavior (AIDS Research, 1990). A case was reported of a heterosexual male becoming

TABLE 8-7   Sexual Activity According to Degree of Risk for Transmitting HIV

Lowest risk	1. Abstinence
	2. Masturbating alone
	3. Hugging/massage/dry kissing
	4. Masturbating with another person but not touching one another
	5. Deep wet kissing
	6. Mutual masturbation with only external touching
	7. Mutual masturbation with internal touching using finger cots or condoms
	8. Frottage (rubbing a person for sexual pleasure)
	9. Intercourse between the thighs
	10. Mutual masturbation with orgasm *on*, not *in* partner
	11. Use of sex toys (dildos) with condoms, or that are not shared by partners and that have been properly sterilized between uses
	12. Cunnilingus
	13. Fellatio without a condom, but never putting the head of the penis inside mouth
	14. Fellatio to orgasm with a condom
	15. Fellatio without a condom putting the head of the penis inside the mouth and withdrawing prior to ejaculation
	16. Fellatio without a condom with ejaculation in mouth
	17. Vaginal intercourse with a condom correctly used and spermicidal foam that kills HIV and withdrawing prior to orgasm
	18. Anal intercourse with a condom correctly used with a lubricant that contains spermicide that kills HIV and withdrawing prior to ejaculation
	19. Vaginal intercourse with internal ejaculation with a condom correctly used and with spermicidal foam that kills HIV
	20. Vaginal intercourse with internal ejaculation with a condom correctly used but no spermicidal foam
	21. Anal intercourse with internal ejaculation with a condom correctly used with spermicide that kills HIV
	22. Brachiovaginal activities (fisting)
	23. Brachioproctic activities (anal fisting)
	24. Use of sex toys by more than one partner without a condom and that have not been sterilized between uses
	25. Vaginal intercourse using spermicidal foam but without a condom and withdrawing prior to ejaculation
	26. Vaginal intercourse without spermicidal foam and without a condom and withdrawing prior to ejaculation
	27. Anal intercourse with a condom and withdrawing prior to ejaculation
	28. Vaginal intercourse with internal ejaculation without a condom but with spermicidal foam
	29. Vaginal intercourse with internal ejaculation without a condom and without any other form of barrier contraception
Highest risk	30. Anal intercourse with internal ejaculation without a condom

(Source: Shernoff, 1988)

HIV-infected after receiving oral sex (fellatio) from a prostitute who was HIV-infected (Fischl et al., 1987). Ireneus Keet and colleagues (1992) reported on several studies on the risk of HIV transmission among gay males. They concluded that the orogenital route of HIV transmission is difficult to assess. Information on questionnaires was frequently contradicted in follow up interviews. For example, of 20 men who denied having receptive anal intercourse, 11 later changed their statements. However, Keet and colleagues concluded that there is sufficient evidence to conclude that orogenital HIV transmission does occur.

Madalene Heng and colleagues (1994) reported that HIV-infected patients with oral herpes simplex lesions are at risk of transmitting HIV to others through oral sex. They tested keratinocytes (live skin cells) from the oral lesions of six men with AIDS and oral herpes infection (HSV-1), and compared those biopsies from six men with HSV-1 but not HIV.

The tissue from the HIV/herpes patients was infected with both viruses, and the number of virus in that tissue was much higher than the number found in samples from the other men—736 particles per skin cell compared to 31 and 0 in the other two groups.

This shows that HIV is capable of infecting epidermal cells when herpes virus is present. Epidermal keratinocytes were thought to be resistant to HIV infection because they lack the CD4 receptor molecule.

Data from this study is similar to that from a previous study of brain cells of people infected with both HIV and cytomegalovirus. The brain tissue also lacks CD4 receptors, yet HIV was able to invade the cells and replicate.

The researchers speculated that the association of HIV envelope proteins with HSV-1 proteins may allow HIV to infect cells without the aid of CD4 molecules.

After reading the six articles, by Jeffrey Lawrence, Alison Quayle, Gerad Ilarca, Alan Lifson, Michael Samuel, and Rebecca Young (1995), adapted from presentations at a seminar "**Oral Sex and Possible HIV Transmission: A Community Discussion**," and after reading *"The Riddle of Oral Sex"* by Robert Marks (1996), the author of this text is convinced that those persons who participate in

oral receptive sex are placing themselves at risk for HIV infection. Periodontal disease, herpes lesions, and other conditions may make an individual more susceptible to transmission. Reported within these and other articles, there are a number of cases where oral sex was the only at risk activity practiced and the oral receptive partner became HIV-positive. The articles listed are recommend reading for those who need to be convinced that orogenital sex places one at risk for HIV infection.

Additional articles are those of G.M. Liuzzi and co-workers (1995) and Omar Bagasra (1996) who determined quantitatively the cell-free HIV RNA molecules in semen, saliva, and plasma from HIV-infected people.

PROSTITUTION (SEX WORKER). There is little if any evidence that prostitutes in pattern I countries (The U.S.A. and other developed nations) play a large role in heterosexual HIV transmission (Cohen et al., 1989).

An unfortunate consequence of the attention prostitutes or sex workers have attracted in relation to AIDS in the United States and other countries, is that they tend to be seen as responsible for the spread of HIV — an attitude reflected in descriptions of prostitutes as reservoirs of infection or high-frequency transmitters. But, the sex worker is only the most "visible" side of a transaction that involves two people: for every sex worker who is HIV-positive there is, somewhere, the partner from whom she or he contracted HIV. Given the fact that the chance of contracting HIV during a single act of unprotected sex is not high, infection in a sex worker is likely to mean that she or he has been repeatedly exposed to HIV by clients who did not or would not wear condoms. Thus the more useful way of reading the statistics of HIV infection in prostitutes or sex workers is to view them as an indication of how strong a foothold the epidemic has gotten within a community.

Risk Estimates for HIV Infection During Sexual Intercourse in the Heterosexual Population— Norman Hearst and Stephen Hulley of the University of California, San Francisco calculated that the odds of heterosexual HIV transmission range from **one in 500 for a single act**

of sexual intercourse with an HIV-infected partner when no condom is used to one in five billion if a condom is used and the sexual partner is HIV-negative at the time.

Table 8-8 presents estimates of the risk of HIV infection from a single heterosexual encounter and after 5 years of frequent heterosexual contact for various types of partners. Risk depends on the following: (1) the probability that the sexual partner carries the virus; (2) the probability of infection given a single sexual exposure to an infected partner; and (3) the reduction in risk by using condoms and spermicides.

The most striking feature of the table is the large variation in the risk of HIV infection under different circumstances. The most important cause of this variation is risk status of sexual partners (Figure 8-12). Choosing a partner who is not in a high-risk group provides almost 5,000-fold protection compared with choosing a partner in the highest-risk category.

Condoms are estimated to provide about 1,250-fold protection. A negative HIV antibody test provides about 2,500-fold protection, against false negatives.

The implication of this analysis is clear: **Choose sex partners carefully and use condoms**.

In a study by Nancy Padian and colleagues (1991), only 1% of HIV-positive women passed HIV by sexual contact to their male partners. In contrast, one of every five uninfected female partners of HIV-infected men acquired the virus

TABLE 8-8   Risk of HIV Infection for Heterosexual Intercourse in the United States

Risk Category of Partner	Estimated Risk of Infection	
	1 Sexual Encounter	500 Sexual Encounters
HIV SEROSTATUS UNKNOWN		
Not in any high-risk group		
Using condoms	1 in 50,000,000	1 in 110,000
Not using condoms	1 in 5,000,000	1 in 16,000
High-risk groups[a]		
Using condoms	1 in 100,000 to 1 in 10,000	1 in 210 to 1 in 21
Not using condoms	1 in 10,000 to 1 in 1,000	1 in 32 to 1 in 3
HIV SERONEGATIVE		
No history of high-risk behavior[b]		
Using condoms	1 in 5,000,000,000	1 in 11,000,000
Not using condoms	1 in 500,000,000	1 in 1,600,000
Continuing high-risk behavior[b]		
Using condoms	1 in 500,000	1 in 1,100
Not using condoms	1 in 50,000	1 in 160
HIV SEROPOSITIVE		
Using condoms	1 in 5000	1 in 11
Not using condoms	1 in 500	2 in 3

[a]High-risk groups with prevalences of HIV infection at the higher end of the range given include homosexual or bisexual men, injection drug users from major metropolitan areas, and hemophiliacs. Groups with prevalences at the lower end of the range include homosexual or bisexual men and injection drug users from other parts of the country, female prostitutes, heterosexuals from countries where heterosexual spread of HIV is common (including Haiti and central Africa), and recipients of multiple blood transfusions between 1983 and 1985 from areas with a high prevalence of HIV infection.

[b]High-risk behavior consists of sexual intercourse or needle sharing with a member of one of the high-risk groups.

(Source: Adapted from Hearst and Hulley, 1988.)

through sex. Overall, the study revealed that women are 17.5 times more likely to become HIV-infected from an infected male than men are to contract the disease from an infected female. The ratio of 18:1 came from a limited study (379 heterosexual couples) and as such may underestimate the relative frequency of female-to-male HIV transmission. But, Padian's findings support the Centers for Disease Control and Prevention figures showing that 90% of the more than 33,000 adults who became HIV-positive through heterosexual contact were women.

Injection Drug Users and HIV Transmission

The hypodermic syringe and needle play an essential role in medical therapy; they also play a role in HIV transmission (Table 8–9). Injection drug use (IDU) is the second high-est risk behavior in the United States and Europe, accounting for about 30% of AIDS cases in 1989. As of June 30, 1997, of 604,176 cases of AIDS reported to CDC, 217,503 (36%) were directly or indirectly associated with injecting-drug use. Injecting-drug-user-associated AIDS cases include persons who are IDUs ($n = 190,431$), their heterosexual sex partners ($n = 22,890$), and children ($n = 4,182$) whose mothers were IDUs or sex partners of IDUs. About half of the females and about one third of the heterosexual males who were diagnosed with AIDS had a sex partner who was an IDU (*HIV/AIDS Surveillance Report*, 1997). State surveillance reports for New York indicate that 60% of IDUs are HIV-infected; in New Jersey, 80% are HIV-infected. Because 70% to 80% of IDUs have sex with non drug users, IDUs are a major source of heterosexual and perinatal HIV infection in the United States and Europe. HIV is also spreading rapidly among IDUs in developing countries such as Brazil, Argentina, and Thailand (Des Jarlais et al., 1989).

Ninety percent of injection drug users in the United States are heterosexuals. Thirty percent are women, of whom 90% are in their childbearing years. From 1988 through 1997, female IDUs made up 45% of all AIDS cases in women. Of those women infected by **heterosexual** contact (39%), (45%) were infected by having sex with a male IDU! During this same period over 6,000 new cases of AIDS in children occurred—40% were from IDU mothers and 18% were from mothers whose sex partners were IDUs (*MMWR*, 1992; *HIV/AIDS Surveillance Report*, 1997). Women drug users and sexual partners of male drug users represent the largest part (61%) of the estimated 100,000 HIV-infected women of childbearing age. Thus, there is a direct correlation between HIV perinatal transmission and pediatric AIDS cases and injection drug use. In addition, 30% to 50% of female injection drug users have engaged in prostitution, and as such represent the largest pool of HIV-infected heterosexuals in the United States and Europe (Drucker, 1986). The use of alcohol (Avins, 1994) and the use of other noninjection drugs such as crack cocaine are believed to play an increasing role in HIV transmission among heterosexuals.

POINT OF INFORMATION 8.7

RAPID SPREAD OF HIV THROUGH INJECTION DRUG USE

Don Des Jarlais (1995) writes that the injection of illegal drugs has now been reported in 118 countries throughout the world, and HIV infection among injecting drug users (IDUs) has been reported in 80 countries. In some areas, the spread of HIV among IDUs due to the multiperson use of drug injection equipment has occurred extremely rapidly. In New York City, HIV seroprevalence among IDUs increased from less than 10% to more than 50% in 5 years; in Edinburgh, Scotland, HIV seroprevalence among IDUs increased from 0 to more than 40% in 1 year; in Bangkok, Thailand, HIV seroprevalence among IDUs increased from 2% to more than 40% in 2 years; and in the Indian state of Manipur, HIV seroprevalence increased from 0 to approximately 50% in 1 year. Clearly, HIV has spread rapidly among some populations of IDUs.

In sharp contrast, however, there are also areas where HIV was introduced into the local population of IDUs, but where HIV seroprevalence has remained low and stable for extended periods. In these areas (for example, Sydney, Australia; Toronto, Canada; Lund, Sweden; Glasgow, Scotland; Tacoma, United States), IDUs have access to sterile injection equipment.

Chance One
Night Encounter

Prostitute

Member
of Low
Risk Group
Population

Injection
Drug User

Bisexual/Homosexual

✪ = sex partner

✪ = HIV infected person

FIGURE 8-12 Risk Transmission of HIV. Sexual transmission can occur among homosexuals or heterosexuals. Prostitutes can be either male or female. The diagram shows possible bridges for transmission of HIV from high-risk groups into low-risk groups. To be safe, *you* must not become part of the chain. Be sure your sexual partner is free of HIV.

Over 80% of reported adult **heterosexual** AIDS cases are associated with people who have a history of injection drug use or have sex with IDUs. Twenty-six percent of *all* AIDS cases in the United States occur in IDUs; 21% of these cases occur where IDU is the only risk factor. Of pediatric AIDS cases, 91% occur perinatally. Of these, 60% are associated with IDU by either the mother or her sexual partner (*HIV/AIDS Surveillance Report*, 1997).

The prevalence of HIV infection in IDUs varies widely with geography. Data from more than 18,000 people tested in nearly 90 surveys consistently show high rates in eastern towns and cities with close proximity to New York City and northern New Jersey. Eighty-two percent of AIDS cases among all **reported** IDUs have been in New York City. It should be noted that most of the surveys were conducted in drug treatment facilities for heroin abuse. Since only 10% to 20% of the estimated 1,100,000 IDUs are currently in treatment, geographical

conclusions based on the surveys may be misleading. More data are needed on HIV prevalence among injection drug users not currently in treatment.

Other Means of HIV Transmission

Other means of HIV infection have been documented. There has been a reported case of HIV transmission via acupuncture. It is believed that HIV-infected body fluids contaminated the acupuncture needles (Vittecoq et al., 1989). Also, artificial insemination can be a means of HIV transmission (Point of Information 8.3). Unlicensed and unregulated tattoo establishments may also present an unrecognized risk for HIV infection to patrons. If the operator does not use new needles or needles which have been autoclaved (steam sterilized), the possibility exists that infection with HIV or a number of other blood-borne pathogens may take place. In addition, single-

TABLE 8-9 Population[a] Risk of HIV Transmission Based on Type of Activity[b]

Activity	Risk	Notes and Sources
Vaginal sexual intercourse	1 infection per 1,000 acts with HIV-positive partner (0.1%)	Mean per-act risk for unprotected intercourse. Source: Isabelle de Vincenzi, European Study Group on Heterosexual Transmission of HIV, 1994
Receptive anal intercourse	5 to 10 infections per 1,000 acts with HIV-positive partner (0.5%–3%)	With no condom use. Source: Victor DeGruttola, Harvard School of Public Health, 1989
Intravenous drug injection with infected needed	10 to 20 infections per 1,000 needle uses (1%–2%)	Source: Don Des Jarlais, Beth Israel Medical Center, New York
Accidental stick in medical setting with infected needle	3 infections per 1,000 sticks (0.3%)	Source: Centers for Disease Control and Prevention
Transfusion of screened blood	1 infection per 450,000 to 650,000 donations (0.0002%–0.00015%)	Source: Centers for Disease Control and Prevention/American National Red Cross

[a]Rough estimates of the relative risks in the United States and Western Europe of the more risky activities that can transmit HIV. **THESE CALCULATIONS CAN NOT BE USED AS A GUIDE TO INDIVIDUAL BEHAVIOR.** Risk to any one person depends on many factors that cannot be reduced to a single number. Recent research, for example, suggests that the infectiousness of HIV can vary greatly over the life of an infected person; infectiousness is likely to be high both at the very outset of the infection, before symptoms have appeared, and several years later. Also, women may be several times more likely than men to be infected during vaginal intercourse, a distinction that the overall risk figure obscures. (Adapted from Bennett et al., 1996)

[b]Risks vary because of differences in genital, anal, and oral mucous membranes. Sex is risk free, with or without a condom **if the partner is known to be uninfected.** Nonpenetrative sex such as mutual masturbation is nearly risk free. Sex involving penetration with fingers is low risk. Sex involving unshared sex toys is risk free. Receiving oral sex is less risky than other penetrative behaviors. Penile-receptive sexual behavior is more risky than its penile-insertive counterpart. Anal or vaginal sex without a condom is far more risky than performing oral sex without a condom. (Source: Voelker, 1996)

service or individual containers of dye or ink should be used for each client.

Human Bites— According to police reports, a Florida woman with a history of arrests for prostitution and who has tested HIV-positive, bit a 93-year-old man on his arm, head, and leg while robbing him. The bites required stitches. The man initially tested HIV-negative but a test several months later was HIV-positive. A complete investigation into his personal life ruled out previous HIV infection.

In October of 1995 the CDC confirmed that a 91-year-old male became HIV-infected when, **being robbed,** he was bitten deeply, inflicting extensive tissue damage to the hand by a prostitute with bleeding gums. The man tested HIV-negative shortly after the bite but tested positive 8 weeks later. There have been other reports in the medical literature in which HIV appeared to have been transmitted by a bite. Severe trauma with extensive tissue tearing and damage and presence of blood were reported in each of these instances. Biting is not a common way of transmitting HIV. In fact, there are numerous reports of bites that did not result in HIV infection.

Sexual Assault— The subject of sexual assault, in all its forms, of children by adults or adult on adult is beyond the scope of this text. However, each time there is a date-rape or any other type of rape there is the chance that the rapist may be HIV-positive. One in five adult women has been the victim of a completed rape at some time in her life (Koss et al., 1991). A **conservative estimate** of the **risk of transmission** of HIV **from sexual assault** (that invoved anal or vaginal penetration and exposure to ejaculate from an HIV-infected assailant) is greater **than two infections per 1,000 contacts,** given a variety of factors, such as clinical stage of the assailant's HIV infection, strength of the strain of HIV and repeated exposure. The per-contact risk is higher if there was violence producing trauma and blood exposure or the presence of inflammatory or ulcerative sexually transmitted diseases (Gostin, 1994). Although 61% of the

——————— BOX 8.7 ———————

PLACING THE RISK OF DEATH DUE TO HIV INFECTION AND AIDS IN PERSPECTIVE IN RELATION TO DEATHS CAUSED BY OTHER DISEASES, ACCIDENTS, AND MURDERS

Before reading this section it might be useful to keep in mind that the line between **risk** and **blame** is very thin. Too often risk figures are used to place or fix blame. Risk figures are used to transmit fact but may give misleading impressions. And misleading impressions can have enormous impact on public policy. Thus the need to place HIV disease in perspective.

In 1996, 555,000 people died from cancer; about 37,000 died from AIDS. In this same year, there were 1,359,000 new cancer cases, there were about 70,000 new AIDS cases (about 6% of the new cancer cases).

An estimated 48 million Americans over age 18 smoke about 24 billion packages of cigarettes each year (*MMWR*, 1994c).

Tobacco use in various forms was associated with the deaths of over 400,000 people **each year** from 1991 through 1997 and most likely will continue at this rate through the year 2000, at an annual cost to the work force of at least $52 billion. Former Surgeon General C. Everett Koop said in early 1989 that smoking was the single most preventable cause of death known. It kills more people than HIV/AIDS, cocaine, heroin, alcohol, fire, automobile accidents, homicide, and suicide combined (Will, 1991). One in six deaths is caused by smoking and smoking-related deaths continue in spite of a 28-year-old warning concerning the risks of smoking. Worldwide, mid-1992, it was reported that about 3 million people a year die due to the Brown Plague, smoking-related diseases (Peto, 1992). In 1993, some 160,000 deaths resulted from various forms of cancer due to tobacco used (Munzer, 1994).

In the United States from 1988 through 1997 some 32,000 to 40,000 people died from AIDS each year—yet 32,000 people died from to-bacco-related diseases every 32 days. Also during each of these years there were about 1.5 million heart attacks resulting in 550,000 deaths; and 1,800,000 people were involved in automobile accidents resulting in 48,700 deaths. In each of these years, between 30,000 and 40,000 people committed suicide and about 30,000 were killed in shootings.

From 1981 to 1990, about a quarter of a million people died because of drunken drivers on American highways. In this same time period about 70,000 people died from AIDS. For the year 1997, over 40,000 men died of prostate cancer and 244,000 new cases were diagnosed. During the same time period 30,000 men died from AIDS and 55,000 new AIDS cases were diagnosed in men.

According to UNICEF, about 39,000 children under age 5 die **each day** in Latin America, Asia, and Africa. They die of starvation, lack of medicine, poor sanitary conditions, and such. Far more children and adults are dying each day from famine than from AIDS. In these countries, HIV infection is not a major concern—their next meal is.

HIV/AIDS is real, it is here, but it is **preventable**. The odds of heterosexual HIV infection after a single penile–vaginal encounter with a low-risk partner when a condom is used are about 1 in 50 million. Without the condom it is about 1 in 5 million. The long-range risk of death from smoking is about 1 in 200; motorcycling, about 1 in 1,000; automobile driving, about 1 in 6,000; canoeing, 1 in 100,000; and having a legal abortion before 9 weeks, 1 in 400,000.

In short, there are many more ways to die than from HIV/AIDS. Worldwide hunger leads the list. AIDS, like so many other diseases, is preventable. Whether you become HIV-infected depends on you.

women stated that physicians should routinely ask about these experiences, only 4% had been asked by their physicians (Walker et al., 1993). Without a complete sexual history that includes questions about rape and so forth, the proper care and medication can be delayed until the onset of HIV disease or AIDS.

Beginning 1998, there were at least 50 cases of purposeful HIV infection of males by HIV-infected females or vice versa. This too should be looked on as a form of **sexual assault**—one partner is being sexually deceived by the other. In some of these cases the jury found the HIV-positive persons who kept this knowledge from their sexual partner guilty of attempted murder.

HIV TRANSMISSION: PREPARATION AND USE OF INJECTION DRUGS

Group use of drug paraphernalia and the type of substance used are factors in transmission of HIV from person to person.

Drugs in powdered form are usually placed in a bottle cap, or "cooker," an item often found on streets or in garbage cans. Water is added and heated to dissolve the powder into a solution.

The solution is withdrawn by needle through a "cotton," or a filter through which the drug solution is drawn into the syringe. Cotton swabs, lint from clothing, cigarette filters, and a variety of other materials are used.

The needle then punctures a vein wherever there is one that can be used. Blood is drawn up into the syringe to mix with the drug solution and the blood–solution mixture is injected into the vein. If the vein is missed, the drug injected subcutaneously (under the skin) hurts and may cause an abscess. Small quantities of a drug may be injected repeatedly—each time blood is drawn up into the syringe. Then, following drug injection(s), the syringe is refilled several times with blood from the vein to wash out any heroin, cocaine, or other drug left in the syringe after the injection(s). If even a tiny, invisible amount of HIV-infected blood is left on the needle or in the syringe, the virus can be transmitted to the next user.

The "works," as the syringe and needle are referred to, are shared and the amount of sharing depends on the number of users present. Everyone after the first user in the "shooting gallery" line receives potentially HIV-infected lymphocytes from all those with HIV infection who used the equipment before them.

It should be noted that in the injection drug culture, the sharing of needles is a sign of comradery, a sign of mutual trust. An unwillingness to share needles may cause others in the group to become suspicious of possible police connections.

Drug paraphernalia are commonly rented in shooting galleries by users who lack the equipment. A set of "works" is usually rented out until the needle is too dull to penetrate the skin. By then the needle has been sharpened often on whatever was available to give it a penetrating edge. Thus, not only is HIV transmitted among those in a "shooting gallery" but other bacteria and viruses that contaminate their surroundings are also shared.

The world of injection drug use is "designed" to transmit infectious agents. However, **it is not**

the drug that is responsible for HIV transmission, rather it is the infected blood shared by each of the users of an HIV contaminated "works." The practice of sharing "works" appears to be equally common among homosexual and heterosexual drug users. Thus it provides a common link between the homosexual and heterosexual population placing both at risk for HIV infection.

Cocaine vs. Heroin— The use of injected cocaine is rising as is exposure to HIV in cocaine IDUs. One major difference between cocaine and heroin abuse is that IV cocaine abusers are binge users or repeat injectors, while the heroin abuser falls asleep after one injection. Studies in New York and San Francisco show that IV cocaine abusers are the more likely to test HIV-positive.

FIGURE 8-13 An Injection Drug User. Note that the arm is tied to force veins to fill with blood making them easier to reach. A candle is used to heat the drug into a solution. This is referred to as "cooking" the drug.

———— BOX 8.9 ————

SEXUAL ASSAULT OF CHILDREN RESULTS IN HIV INFECTION: THREE CASES

Childhood sexual abuse is a common problem that is present in all social and economic groups. Approximately one-half of children who are sexually abused are between 6 and 12 years old, and 30% to 46% have been sexually abused on more than one occasion. Most investigators report a female-to-male ratio of 8:1 or 9:1. These reports, however, come from medical centers and may not reflect the true ratio, because sexual abuse of boys is more often reported only to the police and less likely to be assessed by physicians.

Ninety-eight percent of perpetrators of childhood sexual abuse are male, one of the few common characteristics of pedophiles. No classic profile of a pedophile exists. Little evidence supports the identification of a potential pedophile on the basis of race, religion, income, social class, intelligence, occupation, or education. Forty percent of abusers are family members, and an additional 40% are known to the family. Only 20% of pedophiles are unknown to the child.

SEXUALLY TRANSMITTED DISEASE

Sexually transmitted diseases (STDs) are infrequently encountered in childhood victims of sexual abuse. However, most authorities agree that nonsexual transmission of STDs is rare in children older than 2 years. Routine cultures for STDs are positive in 5% to 12% of sexually abused children. The epithelium and relatively alkaline pH of the prepubertal vagina inhibit the growth of many sexually transmitted organisms (Gibbons, (1994).

CASE I

A woman called from an AIDS organization, asking for someone who could speak to a girl who was HIV-infected at the age of 12. The girl is not a hemophiliac and her father is the only other HIV-infected member of her family. When asked if she had considered sexual abuse as a means of transmission, the wife responded. "The family doesn't talk about that."

CASE II

When I was 13 years old, my mother's boyfriend, who was also a drug supplier, raped me. He infected me with HIV. I was robbed of my teen years and my life. I live knowing I will die soon—yet I have not begun to live.

CASE III

On March 10, 1994, the headline of a local paper read, "Abused Girl with AIDS Dies." This headline says so much yet says so little with regard to this case.

When this physically and mentally tormented young girl came to live with her foster parents in 1992 she was sad, easily frightened, and withdrawn. She had been badly abused sexually. At least a dozen men sexually abused this child. Just one was arrested and given a 10-year sentence.

She was 10 years old and couldn't read or write. She had never heard of Jesus or celebrated Christmas. She also had AIDS. She was close to death.

With the loving care of her foster parents and medications, she rebounded and lived another 2 years. She died at age 11.

The local Department of Health and Rehabilitative Services (HRS) began receiving reports involving this girl in September 1986, when she was 3. At 6, she was treated for herpes and gonorrhea. Her vaginal warts were so enlarged the cervix was not visible. Her collection of sexually transmitted diseases caused such pain that the physician had to render her unconscious to examine her vagina. She was placed on medicine for the virus, for her ears, eyes, tongue, throat, sinus, vagina, itching (which was so intense she would scrape until she bled). She suffered from severe neuropathy in her hands and feet (due to ddI), had Pneumocystis pneumonia, herpes zoster infection, diarrhea, etc. She had four close encounters with death during the 2 years she was with her foster parents.

Although at least two reports were confirmed, HRS didn't permanently remove her from her home until March, 1992.

The foster mother said people were so frightened of her that some physicians "examined" her from across the room—**"they would not touch her!"**

The girl's foster father said their goal was to give her a safe and normal childhood for the time she had left.

She was tutored at home. She went to Disney World. They took her to California to meet Roseanne Arnold. Every occasion was celebrated to the max because she had never had a party.

She had never heard of God or Jesus, so her foster parents had her baptized. When she went

——————— **BOX 8.9** (continued) ———————

up to the altar for her first communion, she put the wafer in her mouth and said in a loud voice. "Oh, that tastes nasty." And everybody broke up.

With regard to Christmas, she told her foster parents, "Santa Claus never found me." Her foster father said he explained that Santa sends parents a bill and if it's not paid, children don't get presents. "And, I told her, 'I have already sent a check to Santa, so you've got to come home.' And she said, 'Oh, boy!'" That Christmas she had seven Christmas trees and 267 gifts. "Most of them were from garage sales, but it didn't make any difference," he said. "She was thankful for anything."

With regard to dying, there were many conversations about God and heaven. She told her foster mother she wanted a God who laughed. And she hoped heaven was like Disney World. She had told her foster mother once that she was afraid to die because she didn't know how to get to heaven. "I told her, 'You'll go to sleep and you won't feel a thing, and when you wake up God will be holding your hand instead of mommy.' And that's exactly how it happened. I believe she said to God, 'This is it. Take me.' And he did."

During the 2 years of making a home for this child, the foster parents lost friends. Even relatives stopped coming to visit. But these people said they would gladly do it over again!

HIV is now the fifth leading cause of death in children under age 15 (Oleske, 1994).

Transplants— On any given day, about 20,000 Americans are waiting for a transplant. There is a small but present risk of receiving HIV along with the transplant tissue. A CDC report revealed that a bone transplant recipient became HIV-infected from an HIV-infected donor. HIV transmission has also occurred in the transplantation of kidneys, liver, heart, pancreas, and skin (*MMWR*, 1988a). In May of 1991, the CDC reported on 56 transplant patients who received organs and tissues from an HIV-infected donor in 1985. A transplantation

service company supplied tissues to 30 hospitals in 16 states. All tissues came from a single young male who was shot to death during a robbery. He twice tested HIV-negative before his heart, kidneys, liver, pancreas, cornea, and other tissues were removed for transplant. By mid-1991, three recipients of these tissues had died of AIDS and six others were HIV-positive. As of mid-1991, 32 other recipients had been located, 11 of whom tested HIV-negative. The others had not yet been tested.

In May of 1994, the CDC published guidelines for preventing HIV transmission through transplantation of human tissue (*MMWR*, 1994b).

Nosocomial

Nosocomial (nos-o-ko-mi-al) refers to hospital-acquired infections. A chain of nosocomial HIV transmission has occurred in southern Russia and among children in Romanian orphanages. In Romania between 1988 and 1990, over 250 children were infected with HIV after exposure to nonsterile needles. By June 1994, 43 of these children had died of AIDS (Bobkov, 1994). Instances of nosocomial HIV transmission have also been reported from industrialized countries such as the United States, where transmission occurred from patient to patient. While nosocomial transmission accounts for a very small fraction of HIV transmission, nosocomial HIV transmission in any country at this time is unacceptable, and underscores defi-

---

——————— **BOX 8.10** ———————

ASSAULT WITH HIV

According to Richard Lacayo (1997), Darnell McGee, through 1995 and 1996, had sex with at least 61 women ranging in age from **12 to 22**. In one of the worst cases on record of a person knowingly transmitting HIV, 13 women with whom McGee had sex have tested HIV-positive. Some are pregnant. At least one has given birth to an infected infant. State public health officials, who are trying to track down and notify his sex partners, expect the tally to climb as more women come forward to be tested.

McGee knew what he was doing. According to the *St. Louis Post-Dispatch*, which broke the story, state records show that he tested positive in 1992 and was told the results.

On January 15, 1997 he was shot and killed, assailant unknown!

ciencies in present medical practices (Heymann et al., 1994).

Influence of Sexually Transmitted Diseases on HIV Transmission and Vice Versa

Sexual intercourse occurs more than 100 million times daily around the world. Results: 910,000 conceptions and over 600,000 cases of sexually transmitted disease. In the United States over 12 million new cases of sexually transmitted diseases occur each year. At current rates at least **one American in four** will contract an STD at some point in his or her life. More than **50 organisms** and syndromes are **transmitted** or occur as a **result of sexual activity** (Hooker, 1996). Worldwide in 1996 and in 1997 there were 333 million mostly curable cases of STDs. STD researchers have long recognized that the behaviors which place individuals at risk for other STDs also increase their risk of becoming infected with HIV.

Infection by sexually transmitted diseases usually occurs through the **mucosal surfaces** of the male and female genital tracts and rectum. The mucosal route also accounts for a large percentage of heterosexual and homosexual transmission of HIV. It is known that STDs increase the number of T4 cells (HIV target cells) in cervical secretions, thereby increasing the chance of HIV infection in women.

Most AIDS researchers agree that treating STDs, which cures genital sores and reduces inflammation, can raise the body's barriers against HIV infection. According to a study by Grosskurth and co-workers (1995), researchers working in rural Tanzania saw the number of new HIV infections plummet by 42% after they improved STD health care.

Because HIV can be sexually transmitted, the association between HIV and other sexually transmitted diseases can be in part attributed to the shared risk of exposure and shared modes of transmission.

For the purpose of understanding which STDs best promote HIV transmission, the sexually transmitted diseases can be divided into **genital ulcer** and **genital nonulcerative diseases**.

Genital Ulcer Disease (GUD)— Signs of genital ulcer disease appear as open sores on the

——— POINT OF VIEW 8.2 ———

PROBABLY THE NUMBER ONE RISK COFACTOR FOR HIV IS A SEXUALLY TRANSMITTED DISEASE (STD)

TIME FOR A WAR ON STDS

According to a report, "The Hidden Epidemic," released in November 1996 by the Institute of Medicine, it is time for a national campaign against sexually transmitted diseases (STDs).

More than 12 million people in the United States, one-fourth of them teenagers, are infected with STDs such as chlamydia, genital herpes, and pelvic inflammatory disease **each year**. The situation is "a national embarrassment," says David Celentano of the Johns Hopkins University School of Hygiene and Public Health. Some of the facts:

- The United States has the highest rate of STDs of any developed country.
- Direct costs of STDs, not including AIDS, are $10 billion annually.
- Women and infants bear a disproportionate burden of complications from STDs, which include infertility and various types of cancers.
- Close to 22% of people over the age of 15 harbor the herpes virus.
- Teens are at an ever-increasing risk: By the 12th grade, 70% have had sexual intercourse—double the rate reported in the early 1970s—and close to 40% of them have had four or more partners.

STDs are "hidden" for a number of reasons, says the report by a committee headed by internist William T. Butler of the Baylor College of Medicine in Houston. They include unwillingness of parents and teachers to talk about sex, physician's ignorance, and the fact that many disorders show no symptoms in the early stages, especially in females.

The report puts special emphasis on the need for health providers to track and treat partners of people who present themselves with STDs. Butler says this recommendation is aimed in particular at easily curable bacterial infections such as gonorrhea, syphilis, and chlamydia, which otherwise will continue to cycle through the population (Figure 8-14).

Committee member Celentano says AIDS is playing a big part in bringing STDs out of the closet: "Probably the number one risk [factor] for HIV is an STD."

To order the $45 report, call 1-800-624-6242.
(Source: *Science*, 274:1473, November 1996)

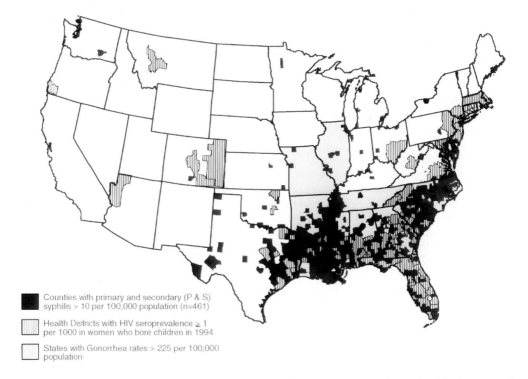

FIGURE 8-14 HIV, Syphilis, and Gonorrhea Rates: United States. Continental U.S. health districts with the highest HIV seroprevalence among childbearing women (1994), counties reporting the highest primary and secondary syphilis rates (1993), and states reporting the highest gonorrhea rates (1993). (*Source:* St. Louis et al., 1997)

penis, vagina, other genital areas and at times elsewhere on the body. The most widespread genital ulcer STDs are syphilis, genital herpes, and chancroid. In the United States, through 1996, these were about 44 million people infected with the Herpes virus (about 1 in 6 people carry the herpes virus).

In early 1997, researchers from the University of Washington showed for the first time that herpes sores contain high levels of HIV, which they believe makes the virus especially easy to spread during sexual contact. We now know that the prevalence of HIV shedding in the genital tracts of both men and women increases substantially in the presence not only of accelerating immunosuppression but also of other STDs. Furthermore, the quantification of viral load in genital secretions indicates that the concentration of HIV shed may increase as much as 7-fold among men who are co-infected with HIV and

STDs such as gonorrhea. Most importantly, both the prevalence and the concentration of HIV shedding can be reduced rapidly to baseline levels with appropriate STD treatment. Together with observations suggesting that HIV susceptibility is increased in women by nonulcerative STDs through recruitment of endocervical CD4 lymphocytes, these data provide a biologically plausible mechanism for the markedly increased risk of HIV transmission associated with other STDs, estimated to range between 3-fold and 50-fold depending on the STD involved (St. Louis et al., 1997).

William Cameron and colleagues (1990) reported on the bidirectional biological interactions between HIV and STDs, especially the genital ulcerative STDs. Bidirectional interaction between HIV and STDs occurs with respect to both transmission and virulence (Table 8-10). HIV transmission is a consequence of both

TABLE 8-10 Bidirectional Interaction between HIV and Sexually Transmitted Genital Ulcer Disease

Types of Biological Transactions	Epidemiological Observation
GUD Increases HIV Prevalence	
Type I interaction:	
Transmission	
GUD increases susceptibility to HIV	Increased incidence of HIV in people with GUD
GUD increases infectiousness of HIV	Increased transmission of HIV with co-exposure to GUD and HIV
HIV Increases GUD Prevalence	
Type II interaction:	
Virulence	
HIV immune disease increases virulence of GUD pathogens	Increased incidence and prevalence of GUD in HIV-infected patients
	Decreased effectiveness of GUD therapy

Two categories of interaction between sexually transmitted genital ulcer disease (GUD) and HIV are relevant to transmission and to disease. Facilitated transmission (type I interaction), in which GUD operates to increase the prevalence of HIV, and enhanced virulence (type II interaction), in which HIV operates to increase the prevalence of GUD, may amplify the prevalence of each in a network of sexual contacts, such as a "core group" of prostitutes and clients, forming an efficient reservoir of high-frequency HIV and sexually transmitted disease transmitters.

(Source: Adapted from Cameron et al., 1990)

infectivity and susceptibility, both of which can be increased by genital ulcer disease. Virulence, the capacity of a pathogen to produce disease, is a consequence of both pathogen and host factors. Thus, HIV infection and associated immune deficiency disease may account for the increased prevalence of genital ulcer disease; and this in turn may further amplify HIV transmission in a network of social contacts.

Evidence that genital ulcer disease may increase the risk of acquiring HIV has been reported from at least one STD clinic in the United States (Quinn et al., 1988). Since 1986, the incidence of primary and secondary

syphilis in the United States has been increasing, especially among minority heterosexuals in urban areas. Between 1986 and 1988, cases of primary and secondary syphilis increased 98%, chancroid cases increased 105%, and herpes simplex increased 78%. In one study at the STD clinic at Kings County Hospital in Brooklyn, the number of GUD cases more than tripled from 1986 to 1988 and by the first half of 1989, 35% of STD clinic visits were for GUDs (Chirgwin et al., 1991).

Worldwide the estimated number of new STD infections for 1997 includes 12 million new cases of syphilis, 62 million new cases of gonorrhea, 89 million new cases of chlamydia, and 170 million new cases of trichomoniasis. Although trichomoniasis does not increase the risk of acquiring HIV as much as does syphilis, the huge number of trichomoniasis infections makes it at least equally important in the context of HIV transmission. All four of these STDs are **curable** - and examples from high- and low-income countries show that it is feasible and affordable to achieve a significant reduction of the STD burden everywhere.

Nonulcerative Disease— The nonulcerative STDs include gonorrhea, chlamydial, and trichomonal infections (also called discharge diseases), and genital warts. There are over 30 million people in the United States infected with genital wart virus. In most populations, these are much more common than genital ulcer diseases. None causes the noticeable open sores that occur in the ulcer diseases but they do cause microscopic breaks in affected tissue, and are associated with HIV transmission (Laga et al., 1993). The most common symptoms are warty growths on the genitals, discharge from the penis or vagina, and painful urination.

Collectively, worldwide there are over 250 million cases a year of just seven major STDs: syphilis, herpes, and chancroid, which cause ulcers; and trichomoniasis, chlamydia, warts, and gonorrhea, which do not (Figure 8-15).

HIV infection and other sexually transmitted diseases (STDs) share the same risk factors. The major difference between HIV/AIDS and the other STDs is the degree of cell and tissue destruction and the mortality of HIV/AIDS.

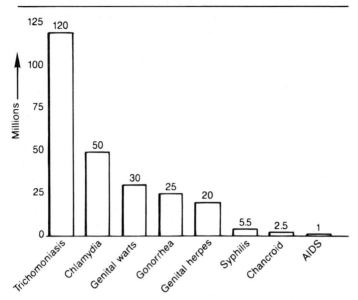

Annual Number of STD Cases Worldwide

(bar chart, "Millions" on vertical axis)

- Trichomoniasis — 120
- Chlamydia — 50
- Genital warts — 30
- Gonorrhea — 25
- Genital herpes — 20
- Syphilis — 5.5
- Chancroid — 2.5
- AIDS — 1

FIGURE 8-15 Global Incidence of Eight Sexually Transmitted Diseases.

HIV is transmitted most often during sexual contact with an infected partner. There is abundant evidence that if a sexual partner has an active STD, especially one that causes an ulcer, he or she is at greater risk of becoming HIV-infected (Laga, 1991).

The types of blood cells, lymphocytes, or macrophages most likely to become infected if exposed to HIV tend to collect in the genital tract of people with STDs. This makes an STD-infected person both more likely to transmit HIV and more vulnerable to it (Laga, 1991). The relationship of STDs to HIV can be seen in Figure 8-16.

Pediatric Transmission

Children can acquire HIV from their mothers in several ways. A pregnant HIV-infected woman can transmit the virus to her fetus in utero (**during gestation**) as the virus crosses over from the mother into the fetal bloodstream (Jovaisas et al., 1985; St. Louis et al., 1993). At least 50% of newborn infections occur **during delivery by ingesting blood or other infected maternal fluids** (Scott et al., 1985; Boyer et al., 1994; Kuhn, et al., 1994). If breast fed, the newborn may also become **infected from breast milk** (Zigler et al., 1985; deMartino et al., 1992; Van DePerre et al., 1993). In case reports, three women who contracted HIV by blood transfusions *immediately after birth* subsequently infected their newborns via breast feeding (Curran et al., 1988). Other studies suggest that the risk of HIV transmission through breast feeding is increased if the mother becomes HIV-infected during lactation (Hu et al., 1992).

The relative efficiency of these three routes of infection is unknown. However, the data on mothers' milk add to the urgency of learning more about mucosal transmission, because the most likely explanation for HIV transmission through breast feeding is that the virus penetrates the mucosal lining of the mouth or gastrointestinal tract of infants. If this occurs in newborns, then what of older children, adolescents, and adults? Does the mucosal lining change with development and become HIV-resistant?

HIV-Infected Babies— One major problem in perinatal transmission is how to determine which babies are truly HIV-infected as opposed to just carrying the mother's HIV antibodies (which would produce a false-positive test). HIV transmission can occur during pregnancy (in utero), as well as at the time of delivery (**intrapartum**) and through breast milk. HIV transmission is more likely if virus can be cultured from the mother's blood, or if she has later stage HIV disease, or if her T4 counts are low; and is more likely to occur in the first born than in the second born of twins. A baby automatically acquires the mother's antibodies and may carry them for 2 or more years. Usually by 18 months of age, most of the mother's antibodies will be gone. The babies may then begin to show signs of clinical AIDS-related illness. But, even at 18 months, a child cannot be unequivocally diagnosed. The most commonly used HIV antibody test is not sufficiently accurate until the child is at least 2 years old. A new antibody test in development shows promise in recognizing newborn infection by examining the **type of HIV antibodies** the infected mother is producing.

Although the rate of perinatal and breast milk HIV transmission is unknown, evidence from 1986 into 1998 indicates that over 90% of pediatric AIDS cases acquired the virus in utero from an HIV-infected mother after the first trimester (12th through 16th weeks) (Marion et al., 1986; DeRossi et al., 1997; Backe et al., 1993). In 1990, researchers concluded that a fetus can become infected as early as the 8th week of gestation (Lewis et al., 1990). HIV has been isolated from a 20-week-old fetus after elective abortion by an HIV-positive female and from a 28-week-old newborn delivered by Caesarean section from a female who was diagnosed with AIDS (Selwyn, 1986).

Reports on the probability of a fetus becoming HIV-infected when the mother carries the virus vary widely. The most often quoted estimate is from 30% to 50%. However, the results of four in-depth follow-up studies on the frequency of HIV transmission by infected mothers to their fetuses gives a range of incidences of from 7% to 65%.

There is little documented information on maternal factors that influence vertical transmission. As with other congenital infections, only one of a pair of twins may be HIV-infected (Newell et al., 1990; Ometto, 1995). A mother's clinical status during pregnancy and the duration of her infection (stage of disease) may be important, but evidence remains circumstantial (see Chapter 11 for update information). Studies to determine mother-to-fetus transmission relative to stage of disease are in progress. One reason that all fetuses of HIV-infected mothers are not HIV-infected during gestation may be because the mothers' antibodies have a high affinity for HIV.

According to the CDC classification, children under 13 years of age are considered pediatric AIDS cases. They make up about 1.3% of all AIDS cases in the United States. Through 1997, about 5% of reported pediatric male AIDS cases occurred due to blood transfusions, 3% received HIV-contaminated blood factor VIII used in treating hemophiliacs, and in 2%, the cause was undetermined (Table 8-11).

The largest number of pediatric AIDS cases through 1997 were in New York, Florida, California and New Jersey, in that order. The highest incidence of all pediatric cases occurs in minority populations. By early 1998, there were

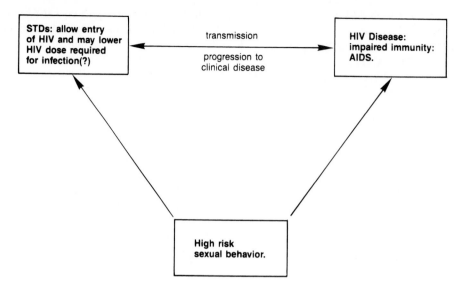

FIGURE 8-16 Bidirectional Interaction Between STDs and HIV. Medical studies support a complex bidirectional interaction between HIV and other sexually transmitted diseases with respect to transmission and virulence. In a group of sexually active, frequently HIV-exposed people with multiple sex partners (e.g., urban prostitutes), a subgroup of efficient, high-frequency HIV transmitters may occur. The epidemiology of HIV dissemination through sexual intercourse may in part be related to regional and demographic differences in the nature and size of sexually active groups and on the patterns of sexual mixing between high-risk groups and low-risk groups in the general population.

over 8,000 pediatric AIDS cases in the United States. Blacks and Hispanics make up 12% and 6% of the United States population, respectively, yet make up 55% and 20%, respectively, of all pediatric AIDS cases. Thus 75% of pediatric AIDS cases occur within two minority populations.

Recent studies demonstrate that HIV seropositivity has reached alarming levels among childbearing women in some major cities. For example, a New York Health Department study conducted in November 1987 indicated that one out of every 61 babies born in New York City was born to a woman infected with HIV. **Approximately 100,000 women of childbearing age are estimated to be infected with HIV in the United States.** The majority of these women may not know they are infected; they are identified as infected only after their children are diagnosed as having an HIV infection or AIDS. It is not uncommon for HIV-infected women to go through several

pregnancies before expressing HIV disease. Also, there are women who become pregnant knowing they are HIV-positive. They want to have a baby regardless (see Chapter 11).

Mother-to-fetus infection or **vertical infection** could be avoided by avoiding pregnancy, but this is possible only in cases where the female is aware of her infection and takes measures to prevent pregnancy (e.g., birth control or tubal ligation). In many cases, pregnancy has occurred before the mother knew she was carrying the virus. In other cases, the mother has become infected after she has become pregnant.

Antiviral Therapy Decreases Perinatal HIV Transmission

Probably the most important step forward in the use of antiviral agents has been the discovery that zidovudine can **decrease the rate of perinatal transmission of HIV**. In a land-

TABLE 8-11 Causes of Pediatric AIDS in the United States Estimates Mid-1997

Pediatric[a] Exposure Category	Totals	(%)
Hemophilia/coagulation disorder	232	(3)
Mother with/at risk for HIV infection:	7,157	(91)
a. Injecting drug use	2,878	
b. Sex with injecting drug user	1,304	
c. Sex with bisexual male	161	
d. Sex with person with hemophilia	27	
e. Sex with transfusion recipient with HIV infection	26	
f. Sex with HIV-infected person, risk not specified	982	
g. Receipt of blood tissue transfusion, blood components, or tissue	150	
h. Has HIV infection, risk not specified	1,629	
Receipt of blood transfusion, blood components, or tissue	375	(5)
Undetermined	138	(1)
Total pediatric AIDS cases (Total adult/adolescent AIDS cases, mid-1997, 604,176	7,902	(100)

[a]CDC classification: Pediatric cases means AIDS cases in children less than 13 years old.

(Adapted CDC *HIV/AIDS Surveillance Report,* June 1997)

mark study by Edward Connor and colleagues (1994) and the interim results of the AIDS Clinical Trials Group (ACTG) Protocol 076 (*MMWR*, 1994d; Goldschmidt et al., 1995; *MMWR*, 1995), the intensive use of zidovudine beginning in the 2nd trimester of pregnancy, incuding intravenous zidovudine during delivery, and 6 weeks of oral therapy in the neonate, decreased the rate of transmission from 25% to 8%. Studies to evaluate the efficacy of oral therapy alone, which may be more appropriate for use in the developing world, have not yet been reported. (For an excellent review of mother-to-child transmission of HIV, see the article by Peckham and College, 1995).

The Impact of ACTG 076 in the United States vs. Developing Countries— In late 1995, magazines and newspapers in the United States began running advertisements that show a baby lying on a quilt with these worlds superimposed over the image: **"The only thing worse than losing a child to AIDS is finding out you didn't have to."** The ad is part of a campaign launched by the Pediatric AIDS Foundation in response to the dramatic finding that the drug zidovudine can reduce the risk of a mother transmitting HIV to her baby by almost 70%. That finding has been heralded by AIDS researchers as their first real breakthrough in a decade-long effort to find a way to prevent HIV infection.

But many physicians and lay people are upset because thousands of HIV-infected pregnant women are not heeding the August 1994 recommendation of the U.S. Public Health Service (PHS) or the July 1995 PHS suggestion that all pregnant women voluntarily receive HIV testing, as there is now an effective means of preventing HIV from being transmitted to their infants.

But a larger problem exists in developing nations as the ACTG 076 findings are relatively meaningless to the majority of HIV-infected pregnant women in the world.

The reasons for this are as follows. **First**, poor nations can't afford the drug zidovudine nor do they have the clinics or other means by which to distribute the drug if they had it. **Second**, the ACTG 076 protocol calls for dosing the women with zidovudine during her pregnancy, and many women in developing countries won't visit medical clinics until they are in labor—if then. What's more, these women most often don't know they are infected with HIV.

Third, ACTG 076 is also out of synch with developing countries because it requires mothers to use infant formula to avoid the possibility of transmitting HIV through breast milk. Not only do most women in poor countries breast-feed, they've been encouraged to do so by the World Health Organization (WHO) and UNICEF, regardless of HIV status, because breast milk reduces infant morbidity and mortality. So, for the moment, although ACTG 076 heralds a long awaited

WHEN THE WONDERFUL NEWS "YOU'RE PREGNANT" BECOMES A TRAGEDY

First Case: Amy Sloan

In 1982, AIDS was a homosexual disease. Amy Sloan became HIV-infected from a blood transfusion. She received the blood because of ulcerative colitis (ulcers in the colon). In 1985, 3 years after her transfusion, and 2 days *after* she learned she was pregnant, Amy was told she had AIDS. She was 24 years old.

By 1985, the general public was being educated to the devastating effects of AIDS; the virus had been named and it was known that blood transfusions were a major route of HIV transmission. Amy Sloan had become pregnant not knowing that she was carrying the AIDS virus. Amy delivered an uninfected son in 1986. She died in January 1987.

Second Case: Elizabeth and Paul Michael Glaser

On March 13, 1990, Elizabeth and Paul Michael Glaser, former star of *Starsky and Hutch*, testified before the House Budget Committee's Human Resource Task Force arguing for increased funding for pediatric AIDS research, education, and treatment.

Elizabeth Glaser was infected with HIV in 1981, after she was given a blood transfusion while giving birth to daughter Ariel. At that time, AIDS did not have a name, and the reporting of cases was just beginning. No one knew about the risk of contracting the virus through transfusions. Elizabeth breast-fed Ariel, unknowingly passing the virus to her daughter. Three years later, Paul and Elizabeth had a son, Jake, who later also tested positive for HIV. Paul is the only one in the family not infected.

Elizabeth testified that she watched her daughter suffer from symptoms that did not seem to affect adults. She watched her daughter's central nervous system atrophy as she became, at age 6, unable to walk, talk, or even sit up.

Ariel Glaser died in 1988, just after her 7th birthday. Elizabeth Glaser died on December 4, 1994.

In November 1996, Jake's viral load began to increase—a sign of a failing immune system. Although the FDA had not yet approved protease inhibitors (PI) for use in children, Paul Glaser took the risk; Jake received PI. Within 2 weeks his viral load dropped below measurement! Jake, now age 13 (1997), is on therapy, and is asymptomatic.

---

breakthrough in Pediatric HIV prevention in developed countries, it makes little if any difference to the economically impoverished nations of the world (Cohen, 1995).

HIV Infection in Older People

Stuart Lichtman and colleagues (1991) reported on 26 patients, aged 60 and over, who were HIV-positive. Twenty were male. Collectively, 58% of the 26 had become HIV-infected via blood transfusions. Other causes were homosexual behavior (19%), heterosexual transmission (15%), injection drug use (4%), and unknown (4%). The means of transmission for one-half of the female patients (three out of six) was heterosexual sex.

In late 1995 Julie Patterson and colleagues reported that now 11% of all new AIDS cases are occurring in persons over age 50. And 3% occur in persons over age 65. For the years 1993 through 1997, there were 398,000 AIDS cases (61% of all AIDS cases occurred during these years!). This means for these years there are about 44,000 people over 50 who have been diagnosed with AIDS, and about 19,000 of these people are over age 65. Prior to 1985, most elderly people became HIV-infected via blood transfusions. Now its through homo- and heterosexual transmission and through IDU and being the partner of an IDUer.

The progression of HIV disease in the elderly appears to be closely related to an age-related **inability** to replace destroyed T4 cells.

HIV Transmission in the Workplace

The idea of contracting HIV from a fellow employee generates fear in many employees regardless of their jobs. It is believed that most people in the United States have been exposed to information on the routes of HIV transmission and on how to practice safer sex. But remote possibilities remain worrisome to many in the job force. In 1997, about one in six companies offered employee HIV/AIDS education. Many still believe that HIV can be transmitted casually via handshakes, coffee cups, and food handling.

It is the anxiety of uncertainty that engenders suspicion about the possibility of HIV infection in the workplace—an anxiety that HIV/AIDS scientists could be wrong about the routes of HIV transmission. As Judith Wilson Ross states, **"We have spent our lives in a culture in which infectious disease does not represent a significant threat. And thus we had consigned living in fear of life-threatening contagious diseases to the pages of history books."** But today, HIV/AIDS forces us to reexamine our faith in the certainty of science. We want to believe, we want to accept—but the fear of death prevents complete surrender to education.

PUBLIC CONFIDENCE: ACCEPTANCE OF CURRENT DOGMA ON ROUTES OF HIV TRANSMISSION

Although no new routes of HIV transmission have surfaced over the last 16 years of this pandemic, **many people still do not believe that's all there is**. People still make the arguments that: (**1**) scientists do not yet know enough about this disease to be certain there are no other routes of transmission; and (**2**) scientists know other routes exist but are either too frightened to tell the truth, or are under political pressure not to do so for fear of creating a public panic. Many thousands of people in the United States firmly believe that in a few years they will look back and say "I told you so": You can get HIV from HIV-infected people if they breathe on you or if you touch their sweat and so on.

Question: How do you get everyone to believe what medical and research scientists say? **Should we get everyone to believe scientific dogma?**

NATIONAL AIDS RESOURCES

AIDS ACTION COUNCIL	1-202-547-3101
COALITION FOR LEADERSHIP ON AIDS	1-202-628-4160

GAY MEN'S HEALTH CRISIS	1-212-807-6655
MOTHERS OF AIDS PATIENTS	1-619-234-3432
NATIONAL AIDS INFORMATION CLEARINGHOUSE	1-301-762-5111
NATIONAL AIDS NETWORK	1-202-546-2424
NATIONAL ASSOCIATION OF PERSONS WITH AIDS	1-202-483-7979
PROJECT INFORM (ALTERNATIVE AIDS INFO.)	1-800-822-7422
PUBLIC HEALTH SERVICE HOTLINE	1-800-342-2437
CENTERS FOR DISEASE CONTROL AND PREVENTION TECHNICAL INFORMATION	1-404-639-2070
AMERICAN RED CROSS, NATIONAL AIDS EDUCATION	1-202-639-3223
GUIDE TO SOCAL SECURITY AND SSI DISABILITY BENEFITS FOR PEOPLE WITH HIV INFECTION	1-800-772-1213

(YOU CAN WRITE OR CALL FOR THIS SOCIAL SECURITY BROCHURE: SOCIAL SECURITY ADMINISTRATION, PUBLIC INFORMATION DISTRIBUTION CENTER, P.O. BOX 17743, BALTIMORE, MARYLAND 21235.)

SUMMARY

The World Health Organization began keeping records of AIDS cases in 1980. By the end of 1997, there were an estimated 9 million AIDS cases in 194 reporting countries and territories. About 16% of these cases occurred in the United States. It has been reported that the first cases of AIDS entered the United States via homosexual men who had vacationed in Haiti in the late 1970s. However, there is evidence of AIDS cases in the United States as early as 1952. While testing West Africans for HIV infection, a second strain of HIV was discovered: HIV-2. Both are transmitted in the same manner and both cause AIDS. However, HIV-2 appears to be less pathogenic than HIV-1.

There are two major variables involved in successful HIV transmission and infection. First is the individual's genetic resistance or susceptibility and second is the route of transmission. Not all modes of HIV exposure are equally apt to cause infection, even in the most susceptible individual. There have been a number of studies and empirical observations that demonstrate that HIV **is not casually acquired.** HIV is difficult to acquire even by means of the recognized routes of transmission.

HIV is transmitted mainly via sexual activities involving the exchange of semen and vaginal fluids, through the exchange of blood and blood products, and from mother to child both prenatally and postnatally (breast milk). Besides a few cases of breast milk transmission, no other body fluids have as yet been implicated in HIV infection.

The current belief is that anal receptive homosexuals have a higher risk than heterosexuals of acquiring HIV because the membrane or mucosal lining of the rectum is more easily torn during anal intercourse. This allows a more direct route for larger numbers of HIVs to enter the vascular system.

Others at high risk for acquiring and transmitting HIV are injection drug users. They infect each other when they share drug paraphernalia. Changes in sexual and injection drug use behavior can virtually stop HIV transmission among these people.

REVIEW QUESTIONS

(Answers to the Review Questions are on page 577.)

1. True or False: Africa makes up the largest percentage of **reported** AIDS cases worldwide. Explain.

2. What evidence is there that HIV may have evolved in the United States and Africa at the same time?

3. Are HIV-1 and HIV-2 related? Explain.

4. True or False: HIV-1 and HIV-2 are transmitted differently and therefore are located in geographically distinct regions of the world. Explain.

5. True or False: HIV is not believed to be casually transmitted. Explain.

6. Name the routes of HIV transmission.

7. True or False: Deep kissing wherein saliva is exchanged is a direct route for efficient HIV transmission. Explain.

8. True or False: Insects that bite or suck have been claimed to be associated with HIV transmission. Explain.

9. True or False: Among heterosexuals, HIV transmission from male to female and from female to male are equally efficient. Explain.

10. True or False: If a person has unprotected intercourse with an HIV-infected partner he or she will become HIV-infected. Explain.

11. What is the percentage of risk that a developing fetus with an HIV-positive mother will be born HIV-positive, with and without zidovudine therapy?

12. Despite the warnings, groups that continue to engage in high-risk sexual activity include:
    a) high school students
    b) black women
    c) injection drug users
    d) all of the above

13. True or False: Prior to 1985, use of blood component therapy put the hemophiliac at risk for contracting HIV.

14. True or False: Relapse to risky sexual behavior can be an important source of new HIV infection in the homosexual community.

15. True or False: The body fluids shown most likely to transmit HIV are blood, semen, vaginal secretions, and breast milk.

16. True or False: Participation in risk behaviors and not identification with particular groups puts an individual at risk of acquiring HIV infection.

17. True or False: Unprotected receptive anal intercourse is the sexual activity with the greatest risk of HIV transmission.

18. True or False: Women who are HIV-infected always transmit the virus to their fetus during pregnancy or delivery.

19. True or False: A person infected with HIV can transmit the virus from the first occurrence of antigemia throughout the rest of his/her life.

20. True or False: Women constitute the fastest growing segment of the population with HIV infection.

21. True or False: The majority of HIV-infected women whose source of infection is known became infected through vaginal intercourse.

22. True or False: HIV infection in children is now a leading cause of death in children between the ages of 1 and 4.

23. True or False: Sexual contact is the major route of HIV transmission among black Americans.

24. True or False: Urine is one body fluid that remains an unproven route of HIV transmission.

REFERENCES

ABBOTT, ALISON. (1995). Murder charges brought in German HIV blood products case. *Nature,* 376:628.

ABBOTT, ALISON. (1996). Japan agrees to pay HIV-blood victims. *Nature,* 380:278.

AIDS Research. (1990). Roundup: Oral sex. *Med. Asp. Human Sexuality,* 24:52.

ALDHOUS, PETER. (1991). France will compensate. *Nature,* 353:425.

ARCHIBALD, D.W., et al. (1990). *In vitro* inhibition of HIV-1 infectivity by human salivas. *AIDS Res. Human Viruses,* 6:1425–1431.

AVINS, ANDREW., et al. (1994). HIV infection and risk behaviors among heterosexuals in alcohol treatment programs. *JAMA,* 271:515–518.

BACKE, E., et al. (1993). Fetal organs infected by HIV-1. *AIDS,* 7:896–897.

BAGASRA, OMAR, et al. (1994). Detection of HIV proviral DNA in sperm from HIV-infected men. *AIDS,* 8:1669–1674.

BAGASRA, OMAR. (1996). Use of in situ PCR for measuring viral burden. *AIDS Reader,* 6:43–47.

BENNETT, AMANDA, et al. (1996). AIDS fight is skewed by Federal campaign exaggerating risks. *Wall Street Journal,* May 1, A1.

BOBKOV, ALEKSEI. (1994). Molecular epidemiology of HIV in the former Soviet Union: analysis of ENV-3 sequences and their correlation with epidemologic data. *AIDS,* 8:619–624.

BOEKELOO, B., et al. (1993). Sexual risk behaviors of STD clinic patients before and after Earvin 'Magic' Johnson's HIV-infection Announcement—Maryland 1991–1992. *MMWR,* 42:45–48.

BOLLING, DAVID R. (1989). Anal intercourse between women and bisexual men. *Med. Asp. Human Sexuality,* 23:34.

BOYER, PAMELA J., et al. (1994). Factors predictive of maternal-fetal transmission of HIV. *JAMA,* 271:1925–1930.

BREO, DENNIS L. (1991). The two major scandals in France's AIDSGATE. *JAMA,* 266:3477–3482.

BURKETT, ELINOR. (1995). The gravest show on earth: America in the age of AIDS. Houghton Miffin: Boston.

BUTLER, DECLAN. (1994a). Allain freed to face new changes. *Nature,* 370:404.

BUTLER, DECLAN. (1994b) Blood scandal raises spectre of Dreyfus case. *Nature,* 371:548.

CAMERON, WILLIAM D., et al. (1990). Sexual transmission of HIV and the epidemiology of other STDs. *AIDS,* 4:S99–S103.

CDC (Centers for Disease Control and Prevention). (1990). *HIV/AIDS Surveillance Report,* Oct.: 1–18.

CHIRGWIN, KEITH, et al. (1991). HIV infection, genital ulcer disease, and crack cocaine use among patients attending a clinic for sexually transmitted diseases. *Am. J. Public Health,* 81:1576–1579.

CHU, S.Y., et al. (1990). Epidemiology of reported cases of AIDS in lesbians, United States 1980–89. *Am. J. Public Health,* 80:1380.

COHEN, J.B., et al. (1989). Heterosexual transmission of HIV. *Immunol. Ser.,* 44:135–137.

COHEN, JON. (1995). Bringing AZT to poor countries. *Science,* 269:624-626.

CONANT, MARCUS. (1995). The current face of the AIDS epidemic. *AIDS Newslink,* 6:14–8.

CONNER, EDWARD, et al. (1994). Reduction of maternal-infant transmission of HIV with zidovudine treatment. *N. Engl. J. Med.,* 331:1173–1180.

COOMBS, ROBERT W., et al. (1989). Plasma viremia in HIV infection. *N. Engl. J. Med.,* 321:1526.

COTTONE, JAMES A., et al. (1990). The Kimberly Bergalis case: An analysis of the data suggesting the possible transmission of HIV infection from a dentist to his patient. *Phys. Assoc. AIDS Care,* 2:267–270.

CURRAN, JAMES W., et al. (1988). Epidemiology of HIV infection and AIDS in the United States. *Science,* 239:610–616.

DANIELS, NORMAN. (1992). HIV-infected Professionals, patient rights, and the switching dilemma. *JAMA,* 267:1368–1371.

DEMARTINO, MAURIZIO, et al. (1992). HIV-1 transmission through breast-milk: Appraisal of risk according to duration of feeding. *AIDS,* 6:991–997.

DEROSSI, ANITA, et al. (1992). Vertical transmission of HIV: Lack of detectable virus in peripheral blood cells of infected children at birth. *AIDS,* 6:1117–1120.

DES JARLAIS, DON C., et al. (1989). AIDS and IV drug use. *Science,* 245:578.

DES JARLAIS, DON, et al. (1995) Maintaining low HIV-seroprevalence in populations of injecting drug users. *JAMA,* 274:1226-1231.

DEVINCENZI, I., et al. (1989). Risk factors for male to female transmission of HIV. *Br. Med. J.,* 298:411–415.

DORFMAN, ANDREA. (1991). Bad blood in France. *Time,* 138:48.

DROTMAN, PETER. (1996). Professional boxing, bleeding, and HIV testing. *JAMA,* 276:193.

DRUCKER, E. (1986). AIDS and addiction in New York City. *Am. J. Drug Alcohol Abuse,* 12:165–181.

ELSON, JOHN. (1991). The dangerous world of wannabes. *Time,* 138:77–80.

Emergency Cardiac Care Committee, American Heart Association. (1990). Risk of infection during CPR training and rescue: Supplemental guidelines. *JAMA,* 262:2714–2715.

FISCHL, M.A., et al. (1987). Evaluation of heterosexual partners, children and household contacts of adults with AIDS. *JAMA,* 257:640–644.

FOX, PHILIP. (1991). Saliva and salivary gland alterations in HIV infection. *J. Am. Dental Assoc.,* 122:46–48.

FRIEDLAND, GERALD H., et al. (1987). Transmission of the human immunodeficiency virus. *N. Engl. J. Med.,* 317:1125–1135.

FRIEDLAND, GERALD H. (1991). HIV transmission from health care workers. *AIDS Clin. Care,* 3:29–30.

GIBBONS, MARY. (1994). Childhood sexual abuse. *Am. Fam. Phys.,* 49:125–136.

Global AIDSNEWS. (1994). A new approach to STD control and AIDS prevention. 4:13-14, 20.

GODDARD, JEROME. (1997). Why mosquitoes cannot transmit the AIDS virus. *Infect, Med.,* 14: 353–354.

GOLDSCHMIDT, RONALD, et al. (1995). Antiretroviral strategies revisited, *J. Am. Board Fam. Pract.,* 8:62–69.

GOSTIN, LAWRENCE. (1994). HIV testing, counseling and prophylaxis after sexual assault. *JAMA,* 271:1436–1444.

GOTO, Y., et al. (1991). Detection of proviral sequences in saliva of patients infected with human immunodeficiency virus type 1. *AIDS Res. Hum. Retroviruses,* 7:343–347.

GROSSKURTH, HEINER, et al. (1995). Impact of improved treatment of sexually transmitted diseases on HIV infection in rural Tanzania. *Lancet,* 346: 530–536.

GUINAN, MARY (1995). Artificial Insemination by Donor: safety and secrecy. *JAMA,* 273:890–891.

HEARST, NORMAN, AND HULLEY, STEPHEN B. (1988). Preventing the heterosexual spread of AIDS: Are we giving our patients the best advice? *JAMA,* 259:2428.

HENG, MADALENE, et al. (1994). Co-Infection and synergy of human immunodeficiency virus-I and herpes simplex virus-I. *Lancet,* 343: 255–258.

HEYMANN, DAVID, et al. (1994). The laboratory, epidemiology, nosocomial infection and HIV. *AIDS,* 8:705–706.

HIV/AIDS Survailance Report. (1996). December 8:1–39.

HIV/AIDS Surveillance Report. (1997). June 9:1–39.

HOLDEN, CONSTANCE. (1994). Switzerland has its own blood scandal. *Science,* 264:1254.

HOLMSTROM, PAUL, et al. (1992). HIV antigen detected in gingival fluid. *AIDS,* 6:738–739.

HOOKER, TRACEY. (1996). HIV/AIDS: facts to consider: 1996 National Conference of State Legislators, Denver, Colorado, February. 1–64.

HU, DALE J., et al. (1992). HIV infection and breastfeeding: Policy implications through a decision analysis model. *AIDS,* 6:1505–1513.

ILARIA, GERARD, et al. (1995). Detection of HIV DNA in pre-ejaculate. *Primary Care Rev.: Update Urol.,* 29:8–9.

IPPILITO, GIUSEPPE, et al. (1994). Transmission of zidorudine-resistant HIV during a bloody fight. *JAMA,* 272:433–434.

JAYARAMAN, KRISHNAMUNTHY. (1995). HIV scandal hits Bombay blood centre. *Nature,* 376:285.

JOSEPH, STEPHEN C. (1993). Dragon within the gates: The once and future AIDS epidemic. *Med. Doctor,* 37:92–104.

JOVAISAS, E., et al. (1985). LAV/HTLV III in 20-week fetus. *Lancet,* 2:1129.

KAISER, JOCELYN. (1996). Pasteur implicated in blood scandal? *Science,* 272:185.

KATNER, H.P., et al. (1987). Evidence for a Euro-American origin of human immunodeficiency virus. *J. Natl. Med. Assoc.,* 79:1068–1072.

KEET, IRENEUS, et al. (1992). Orogenital sex and the transmission of HIV among homosexual men. *AIDS,* 6:223–226.

KINGSLEY, L.A., et al. (1990). Sexual transmission efficiency of hepatitis B virus and human immunodeficiency virus among homosexual men. *JAMA,* 264:230–234.

KOSS, M.P., et al. (1991). Deleterious effects of criminal victimization on women's health and medical utilization. *Arch. Intern. Med.,* 151: 342–347.

KUHN, LOUISE, et al. (1994). Maternal-infant HIV transmission and circumstances of delivery. *Am. J. Public Health,* 84:1110–1115.

LAGA, MARIE. (1991). HIV infection and sexually transmitted diseases. *Sexually Transmitted Dis. Bull.,* 10:3–10.

LACAYO, RICHARD. (1997). Assult with a deadly virus. *Time Magazine,* 149:82.

LAGA, MARIE, et al. (1993). Non-ulcerative STDs as risk factors for HIV transmission in women: Results from a cohort study. *AIDS,* 7:95–102.

LAURENCE, JEFFREY. (1995). The mechanics of HIV transmission. *Primary Care Rev: Update Urol.,* 29:4–5.

LEVY, JAY A. (1989). Human immunodeficiency viruses and the pathogenesis of AIDS. *JAMA,* 261:2997–3006.

LEWIS, S.H., et al. (1990). HIV-1 introphoblastic villous Hofbauer cells and haematological precursors in eight-week fetuses. *Lancet,* 335:565.

LICHTMAN, STUART M., et al. (1991). Greater attention urged for HIV in older patients. *Infect. Dis. Update,* 2:5.

LIFSON, ALAN. (1995). HIV transmission through specific oral-genital sexual practices. *Primary Care Rev.: Update Urol.,* 29:9–11.

LIUZZI, G.M. (1995). Quantitation of HIV genome copy number in semen and saliva. *AIDS,* 9:651–653.

MARION, R.W., et al. (1986). Human T cell lymphotropic virus type III embryopathy: A new dysmorphic syndrome associated with intrauterine HTLV III infection. *Am. J. Dis. Child,* 140:638–640.

MARKS, ROBERT. (1996). The riddle of oral sex. *Focus,* 5:5–8.

MARLINK, RICHARD, et al.(1994). Reduced rate of disease development after HIV infection as compared to HIV-1.*Science,* 265:1587–1590.

MERIMAN, J.H., et al. (1991). Detection of HIV DNA and RNA in semen by the polymerase chain reaction. *J. Infect. Dis.,* 164:769–772.

MIIKE, LAWRENCE. (1987). Do insects transmit AIDS? Office of Technological Assessment, Sept. 1:43.

MONZON, O.T., et al. (1987). Female to female transmission of HIV. *Lancet,* 2:40–41.

Morbidity and Mortality Weekly Report. (1988a). Update: Universal precautions for prevention of transmission of human immunodeficiency virus, hepatitis B virus, and other bloodborne pathogens in health-care settings. 37:377–382,387–388.

Morbidity and Mortality Weekly Report. (1988b). Transmission of HIV through bone transplantation: Case report and public health recommendations. 37:597–599.

Morbidity and Mortality Weekly Report. (1990a). Possible transmission of HIV to a patient during an invasive dental procedure. 39:489–493.

Morbidity and Mortality Weekly Report. (1990b). HIV infection and artificial insemination with processed semen. 39:249–256.

Morbidity and Mortality Weekly Report. (1991a). Update: Transmission of HIV infection during an invasive dental procedure—Florida. 40:21–27,33.

Morbidity and Mortality Weekly Report. (1991b). Drug use and sexual behaviors among sex partners of injecting-drug users—U.S. 40:855–860.

Morbidity and Mortality Weekly Report. (1992). Childbearing and contraceptive-use plans among women at high risk for HIV infection—Selected U.S. sites, 1989–1991. 41:135–144.

Morbidity and Morality Weekley Report. (1994a). Human immunodeficiency virus transmission in household settings—United States. 43:347, 353–357.

Morbidity and Morality Weekley Report. (1994b), Guidelines for preventing transmission of HIV through transplantation of human tissue and organs. 43:1–15.

Morbidity and Mortality Weekley Report. (1994c) Medical-care expenditures attributable to cigarette smoking—United States, 1993. 43:469– 472.

Morbidity and Mortality Weekly Report. (1994d). Zidovudine for the prevention of HIV transmission from mother to infant. 43:285–287.

Morbidity and Mortality Weekly Report. (1995). Use of AZT to prevent perinatal transmission (ACTG 076): workshop on implications for treatment, counseling, and HIV testing. 44:1–12.

Morbidity and Martality Weekly Report.(1997). Transmission of HIV possibly associated with exposure of mucous membrane to contaminated blood. 46:620–623.

MUNZER, ALFRED. (1994). The threat of secondhand smoke. *Menopause Manage.,* 3:14–17.

NAFTALIN, RICHARD J. (1992). Anal sex and AIDS. *Nature,* 360:10.

NEWELL, MARIE-LOUISE, et al. (1990). HIV-1 infection in pregnancy: Implications for women and children. *AIDS,* 4:S111–S117.

NOWAK, RACHEL. (1995). Rockefeller's big prize for STD test. *Science,* 269:782.

OLESKE, JAMES M. (1994).The many needs of HIV-infected children. *Hosp Pract.* 29:81–87.

OMETTO, LUCIA et al. (1995) Viral phenotype and host-cell susceptibility to HIV infection as risk factors for mother-to-child HIV transmission. *AIDS,* 9:427-434.

PADIAN, NANCY S., et al. (1991). Female to male transmission of HIV. *JAMA,* 266:1664–1667.

PATTERSON, JULIE, et al. (1995). Basic and Clinical Considerations of HIV infection in the elderly. *Infect. Dis.,* 3:21–34.

PECKHAM, CATHERINE, et al. (1995). Mother-to-child transmission of HIV. *N. Engl. J. Med.,* 333:298–302.

PETERMAN, THOMAS A.,et al. (1988). Risk of human immunodeficiency virus transmission from heterosexual adults with transfusion-associated infections. *JAMA,* 259:55–58.

PETO, RICHARD. (1992). Statistics of chronic disease control. *Nature,* 356:557–558.

PHILLIPS, DAVID. (1994). The roll of cell-to-cell transmission in HIV infection. *AIDS,* 8:719–731.

PHILLIPS, KATHRYN, et al. (1994). The cost effectiveness of HIV testing of physicians and dentists in the United States. *JAMA,* 271:851–858.

POURTOIS, M., et al. (1991). Saliva can contribute in quick inhibition of HIV infectivity. *AIDS,* 5:598–599.

PUDNEY, J., et al. (1991). White blood cells and HIV in semen from vasectomized seropositive men. *Lancet,* 338:573.

QUAYLE, ALISON. (1995). Mucous membrane susceptibility to HIV infection. *Primary Care Rev.: Update Urol.*, 29:6–8.

QUINN, THOMAS C., et al. (1988). HIV infection among patients attending clinics for sexually transmitted diseases. *N. Engl. J. Med.*, 318:197–203.

REICHHARDT, TONY. (1995). Top aide to face charges in French HIV blood scandal. *Nature*, 375:349.

ROGERS, DAVID, et al. (1993). AIDS policy: Two divisive issues. *JAMA*, 270:494–495.

ROYCE, RACHEL, et al. (1997). Sexual transmission of HIV. *N. Eng. J. Med.* 336:1072–1078.

ROZENBAUM, W. et al. (1988). HIV transmission by oral sex. *Lancet*, 1:1395.

SADOVSKY, RICHARD. (1989). HIV-infected patients: A primary care challenge. *Am. Fam. Pract.*, 40:121–128.

SAMUEL, MICHAEL. (1995). What does risk mean? Prospective and cross-sectional studies. *Primary Care Rev.: Update Urol.* 29:11–13.

SATO, HIRONORI, et al. (1992). Cell to cell spread of HIV occurs within minutes and may not involve the participation of virus particles. *Virology*, 186:712–724.

Science in California. (1993). AIDS: I want a new drug. *Nature*, 362:396.

SCOTT, G.B., et al. (1985). Mothers of infants with the acquired immunodeficiency syndrome: Evidence for both symptomatic and asymptomatic carriers. *JAMA*, 253:363–366.

SEGARS, JAMES H. (1989). Heterosexual anal sex. *Med. Asp. Human Sexuality*, 23:6.

SELWYN, PETER A. (1986). AIDS: What is now known. *Hosp. Pract.*, 21:127–164.

SHERNOFF, MICHAEL. (1988). Integrating safer-sex counseling into social work practice. *Social Casework: J. Contemp. Social Work*, 69:334–339.

SPITZER, P.G., et al. (1989). Transmission of HIV infection from a woman to a man by oral sex. *N. Engl. J. Med.*, 320:251.

SPURGEON, DAVID. (1994). Canadian AIDS suit raises hope for HIV-blood victims. *Nature*, 368–281.

SPURGEON, DAVID. (1996). Canadian inquiry points the finger. *Nature*, 379–663.

ST. LOUIS, MICHAEL E., et al. (1993). Risk for perinatal HIV transmission according to maternal immunologic, virologic and placental factors. *JAMA*, 269:2853–2860.

ST. LOUIS, MICHAEL E., et al. (1997). Editorial: Janus considers the HIV pandemic—harnessing recent advances to enhance AIDS prevention. *Am. J. Public Health*, 87:10–11.

STRYKER, JEFF, et al. (1993). AIDS policy: Two divisive issues. *JAMA*, 270:2436–2437.

SWENSON, ROBERT M. (1988). Plagues, History and AIDS. *Am. Scholar*, 57:183–200.

SWINBANKS, DAVID. (1993). American witnesses: Testify in Japan about AIDS risks. *Nature*, 364:181.

UNAIDS. (1997). Inplications of HIV variability for transmission: Scientific and policy issues. *AIDS*, 11:S1–S15.

VAN DE PERRE, PHILIPPE, et al. (1993). Infective and anti-infective properties of breast milk from HIV-infected women. *Lancet*, 341:914–918.

VITTECOQ, D., et al. (1989). Acute HIV infection after acupuncture treatments. *N. Engl. J. Med.*, 320:250–251.

VOELKER, REBECCA. (1996). HIV guide for primary care physicians stresses patient-centered prevention. *JAMA*, 276:85–86.

WALKER, EDWARD A., et al. (1993). The prevalence rate of sexual trauma in a primary care clinic. *J. Am. Board Fam. Pract.*, 6:465–471.

WEBB, PATRICA, et al. (1989). Potential for insect transmission of HIV: Experimental exposure of *Cimex hemipterous* and *Toxorhynchites amboinensis* to human immunodeficiency virus. *J. Infect. Dis.*, 160:970–977.

WILL, GEORGE F. (1991). Foolish choices still jeopardize public health. *Private Pract.*, 24:46–48.

Women's AIDS Network. (1988). Lesbians and AIDS: What's the connection? San Francisco AIDS Foundation, 333 Valencia St., 4th Floor, P.O. Box 6182, San Francisco, CA 94101-6182.

WOOLLEY, ROBERT J. (1989). The biologic possibility of HIV transmission during passionate kissing. *JAMA*, 262:2230.

YOUNG, REBECCA. (1995). The scarcity of data on cunnilingus *Primary Care Rev.: Update Urol.*, 29:13–14.

ZIGLER, J.B., et al. (1985). Postnatal transmission of AIDS-associated retrovirus from mother to infant. *Lancet*, 1:896–897.

CHAPTER

9

General Preventive Measures to Stop HIV Transmission

CHAPTER CONCEPTS

♦ HIV transmission can be prevented; the responsibility rests with the individual.

♦ No new routes of HIV transmission have been found after 17 years.

♦ Safer sex essentially means using condoms and not having intercourse with an HIV-infected person.

♦ New female condom (vaginal pouch) was FDA approved in 1993.

♦ Oil based lubricants must not be used with latex condoms.

♦ Plastic condoms are now available.

♦ Free syringe and needle exchange programs may help lower the incidence of HIV transmission.

♦ Blood bank screening to detect HIV antibodies began in 1985.

♦ Universal precautions and blood and body substance isolation are techniques to help health care workers prevent infection.

♦ Under universal precautions certain body fluids from all patients are to be considered potentially infectious.

♦ Partner notification is a means of notifying at risk partners of HIV-infected individuals.

♦ Vaccines are made from whole or parts of dead microorganisms, inactivated viruses, or attenuated viruses and microorganisms.

♦ Experimental subunit vaccines are prepared using recombinant DNA techniques.

♦ Animal models are being prepared for vaccine trial studies.

♦ Why Isn't there a vaccine for HIV disease?

♦ A moral problem exists in attempting to get human volunteers for AIDS vaccine testing.

PREVENTION OF INFECTIOUS DISEASES

While the hope of eradicating HIV is universal, the universe of AIDS comprises many worlds, and the goal can only be achieved if methods of prevention are designed and implemented in the context of each of these

247

worlds. Infectious agents have persisted over the centuries through transmission from one infected person to another. To combat these infections, **prevention programs have attempted to interrupt the chain of transmission.** While some methods focus on stopping transmission from person-to-person contact by using vaccines or prophylactic (preventative) therapy, other methods focus on stopping the transmission that occurs through environmental contamination by sanitary improvements.

With regard to HIV infection, there is no available vaccine against the virus, but effective methods for preventing it do exist. The leading preventative is education: teaching people how to adjust their behavior to reduce or eliminate HIV exposure. Because the vast majority of HIV infections are transmitted through consensual acts between adolescents and adults, the individual has a choice as to whether to risk infection or not.

Despite widely supported educational efforts at both institutional and street levels, a large number of gay males, drug abusers, and heterosexuals, continue to participate in *unsafe* sexual practices. **Unsafe sex is defined as having sex without using a condom.** This allows the exchange of potentially infectious body fluids such as blood, semen, and vaginal secretions. Unsafe sex most often occurs with injection drug users, bartering sex for drugs, and having sex with multiple partners. The sharp increase in the use of crack cocaine and its connection to trading sex for drugs has led to a dramatic rise in almost all of the sexually transmitted diseases. **The idea of *safer* sexual practices began in the early 1980s and now refers almost exclusively to the use of a latex or plastic condom with or without a spermicide.**

Among the severely addicted, concerns about personal safety and survival are secondary to drug procurement and use. Thus their range of acceptable unsafe behaviors leads to random sex and sex without condoms. These behaviors are in part responsible for the increased incidence of HIV and other sexually transmitted diseases (Weinstein et al., 1990). **Eliminating all unsafe sex is not a reasonable goal. Preventing all future HIV infections is impossible, but striving for anything less is unacceptable.**

---— BOX 9.1 ———

HIV PREVENTION EDUCATION— UNITED STATES

Since 1988, CDC has provided fiscal and technical assistance to state and local education agencies and national health and education organizations to assist schools in implementing effective HIV prevention education for youth. These agencies and organizations develop, implement, and evaluate HIV prevention policies and programs and train teachers to initiate effective prevention efforts and implement curricula in classrooms. As a result of these and other efforts, school-based HIV education is widely implemented in the United States. From 1987 to 1994, the number of states requiring HIV prevention education in schools increased from 13 states to 39 states plus the District of Columbia. This high level of policy support is consistent with public support; 95% of U.S. residents in a 1996 survey reported that information about AIDS should be provided in school.

The findings in this survey indicate that, despite wide implementation of HIV prevention education in U.S. schools, improvements in HIV prevention programs are still needed. In particular, **efforts are needed to increase the percentage of teachers who teach HIV prevention in a health education setting and who receive in-service training on HIV prevention**. A national health objective for the year 2000 is to increase to at least 95% the proportion of schools that provide age-appropriate HIV and other sexually transmitted disease (STD) curricula for students **in 4th through 12th grades**, preferably as part of comprehensive school health education, based on scientific information that includes the way HIV and other STDs are prevented and transmitted. Based on the findings, an 11% increase is needed in the percentage of middle/junior and senior high schools that implement HIV and STD prevention education programs.

AIDS prevention is, in a sense, more essential than, say, cancer prevention. Preventing one HIV infection now will not simply prevent one death from AIDS, as preventing one incurable cancer would prevent one cancer death. Preventing an HIV infection now will help break the chain of transmission, averting

HIV PREVENTION HELP IS AVAILABLE

The Centers for Disease Control and Prevention (CDC) manages a national AIDS public information system, consisting of mass media educational efforts, the CDC National AIDS Hotline, the CDC National AIDS Clearinghouse (see telephone numbers, page 18), and partnerships with national organizations. This system helps ensure public and professional access to information about HIV and improve social support at the community level for people to maintain or adopt behaviors that will keep them from acquiring HIV. CDC-approved HIV prevention budget for fiscal year 1997 was 617 million dollars.

the risk that the infected person will knowingly or unknowingly pass the virus on to others who in turn might infect a still wider circle of people.

PREVENTING THE TRANSMISSION OF HIV

HIV/AIDS: The News Is Mostly Bad

We are now into the 17th year of an epidemic that has touched—directly or indirectly—virtually every person on the planet. We know so much about the virus, yet despite our knowledge, our only option is to **prevent** the initial infection. Prevention is foremost because there are **no vaccines, no cure** and, even using the best AIDS drug cocktails available, long-term survival remains questionable, even for those who can afford the drugs. **MOST HIV-INFECTED PEOPLE CANNOT AFFORD THESE DRUGS!** As we face this realization, alarming statistics continue to emerge about the spread of HIV infection.

For 1994and 1995, HIV disease/AIDS was the leading cause of death among men and women ages 25 to 44 in the United States. It is now second. In San Francisco, estimates suggest that at least 50% of homosexual African-American men are infected with HIV. Unsafe sexual practices that could lead to HIV transmission are common among adolescents and young adults, as evidenced by the epidemic of other sexually transmitted diseases in this pop-

ulation. And tens of millions of persons in developing countries will become HIV-infected and most likely die. Entire generations are threatened with extinction in these countries.

The Hard Questions

The political, social, cultural, economic and biological factors that have led to the HIV pandemic seem overwhelming. How can a drug user be convinced to use clean needles to prevent an infection that may kill him in 10 years, when he faces an immediate struggle in a violent environment every day? How can condom use be promoted in countries with inadequate supplies of condoms or resources to provide even basic immunizations? Why should young women on the streets of New York, San Francisco, New Delhi, or Bangkok who depend on the sex industry for daily survival care about safer sex when it might lead to rejection by their customers and an end to their livelihood?

In many societies, there is a large power differential between men and women. Socially and culturally determined gender roles bestow control and authority on males. The subordinate status of women is reinforced by the fact that men are the main or only wage earners in the majority of families. This is compounded further by age differences: in most heterosexual relationships, the man is the older partner.

Wives in many cultures are expected to tolerate infidelity by their husbands, while remaining totally faithful themselves. **But AIDS has raised the price of such tolerance, as it puts women at great risk of infection by their husbands.** Many women feel powerless to ask their husbands to use condoms at home. Even when they can do this, their need to protect themselves may conflict with a social or personal imperative to have children.

Is There Hope?

Hopelessness threatens reason. But there is reason to believe that education may reduce the number of new HIV infections. In San Francisco, gay men organized grassroots efforts to educate themselves about HIV transmission, and the results are impressive: less than 1% of the gay male population was infected with HIV after 1985, compared to 10%

to 20% in the preceding years. People **can** change their behavior when educated about the risks of transmission (Clement, 1993).

But, if these successes were known in the mid-1980s, why the continued delay in educating the general population, especially sexually active adolescents? Most likely because early efforts to describe the HIV epidemic focused on risk groups rather than the **behaviors** associated with HIV transmission. The epidemic was and still is described with labels—the gay, bisexual, injection drug user, hemophiliac, and heterosexual.

Educators Given the Job of Prevention

Former Surgeon General Joycelyn Elders (1994), Patsy Fleming, past Director of National AIDS Policy, and Sandy Thurman, current Director of National AIDS Policy (Figure 9-1) placed prevention and education at the top of their list of priorities in fighting this epidemic.

The importance of prevention is especially clear as one comes to understand the state of the art in HIV/AIDS therapy. Regardless of what can be medically done for patients with HIV disease, there is no cure. Thus officials from the Centers for Disease Control and Prevention (CDC), the World Health Organization (WHO), and the American Health Organization (AHO) have placed the responsibility of prevention in the hands of the educators, which include health care professionals, parents, and teachers.

Grim Reality

Steven Findlay (1991) wrote that burying those who have died from AIDS has become almost routine. With over 400,000 AIDS deaths expected by the end of 1997 and over 440,000 ending 1998, most Americans are indeed becoming accustomed to HIV/AIDS related deaths. But how many will die, say, by the year 2000 or 2010? Will a cure or preventive and therapeutic vaccines be produced? Will our health care system become swamped and ineffective? The best guess by scientists is that neither an effective vaccine nor cure will be found by the end of this century. By the year 2000 it is projected that, worldwide over 12 million people will have died of AIDS, about 1 million

FIGURE 9-1 Photograph of Sandra Thurman, current Director of National AIDS Policy–United States.

of them in the United States. San Francisco may lose 4% of its population; New York 3%; Central Africa 15%. To avoid the realization of these projections, people of the world must work on HIV/AIDS **PREVENTION**.

Based on over 16 years of intensive epidemiological surveys, scientific research, and empirical observations, it is reasonable to conclude that HIV is not a highly contagious disease. HIV transmission occurs mainly through an exchange of body fluids via various sexual activities, HIV-contaminated blood or blood products, prenatal events, and in relatively few cases post-natally through breast milk. **Since 1981, no new route of HIV transmission has been discovered.** The virus is fragile and, with time, self-destructs outside the human body. The most recent data show that HIV remains active for up to 5 days in dried blood, although the number of virus particles (titer) drops dramatically. But it is dangerous to assume that there are no infectious viruses remaining in the dried blood or stored body fluids from an HIV/AIDS patient. In cell-free tissue culture medium, the virus retains activity for up to 14 days at room temperature (Sattar et al., 1991). According to a recent study, HIV was found to survive between 2 and 4 days in glutaraldehyde (Table 9-1), a lubricant used to clean surgical instruments. This finding has serious implications when instruments too delicate for autoclaving: (high-pressure steam sterilization), such as endoscopes, must be used (Lewis, 1995).

Joseph Burnett (1995) reported that HIV can survive 7 days storage at room temperature, 11 days at 37°C in tissue culture extracellular fluid, and can still be infectious in refrigerated postmortem tissue cadavers for 6 to 14 days. The bottom line is that, HIV is more resistant to the environment than originally believed. Chemical agents used to destroy or inactivate the virus are listed in Table 9-1.

It appears that HIV transmission can be prevented by individual action but it will require change in social behaviors. The best way to protect against all sexually transmitted diseases is **sexual abstinence**. The next best way is a mutually monogamous sexual relationship. Following these two options is the use of a barrier method during sexual activities—male and female condoms or rubber dams.

Over 90% of **new** HIV infections now occur in the developing world. For the foreseeable future, prevention through behavioral change is the only way to slow this epidemic. In fact, **history shows that prophylaxis and immunization for any disease will only be partially effective in the absense of behavioral change**.

Sexual transmission accounts for the majority of HIV infection in the developing world; but, this is the most difficult type of transmission to prevent. The use of condoms, reducing numbers of partners and abstinence remain the mainstays of preventing sexual transmission of HIV, but they will not be enthusiastically adopted anywhere just because health authorities tell people to do so.

Behavior has changed in many populations: among gay men in San Francisco, among injecting drug users in Amsterdam and New Haven, Connecticut, and among sex workers

TABLE 9-1 Agents Effective Against Human Immunodeficiency Virus

Agents (freshly prepared)	Recommended Concentration
Sodium hypochlorite (household bleach)[a]	Full strength (no dilution)
Chloramine-T	2%
Sodium oxychlorosene	4 mg/mL
Sodium hydroxide	30 mm
Glutaraldehyde	2%
Formalin	4%
Paraformaldehyde	1%
Hydrogen peroxide	6%
Propiolactone dilution	1:400
Nonoxynol-9	1%
Ethyl alcohol	70%
Isopropyl alcohol	30%–50%
Lysol	0.5%–1%
NP-40 detergent[b]	1%
Chlorhexidine gluconate/ethanol mix	4/25%
Chlorhexidine gluconate/isopropyl mix	0.5%/70%
Tincture of iodine/isopropyl	1/30%–70%
Betadine	0.5%
Quarternary ammonium chloride	0.1%–1%
Acetone/alcohol mix	1:1
pH of 1 or 13	
Heat[c] 56°C for 10 minutes	

[a]In 1993, the CDC and Public Health Association recommended that household bleach (e.g., Clorox) be used at full strength.

[b]To be used at 1% solution at room temperature for 2 to 10 minutes.

[c]Dried HIV is ineffective at room temperature after 3 or more days. HIV at high concentration in liquid at room temperature remained ineffective for over 1 week.

Isopropanol (35%), ethanol (50%), Lysol (0.5%), hydrogen peroxide (0.3%), paraformaldehyde (0.5%), and detergent NP-40 (1%) effectively inactivate HIV when incubated at room temperature for 2 to 10 minutes.

(Adapted from Tierno, 1988)

and their clients in Nairobi, to name a few. In none of these examples is it clear how the behavioral change took place. Even so, success stories in HIV/AIDS prevention seem to have some elements in common, including consistent and persistent intervention measures over a period of time, a clear understanding of the realities of the target population and involvement of members of that population in prevention efforts. Successful interventions do far more than provide information: they teach communication and behavioral skills, change perceptions of what is **preventive behavior** and ensure that the means of prevention, such as condoms or clean needles, are readily available. (Hearst et al., 1995)

Table 9-2 provides a number of recommendations for preventing the spread of HIV. These recommendations place the responsibility for avoiding HIV infection on both adults and adolescents. **Lifestyles must be reviewed, choices made, and risky behavior stopped**. The public health service and the CDC have established guidelines that, if followed, will prevent HIV transmission while still allowing individuals to be somewhat flexible in their personal behaviors (*MMWR*, 1989a).

Quarantine

With few exceptions, proposals to quarantine all individuals with HIV infection have virtually no public support in the United States. Given the civil liberties implications of quarantine, its potential cost, and the realization that alternative, less repressive strategies can be effective in limiting the spread of HIV infection, quarantine proposals in most countries have been dismissed. Despite claims that AIDS is similar to other diseases for which quarantine has been used, public health officials have insisted on distinguishing between behaviorally transmitted infections and those that are airborne. AIDS is not tuberculosis. The CDC and Public Health Association believe that strategies less repressive than quarantine are more effective, for example, effective education and counseling. But many

─────── **POINT OF INFORMATION 9.2** ───────

EXAMPLE OF STATE LAWS TO DETAIN AND/OR QUARANTINE FOR A DISEASE

In 1993, a 50-state survey of tuberculosis (TB)-related legislation by the American Society of Law and Medicine found that **36 states** have given public health officials the **power to order examinations**, **24 states and the District of Columbia** have given them the **power to order treatment**, and **more than 40 states** permit health officials to order **civil commitment** of a person with TB. Based on past practices, **33 states can quarantine** or isolate individuals who endanger public health, and **19 states** have provisions for **emergency detention**.

people believe that less repressive strategies are inadequate.

In the first 10 years of the epidemic 25 states enacted revised public health statutes providing for conditions under which individuals who engaged in behaviors that could spread disease could be restricted or quarantined (Bayer et al., 1993). In 19 of these states, statutes criminalizing HIV transmission-related behavior were also enacted. Framed broadly to cover public health threats, such legislative action was clearly inspired by the AIDS epidemic. However, neither California nor New York, states that together account for close to 40% of AIDS cases in the United States, enacted criminal laws or revised public health statutes to cover the sexual transmission of HIV. Despite the extended and often acrimonious debate over the use of the power to quarantine in the context of AIDS, little is known about how such powers have been used in states where they have been granted to public health officials. **Through early 1998, the official policy of the United States for HIV prevention remained education, counseling, voluntary testing and partner notification, drug abuse treatment, and syringe exchange programs.** To date, the power to quarantine, for any disease, has rarely been used in the United States. In fact, only one country, Cuba, officially used the power of quarantine to stem the spread of HIV. Data to date indicate that the use of quarantine of HIV-infected and AIDS persons in Cuba had been very effective. Cuba had 13 sanatoriums holding some 900 persons of which about 200 have AIDS. Cuba stopped the quarantine of HIV infected persons in mid-1994 for a variety of reasons.

NEW RULES TO AN OLD GAME : PROMOTING SAFER SEX

Barriers to HIV Infection

The two most effective barriers to HIV infection and other sexually transmitted diseases are (1) **abstinence**, which can be achieved by saying *NO* emphatically and consistently; and (2) **forming a no-cheating relationship with one individual, preferably for life**. These solutions to the danger of HIV infection may not

TABLE 9-2 Guidelines for Prevention of HIV Infection

I. For the General Public:

1. Sexual abstinence
2. Have a mutual monogamous relationship with an HIV-negative partner (the greater the number of sexual partners, the greater the risk of meeting someone who is HIV-infected).
3. If the sex partner is other than a monogamous partner, use a condom.
4. Do not frequent prostitutes—too many have been found to be HIV-infected and are still 'working' the streets.
5. Do not have sex with people who you know are HIV-infected or are from a high-risk group. If you do, prevent contact with their body fluids. (Use a condom and a spermicide from start to finish.)
6. Avoid sexual practices that may result in the tearing of body tissues (e.g., penile–anal intercourse).
7. Avoid oral–penile sex unless a condom[a] is used to cover the penis.
8. If you use injection drugs, use sterile or bleach cleaned needles and syringes and *never* share them.
9. Exercise caution regarding procedures such as acupuncture, tattooing, ear piercing, and so on, in which needles or other unsterile instruments may be used repeatedly to pierce the skin and/or mucous membranes. Such procedures are safe if proper sterilization methods are employed or disposable needles are used. Ask what precautions are being taken before undergoing such procedures.
10. If you are planning to undergo artificial insemination, insist on frozen sperm obtained from a laboratory that tests all donors for infection with the AIDS virus. Donors should be tested twice before the sperm is used— once at the time of donation and again 6 months later.
11. If you know that you will be having surgery in the near future and you are able to do so, consider donating blood for your own use. This will eliminate the small but real risk of HIV infection through a blood transfusion. It will also eliminate the more substantial risk of contracting other transfusion blood-borne diseases, such as hepatitis B.
12. Don't share toothbrushes, razors, or other implements that could become contaminated with blood with anyone who is HIV-infected, demonstrates HIV disease, or has AIDS.

II. For Health Care Workers:

1. *All* sharp instruments should be considered as potentially infective and be handled with extraordinary care to prevent accidental injuries.
2. Sharp items should be placed into puncture-resistant containers located as close as practical to the area in which they are used. To prevent needlestick injuries, needles should not be recapped, purposefully bent, broken, removed from disposable syringes, or otherwise manipulated.
3. Gloves, gowns, masks, and eye-coverings should be worn when performing procedures involving extensive contact with blood or potentially infective body fluids. Hands should be washed thoroughly and immediately if they accidentally become contaminated with blood. When a patient requires a vaginal or rectal examination, gloves must always be worn. If a specimen is obtained during an examination, the nurse or individual who assists and processes the specimen must always wear gloves. Blood should be drawn from all patients—regardless of HIV status—only while wearing gloves.
4. To minimize the need for emergency mouth-to-mouth resuscitation, mouthpieces, resuscitation bags, or other ventilation devices should be strategically located and available for use where the need for resuscitation is predictable.

III. People at Risk of HIV Infection:

1. See recommendations for general public.
2. Consider taking the HIV antibody screening test.
3. Protect your partner from body fluids during sexual intercourse.
4. Do not donate any body tissues.
5. If female, have an HIV test before becoming pregnant.
6. If you are an injection drug user, seek professional help in terminating the drug habit.
7. If you cannot get off drugs, do not share drug equipment.

IV. People Who Are HIV-Positive:

The prevention of transmission of HIV by an HIV-infected person is probably lifelong, and patients must avoid infecting others. HIV seropositive persons must understand that the virus can be transmitted by intimate sexual contact, transfusion of infected blood, and sharing needles among injection drug users. They should refrain from donating blood, plasma, sperm, body organs, or other tissues. HIV-infected people should:

(continued)

TABLE 9-2 *Continued*

1. Seek continued counseling and medical examinations.
2. Do not exchange body fluids with your sex partner.
3. Notify your former and current sex partners, encourage them to be tested.
4. If an injection drug user, do not share drug equipment and enroll in a drug treatment program.
5. Do not share razors, toothbrushes, and other items that may contain traces of blood.
6. Do not donate any body tissues.
7. Clean any body fluids spilled with undiluted household bleach.
8. If female, avoid pregnancy.
9. Inform health care workers on a need-to-know basis.

V. Practice of Safer Sex:

Safer sex is body massage, hugging, mutual masturbation, and closed mouth kissing. HIV seropositive patients must protect their sexual partners from coming into contact with infected blood or bodily secretions. Although consistent use of latex condoms with spermicide containing nonoxynol-9 can decrease the chance of HIV transmission, condoms do break. If engaging in sexual intercourse with an HIV-positive person use two condoms. But even this is no guarantee. (also see 1 through 6 under "For the General Public" in this table.)

[a]Tests show that HIV can sometimes pass through a latex condom. Experts believe that natural-skin condoms are more porous than latex and therefore offer less effective protection. Never use oil-based products such as Vaseline, Crisco, or baby oil with a latex condom, because they make the latex porous, cause latex deterioration and breakage thus nullify the protection the condom provides against the virus. The use of condoms containing a spermicide is recommended.

be "cool," but they do work. These two completely safe approaches are endorsed by the Surgeon General as the **preferred** methods. For those who do not practice abstinence, barrier methods are necessary to prevent HIV infection/transmission.

The barrier methods used to prevent HIV infection are the same methods used to prevent other sexually transmitted diseases (STDs) and often pregnancy. They include latex condoms, plastic condoms (new in 1995), and latex dams, and diaphragms, used in conjunction with a spermicide. Barrier dams or dental dams are thin sheets of latex or similar material placed over the vagina, clitoris, and anus during oral sex. (Ask your dentist to show you a dental dam.) **Spermicides are chemicals that kill sperm.** These same chemicals have also been shown to

--- **POINT OF INFORMATION 9.3** ---

A LESSON ON CONDOM USE FROM WORLD WARS I AND II

In his social history of venereal disease, *No Magic Bullet*, Allan M. Brandt describes the controversy in the U.S. military about preventing sexually transmitted disease among soldiers during World War I. Should there be an STD **prevention effort** that recognized that many young American men would succumb to the charms of French prostitutes, or should there be a more **punitive approach** to discourage sexual contact? Unlike the New Zealand Expeditionary forces, which gave condoms to their soldiers, the United States decided to give American soldiers after-the-fact, and largely ineffective, chemical prophylaxis. American soldiers were subject to court martial if they contracted a venereal disease. These measures failed. More than 383,000 soldiers were diagnosed with venereal diseases between April 1917 and December 1919 and lost 7 million days of active duty. Only the influenza epidemic was a more common illness among servicemen at that time!

This grim lesson was lost on Americans back home, and campaigns against syphilis continued to emphasize abstinence. **By the 1930s, almost 1 in 10 Americans was infected with syphilis.**

During World War II, however, the American armed forces took a more realistic approach and distributed 50 million condoms each month during the war. The military's new motto—**"If you can't say no, take a pro"**—recognized that abstinence is the best way to prevent STDs, but for those who don't say no, the next best option is to use a condom (Glantz, 1996).

CLARIFYING THE ISSUES OVER CONDOM USE

Two major issues surface in the debate over advocating condom use in the prevention of HIV infection: One concerns the concept of efficacy, the condoms ability to stop the virus from passing through, and the other, the fear that making condoms available will encourage early sexual activity among adolescents and extramarital sex among adults.

EFFICACY (DO THEY WORK?)

All condoms are not 100% impermeable; they are not all of the same quality. Investigators using different testing methods have reported that latex condoms are effective physical barriers to high concentrations of *Chlamydia trachomatis, Neisseria gonorrhoeae,* the herpes and hepatitis viruses, cytomegalovirus, and HIV (Judson, 1989). But for maximum effectiveness condoms must be properly and consistently used from start to finish (Table 9-3).

To be effective, a condom must be worn on the penis during the entire time that the sex organ is in contact with the partner's genital area, anus, or mouth. Care must be taken that the condom is on before vaginal, anal, or oral penetration, and that it does not slip off. If properly used, the condom provides protection against most of the STDs that occur within the vagina, on the glans penis, within the urethra or along the penile shaft.

Because the condom covers only the head and shaft of the penis, it does not provide protection for the pubic or thigh areas, which may come in contact with body secretions during sexual activity.

Margret Fischel reported in 1987 that 17% of women whose husbands were HIV-positive became HIV-infected while using condoms properly and consistently.

Susan Weller (1993) reported on the use of condoms as a barrier to HIV transmission. She analyzed the data from 11 studies involving 593 partners of HIV-infected people. The resulting data showed that condoms are only 69% effective in preventing HIV transmission in heterosexual couples. These data surprise people because earlier contraceptive research indicated that condoms are about 90% effective in preventing pregnancy. Thus many people assume condoms prevent HIV transmission with the same degree of effectiveness. However, transmission studies by Weller do not show that to be true. Weller states that condom effectiveness in blocking HIV transmission may be as low as 46% or as high as 82%!

TABLE 9-3 Proper Placement of a Condom[a] on the Penis

1. Open the packaged condom with care; avoid making small fingernail tears or breaks in the condom.
2. Place a drop of a water based lubricant inside the condom tip before placing it on the head of the penis. Be sure none of the lubricant rolls down the penis shaft as it may cause the condom to slide off during intercourse.
3. Hold about a half an inch of the condom tip between your thumb and finger—this is to allow space for semen after ejaculation. Then place the condom against the glans penis (if uncircumcised, pull the foreskin back).
4. Unroll the condom down the penis shaft to the base of the penis. Squeeze out any air as you roll the condom toward the base.
5. After ejaculation, hold the condom at the base and withdraw the penis while it is still firm.
6. Carefully take the condom off by gently rolling and pulling so as not to leak semen.
7. Discard the condom into the trash.
8. Wash your hands after the procedure.
9. Never use the same condom twice.
10. Condoms should not be stored in extremely hot or cold environments.

[a]Males should practice putting on and removing a condom prior to engaging in sexual intercourse.

Isabelle deVincenzi (1994) reported on HIV transmission among heterosexual sexual couples in which one partner was known to be HIV-positive. Study participants were advised to use condoms during intercourse, and among the 124 (or 48%) of couples who followed that advice consistently, no seronegative partner became HIV infected during roughly 24 months of follow-up. However, despite knowledge about HIV transmission, more than 50% of the couples failed to use condoms consistently. Twelve of the seronegative individuals in that group became HIV-positive during the study.

The importance of compliance is illuminated by an analogy with pregnancy prevention programs. Although typical pregnancy rates for couples who use condoms are as high as 10% to 15%, rates are estimated to be as low as 2% for couples who use condoms correctly and consistently.

A mathematical model predicts that consistent condom use could prevent nearly half of the sexually transmitted HIV infections in persons with one sexual partner and over half of HIV infections in persons with multiple partners. A reduction of this magnitude could help interrupt the propagation of the epidemic. Therefore, promoting more widespread understanding of condom efficacy or effectiveness, and advocating their consistent use by those who choose to be sexually active, is crucial to protecting people from HIV infection and to slowing the spread of the HIV and sexually transmitted disease epidemic.

DO CONDOMS ENCOURAGE SEXUAL ACTIVITY?

Many persons assert that those who promote condom use to prevent HIV infection appear to be condoning sexual intercourse outside of marriage among adolescents as well as among adults. Recent data from Switzerland suggest that a public education campaign promoting condom use can be effective without increasing the proportion of adolescents who are sexually active. A 3-year, 10-month study showed condom use among persons aged 17 to 30 years increased from 8% to 52%. By contrast the proportion of adolescents (aged 16 to 19 years) who had sexual intercourse did not increase over that same period. A report from Deborah Sellers and colleagues (1994) and Sally Guttmacher et al. (1997) also concluded that the promotion and distribution of condoms did not increase sexual activity among adolescents. The study involved 586 adolescents who were 14 to 20 years of age.

The AIDS epidemic has brought new dimensions of complexity and urgency to the debate over adolescent sexual activity. Some have urged abstinence as the only solution; while others champion condom use as the most practical public health approach. Thus a clear message about condoms may have been obscured by controversy over providing condoms for adolescents in schools while at the same time trying to discourage these same young people from initiating sexual activity.

There must be a common ground: People should be able to agree that premature initiation of sexual activity carries health risks. Therefore, young people must be encouraged to postpone sexual activity. Parents, clergy, and educators must strive for a climate supportive of young people who are not having sex. Let them know it is a very positive and intelligent decision, and so help to create a new health-oriented social norm for adolescents and teenagers about sexuality.

The message that those who initiate or continue sexual activity must reduce their risk through correct and consistent condom use needs to be delivered as strongly and persuasively as the message, "Don't do it." Protection of the individual and the public health will depend on our ability to combine these messages effectively (Roper et al., 1993).

ANECDOTE

Presenting facts without understanding won't work! Here is a simple story to emphasize the point: A minister following his custom, paid a monthly call on two spinster sisters. While he was standing in their parlor, holding his cup of tea, engaged in their usual chit chat, he was startled by something that caught his eye. There on the piano was a condom! 'Ladies, in all the years we've known each other I have never intruded into your private lives, and never felt the need to. But now I am forced to ask what is that thing doing there?' 'One of the ladies replied, 'Oh, that's a wonderful thing, pastor, and they really work!' 'The minister was agitated: I'm not talking about their value or effectiveness. I just want to know what that thing is doing on your piano?'

'Well, my sister and I were watching television. We heard this lovely man, the Surgeon General of the whole United States. He said that if you put one of those on your organ, you'll never get sick. Well, as you know we don't have an organ, but we bought one and put it on the piano, and we haven't had a day's sickness since!'

kill bacteria and inactivate viruses that cause STDs (Bolch et al., 1973; Singh, 1982; Amortegui et al., 1984; Hicks et al., 1985). Spermicides are commercially available in foams, creams, jellies, suppositories, and sponges. **Use of these products may provide protection against the transmission of STDs, but the only recommended barrier protection against HIV infection is a condom with a spermicide.** National Condom Week is the week of February 14–21.

Condom—A Medical Device?

Condoms are classified as medical devices. Every condom made in the U.S. is tested for defects and must meet quality control guidelines enforced by the federal Food and Drug Administration (FDA).

Condoms are intended to provide a physical barrier that prevents contact between vaginal, anal, penile, and oral lesions and secretions and ejaculate.

At least 50 brands of condoms are manufactured in the United States. They are produced to fit every fancy. There are colored condoms—pink, yellow, and gold; flavored condoms; and condoms that are perfumed, ribbed, stippled, and phosphorescent (glow in the dark). This assortment of condoms exposes the user and his partner not only to rubber but also to a variety of different chemicals—some that can cause allergic skin reactions (contact dermatitis). One to two percent of people are sensitive to latex rubber a demonstrate contact dermatitis.

Condoms are also called rubbers, prophylactics, bags, skins, raincoats, sheaths, and French letters. They can be lubricated or not, have reservoir tips or not, and can contain spermicide.

Over the years people have been told to use condoms to prevent STDs and pregnancy. Today people are told that an additional use of the condom is to save lives.

History of Condoms

It has been reported that early Egyptian men used animal membranes as a sheath to cover their penises (Barber, 1990). Animal intestines were flushed clean with water, sewn shut at one end and cut to the length of the erect penis. In 1504, Gabriel Fallopius designed a medicated linen sheath that was pulled on over the penis. A Japanese novel written in the 10th century refers to the uncomfortable use of a tortoise shell or horn to cover the penis.

It is interesting to note that condoms were used far more often throughout history as protection against STDs than as contraceptives. For example, an 18th century writer recommended that men protect themselves against disease by placing a linen sheath over the penis during intercourse.

The term condom came into common usage in the 1700s. According to accounts, in the early 1700s, condoms were sold and even exported from a London shop whose propri-

etress laundered and "recycled" them in a back room (Barber, 1990). Condoms became more widely available after 1854 when the method for making rubber was invented by Charles Goodyear (as in Goodyear tires). The latex condom was first manufactured in the 1930s.

Condoms have been available in the United States for over 130 years, but have never been as openly accepted as they are now. Their sale for contraceptive use was outlawed by many state legislatures beginning in 1868 and by Congress in 1873. Although most of these laws were eventually repealed, condom packages and dispensers until only a few years ago continued to bear the label **"Sold only for the prevention of disease,"** even though they were being used mainly for the prevention of pregnancy.

After the advent of nonbarrier methods of contraception during the 1960s (mainly the use of the birth control pill) there was an ensuing epidemic increase in most sexually transmitted infections. Condoms once again are being marketed for the prevention of disease (Judson, 1989).

In 1979, only 8% of respondents to a *Consumer Reports* survey on condoms said they used condoms for the prevention of STDs. However, in *Consumer Reports'* 1989 study, 26% said they used condoms to prevent STDs, especially HIV infection (Figure 9-2, A and B).

Safer Sex, the Choice of Condom

Although a variety of preventative behaviors have been recommended (Table 9-2), the responsibility of **safer sex**, with a condom, is a personal choice. If one decides to use a condom, then the choice is what kind, and whether or not to use a spermicide.

The Male Condom— The American- made condom most often sold is made of latex, is about 8 inches long, and in general, one size fits all. About 500 million condoms were sold in the United States in 1992. Over five billion are sold annually worldwide (Grimes, 1992).

Intact latex condoms provide a continuous mechanical barrier to HIV, herpes virus (HSV), hepatitis B virus (HBV), *Chlamydia trachomatis*, and *Neisseria gonorrhoeae*. A recent laboratory study indicated that latex and the **new polyure-**

A

B

FIGURE 9-2 Advertisements for Condoms. **A,** A common theme centered around the use of a condom to protect against sexually transmitted diseases. **B,** A specific type of condom in a comic book style advertisement.

thane condoms are the most effective mechanical barrier to fluid containing HIV-sized particles (0.1 μm in diameter)available (Figure 9-3).

In a study of heterosexual couples—in which only one partner was HIV-positive—none of the 123 uninfected partners who used latex condoms consistently and correctly contracted the disease. Among a similar group who were less conscientious, 10% became infected (*MMWR*, 1993a; *Office Nurse*, 1995).

Three prospective studies in developed countries indicated that condoms are unlikely to break or slip during proper use. Reported breakage rates in the studies with latex condoms were 2% or less for vaginal or anal intercourse (*MMWR*, 1993a).

There is another kind of condom made from **lamb's intestine**. It is commonly called a "skin." It is believed that it may allow viruses to slip through and is **not recommended** for use. Animal-derived condoms are used mainly because they allow greater passage of body heat, provide better tactile sensation, and can be reused.

Choice— The best choice for preventing STDs and pregnancy is condoms that are made of latex or polyurethane (plastic) and contain a **spermicide**. The spermicide is added protection in case the condom ruptures or spills as it is taken off. During in vitro studies, condoms were artificially ruptured in a medium containing nonoxynol-9 or N-9 (*p*-diisobutylphenoxypolyethoxethanol). On examination, no virus capable of reproduction was found. Tests done without the spermicide resulted in viruses capable of reproducing (Connell, 1989). It must be mentioned, however, that there is no evidence that N-9 has any effect on HIVs that are carried within lymphocyte cells in the semen.

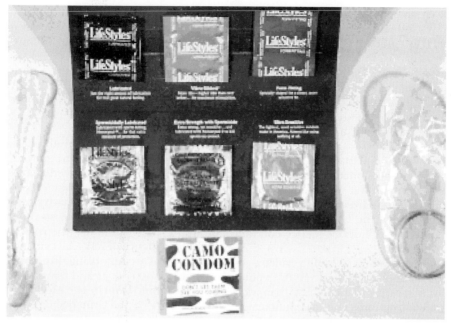

FIGURE 9-3 A Collection of Condoms. The condom is sealed in an aluminum foil package, sometimes along with a spermicide. On the left side is an unfolded or unrolled male condom; on the right side is a vaginal pouch (female condom) (see Figure 9-4).

Nonoxynol-9— Evidence from the mid-1970s has lent support to the prophylactic use of N-9 as a spermicide against sexually transmitted diseases (Bird, 1991). There are reports, however, that some males and females are sensitive to it. N-9 has been shown to variably inactivate *Neisseria gonorrhoeae, Trichomonas vaginalis, Ureaplasma urealyticum, Treponema pallidum, Candida albicans,* herpes and hepatitis B viruses, and cytomegalovirus and HIV. There is some question about its effectiveness against *Chlamydia trachomatis,* and it has been reported to be ineffective against the genital wart virus (Stone et al., 1986; Rosenberg et al., 1992). More recently, concern has been raised that N-9 may serve to digest nonspecific protective mucosal coatings and induce the increased presence of lymphocytes and bleeding, which by itself might promote HIV and other viral and bacterial infections (Fisher, 1991). However, Knut Wittkowski (1995) points out that there is now sufficient evidence to conclude that possible minor abrasions of the multilayered vaginal

skin, from the use of N-9, are more than compensated by the protective effect of the chemical barrier. If N-9 were less effective than condoms, but more simple to use, some couples might switch to N-9 and consequently increase their risk of HIV infection.

Condom Advertising on American Television— On January 4, 1994, condoms danced into America's living rooms as part of the most explicit HIV prevention campaign the nation has even seen. Previously, condoms were rarely seen or even mentioned on American television. But the Centers for Disease Control and Prevention (CDC) launched a series of radio and television public service announcements targeting sexually active young adults, a group at high risk for HIV infection.

One of the television ads, entitled *Automatic,* features a condom making its way from the top drawer of a dresser across the room and into bed with a couple about to make love. The voice-over says, "It would be nice if latex condoms were automatics. But since they're not, using them should be. Simply because a latex condom, used consistently and correctly, will prevent the spread of HIV." Another, entitled *Turned Down*, features a man and woman kissing, when the woman asks the man, "Did you bring it?" When he says he **forgot it**, she replies, "Then **forget it**," and turns on the light. There is also a pair of abstinence ads, in which condom use is not mentioned. The ads feature a man and woman talking. She says, "There is a time for us to be lovers. We will wait until that time comes."

Language that was once forbidden on TV has now become routine. Will it prevent HIV infection? **Will it save lives?**

Beginning 1996, the CDC began another series of radio and TV public service condom announcements.

The spots reel along like MTV videos, interspersing personal advice from young people with scenes from dance clubs, Greenwich Village, and a drugstore. They are punctuated by headlines that scream, "Put It On," "Talk About It," and "It's O.K. to Wait to Have Sex."

The bottom line to the new announcements is: **"Respect Yourself, Protect Yourself."**

The advertising campaigns are hailed as a milestone, marking a high point of visibility for the condom on network television and introducing a new level of explicitness to the Centers for Disease Control and Prevention's public pronouncements about AIDS prevention.

Class Discussion: What is your opinion on condom advertising?

Buying Condoms— Women are taking a more active role in buying condoms. In 1985, women bought about 10% of the condoms sold. In 1989, they purchased 40% to 50%. According to surveys, most women buying condoms are single, and their concern is about HIV infection rather than pregnancy. The fact that more women are willing to buy condoms is evidence that HIV education is working to some degree.

Many condoms are purchased from vending machines. The FDA recommends the following guidelines when purchasing condoms from a vending machine:

1. Is the condom made of latex or polyurethane?
2. Is the condom labeled for disease prevention?

3. Is the spermicide (if any) outdated?
4. Is the machine exposed to extreme temperatures or direct sunlight?

In mid-1992, the first drive-up "Condom Hut" opened in Cranston, Rhode Island. With each purchase the customer receives a brochure on safer sex.

Free Condoms— In the south of France, the regional tourism authority announced, in 1991, that condoms would be placed alongside soap and shampoo in all hotel rooms and would be supplied free to all people using campsites in the area. Some 8 million tourists visit the south of France every summer—the region has the highest incidence of HIV/AIDS in the country.

Condoms are now being dispensed without charge in most college and university and public health clinics, and in at least 336 high school health offices in the United States. Some cities in Canada have been providing access to free condoms in high schools since 1984.

Regardless of educational programs on safer sex and condom usage, recent studies indicate that teenagers still refuse to use condoms. **What they know is not equal to what they do!** Based on their findings, the researchers said information-oriented school- and community-based AIDS prevention programs will not succeed in getting adolescents to use condoms, because there is no association between knowledge and preventive behavior.

Condom Availability in Developing Nations

Access to condoms in developing nations, although crucial, is poor even though over **1 billion** condoms are distributed in developing nations each year. The World Health Organization spends some $70 million a year for condoms distributed in 14 countries. But, it would cost $460 million to provide just Africa with an adequate condom program. The United Kingdom, in 1992, purchased 66 million condoms for Zimbabwe but the country needs at least 120 million condoms per year. And it must be recognized that a number of cultures in developing nations prohibit the use of condoms.

———— BOX 9.2 ————

CONDOMS: A LIFE OR DEATH ISSUE

ADULTS

Some males argue that they want to feel the *real you*, others argue that they don't make condoms *large* enough, while others say they are an inconvenience and putting one on takes away the pleasure of the moment. But not to use a condom or insist on the use of a condom *invites* infection. And if it's an HIV infection, the invitation will, most likely, lead to death.

There are many men and women who want to practice safer sex and are willing to use a condom. The problem is, many do not carry condoms with them 100% of the time. If they happen to have a condom available, they might be thought of as promiscuous. If they do not have a condom, they may not get the chance to have sex, especially if their potential partner is `safe sex' conscious. In other words, to demand one's sexual partner to use a condom may be taken as an accusation, while an offer to use a condom may be viewed as a confession. This is a kind of "Catch-22" scenario—damned if they do and damned if they do not.

TEENAGERS

Part of being a teenager is taking risks. Too many teens act as though they're invincible. They test limits and question authority. But now, the impact of unsafe sex can be irreversible. It's like playing a game of Russian roulette: **maybe they won't get infected, but maybe they will**. Most

STDs can be treated. But **no one** has yet been cured of HIV / AIDS.

Although information alone does not keep young people from having sex, becoming infected with HIV, or getting pregnant, accurate information about the consequences of unsafe sex may strengthen a youth's resolve not to have sex or not to have it without protection. Knowing that many of their peers do not have sex also helps youth understand they have the option to abstain.

In order for information to influence decisions, teenagers must understand that the information is about them.

According to data from the CDC's national school-based Youth Risk Behavior Survey, at least half of all high school students have had sexual intercourse. By the age of 17, 72% were sexually active. The survey, based on a questionnaire given to 12,272 students at 137 schools in the United States, revealed that 48% said they used a condom the last time they had sex, but that figure dropped to 19% for couples using birth control pills to prevent pregnancy.

That suggests students understand the importance of using birth control but do not understand the value of condoms in preventing HIV infection.

In another study, the CDC found that 88% to 98% of teenagers in homeless shelters, medical clinics, and correctional institutions were sexually active.

Condom Quality

Some have touted condoms as a bulletproof vest for preventing HIV infection. This is simplistic and inaccurate because condoms may break or be used improperly. Condoms have been shown to **reduce** significantly but **not eliminate** the transmission of HIV. **Condom use is a form of safer sex but not absolutely safe sex.** The March 1989 issue of *Consumer Reports* did a rather extensive study on the quality of different brands of condoms. The reader survey revealed that one in eight people who used condoms had two condoms break in one year of sexual activity; one in four said one condom had broken. Calculated from its data, about one in 140 condoms broke, with condom breakage occurring more often during

some sexual activities than others. For example, the breakage rate during anal sex was calculated at one in 105 compared to one in 165 for vaginal sex. One in 10 heterosexual men admitted to engaging in anal sex using condoms (*Consumer Reports*, 1989).

In a separate United States Public Health Service study (1994), if a couple used male condoms consistently and correctly, there was a 3% chance of unintentional pregnancy. Other studies have found that condoms reduce the risk of gonorrhea by as much as 66% in men, but by no more than 34% in women. It doesn't appear as though they prevent papilloma virus infection—which causes genital warts—in either sex (Stratton et al., 1993). Table 9-4 presents the results on **latex** condom efficacy in preventing HIV infection.

TABLE 9-4   Efficacy of Latex Condoms to Stop HIV Transmission

Study	Subjects	HIV-Positive
Fischl et al., 1987	Partners of HIV-positive individuals	Without barrier, 86%
		With barrier, 10%
Mann et al., 1987	Prostitutes, Zaire	No condom use, 26%
		Up to 25% use, 35%
		26%–49% use, 32%
		50%–74% use, 0%
		75%–100% use, 0%
Ngugi et al., 1986	Prostitutes, Kenya	No condom use, 72%
		Less than 50% use, 56%
		50% use or more, 33%
		100% use, 0%
CDC, 1987	Prostitutes, United States	No or some condom use, 11%
		100% use, 0%
Padian, 1987	Female partners of HIV-positive males	Relative risk, 0.6[a] (95% CI, 0.3–1.3)
Laurian et al., 1989	Female partners of HIV-positive males	No or some condom use, 17%
		100% use, 0%

CDC, Centers for Disease Control and Prevention; CI, confidence interval.

[a]Extensive condom use likely to have begun after seroconversion.

(Adapted from Stratton et al., 1993.)

In 1987, FDA inspectors began making spot checks for condom quality. They fill the condom with 10 ounces (about 300 mL) of water to check for leaks. If leaks are found in more than four per 1,000 condoms, that entire batch is destroyed. Over the first 15 months of spot inspections, one lot in 10 was rejected. Import condoms failed twice as often—one lot in five.

The New Polyurethane (Plastic) Condoms—For the 1% of the general population that is sensitive to latex and for those who have a variety of other reasons not to use a latex condom, there is now a clear, thin, strong, FDA approved polyurethane (plastic) condom for sale in the United States. The condoms are colorless, odorless, and **can** be used with **any** lubricant. The current cost is about $1.80 each. Manufacturers of at least five other plastic condoms are waiting FDA approval.

The Female Condom (Vaginal Pouch)— The female condom was FDA approved in May of 1993, and has become available to the general public. Before giving the Reality condom final approval, the FDA asked that two caveats be put into the labeling. First, the agency required a statement on the package label that male condoms are still the best protection against disease, and second, that the label compare the effectiveness of female condoms with that of other barrier methods of birth control. According to the FDA, in a study of 150 women who used the female condom for 6 months, 26% became pregnant. The manufacturer contends that the pregnancy rate was 21%—and only because many women did not use the condom every time they had sex. With **"perfect use,"** company officials say, the rate is 5%, in contrast to 2% for male condoms. Both conditions were met to the FDA's satisfaction. Gaston Farr and co-workers (1994) concluded that the female condom provided contraceptive efficacy in the same range as other barrier methods, particularly when used consistently and correctly, and has the added advantage of helping protect against sexually transmitted diseases.

The female condom is now called the **vaginal pouch**. It is 17 cm long and it consists of a 15-cm polyurethane sheath with rings at each end (Figure 9-4). The closed end fits into the vagina like a diaphragm. The outer portion is designed to cover the base of the penis and a large portion of the female perineum (the area of tissue between the anus and the beginning of the vaginal opening) to provide a greater surface barrier against microorganisms. Studies of acceptability, contraceptive effectiveness, and STD prevention are currently underway. Potential advantages of this

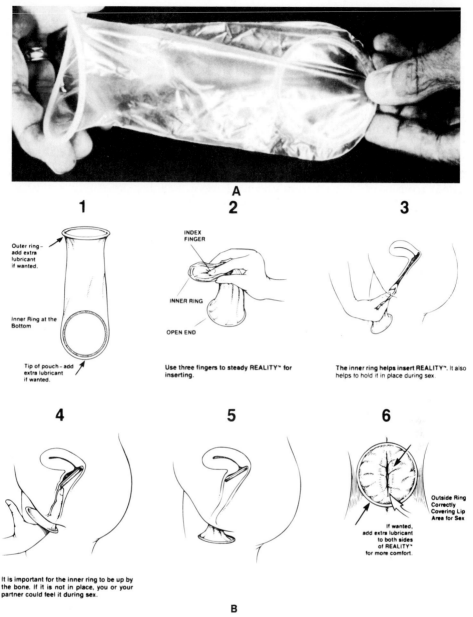

A

1

Outer ring – add extra lubricant if wanted.

Inner Ring at the Bottom

Tip of pouch – add extra lubricant if wanted.

2

INDEX FINGER

INNER RING

OPEN END

Use three fingers to steady REALITY™ for inserting.

3

The inner ring helps insert REALITY™. It also helps to hold it in place during sex.

4

It is important for the inner ring to be up by the bone. If it is not in place, you or your partner could feel it during sex.

5

6

Outside Ring Correctly Covering Lip Area for Sex

If wanted, add extra lubricant to both sides of REALITY™ for more comfort.

B

FIGURE 9-4 A, The Vaginal Pouch. **B,** The 7-inch female condom or vaginal pouch is made of lightweight, lubricated polyurethane and has two flexible rings (1), one at either end. It is twice the thickness of the male latex condom. The inner ring (2) is used to help insert the device and fits behind the pubic bone. The outer ring remains outside the body. Unlike the diaphragm, the vaginal condom protects against the transmission of HIV, which can penetrate the vaginal tissues. The pouch can be inserted anytime from several hours to minutes prior to intercourse. The vaginal pouch is inserted like a diaphragm and removed after sex. FDA approved in May, 1993. (*Courtesy of Wisconsin Pharmacal Co.*)

product are: (1) it provides women with the opportunity to protect themselves from pregnancy and STDs; (2) it provides a broader coverage of the labia and base of the penis than a male condom; and (3) its polyurethane membrane is stronger than latex.

At least three versions of the female vaginal pouch are currently undergoing testing and awaiting Food and Drug Administration approval—one developed by a Wisconsin company, another by a father and son doctor team in California, and a third by a Wyoming physician. The Wisconsin version has recently been named *Reality*. The cost for the Reality condom is about $2.50 each. The female condom has been sold in Switzerland since 1992 and in France and Britain since mid-1993.

The Wyoming pouch is folded into the crotch of a latex G-string. The three products all perform in essentially the same way. They are disposable, contain protective sheaths of rubber or plastic, and are worn on the inside of a woman instead of on the outside of a man.

Redressing the Balance of Power

The symbolic importance of the female condom should not be understated: **it is the first woman-controlled barrier method officially recognized as a means for the prevention of sexually transmitted disease**. The female condom allows women to be able to deal with the twin anxieties—AIDS and unwanted pregnancy— with a method that is under their own control.

Many women become HIV infected due not to their own behavior, but to their partner's behavior. And, because of the nature of gender relations, women may have little influence over their partner's sexual behavior.

As the number of women infected with HIV escalates and the ratio of female to male infection increases, the way contraceptives affect HIV transmission becomes an even more urgent concern for women. Medical, cultural, political, and socioeconomic conditions affect which contraceptive method a woman will choose, or whether she will have access to contraception at all.

Of female-controlled contraceptives in use today, only the female condom provides any definite preventive effect against HIV transmission.

POINT OF INFORMATION 9.5

FRENCH BISHOP SUPPORTS SOME USE OF CONDOMS TO PREVENT HIV INFECTION/AIDS

In February 1996 Bishop Albert Rouet of Poitiers, the chairman of a French Roman Catholic bishops committee, suggested in their report that the use of condoms could be justified in some cases to prevent the spread of AIDS, contradicting the Vatican's general condemnation of most methods of birth control. The 235 pages of Bishop Rouet's discussion and the committee's report, called "AIDS: Society in Question," broadly conformed to the church's emphasis on abstinence and its condemnation of most birth control. The report noted that public health campaigns sponsored by French Government authorities have gone to great lengths to expose young people to the idea that using condoms could help keep them from being infected with HIV.

After a very long reaction time, it appears that young people are using them more often. Public health authorities endorse this use. The church, thought to be opposed to it, sees itself accused of promoting death. The issue is badly posed, because it confuses several domains that are not on the same moral level. To think that a generalization of the use of condoms will remove all risk is to look only at the consequences without examining the causes and conditions of the spread of AIDS. Advising young adolescents to use condoms, far from helping them to understand their sexual identity, confines them to the power of their desires.

Although there have been no clinical studies of the effectiveness of female condoms in preventing HIV transmission, in vitro studies have found that the polyurethane sheath may provide an effective barrier against the virus. Clinical studies suggest that the female condom is more durable and less likely to break than male condoms. Yet female condoms are unavailable to most women worldwide and are much more expensive than male condoms and more difficult to use.

Condom Lubricants

It has been demonstrated that petroleum or vegetable oil based lubricants should not be used with latex condoms. Nick White and col-

TABLE 9-5 Water-Based[a] and Oil-Based[b] Lubricants Often Used with Latex Condoms

Lubricants Recommended	Lubricants Not Recommended
Aqualube	Petroleum jellies
Astroglide	Mineral oils
Cornhuskers Lotion	Vegetable oils
Forplay	Baby oil
H-R Jelly	Massage oil
K-Y Brand Jelly	Lard
RePair	Cold creams
Probe	Hair oils
Today Personal Lube	Hand lotions containing vegetable oils
	Shaft
	Elbow Grease
	Natural Lube

[a]Water-based lubricants can be used with latex condoms.

[b]Oil-based lubricants will chemically weaken latex, causing it to break.

The above lists are not exhaustive of all available lubricants used by consumers.

(Source: The STD Education Unit of the San Francisco Department of Public Health)

leagues (1988) have reported that these lubricants weaken latex condoms. Latex condoms exposed to mineral oil for 60 seconds demonstrated a 90% decrease in strength (Anderson, 1993). There are a number of water based lubricants that do not adversely affect latex condoms; these should be the lubricants of choice (Table 9-5).

An Alternative: Chemical Barrier Protection—Vaginal Microbicides: A Protection Method That Women Can Control

While condoms, when used consistently and correctly, are effective in preventing the sexual spread of HIV, there is an urgent need for chemical barrier methods that women can use for HIV prophylaxis, such as vaginal microbicides. Vaginal microbicides are products for vaginal administration that can be used to prevent HIV infection and/or other sexually transmitted diseases (STD). An ideal vaginal microbicide would be safe and effective, and also tasteless, colorless,

odorless, nontoxic, stable in most climates, and affordable.

It takes two people to have sex, but only one to slow the spread of sexually transmitted diseases and HIV/AIDS. A man can use condoms, but a woman's choices are limited. The most glaring gap in HIV/AIDS prevention is the lack of a method a woman can use when she suspects her partner may have a sexually transmitted disease or HIV infection and she cannot compel him to use a condom.

The risks of AIDS and other sexually transmitted diseases are stacked against women. Sexually transmitted diseases present fewer symptoms but cause more long-term damage in women than in men; sexualy transmitted diseases and HIV pass more easily from men to women than vice versa, so even though the average man has more sexual partners than most women, women acquire HIV at an earlier mean age than men; and women can pass sexually acquired infections and HIV to the next generation during pregnancy, delivery, or breast feeding. HIV and other sexually transmitted diseases spread most rapidly where women are most disadvantaged: among prostitutes it is those who charge least who are most likely to get infected. The female condom is a new choice for women that should slow HIV transmission, but it cannot be used without the man's knowledge.

Chemical Barriers

Chemical methods that can be controlled by women are likely to have a powerful effect on the spread of HIV for several reasons. They could be distributed rapidly and cheaply by well understood social marketing techniques. They have the potential to slow HIV transmission directly and to reduce other sexually transmitted diseases that are cofactors in transmission.

In the United States, HIV-infected women are among the most rapidly growing groups affected by the disease. Globally, the largest number of cases are the result of heterosexual transmission. From a public health perspective, a modest reduction in HIV transmission brought about by a vaginal microbicide made available today might save as many lives as a more effective method (e.g., a vaccine) made avail-

QUESTIONS AND ANSWERS ABOUT THE FEMALE CONDOM

1. **Does one have to be fitted for use of a female condom?** The female condom is offered in one size and is available without prescription. Unlike using a diaphragm, the female condom covers not only the cervix but also the vagina, thereby containing the man's ejaculate.

2. **Should a lubricant be used with the female condom?** A lubricant is recommended for use with the female condom to increase comfort and ease the entry and withdrawal of the penis. The female condom is prelubricated on the inside with a silicone-based, nonspermicidal lubricant. Additional water-based lubrication is included. The lubricant can be placed either inside the female condom or on the penis.

3. **Can oil-based lubricants be used with the female condom?** The female condom is made of polyurethane which is not reported to be damaged by oil-based lubricants.

4. **Can a spermicide be used with the female condom?** Use of a spermicide has not been reported to damage the female condom. It is recommended that a spermicide containing nonoxynol-9 be used with the female condom for additional protection against HIV in the event of displacement, breakage, or leakage.

5. **How far in advance of sexual intercourse can the female condom be inserted?** The female condom may be inserted up to 8 hours before sexual intercourse. Most women insert it 2 to 20 minutes before engaging in vaginal intercourse.

6. **Can the female condom be reused?** No. A new female condom must be used for each act of vaginal intercourse. After intercourse, the condom must be removed before the women stands, to ensure that semen remains inside the pouch.

7. **Should a female condom and a male condom be used at the same time?** The female condom and male condom can be used at the same time but it is not recommended because the condoms may not stay in place due to friction between the latex in the male condom and the polyurethane in the female condom.

8. **Does Medicaid cover the female condom?** Currently Medicaid does not cover this device, as it does the male condom, spermicide, and other barriers. However, Medicaid coverage is expected in 1995. (*Information provided by the New York State Department of Health AIDS Institute Division of HIV Prevention*, Info Bulletin, *Jan. 1994, Number Five.*)

able in 10 years' time, when there might be 5 or 10 times as many infected people (Potts, 1994).

Chemical Barriers Used in Foam, Gel, or Sponge

In November of 1993, the WHO began a strategy to identify a safe and effective substance that can be inserted into the vagina in a **foam**, **gel**, **sponge**, or other form to destroy HIV or prevent it from infecting cells in the body. Researchers hope that it can be used by a woman without her partner's knowledge. WHO scientists believe that if there is one thing which truly can make a difference to the epidemic, it is a vaginal microbicide.

In developing a vaginal microbicide, **scientists must be sure that the substance is safe, does not kill microbes naturally present in the vagina that benefit female hygiene, and does not impair a woman's ability to conceive**. Any microbicide will have to be tested to determine whether it damages spermatozoa, which could result in birth defects. Currently 10 substances are being explored as potential microbicides. The earliest expected success is some years off. However, even if an early vaginal microbicide proves to be far less than 100% effective, it still can make a major impact on the HIV/AIDS epidemic. The prevalence of HIV infection in some populations, particularly in the developing countries, is so high that even something that was 50% effective would be a great advance.

Update on Vaginal Microbicide Research

In July of 1996 the United States government pledged $100 million to help develop virus-inactivating creams that would let women protect themselves from HIV infection without relying on their partners. The goal is to create alternatives to condoms that women can use without men's permission—especially creams that protect against HIV but would still allow them to get pregnant.

Beginning 1997, **sulfated polysaccharides** (PS) (a sugar molecule with sulfur groups attached) should enter Phase II safety trials. It appears that PS offers protection of the cervical epithelial (surface) cells by coating the HIV-infected lymphocytes, free HIV, and uninfected epithelial cells with a negative charge. Thus the different cell types and free HIV repell each other, attachment of virus to cells is blocked, and infection is prevented.

Four surfactant products are available: nonoxynol-9, octoxynol-9, benzalkonium chloride, and menfegel, but only the first two are approved for use in the United States. They are all detergent-based, disrupting both cell and viral membranes. But they are also irritating to normal genital mucosa. This has led to the suggestion that such compounds might actually facilitate HIV spread in certain instances.

A **second avenue** of prevention is a study using thermoreversible gels. The gels, hopefully, will block HIV entry into cervical, vaginal, or anorectal mucosa. The chemical composition of the gel allows it to behave like water at 4°C, but it becomes toothpaste-like at body temperature, blocking HIV penetration (Voelker, 1995).

A **third approach**, and one currently being tested, is to place drugs like zidovudine, which inhibit HIV reverse transcriptase from making new viral strands, into vaginal gels. Early test results on monkeys show promising results and phase I trials in humans began in late 1996.

Ending 1997, 20 vaginal microbicide products are in preclinical, 13 in early clinical, and two in advanced clinical trials. However, there is little private-sector involvement, and it is unlikely that any product will be approved before the year 2000. There are few clinical-trial infrastructures for such studies, with a limited number of places in the world where a high enough incidence of sexual transmission occurs to make such trials feasible within a short time period.

INJECTION DRUG USE AND HIV TRANSMISSION: THE TWIN EPIDEMICS

About 36%, almost 245,000 of the 680,500 (through mid-1998) U. S. AIDS cases recorded since 1981 were transmitted through injection drug use.

Syringes and needles used to inject drugs or steroids, or to tattoo the body, or to pierce the ears, should never be shared. If an individual is going to assume the risk of HIV transmission through needle sharing, the risk can be reduced by sterilizing the needle, and the syringe, if one is used, in undiluted chlorine bleach. The needle and syringe should be flushed through twice with bleach and rinsed thoroughly with water. (**NOTE: FROM THIS POINT FORWARD, "SYRINGE" INCLUDES *BOTH* SYRINGE AND NEEDLE.**)

Both injection drug use (IDU) and HIV infection are on the increase. They are twin epidemics in the United States and Europe because the virus is readily transmitted by injection drug users and then from infected drug users to their noninfected sexual partners. Stopping injection drug-associated HIV transmission in theory is easy—just avoid injection drugs use. But, that is a difficult proposition for most of the over 1.5 million IDUs in the United States. IDUs will remain a major HIV connection to the homosexual, heterosexual, and pediatric populations.

HIV PREVENTION FOR INJECTION DRUG USERS

What can be done and what is being done to prevent HIV transmission by this population? Available drug rehabilitation programs are far too few. It is estimated that only 15% of injection drug users in the United States are receiving treatment at any given time. Many addicts want to quit their habit but may become discouraged because of having to wait long periods of time before getting treatment because of lack

THE MAGNITUDE OF THE EPIDEMICS OF DRUG USE AND BLOOD-BORNE DISEASES

The dual epidemics of drug use and HIV/AIDS are highly destructive of public health and social life in America. Drug-related health problems of the estimated 1.5 million injection drug users (IDUs) in the United States range from blood-borne infections such as hepatitis B and C, HIV/AIDS, endocarditis, and malaria to physical deterioration and death. Illegal drug use and the drug industry that fuels it are associated with a multitude of crimes against persons and property. Drug use induces family disintegration, child neglect, economic ruin, and social decay. **Drug use exacts an estimated annual social cost of $58.3 billion—in lost productivity, motor vehicle crashes, crime, stolen property, and drug treatment.**

IDU is the second most frequently reported risk for adolescent/adult AIDS since the beginning of the United States epidemic in 1981. It now accounts for about half of all new HIV infections, each year. From 1994 through early 1998, 36% of all AIDs cases occurred among IDUs, their heterosexual sex partners, and children whose mothers were IDUs or sex partners of IDUs. In contrast, in 1981, only 12% of all re-ported AIDS cases were associated with injection drug use. In some areas, seroprevalence among IDUs is now as high as 65%; in other areas, the rates are significantly lower. Minorities bear a disproportionately high burden. The rate of **IDU-associated AIDS** per 100,000 population is 3.5 for whites, 21.9 for Hispanics, and 50.9 for African Americans.

Transmission of HIV infection through injection drug use has a cascading effect; infections spread from IDUs to their sexual and syringe-sharing partners and from HIV-infected mothers to their children. Of the **99,000** AIDS cases among women reported through December 1997, nearly 65% were IDUs or were sexual partners of an IDU. Further, of the **8,279** perinatally acquired AIDS cases in early 1998, 60% had mothers who were IDUs or had sex with an IDU. These data suggest that drug use and related behaviors are strong catalysts for spreading HIV throughout the population. **It has been estimated that approximately half of all new HIV infections in the United States occur among IDUs** (Gostin et al., 1997).

of money. Even if there were a sufficient number of treatment centers, there will always be the hard core IDUs who will not enter a program.

A massive education program on how to clean drug equipment and not sharing such equipment has for the most part failed. IDUs have an economic motive to share equipment (Mandell et al., 1994). In addition, it takes time and effort to clean the syringe and it takes time to find and purchase cleansing chemicals (detergents or bleach). Beginning 1998, several studies have shown that over 50% of IDUs continue to share drug injection equipment. Also, less than half clean their injection drug equipment! Perhaps the most important drawback may be that IDUs have little interest in health care or changing their behaviors. In addition, there is always the problem of legality. **IDU is illegal throughout the United States** (see Point of Information 9.7 and Box 9.4).

IDUs know this and fear incarceration without the possibility of a "fix." A "Catch-22" situation also exists for those who want to help make injection drug use safer: **many governmental agencies and law enforcement officers interpret the intention of making drug use safer as advocating drug use.** As a result, many proponents of safer drug use have avoided becoming involved in the issue. A recent public opinion poll showed that 55% of those polled were in favor of syringe exchange programs (Marwrck, 1995). Through 1997 federal money could **not** be used to fund syringe exchange programs.

The Syringe Exchange Program Strategy

The idea of syringe-needle exchange programs (SEPs) is based on the established public health policy of eliminating from any system potentially infectious agents or, where possible, carriers of infectious agents. The rationale of SEPs is similar, wherein active injection drug users exchange used, potentially contaminated syringes for new, sterile syringes. In general, these exchanges are done on a one-used-syringe for one-new-syringe basis, though some programs will add an additional number of syringes on top of those already exchanged. SEPs also provide other paraphernalia and supplies, including cotton, cookers, water, and sterile alcohol prep pads. In addition, SEPs offer a variety of other services to IDUs including education, HIV testing and counseling, referrals to primary medical care, substance abuse treatment, and case management.

Free Syringe Exchange Programs in the United States

Tacoma, Washington— The nation's **first** syringe exchange program began in August 1988. It began as a one-man program. Dave Purchase, a 20-year drug counselor, between August 1988 and April 1989, traded out over 19,000 syringe packages. The following conversation between Purchase and an IDU offers a sense of what happens daily at the Tacoma syringe exchange site:

> Many of the 40 or so clients to use the needle exchange one day last month were regulars. They knew the drill. If they dropped five syringes into

FIGURE 9-5 Syringe Exchange. The injection drug user drops the used syringe into the collection box. For each deposit, the user receives a new syringe. The use of clean equipment prevents the spread of HIV. (Through 1997 federal money could not be used for syringe exchange programs.)

the red box marked **BIOHAZARD**, they got five clean ones in return (Figure 9-5). Soon two new clients appear. One leans close to Purchase and quietly asks for a syringe. They have none to trade.

"You've got to give me one to get one," Purchase says loudly. "It's an absolute rule."

"But he's going by this girl's," says the spokesman, leaning closer. "She doesn't know nothin' about these. I didn't know nothin' about it either."

"It pisses me off that I can't do it. But this is an exchange program. I can't do it. I'm under too much pressure to shut this place down. Go down to Bimbo's, man, and get the ones they throw away," Purchase advises. "I don't care where you get it, just get me one."

They leave in the direction of Bimbo's, a nearby restaurant, across the street from which junkies often shoot up, but they never come back (Perrone, 1989).

The SEP in Tacoma held the HIV infection rate to under 5% over a 5-year study period (1988–1992). During that same 5-year study period, the prevalence of HIV infection among IDUs in New York City, with few syringe exchange programs, increased from 10% to 50%!

Evaluation of Syringe Exchange Programs

Entering 1998, there were 101 known SEPs operating in 71 American cities exchanging about 8 to 9 million syringes annually.

New York City— In November 1988, after many delays, New York City began its syringe exchange program. The program was canceled in early 1990—the reason: because over 50% of NYC's 240,000 IDUs were HIV-infected, the program offered too little too late to have an impact. IDUs make up about 38% to 40% of NYC AIDS cases. Beginning 1998 there were at least five SEPs operating in New York City.

New Haven, Connecticut— Their 6-year-old program has demonstrated that SEPs dramatically slows the rate of infection without encouraging new injection drug use. Some indicators even suggest that the program has been responsible for a decrease in both crime and the amount of drugs used illegally. The city's police chief claims that crime actually dropped over 20% over the past 5 years, per-

THE CONTROVERSY: PROVIDING STERILE SYRINGES AND NEEDLES TO INJECTION DRUG USERS (IDUs)

As the HIV pandemic enters the late 1990s in the United States, the profile of those affected is beginning to change. HIV is slowly changing from a disease of men who have sex with men to a disease of injection drug users, their sexual partners and children. In 1997, 50% of all new HIV infections occurred among IDUs with an additional 10% to 20% of new infections occurring among their sexual partners. **THE SYRINGE IS THE TYPHOID MARY OF THE 1990s!** Accordingly, should IDUs be provided at public expense, with free syringe and needles to help stop the spread of HIV?

There has been no other HIV prevention activity, with the possible exception of condom distribution in public schools, that has generated as much controversy as syringe exchange programs (SEPs.) **Pro forces** believe that it is impossible to eliminate injection drug use. Providing IDUs with free sterile equipment is an attempt at slowing the spread of HIV among drug users and their sexual partners, subsequently reducing the number of people in the general population that will become infected. In support of the Pro forces, the CDC reviewed the 37 SEPs operating in the United States in 1993 and 1997 (Beginning 1998 there were 101 in 71 cities) and others in Canada and Europe. **The most important conclusion is that SEPs are preventing HIV infections in drug users, their sex partners, and their children.** That finding was based, in part, on evidence collected in Tacoma and Seattle, Washington and in New Haven, Connecticut where there was a 33% reduction in the rate of new infections among SEP clients. In another key finding, they found no evidence that *distributing syringes leads to an increase in drug use.*

Besides saving lives, these syringe exchanges deliver a huge financial payoff. Consider the case of an HIV-positive addict who infects eight others in a 1-year period (a reasonable estimate). If each turns to Medicaid to pay his or her lifetime medical costs (at an average $119,000 plus), that's about a $1 million burden for taxpayers—money that could have been saved if the one addict had been in a syringe exchange program.

Con forces feel that to provide free sterile equipment is to condone drug addiction and perhaps promote injection drug use among those who would not otherwise participate. Some feel that free syringe programs are just a Band-Aid that attempts to prevent HIV infection but does nothing to cope with the underlying drug addiction problem. (**These people may feel its too little, too late.**)

A side issue of course is the fact that it is **illegal to sell** syringes over the counter in 10 of the 50 states and the District of Columbia. Statutes in 44 states and the District of Columbia place criminal penalties on the possession and distribution of syringes (drug paraphernalia laws) (*MMWR,* 1993b) in 28 states and Puerto Rico (*MMWR,* 1997). Laws restricting these sales were intended to discourage drug use, (Fisher, 1990). (Gostin et al., 1997). Law enforcement and community leaders (e.g., police, churches, businesses, parents, teachers, and residents) are concerned that allowing access to syringes sends the wrong message, encourages initiation into drug use, and accelerates the disintegration of families. Residents and business owners fear increased street crime, lower property values, and health risks from discarded syringes.

There is a **third force** of people who take the middle ground. They advocate providing free bleach to IDUs to clean their drug equipment. People from many AIDS-action groups in metropolitan areas are involved in the free bleach dispensing program. With each bottle of bleach is a set of directions. But as many IDUs can not read, they are given verbal instructions, though some are too "spaced out" to listen or too uncomfortable to care. Third force people have to understand that SEPs and distribution of bleach kits have to be accessible privately, off the street and out of sight, as well as publicly. Use of a public, streetcorner SEP is a statement to the entire community that the person exchanging a syringe is an IDU. This has potentially very different consequences for women than for men. Women who have children have good reason to try to conceal their addiction as they risk losing custody or contact with their children if the state finds out they are actively using drugs—and if they are using a public SEP the child welfare bureaucracy is more likely to find out than if they are not getting syringes in public. Perhaps SEPs should provide some type of informal child care so that a mother doesn't have to literally exchange syringes in front of her children.

Addiction among women is often taken as a statement of sexual availability.

A **fourth force** suggests that drugs be legalized so that they can be used openly, thereby reducing the threat of HIV transmission through illegal "shooting galleries." Discussion of the fourth force's position is beyond the scope of this text. However, a quasi-fourth force situation did exist in Zurich, Switzerland until 1992.

Zurich gained notoriety for its vast amounts of gold but in 1988 it gained a new image—that of an open Syringe Park. The city of 250,000 people experimented in setting aside a park where cocaine and heroin addicts could openly buy, sell, and use injection drugs. The park attracted up to 4,000 drug users/day.

Next to the United States, Switzerland has the highest incidence of HIV/AIDS in the developed world. The city has tried to stop the spread of the disease among addicts sharing contaminated syringes by isolating them and giving them free new syringes. A cart laboratory has been converted for this purpose. For every used syringe an addict turns in, he or she will get a free, sterile one. About half of the young people in the park are HIV-infected. All of them are slowly killing themselves. At the end of each day, some 7,000 dirty syringes have been turned in. The syringe park was not run to prevent drug use but to prevent the spread of HIV/AIDS. The program appeared to be working. The incidence of AIDS cases dropped from 50% to 5% (*Time*, 1992). An example of the people in the park are Reno, age 28, and Sophie, age 24. She has not only tested HIV-positive, she is suffering the first stages of the disease. For both of them their main concern now is not AIDS but getting the $400 or $500 a day they need to support their drug addiction.

There are no figures on how many of these addicts in the park die from AIDS. Many just drift away. It is known that more than 250 died in 1991 from addiction alone. And the rate of addiction is increasing, the population of the park is increasing, and the number overdosing is increasing. The medical staff tries to help, and the addicts, many of whom have lost hope for themselves, try to help each other. One man tries to keep the other who has overdosed upright and moving, trying to stop death. The fight is for life. A social worker volunteer says she has watched life and death in Syringe Park for 4 years. She feels that death may be the best alternative. She does not make that statement lightly. Her own 22-year-old son has been in the park for almost 5 years—one who lives from fix to fix, one of the players in the drama that is played out each day in one of the world's financial capitals. But in early 1992, the park was closed because the park became a magnet for professional dealers, especially Lebanese, Yugoslav, and Turkish gangs that overran small dealers in a violent price war. Some of the park's inhabitants clustered around the central train station, others headed off in search of methadone. Others went back to the alleys and shelters from which they came. With sales suddenly back underground, addicts complained that the price of heroin had doubled overnight to $214 a gram (454 grams/pound = $97,156). Health workers said efforts to prevent the spread of HIV/ AIDS will now be much more difficult.

COMMENTARY

It is hard to avoid the suspicion that the concerns about free syringe programs have less to do with science or public health than with politics: specifically, a reluctance to **detract** or **distract** the "**JUST SAY NO**" message. But there is another message that both sides would agree on—that no one should die needlessly! A leading University of California researcher estimates that nearly 10,000 lives could have been saved over the past few years by an aggressive expansion of syringe exchange programs. Wasn't the war on drugs supposed to be about saving lives? Isn't a part of government about saving lives? (**Class Discussion**)

haps because of the improved relationship between city workers and the community. Meanwhile, referrals to drug treatment centers increased. These results have enabled policymakers elsewhere to call for SEPs. Edward Kaplan (1993) of Yale University reported at the Eighth International AIDS Conference that the New Haven syringe program cut the rate of new HIV infections by 33% to 50%. His data come from comparing the number of HIV-contaminated syringes found on the streets versus those turned in at syringe exchange points.

After passing a 1992 law permitting pharmacies to sell syringes without a prescription, syringe sharing has dropped 40% in the state of Connecticut. Seventy-five percent of AIDS

SYRINGE LAWS—UNITED STATES

Early in this century, increasing numbers of individuals began using the more potent and easily transportable, injectable opiates instead of smoking opium. It was believed, not unreasonably, that the use of these drugs could be curtailed by limiting access to the tools necessary to inject them; therefore, all states introduced laws to govern the sale and distribution of hypodermic syringes.

Lawrence Gostin and colleagues (1997) reported on the results of a national survey of laws and regulation governing the sale and possession of syringes in the United States and its territories. They reported that every state, the District of Columbia (DC), and the Virgin Islands (VI) have enacted state or local laws or regulations that restrict the sale, distribution, or possession of syringes. Drug paraphernalia laws prohibiting the sale, distribution, and/or possession of syringes known to be used to introduce illicit drugs into the body exist in 47 states, DC, and VI. Syringe prescription laws prohibiting the sale, distribution, and possession of syringes without a valid medical prescription exist in eight states and VI. Pharmacy regulations and practice guidelines restrict access to syringes in 23 states. However, ending 1997, legislatures in eight states (Connecticut, Hawaii, Maryland, Massachusetts, Rhode Island, Maine, Minnesota, New Hampshire, and the District of Columbia) either enacted or removed laws that barred the **establishment of syringe exchange programs**. For additional source material on regulations on the sale and possession of syringes on a state-by-state basis, read Scott Burris and colleagues (1996), "Legal strategies used in operating syringe-exchange programs in the United States" and Luric Drucker et al. (1997), "An opportunity lost: HIV infection associated with lack of a national needle-exchange program in the USA."

THE IMPACT—Existing laws make it difficult for injecting drug users to obtain sterile syringe.

In April 1996, the governor of New Jersey, the state with one of the highest rate of injection drug-related AIDS cases, rejected the recommendation of her Advisory Council on AIDS to distribute clean syringes to intravenous drug users (Glantz, 1996). Many syringe exchange programs in this country operate in a gray area of the law.

Question: Would changing the laws make a significant difference?

SOMETHING TO THINK ABOUT

Researchers at St. Louis University School of Public Health, Missouri, have concluded in a recent study that loosening restrictions on the sale of clean syringes may lower HIV transmission rates.

The study found that states with strict laws banning the public sale of syringes have the highest rate of HIV/AIDS transmission among intravenous drug users.

All 50 states and the District of Columbia were placed into three categories. The **first** were states that had **no laws** (no barriers) to obtaining clean needles. The **second** category included states that **had paraphernalia laws** (laws that make it a felony to have a syringe). And **third**, states that **had paraphernalia and prescription laws** (only able to get a syringe through prescription).

The research results came up with the following conclusions:

- **No law—HIV transmission rate: 0.83 per 100,000 people.**
- **Paraphernalia law—AIDS rate: 1.63 per 100,000.**
- **Paraphernalia and prescription law—AIDS rate: 5.78 per 100,000.**

Their conclusion is that the government should be involved in preventing drug use. But in the interim, there should be a means for reducing the potential for harm. Because the percentage increase in numbers of newly HIV-infected people will be highest among IDUs and their sexual partners by the year 2000, changing state statutes regarding the distribution and use of clean syringes could, most probably, significantly lower the rate of new HIV infections among this population.

Finally, many public health, medical, and legal organizations have supported the deregulation of syringes as a strategy to prevent HIV/AIDS and other blood-borne diseases among IDUs. Most laws, regulations, and practice guidelines that restrict the sale, possession, or distribution of syringes were promulgated before HIV/AIDS among IDUs was recognized as a pressing public health problem and without carefully contemplating the health implications. Since that time, the interconnected epidemics of drug use and HIV/AIDS have produced illness and death, particularly among poor, urban, minority communities.

cases in Connecticut occur among IDUs, their sex partners, and their children. Going into 1998, Connecticut, North Dakota, Alaska, Iowa, and South Carolina allow nonprescription sales of syringes and have no drug paraphernalia law against their possession. Nine states and the District of Columbia require prescriptions both to buy syringes and to possess them. Six of the nine states (California, New York, New Jersey, Illinois, Pennsylvania, and Massachusetts) have the largest numbers of IDUs and the highest incidence of AIDS among them.

The mayor of Washington has called for syringe exchange for addicts, as well as the distribution of free condoms in city schools and jails. Movements are underway in New Jersey, California, and Massachusetts to remove legal barriers and begin officially sanctioned syringe programs. Even in the U.S. Congress, Charles Rangel, who has led the opposition to syringe exchange on the ground that it threatens blacks, has asked the General Accounting Office to reevaluate the effects of such programs.

The most important catalyst for this change has been the experiment conducted in New Haven (Thompson, 1992; *Time*, 1992).

Hawaii— In 1990, Hawaii became the first state to legalize a statewide SEP. The state legislature felt it was necessary to stem the rate of HIV infection in women and newborns. The results of this program will have an impact on decisions to be made in other states. In Hawaii, a drug user comes in, drops a dirty syringe into a plastic bucket, and receives a fresh sterile syringe and syringe in exchange. No name is given, no questions are asked. Under the 2-year pilot project, an addict can swap a used syringe for a new one supplied by the nonprofit Life Foundation up to 5 times a day 5 days a week.

Alaska—A clinical trial SEP is underway at the University of Alaska, Anchorage. The trial, supported by the National Institute on Drug Abuse (NIDA), is a 3-year, $2.4 million study that will compare the incidence of hepatitis B virus (HBV) among participants who obtain clean syringes through syringe exchange centers and among those who purchase them at pharmacies. It will attempt to determine if one method of syringe distribution is more effective than the other at stopping the spread of disease. It will also attempt to determine if access to clean syringes encourages drug use.

--------- SIDEBAR 9.1 ---------

SYRINGE EXCHANGE SURVEY: HOW MANY SYRINGES ARE BEING EXCHANGED?

In November 1996, the Beth Israel Medical Center in New York City, in collaboration with the North American Syringe Exchange Network (NASEN), mailed questionnaires to the directors of 101 SEPs in the United States that were members of NASEN. Although the total number of SEPs in the United States is unknown, most are believed to be members of NASEN. From November 1996 through April 1997, SEP directors were asked about when their SEP began; the number of syringes exchanged during 1995; and, for 1996, legal status, services provided, and the **number of syringes exchanged**.

Of 101 SEPs, 87 (86%) participated in this survey. Of these, 51 began operating before 1995; 22, in 1995; and 14, in 1996. These 87 SEPs reported operating in 71 cities in 28 states and one territory; 44 (51%) of the SEPs were located in four states (California [17], Washington [11],

New York [10], and Connecticut [six]). In eight cities, at least two SEPs were reported operating. In the 1994–1995 survey, 60 SEPs reported operating in 46 cities and in 21 states.

Of the 73 SEPs operating in 1995, 70 reported exchanging approximately **11 million** syringes. In 1996, of the 87 SEPs that provided information about the number of syringes exchanged, 84 reported exchanging approximately **14 million syringes** (median: 36,017 syringes per SEP). The 10 most active SEPs (i.e., those that exchanged ≥500,000 syringes) exchanged approximately 9.4 million (69%) of all syringes exchanged. The SEP in San Francisco reported exchanging the largest number of syringes (1,461,096) in 1996. During 1996, a total of 50 SEPs (57%) reported exchanging ≤55,000 syringes each; of these, 23 (46%) exchanged 10,000 syringes each (*MMWR*, 1997).

While the study is funded by government money, because of the federal ban, the actual SEP is supported separately by the nonprofit Alaska Science and Technology Foundation (Benowitz, 1997).

Syringe Exchange Programs in Other Countries

Syringe exchange program results from England, Austria, the Netherlands, Sweden, and Scotland, presented at the Fourth International AIDS Conference (1988) suggest that the European programs attracted IDUs who had no previous contact with drug treatment programs; and that IDUs were drawn from clean syringe programs into treatment programs, thus the decrease in drug use. There was no indication in these studies of an increase in injection drug use in cities with exchange programs. Where HIV testing had been done, the rate of HIV infection showed a marked decline after the introduction of the exchange program. Furthermore, self-reported instances of syringe sharing and sexual intercourse without condoms, to the extent that they are reliable, also showed a downward trend (Raymond, 1988; Hagen, 1991).

Some of the countries with active SEPs are:

Canada— In 1989, Montreal, Toronto, and Vancouver began SEPs.

England— Over 2 million syringes and needles were exchanged in 120 programs each year. Needles and syringes can be legally purchased throughout England. Free distribution and exchange remains a relatively nonpolitical and noncontroversial issue (Stimson et al., 1989). Overall, the programs in England indicate that although changes in IDUs' behavior are slight, they are encouraging and may be important in reducing the spread of HIV (Hart et al., 1991). One problem found in England, the United States, and elsewhere is that these exchange programs attract IDUs who are at *lower risk* for HIV infection while *high-risk* IDUs are less likely to participate.

Netherlands— SEPs are available in 40 municipalities. Data from these programs suggest that the staff operating the syringe exchange centers should be multilingual and the centers should be operational 24 hours a day.

Australia— Australia has 10% of the population of the United States but has 2,000 syringe exchange programs in five states and one territory. The remaining state and one jurisdiction may have since joined the program. An evaluation concluded that a substantial number of IDUs have made appropriate changes in their behavior to support the continuation of these programs (Wodak, 1990, updated).

An assessment of Sydney's program in 1989 suggested that some 9 to 12 million needles and syringes a year would have to be distributed to meet the need for sterile equipment. By 1994 the program was distributing around 3 million syringes, and some exchanges in the suburbs of Sydney as well as in the city center were seeing attendances rise by 1,000 clients per month from late 1992.

New Zealand—A nationwide syringe exchange program began in 1988. The overall rate of HIV-infected IDUs remains low. In 1995, less than 1% of IDU men and no women tested at the syringe exchange centers were HIV-positive. There were about four to six new cases each year since 1987. Their data are too few to make statistically significant claims to support the syringe program (Lichtenstein, 1996).

Italy— Only a few limited exchange programs have been reported. However, between 1983 and 1988, the sale of syringes and needles, which is legal, increased by 50%.

Advocates for and against safe drug use activities present forceful arguments. The major problem is that HIV infection is now increasing rapidly among the IDU population. The proportion of AIDS cases involving adult/adolescent males with a history of homosexual/bisexual activity as the only risk factor decreased from 70% in 1987 to 56% in 1991. But in the same time period, the proportion of AIDS cases in adult/adolescent males with a history of IDU as the only risk factor increased from 14% to 20%. In adult/adolescent single risk female AIDS cases the proportion of IDUs was 49% in 1987 and 49% in 1991. The proportion of AIDS cases in children whose mothers had sexual intercourse with IDUs rose from 11% before 1985 to 21% through 1991 (*MMWR*, 1989b; 1992a).

Through 1995, 84% of IDUs in Glasgow, 82% in Lund, 84% in Sydney, 73% in Tacoma, and 87% in Toronto reported they had changed their behavior in order to avoid HIV/AIDS. The most commonly mentioned specific behavior change: reducing sharing of injection equipment (Des Jarlais, 1995).

PREVENTION OF BLOOD AND BLOOD PRODUCT HIV TRANSMISSION

Blood Donors

There is **no risk** in the United States or in other **developed nations** of contracting HIV **by donating blood**. Blood centers use a new, sterile needle for **each** donation, yet a 1993 survey revealed that 25% of those polled believed that they could become HIV-infected by donating blood. In Third World nations, it is important to make certain that a new, sterile needle is used before donating blood.

Over 8 million people are donating some 20 million units of blood which are transfused into 4 million people annually in the United States. Blood can carry HIV in a cell-free state or HIV may be carried within cells of the blood. The amount of virus taken in (**dose**) and a person's biological susceptibility determines whether infection will occur after HIV exposure. A large dose of HIV received via blood transfusion almost universally results in HIV infection. A small dose of HIV-contaminated blood, such as the blood received by a needlestick seldom results in infection (Francis et al., 1987). The mean volume of blood injected by a needlestick has been calculated to be 1.4 μL (1.4 millionths of a liter). It is difficult to determine exactly how large a viral dose is necessary to cause infection. However, it is known that infection is more likely to occur if blood is donated close to the time the HIV-infected donor becomes symptomatic. Entering 1998, 6% of HIV-infected adults and

--- BOX 9.5 ---

BLOOD TRANSFUSIONS: EARLY HISTORY

Transferring blood products from one person to another dates back 500 years. The **first recorded blood transfusion** was administered to Pope Innocent VIII in 1492. It did little to reverse the Pope's altered mental status and cost the lives of three young donors. In 1667, the English team of Wren, Lower, and King, along with the Frenchman Jean Baptiste Denys, simultaneously claimed the first successful transfusion of blood from animal to human. Further work done by Denys was halted by the untimely death of a patient; initially attributed to the transfusion, this death was later determined to be the result of poisoning by an abused wife.

As a result of this scandal, the practice of blood transfusion was halted in Europe. Transfusions were not attempted again until 1818, when Blundell, an American obstetrician, successfully revived the practice for the treatment of postpartum hemorrhage. Since that time, a better understanding of blood transfusion and storage, blood group incompatibility, and detection of infectious agents has greatly reduced the risk of post-transfusion illness and death. Not all complications are unavoidable, however, and risks still persist.

RISKS OF BLOOD PRODUCT TRANSFUSION

More than 12 million units of red blood cells (RBCs), 5 million units of platelets, and 2 million units of plasma are administered annually in the United States. About 10% to 15% of recipients experience an adverse reaction, and 1% experience a serious side effect. Approximately 30 people die each year in the United States as a direct result of blood product transfusion. This estimate is conservative because transfusion reactions can mimic common postsurgical or intensive care unit problems. For example, bacterial infection occurs commonly in these patients, and the association with a blood transfusion may be overlooked. The delayed effects associated with the infectious process are another reason for the under-reporting of blood product transfusion reactions. Examples are the transmission of hepatitis and other viruses, which may not be discovered until weeks, months, or years after the transfusion (Greene et al., 1996).

10% of HIV-infected children in the United States are believed to have become infected via blood transfusions or by the use of contaminated blood products. The majority of HIV infections occurred prior to the initiation of the blood screening program. To date **only** whole blood, blood cellular components, plasma, and blood clotting factors have been involved in transmitting HIV.

Blood Collection and Blood Screening for HIV

Regardless of whether blood comes from volunteer donors or is purchased, it is now screened for antibodies to HIV-1 and HIV-2. If the test

indicates that the blood carries antibodies to either HIV, it is treated to destroy the HIV and then discarded. Current blood screening procedures have significantly reduced the number of blood transfusion-associated HIV infections.

Blood Screening for HIV— In March of 1983, the major United States blood banking organizations instituted procedures to reduce the likelihood of HIV transmission through blood transfusions. People with signs or symptoms suggestive of HIV disease/AIDS, sexually active homosexual and bisexual men with multiple partners, recent Haitian immigrants to the United States, past or present IDUs, men and women who have engaged in prostitution since 1977 or have patronized a prostitute within the past 6 months, and sexual partners of individuals at increased risk of HIV infection were asked to refrain from donating blood.

In March of 1985, the FDA approved the ELISA test for use in commercial blood banks, plasma centers, and public health clinics to screen blood for antibodies to HIV. This test did not and still does not diagnose AIDS. It merely indicates whether or not a blood donor has antibodies against HIV (has been infected with HIV).

All blood that tests positive for antibody to the HIV virus is rejected. This test, in conjunction with current measures to exclude blood donations by members of behavioral high-risk groups, has substantially reduced the chance of transmitting HIV through blood transfusion (ELISA and other test procedures are presented in Chapter 13). The risk of becoming HIV-infected from a blood transfusion has dropped by more than 99% from 1983 to 1991.

Blood Transfusions Worldwide— Ten years after the industrialized world began to screen all blood used in transfusions for HIV, as many as 1 in 10 seropositives in developing countries are still being infected through this route.

A combination of the lack of screening with high levels of infected donors turns transfusion into a form of Russian roulette. A survey carried out by WHO in 1990, for example, showed that centres in Kinshasa, Zaïre, screened fewer than a quarter of blood units for HIV, even

---

———— **BOX 9.6** ————

EXAMPLE OF BLOOD SUPPLY HIV PREVENTION

Testimonial: I'm 56 and have donated over 90 pints of blood. After my last donation, I received a letter that read, in part: "Unfortunately, we can no longer accept you as a donor because there was something in your blood detected in our HIV antibody screening test. . . . However, we did additional testing by a more specific method and the final result was negative for antibody to HIV. . . . It is our policy, based on current federal and state guidelines, not to accept blood donors whose blood has been found to be falsely positive for anti-HIV." (State of California)

Explanation: The first screening test his blood bank used was probably the ELISA test, a quick, relatively cheap screening method that occasionally yields false-positive results (see Chapter 13). Blood that tests positive for HIV in the ELISA test is then put through a more specific test called the Western blot (WB). Even though the WB showed no HIV antibodies in his blood, the blood bank's rules required it to reject his blood—on the theoretical but unlikely possibility that the first test could be right and the second one wrong. This person can request a more specific HIV test that is less likely to give a false-positive result. If that test is negative and he wants to resume blood donations, he can check to see if the blood bank has a donor re-entry program. He will have to wait 6 months and then get negative results on both the ELISA and Western blot tests before being allowed to donate.

---

though about 5% of donors were HIV-infected. Beginning 1998, blood transfusions accounted for 5% to 10% of HIV infections worldwide.

Blood Safety— From 1985 through 1997, over 170 million blood or plasma donations had been screened for HIV antibody in the United States. By excluding those who test HIV-positive and by asking people from high-risk behavior groups not to donate blood, the incidence of HIV transmission from the current blood supply is relatively low. And with faster and more accurate testing procedures now in use, the risk is becoming even lower. **However, the probability or risk of receiving HIV-contaminated blood will never be zero.** The reason a small risk still exists is because some people infected with HIV may donate blood during what is known as the "**window period.**" **During that period, a person may be infected with the HIV, but the test can not yet detect the infection.** And, the test is not 100% accurate.

In 1991, the CDC estimated the risk of receiving HIV-infected blood at 1 in 39,000 to 1 in 250,000. That is, for every 39,000 to 250,000 units of whole blood used in transfusions, one patient would receive HIV-infected blood. On average, a blood transfusion requires five or more units of whole blood (Pines, 1993).

Eve Lackritz and eight colleagues (1995) reported that, of 4.1 million blood donations from 19 regions served by The American Red Cross, one donation in every 360,000 was made during The Window Period. They further estimated that one in 2,600,000 donations contained HIV but was not identified (**false negative**) because of laboratory error. Their report states that collectively, of 42 Red Cross regions collecting 9 million units of blood, the risk of HIV transmission was one transmission for every 450,000 to 660,000 available units of screened blood. Based on their data they conclude that there are about 18 to 27 infectious units of blood available for transfusion each year. This is about half the previous estimates. (The American Red Cross collects about half the donated blood in the United States annually.)

PLAYING THE ODDS. For comparison, the odds of dying in a highway accident are 1 in 5,960

─────── BOX 9.7 ───────

BLOOD TRANSFUSIONS: A GIFT OF LIFE OR THE CARRIER OF DEATH?

In 1987, a grief-stricken mother wrote an open letter to her neighbors thanking them for their compassion when her oldest son, a hemophiliac, died of AIDS. In 1989, this mother was to experience the loss of her second son to AIDS. He was also a hemophiliac. Her letter was to thank her community for caring for one of its members as a family cares for its child. It was an example of compassion to a nation demonstrating mixed emotions about those with AIDS.

In contrast, vandals burned down the home of Clifford and Cynthia Ray of Arcadia, Florida in 1987. Their three young boys, all hemophiliacs, acquired HIV from blood products used to stop life-threatening bleeding episodes. They also developed AIDS. Unlike the first family's experience, the Rays lost their friends, became the targets of hate mail, received threats of physical violence, were recipients of verbal abuse, and their children were not permitted to attend school. The Desoto County School Board, after threat of lawsuit, offered to let the boys attend class in a portable trailer in isolation from other children. Food would be served using disposable plates, cups, and utensils. The playground and library could be used only when other children were in class. Pickets again marched at the school and verbally abused the Ray family. Finally, their home was burned down and the Rays moved to Sarasota, Florida where the boys were enrolled in school without incident.

in a lifetime of driving. The CDC calculates that, **at worst,** with a risk factor of 1 HIV infection in 39,000 transfusions, there will be about 540 new HIV infections per year. (Eighteen million units of blood transfused each year means that three one thousandths of one percent (.00003%) of the 18 million units of blood are infected or 540 units.) By contrast, the CDC estimates that 10 times the number (5,400) will become infected with hepatitis C, which can be fatal.

Blood Supply Shortages— For over 50 years American blood collection centers have been buying and selling blood and blood products. But today, subtle trends are altering the nation's ability to provide a safe and adequate blood and plasma supply.

Because of HIV infection, fewer people can give blood now than gave in 1980. Today donated blood must pass seven laboratory tests that screen for HIV antibody, HTLV I (the virus associated with tropical spastic paraparesis and some forms of leukemia), Non-A Non-B hepatitis, syphilis, hepatitis B and hepatitis C antigens, and HIV-2.

New screening criteria are reducing the donor pool by 10% to 15%. Many former blood donors, some of whom routinely donated several times each year, are no longer eligible. In addition, some states have outlawed paid blood donations.

Blood banks in New York, Miami, Los Angeles, and San Francisco have, at times, had to issue urgent pleas for blood donations. Recent blood shortages have been the most severe in the nation's history and the situation is expected to get much worse. The reasons for the shortages are: (1) the additional transfusions necessary for the ever increasing number of symptomatic HIV and AIDS patients; (2) the restrictions on who may now donate blood; and (3) the loss of a significant percentage of potential blood donors who still believe they can become HIV-infected by donating blood.

Autologous Transfusions— These are transfusions using "**self**" (your own) blood. It has been suggested that the two groups that benefit most from autologous blood storage are: expectant mothers facing Caesarean section and certain elective surgical candidates where substantial loss of blood is anticipated. A person's blood is drawn and refrigerated for transfusion back into his or her own body when needed. (Stored whole blood remains usable for a maximum of 42 days.) This is the safest blood available. A healthy person taking iron supplements can donate one unit of blood a week, generally, for up to 6 weeks. In emergency situations, including some surgeries, it may be necessary to receive another person's blood through transfusion. If a transfusion is necessary to sustain life, the risk of contracting HIV from the transfusion is outweighed by the risk of refusing the transfusion and suffering further consequences from the emergency.

INFECTION CONTROL PROCEDURES

With no cure or vaccine for HIV/AIDS, prevention of infection is of paramount importance. With the advent of the HIV/AIDS epidemic, health care workers and others who are occupationally exposed to body fluids, especially blood, are understandably concerned about the risk of contracting HIV disease/AIDS. However, when precautions are observed, the risk is very small, even for those treating HIV/AIDS patients.

Two sets of infection control procedures are in use in hospitals, medical centers, physicians' offices, and units that deal with people in medical emergencies. One is called **universal precautions, the** other blood **and body substance isolation.**

Universal Precautions

Universal precautions (Table 9-6) are standard practices that workers observe on the job to protect themselves from infections and injuries. These precautions or safety practices are called "universal" because they are used in all situations

———— **POINT OF INFORMATION 9.8** ————

UNIVERSAL PRECAUTIONS

The standards from the United States office of **Occupational Safety** and **Health Administration** (OSHA) say that employers shall protect their employees from the hazards of blood-borne pathogens and comply with the standard through the use of **universal precautions**, engineering controls, work practice controls, personal protective equipment, proper housekeeping, and handling of regulated waste. This section pertains to the universal precautions which are implemented at the employer's facility.

Universal precautions is OSHA's accepted method of control to protect employees from exposure to **all human blood and other potentially infectious materials** (OPIM). The term refers to a concept that all human blood and OPIM be treated as if known to be infectious for HIV, HBV, or other blood-borne pathogens, regardless of the perceived "low risk" of a patient or patient population.

even if there seems to be no risk. Universal precautions had their beginnings in 1976 when barrier techniques were first recommended for the prevention of hepatitis B infection. Precautions required the use of protective eyewear, gloves, and gowns, and careful handling of needles and other sharp instruments. In 1977, hepatitis B immune globulin was recommended for those exposed to hepatitis B through needlesticks. In 1982, hepatitis B vaccine became commercially available and recommended for all health care workers exposed to human blood.

In 1983, the CDC published "Guidelines for Isolation Precautions in Hospitals." It contained a section that recommended specific blood and body fluid precautions to be followed when a patient was known or suspected to be infected with blood-borne pathogens. In 1987, the CDC published "Recommendations for Prevention of HIV Transmission in Health-Care Settings." It recommended that blood and body fluid precautions be consistently followed for all patients regardless of their blood-borne infection status. This extension

TABLE 9-6 Universal Precautions

DEFINITION

Universal precautions (UP) are a set of infection control practices, developed by the Centers for Disease Control and Prevention (CDC), in which health care workers (HCWs) appropriately utilize barrier protection (gloves, gowns, masks, eyewear, etc.) for anticipated contact with blood and certain body fluids of *all* patients.

1. The hands and skin must be carefully washed when contaminated with blood or certain body fluids.
2. Particular care is taken to prevent injuries caused by sharp instruments.
3. Resuscitation devices should be available where the need is predictable.
4. HCWs with exudative lesions or weeping dermatitis should refrain from patient care until the condition resolves.

BLOOD AND BODY FLUIDS TO WHICH UP APPLY

Blood is the single most important risk source of HIV, HBV, and other blood-borne pathogens in the occupational setting. Thus prevention of transmission must focus on reducing the risk of exposure to blood and other body fluids or potentially infectious materials containing visible blood.

1. UP should be used when exposure to the following body fluids may be anticipated:
   a. Blood
   b. Serum plasma
   c. Semen
   d. Vaginal secretions
   e. Amniotic fluid
   f. Cerebrospinal fluid (CSF)
   g. Synovial fluid
   h. Pleural fluid
   i. Vitneous fluid
   j. Peritoneal fluid
   k. Pericardial fluid
   l. Wound exudates
   m. Any other body fluid containing visible blood (but not feces, urine, saliva, sputum, tears, nasal secretions, or sweat, unless they contain visible blood).
2. Note: Blood, semen, and vaginal secretions have been shown to transmit HIV. The others, with the exception of fluids containing visible blood, remain a theoretical risk.

RATIONALE

1. UP reduce the risk of parenteral, mucous membrane, and skin exposure to blood-borne pathogens such as, but not limited to, HIV and HBV.
2. For several reasons, focusing precautions only on diagnosed cases misses the vast majority of persons who are infected (many of whom are asymptomatic or subclinical) and who may be as infectious as the diagnosed cases. Persons who have seen a physician and have been diagnosed with acute or active disease represent only a small proportion of all persons with infection. Infectivity always precedes the diagnosis, which often is made once symptoms develop.

(Adapted from Mountain-Plains Regional AIDS Education Training Center. *HIV/AIDS Curriculum*, Nov. 1994.)

DOES THE PATIENT HAVE HIV? I CAN'T TELL

Treating disease can be difficult. Dealing with the legal system and the politics of disease can be a conundrum.

Recently, a nurse in California brought charges against a patient after the nurse accidentally cut herself with a contaminated scalpel and subsequently learned that the patient had AIDS. The prosecution based its case on the patient's failure to fully disclose information relevant to her care. The defense case centered on the failure of medical personnel to use **universal precautions** for treating all patients regardless of their health history.

I side with the nurse and so did the Los Angeles jury who convicted the patient of fraud for failing to disclose that she had AIDS.

Yes, **universal precautions** are required for all patients regardless of health history, but the practical fact is that different situations in medicine require different levels of attentiveness. Care for a young man with a simple cough will and should differ from care for a young man who has a cough and mentions he has AIDS and has had pneumocystis pneumonia in the past. In an emergency department, activity levels vary from dull and routine to harried and panicked. If medical personnel put on gloves, gowns, and masks and slowed their activities to the safest pace for every patient, regardless of known or suspected risk, gridlock would result.

Medical history is critical to proper patient care. When a patient comes to a hospital and is unable to provide a detailed history, medical records are often enormously helpful in providing proper treatment. Therefore, I was surprised recently when a new directive was tacked to the bulletin board in one of the emergency departments where I work. It said that a patient's HIV status could not be recorded on the emergency department chart. I can document syphilis, cancer, schizophrenia, or violent or suicidal behavior, which are all pertinent to a patient's history. Such documentation may help other healthcare professionals provide proper care or take "more attentive" precautions. But I cannot document HIV status. I asked why and was told that this was an effort to comply with a new part of the state of California's Health and Safety Code.

I understand the rationale for this directive. Not only do those who are HIV-positive live with the threat of a terminal disease, but they are discriminated against in the workplace and by insurance carriers, even while they are healthy. The state code is an effort to prevent paranoid discrimination. But I believe the effort to preserve a patient's privacy may put healthcare workers at greater risk.

AIDS is a terrible disease, and paranoia about it is rampant., But protecting patient privacy by putting blinders on healthcare workers is not good medicine.

(Reprinted, with permission, from Pollack B. (1994). Does the patient have HIV? I can't tell. *Postgrad Med* 96(3):19. Copyright © 1994 McGraw-Hill Inc.)

Class Discussion: Your Assessment of Dr. Pollack's concerns?

---

of blood and body fluid precautions to all patients is referred to as **Universal Precautions**.

Under universal precautions, the blood and certain body fluids of all patients are considered potentially infectious for HIV, hepatitis B virus (HBV), and other blood-borne pathogens.

Universal precautions are intended to prevent parenteral (introduction of a substance into the body by injection), mucous membrane, and broken skin exposure of health care workers (HCWs), teachers, or any other person who may become exposed to blood-borne pathogens. In 1987, the CDC also published a report that got the immediate attention of most, if not all, informed health care workers. The report stated that three health care workers who were exposed to the blood of AIDS patients tested positive for HIV. What was so startling was that until that time, needle punctures and cuts were thought to be the only dangers in a clinical setting. These three cases appeared to involve only skin exposure to HIV-contaminated blood. One of the three cases involved a nurse whose chapped and ungloved hands were exposed to an AIDS patient's blood.

The second case involved a nurse who broke a vacuum tube during a routine phlebotomy on an outpatient. The blood splashed on her face and into her mouth. A blood splash was also involved in the third case. The worker's ungloved hands and forearms were exposed to HIV-contaminated blood (Ezzell, 1987).

The importance of these three cases of HIV infection is that they informed health care workers in the most dramatic way that they were all **vulnerable**. In addition to hepatitis and other infections, they could now add a more lethal virus to their occupational hazards. Perhaps these three cases produced a fear among health care workers out of proportion to the actual risk of their becoming infected. However, the fear of an individual and the actual reason he or she has for it are very difficult to judge. **Although calculations show that the risk of HIV infection after exposure to blood from an HIV/AIDS patient is about one in 200**, if **you are that one**, **probability is meaningless**. Some health care workers have used, and still use, such data to support their decisions to avoid caring for HIV/AIDS patients.

The universal precautions as published by the CDC currently apply to some 5.3 million health care workers at 620,000 work sites across the United States and another 700,000

Americans who routinely come in contact with blood as part of their job, for example, people in law enforcement, education, fire fighting and rescue, corrections, laboratory research, and the funeral industry.

In July of 1991, the CDC published an additional set of recommendations. These recommendations are also for preventing the transmission of HIV and hepatitis B virus to patients during exposure-prone procedures.

In summary, the concept of universal precautions assumes that all blood is infectious, no matter from whom and no matter whether a test is negative, positive, or not done at all. Rigorous adherence to universal precautions is the surest way of preventing accidental transmission of HIV and other blood-borne pathogens.

Blood and Body Substance Isolation (BBSI)

An alternative, and some believe superior, approach to the CDC's universal precautions in areas of high HIV prevalence is the system referred to as **body substance precautions or Blood Body Substance Isolation (BBSI)** (Gerberding, 1991).

In practice, these precautions are similar to universal precautions, in that prevention of needlestick injury and use of barrier methods of infection control are emphasized. Philosophically, however, the two are quite different. Whereas universal precautions place a clear emphasis on avoidance of blood-borne infection, body substance precautions take a more global view. **Body substance isolation (BSI) requires barrier precautions for all body substances (including feces, respiratory secretions, urine, emesis, etc.) and moist body surfaces (including mucous membranes and open wounds).** BSI is designed as a system to reduce the risk of transmission of all nosocomial pathogens, not just blood-borne pathogens. Gloves are worn for any anticipated or known contact with mucous membranes, or nonintact skin and moist body substances of all patients.

The degree of contact with the blood and body fluids or tissues of each patient is considered to determine the type of precaution (if any) required. Unlike the CDC system in which precautions are based on the premise that all

---

──────── BOX 9.9 ────────

WHAT TO ASK YOUR DOCTOR

Few health care workers (HCWs) will willingly disclose their HIV status, but the chances of your becoming HIV-infected are slim if HCWs follow standard procedures. Here are a few examples of what to look for:

1. Do the doctors and nurses wear gloves when doing invasive exams, such as dental, vaginal, or rectal exams?

2. Do they use a new set of gloves and freshly disinfected instruments with each patient?

3. Do they routinely wash their hands before seeing every patient?

4. Do all health care workers follow universal precautions, wearing masks, protective eyewear, and gowns in addition to gloves when there's a risk of being sprayed with blood or other body fluids?

5. How often does the clinic or hospital make sure its staff is actually following universal precautions?

blood is infectious, body substance precautions are procedure-specific, that is, based on the degree of anticipated contact. Users of the BBSI system find that this approach is actually easier to teach and implement than universal precautions, although the end result is much the same: the prevention of HIV infection.

PARTNER NOTIFICATION

Partner notification, formerly called contact tracing, is the practice of **identifying** and **treating** people exposed to certain communicable diseases. The term *partner notification* is used by the CDC and some health care providers because it more comprehensively describes the process by which the physician, other health care workers such as Disease Intervention Specialists (DIS, someone who is specially trained in STD work), and the infected person may provide information to at- risk partners.

There are two very different approaches to informing unsuspecting third parties about their potential exposure to medical risk.

Each approach has its own history, including a unique set of practical problems in its implementation, and provokes its own ethical dilemmas. The **first approach**, involving the moral **duty to warn**, arose out of the clinical setting in which the physician knew the identity of the person deemed to be at risk. This approach provided a warrant for disclosure to endangered persons without the consent of the patient and could involve revealing the identity of the patient. The **second approach**—that of contact tracing—emerged from sexually transmitted disease control programs in which the clinician typically did not know the identity of those who might have been exposed. This approach was founded on the voluntary cooperation of the patient in providing the names of contacts. It never involved the disclosure of the identity of the patient. The entire process of notification was kept confidential (Bayer, 1992).

History of Partner Notification

The concept of partner notification was proposed in 1937 by Surgeon General Thomas Parran for the control of syphilis (Parran, 1937). By tracing and treating all known contacts of a syphilitic patient, the chain of transmission could be interrupted. According to George Rutherford (1988), contact tracing has been successfully used in a number of STDs beginning in the 1950s. It is still used in cases of syphilis, endemic gonorrhea, chlamydia, hepatitis B, STD enteric infections, and particularly in cases of antibiotic-resistant gonorrhea.

In 1985, when the HIV antibody was first used in screening the blood supply, notification of blood donors and other HIV-infected individuals and their contacts became possible. The strategy in HIV partner notification is the same as that used for the other STDs: to identify HIV-infected individuals, counsel them, and offer whatever treatment is available. In asymptomatic HIV-infected people only counseling is given. But, symptomatic HIV-infected patients receive counseling and treatment, if available, for their signs and symptoms. Partner notification depends on HIV-positive people to give the names of their partners; but, they may be reluctant to do so fearing that their identification may result in physical abuse and loss of their jobs and housing.

The Use of Partner Notification: An Example

In April 1993 an incarcerated male asked for an HIV test. The diagnosis was HIV-positive. Contact tracing turned up a network of 124 persons, all were linked by syringe-sharing and syringe-sharing with sex. One hundred and twenty-one were contacted and offered an HIV test; 118 accepted the test; 44 were HIV-positive. One hundred and thirteen of the 124 lived in the same county. The estimated cost for partner notification in this network was $13,969. (*MMWR*, 1995).

Opposition to Partner Notification for HIV Disease

There is currently wide opposition to partner notification on the grounds that: (**1**) nothing can be done medically for the HIV-positive asymptomatic person, nor can he or she be segregated from the noninfected population; (**2**) it is not cost effective; (**3**) there is little evidence that those who are informed of their infection will do anything about changing the high-risk behaviors that got them infected in the first place; (**4**) the threat of social discrimination undermines the intent of contact tracing; (**5**) the unintended consequences of partner notification may include violence and even death from an abusive partner (Rothenberg, 1995); and (**6**) in 24 states homosexuality is a crime, and HIV-infected homosexuals fear prosecution if they acknowledge same-sex contacts and be responsible for having their sexual partner(s) prosecuted.

By the end of 1985, five states, Colorado, Idaho, South Carolina, North Carolina, and Virginia, had reported data to the CDC from their partner notification programs. The first four states emphasize provider referral as the best method for notifying sexual and needle-sharing partners of HIV-infected individuals. Virginia provides contact tracing services to HIV-infected patients who **request assistance** with notifying their sexual and needle-sharing partners (*MMWR*, 1988). Beginning 1995, 32 states enacted partner notification laws. At least 12 states specifically allow disclosure of HIV-related information to spouses. And, by 1995, at least 44 states passed laws requiring or permitting workers (mostly health care workers or public safety employees) to be notified of potential exposure of HIV. In some cases, the laws allow testing of the source patient. To date, Arkansas and Missouri are the only states that require patients to notify health care providers of their HIV status before receiving care (Hooker, 1996). All 50 states are now somewhere in the process of establishing the capacity for contact tracing at the request of a patient.

In Support of Partner Notification

The following discussion is from Stephen J. Josephs' article, "The Once and Future AIDS Epidemic," *Medical Doctor*, 37:92—104. Mr. Joseph is the past Commissioner of Health of New York City, 1986–1990.

The New York City Medical Examiner looked at a large sample of dead persons who were tested postmortem and found to be HIV-positive, but who had no notification in their medical records of having been diagnosed as infected. Over 35% of those persons had a readily identifiable spouse or steady sexual partner. Josephs asks,

> How can one justify, on clinical, public health or humanitarian grounds, *not* **notifying that surviving partner, who might be the source of the infection in the deceased, or the recipient of infection**? Arguments against this procedure border on the absurd; one has to start with the premise that increased medical knowledge is more dangerous than helpful to the individual, and that the rights of the uninfected count for nothing against the rights of the infected.

Josephs states that vigorous contact tracing, under conditions of strict public health confidentiality, is the most important step we can now take to reduce the further progress of HIV and to protect those who, unsuspecting, are at greatest risk of infection or in greatest need of early medical management.

What is your response to Stephen Josephs' point of view on partner notification?

HIV VACCINE DEVELOPMENT

Goal of HIV Vaccination

The ultimate goal of an HIV vaccine is to prevent HIV infection. Realistically, this means that vaccine-induced immune responses should clear all HIV-infected cells quickly, before secondary spread occurs and persistent viral infection is established. Therefore, more than with any previous vaccine, the development of a vaccine against HIV infection must be driven by a detailed understanding of viral pathogenesis and immunity.

What the World Needs NOW Is a Vaccine for HIV Disease—Why Isn't There One?

On April 24, 1984, Margaret M. Heckler, who was then Secretary of the Department of Health and Human Services, announced the discovery of the AIDS virus. **She predicted an AIDS vaccine within 2 years.** Even though the prediction proved wrong, research has remained guided by the idea that finding the virus was the hard part, and vaccines could be made by simply injecting people with crucial viral proteins. Her optimism

PRO AND CON OF PARTNER NOTIFICATION

CON: HIV testing and contact tracing or partner notification amount to a cruel hoax. A gay representative of Act Up Now from the West Coast said, "There are not enough beds to take care of known AIDS patients. Why identify more?"

PRO: Amitai Etzioni (1993) said that "testing is cruel only in a world where captains of sinking ships do not warn passengers because the captains cannot get off. We must marshall the moral courage to tell those infected with HIV: It is truly tragic that currently we have no way to save your life, but surely you recognize your duty to try to help save the lives of others."

CON: Telling others that you are HIV positive is unnecessary because everybody **should** behave safely **all the time**.

PRO: Collective data indicate that most people will not act safely all the time. Warning people that they are about to enter a highly dangerous situation may help them take special precautions. The moral duty of those already infected is clear. They must not become intimate without prior disclosure. Not to do so is like serving poisoned candy. Not informing previous contacts (or not helping public authorities trace them without disclosing your name) leaves them, unwittingly, to transmit the virus to others.

CON: Testing and partner notification may lead to a person's being deprived of a job, health insurance, housing and privacy, and many other types of discrimination.

PRO: This is true today, but ways must be found to protect civil rights without sacrificing public health. It may seem mean spirited but the fact that an individual may suffer as a result of doing what is right does not make doing so less of an imperative. Recognize that the first victims of nondisclosure are the loved ones of those already infected with HIV, in the case of infected women—their children.

CON: It is not cost effective to trace sexual partners of HIV-infected persons.

PRO: A nonclinic HIV test costs, on average, between $60 and $70 (most HIV/AIDS clinic HIV/AIDS tests are free). Etzioni (1993) estimates that if those who were HIV-positive were to transmit the disease to only one less person on average, the suggested tests would pay for themselves much more readily than various surgical operations like coronary bypasses, and so forth. Etzioni states that there are many other excesses and rationalizations being put forth to prevent HIV partner notification programs. But, he says, "If AIDS were any other disease—say, hepatitis B or tuberculosis—we would have no trouble (and indeed we have had none) introducing the necessary preventive measures. Moreover, we should make it clear that doing all you can to prevent the spread of AIDS or any other fatal disease is part and parcel of an unambiguous commandment: Thou shalt not kill."

Whose side do you favor in this discussion? What are your reasons? (Class Discussion)

was most likely based on the success of the polio, measles, and flu vaccines. **The approach to combating these diseases was: isolate the virus, develop a vaccine, and prevent the disease!** Since then, in the rush to develop new vaccines, sci-

entists have only belatedly understood that their technical ability to mass-produce vaccines has failed to match their knowledge about the cellular and molecular processes used by the body to protect itself from invading pathogens.

THE GOAL OF DEVELOPING AN HIV VACCINE

The ideal HIV vaccine would eradicate HIV infection. But ideals are seldom realized in biology and this ideal in particular does not seem likely. For all of the infectious agent vaccines that have been marketed, **only smallpox has been eradicated**!

For an infectious agent to be a good candidate for eradication, several conditions must exist. The most important of these are: (**1**) that only humans are affected, (**2**) that infection is easily recognized, and (**3**) that infected persons do not remain asymptomatic for long periods of time. HIV meets only the first of these conditions, and even this is questionable as it may have mutated from closely related monkey viruses. Thus a realistic HIV vaccine goal would be to develop candidate vaccines that demonstrate some percent of efficacy, with fewest side effects, and begin their distribution. Saving some lives is better than a complete loss. Because there are an increasing number of HIV strains evolving, no one vaccine is expected to be effective in everyone.

In 1984, Mrs. Margaret Heckler, then the U.S. Secretary of Health and Human Services, spoke convincingly of the immediate production of an HIV vaccine. Is it surprising that both the scientists and public are disappointed with this work to date?

The ideal HIV vaccine has to be safe, orally administered, single dose, stable, inexpensive, confer permanent life-time immunity, and be effective against all HIV strains. This is an unrealistic expectation, at least in the next 5 to 10 years.

UPDATE 1997

Speaking to the graduating class at Morgan State University on May 18, 1997, President Clinton invoked the legacy of John F. Kennedy's 1960s race to the moon and set a national target of developing an AIDS vaccine within the next 10 years. The President said, "We dare not be complacent in meeting the challenge of HIV, the virus that causes AIDS." He then announced the creation of a research center at the National Institutes of Health in Bethesda, Maryland, to complete the task.

Up to 50 researchers will staff the suburban Washington facility, drawn from existing NIH programs, but no new money was earmarked for the project!

Robert Gallo stated, after the President's announcement, that "it is a serious possibility that we may never develop a vaccine for HIV."

SOUND OFF

Following President Clinton's announcement about developing an HIV vaccine in 10 years, the telephone at a large Northeastern newspaper rang nonstop that day. Here are but a few of the callers' comments concerning what the government can do to find a cure for AIDS (names are withheld).

"What is President Clinton doing with people dying of cancer who had nothing to do with getting their disease?"

"Let's use the research money on the big killers, cancer and heart disease. Stop the spread of AIDS by prohibiting blood donations from drug users and homosexuals and quarantine those who are HIV positive or have AIDS."

"The government has to be really serious about it. I can compare this to the 400 blacks down south who had syphilis in the 1920s and 30s. Our government did nothing for them. AIDS is just a disease that's been made by our government to get rid of a segment of society. A form of genocide."

"Presently, there is a 100 percent cure for AIDS. It's called abstinence and that's what the government should be teaching."

"The government can't do much, but the thousands of researchers already working hard on AIDS must really have appreciated his telling them to get busy."

"The government cannot do enough. We need around-the-clock research."

"I don't know what the government can do, but in the meantime, I know what people can do. Men, keep your zippers up and women, keep your pants on and try to use "some self control. This way, a million more lives will not be affected with this horrible virus."

"There will be no cure for AIDS because no viral infections has ever been cured. As far as a vaccine goes, it's possible but extremely difficult since we're dealing with a retrovirus. The best thing is abstinence and chastity, as unpopular as those words are today."

"Contact the Nation of Islam. We, as Muslims, can sit down with the government and come up with a cure for AIDS if the government has decided to rectify the difference with us so we can sit down and talk."

"They should set up a program where everyone in the United States can get an AIDS-HIV test, starting at age 15 and 16, just to know where it is heavily exposed."

Vaccines are designed to provoke the immune system into making antibodies against a disease-causing agent. Most are made of killed or attenuated (genetically weakened) viruses and, in the case of some newer vaccines, extracts of viral coat proteins. In some cases, vaccination may result in worsening the disease. The distinction between protective, useless, and dangerous responses is essential for vaccine design.

Vaccines that work well are the most cost-effective medical invention known to prevent disease.

What Is a Vaccine?

A vaccine is a suspension of whole microorganisms, or viruses, or a suspension of some structural component or product of them that will elicit an immune response after entering a host. In brief, vaccines mimic the organisms or virus that cause disease, alerting the immune system to be aware of certain viruses or bacteria. Because of this advance warning system, when the real organism or virus invades the body, the immune system marshals a response before the disease has time to develop.

Ideally, the body will make antibodies that bind to and disable the foreign invader (humoral immunity) and trigger white blood cells called T cells to organize attack cells in the body to destroy those cells that have been infected by viruses (cellular immunity). Once the immune system's T cells and B cells, which make antibodies, are activated, some of them turn into **memory cells.** The more memory cells the body forms, the faster its response to a future infection.

Vaccines can trigger these responses in three ways. Some vaccines, such as those against smallpox, polio (Sabins), measles, mumps, and tuberculosis, contain genetically altered or weakened organisms or viruses that are reproduced in the body after being administered but do not generally produce disease. Yet since the virus or bacterium is still alive, there is a small risk of developing the disease.

Whooping cough, cholera, and influenza vaccines are made of inactivated (killed) whole organisms and virus or pieces of them. Because killed organisms and virus do not replicate inside the recipient, the vaccines confer only humoral immunity, (the production of antibody) which may be short-lived.

Finally, vaccines can be made against toxic products produced by microorganisms. In diseases like tetanus, it is not the bacteria that kill, but the toxins they release into the bloodstream (Christensen, 1994a).

An effective viral vaccine usually blocks viral entry into a cell. **But vaccines are generally not 100% effective.** Because HIV, once inside the cell, is capable of integrating itself into the genetic material of infected cells, a vaccine would have to produce a constant state of immune protection, which not only would have to block viral entry to most cells, but also would continue to block newly produced viruses over the lifetime of the infected person. Such complete and constant protection has never before been accomplished in humans, but it has been accomplished to some degree in cats who are vaccinated against the feline leukemia virus, also a retrovirus (Voelker, 1995b). But, perhaps more pertinent explanations for why there is still no HIV vaccine nor is one likely to be available soon are the facts that scientists lack sufficient understanding of HIV infection and the biology of HIV disease/AIDS is very complex.

Scientists know that the body defends itself against HIV in the early years of infection. But the great mystery has always been why it cannot neutralize HIV completely. One possibility is that the body has trouble seeing all of the variant viruses. Like a Stealth fighter plane, some HIV may have hidden parts that do not show up on the immune system scanner. As a result, the immune system may not produce the right kind of antibody to neutralize all the variant HIVs.

Types of HIV Vaccines

Scientists are attempting to design three types of vaccines: (1) a **preventive** or **prophylactic vaccine** to protect people from becoming HIV-infected, analogous to classic virus vaccines such as those for measles and polio; (2) a **therapeutic vaccine** (this is not a true vaccination, but a postinfection therapy to stimulate the immune system; the term vaccination is reserved for preventive strategies) for those who are already infected with HIV to prevent them from progressing to AIDS (with recent findings that within days of infection massive quantities of HIV has seeded the lymph nodes, a therapeutic vaccine may be too little, too late); and (3) a **perinatal vaccine** for administration to pregnant HIV-infected women to prevent transmission of the virus to the fetus. Stephen Straus and co-workers (1994) reported that researchers have developed a therapeutic vaccine for the herpes virus. The new, therapeutic vaccine reduces the frequency with which genital sores appear in patients infected with the herpesvirus. While it fails to outperform the existing antiherpes drug, acyclovir, it sets the stage for a more effective treatment in the future. Over 40 million people in the United States are infected with the herpes virus, which stays in the body for life.

The ability to influence the frequency of genital herpres outbreaks with this vaccine inspires optimism that similar successes may be possible with other chronic viral diseases, such as AIDS.

TABLE 9-7 Problems with Vaccine Development Against HIV

1. HIV integrates its genetic material into cellular DNA.
2. Regulatory genes are responsible for controlled, low-level viral expression.
3. Cells of the immune system serve as both targets of viral infection and vehicles of immune protection.
4. Mimicry between viral envelope proteins and MHC II (HLA) molecules.
5. Rapid rate of HIV mutations.
6. HIV antigens may act as decoys to antibody-producing cells.
7. Viral envelope proteins are poor antigens due to high carbohydrate content.
8. HIV rapidly sheds its viral envelope glycoproteins.
9. Cell-to-cell fusion may result in transmission of HIV RNA without complete assembly of virus particles.
10. Presence of HIV antibody may induce viral latency.
11. Vaccines have not been developed for any lentiviral infections.
12. The need to maintain a constant level of protective immune activation in the face of an immune system suppressor network.

(Adapted from Peter Nara, *Los Alamos Science,* 1989)

Scientists are confronted with a number of perplexing problems (Table 9-7). One is that people infected with HIV develop antibodies that inactivate the virus in laboratory tests, yet they become sick and die anyway. Why don't these patients' antibodies work against the virus? Researchers are in the difficult position of trying to design a vaccine without even knowing what kinds of immune responses will protect a person from HIV infection. This uncertainty has prompted some researchers to question whether a protein from HIV or the entire virus should be used to make a vaccine.

Recent reports by David Ho (1995) and Xiping Wei (1995) state that HIV and the immune system engage in a desperate struggle of survival that begins with HIV infection. From early on, a billion or more new viruses are released each day into the bloodstream and a billion or more white blood cells die each day in the battle to keep the infection under control. The body, in the meantime, attempts to replace the billion white blood cells lost each day. The virus wins, in the end, because it has an edge in the fight. This edge is not yet completely understood. But, an important component of that "edge" has to be the ability of HIV to mutate, i.e., to produce immune and drug-resistant variants within the first 2 to 4 weeks after infection.

VACCINE PRODUCTION

To make vaccines, scientists use either **dead microorganisms** and **inactivated viruses** or **attenuated viruses** and **microorganisms**. Attenuated means that viruses and other microorganisms are modified; they are capable of reproducing and invoking the immune response but lack the ability to cause a disease.

Attenuated Viruses

Attenuated viruses in vaccines provide a better immunity than inactivated viruses because attenuated viruses continue to reproduce, thereby acting as a constant source of antigenic stimulus to the immune system. Thus attenuated vaccines appear to provide lifelong immunity **without** requiring periodic boosters. One of the major concerns with using attenuated virus vaccine is the fear that first, all the virus may **not be attenuated** and second, the attenuated virus may revert to the virulent form. For example, approximately 10 cases of polio using attenuated polio virus vaccine, occur in the United States per year which represents 1 case per 2.4 million doses of vaccine administered (Stoeckle et al., 1996). This is a major reason that attenuated HIV is not used in government-sponsored experimental vaccine preparations. There is, however, an equally great fear that has not received proper attention; that is, no one knows the long-term consequences of having an attenuated **retrovirus** (HIV) inside the body for 20 to 50 years. **Such viruses inserted into human DNA may turn genes off and on at the wrong time causing cancer and other types of disease** (see Figure 6–14).

In July of 1996, to improve the safety of experimental AIDS vaccines based on live but weakened HIV, scientists at the National Institute of Allergy and Infectious Diseases (NIAID) made a prototype of such a vaccine drug-susceptible so it can be eliminated from the body soon after use. This off switch will make attenuated vaccines safer to use— perhaps safe enough for use against HIV.

In March 1995, the FDA approved the use of an attenuated chickenpox vaccine (VARIVAX) stating that it is 90% effective at preventing chickenpox. This vaccine has been under development since 1981 and tested on 11,000 people across the United States. About 7 million people in the United States get chickenpox each year—some die from it, about 100 people a year and about 10,000 people are hospitalized with complications. On May 1, 1995 Merck and company began shipping millions of doses of VARIVAX to physicians nationwide.

Inactivated Viruses

To inactivate viruses for use in vaccines, the viruses are treated with formalin or another chemical. There is a danger in using inactivated viruses—**they may not all be inactivated**. Inactivated virus vaccines have been made against hepatitis B, rabies, influenza, and polio (Salk vaccine). Salk's first vaccine killed a number of recipients in the late 1950s because not all the polio viruses were destroyed, that is, some could still replicate.

Jonas Salk announced at the Fifth International Conference on AIDS (1989) the development of a new HIV vaccine. He used gamma radiation to destroy the virulence of HIVs and stripped them of their outer envelope. Salk's vaccine was injected into three chimpanzees. After reasonable success in protecting the chimpanzees, Salk asked for and received permission to inject volunteer priests and nuns over age 65 with his vaccine. The project was suspended in 1993, as there were little if any observable beneficial effects of his vaccine, e.g., specific neutralizing antibody to HIV was not found.

ROLE OF GENETIC DIVERSITY IN VACCINE DEVELOPMENT

Genetic diversity, or the production of HIV variants, is a major problem in vaccine development. In 1988, Robert Gallo, reported that **every** HIV isolate has been different. And, different subtypes of HIV can swap or exchange genetic information producing new subtypes of HIV. Even sequential HIV isolates from the same patient differ and demonstrate different susceptibilities to a standard neutralizing antibody. The problem can be underscored by a report from Gallo's laboratory that even a **single amino acid** change in the HIV envelope can result in a virus that resists the same neutralization antibodies that had previously neutralized parent HIV. Further, it has been reported that at least 25% of the amino acids in HIV envelope protein are subject to change at any time during the production of HIV.

Subunit Vaccines

Subunit vaccines are made from antigenic fragments of an organism or virus most suitable for evoking a strong immune response. The genetic code for producing particular components, such as proteins found in the HIV envelope, an internal core protein, or the reverse transcriptase enzyme, can be genetically engineered in a bacterium, fungus (yeast) or another virus. These subunits can then be mass produced and used in pure form to make a specific vaccine. Vaccine against hepatitis B is made from a subunit of the hepatitis B virus and produced in quantity in yeast.

In the United States, researchers are currently basing their vaccine strategies on the use of proteins found in the envelope of HIV. Most HIV vaccines developed through 1996 are those made by Genentech, Chiron, and Micro GeneSys of the United States and Austria's Immuno. All are genetically engineered versions of HIV's surface protein.

PROBLEMS IN THE SEARCH FOR HIV VACCINE

HIV poses some unique problems for making a human vaccine. **First,** scientists have not established what immune responses are crucial for protecting the body against HIV infection. Without this information, they cannot tailor the vaccine to produce those particular responses. **Second,** it is too risky to use the entire weakened or inactive HIV.

Third, HIV undergoes a high rate of mutation as it replicates, and strains from different parts of the world vary by as much as 35% in terms of the proteins that comprise the outer coat of the virus. Even within an infected individual, over a period of years, the virus may change its proteins by as much as 10%. This degree of antigenic drift or variation means that a vaccine made from one strain of HIV may not protect against a different strain. To prove effectiveness, vaccines may have to be tested in geographic areas where the prevalent strains are the same as the strain used in the vaccine.

Fourth, the immune response raised by the vaccine may be protective for only a short period of time. In such cases, booster vaccinations would be required too frequently to be practical.

Fifth, it is possible that the vaccine may make people more susceptible to HIV infection. That is, vaccine producers are concerned that if they are unable to make a completely HIV–neutralizing vaccine, the vaccine when taken might make the disease worse by **boosting the number of antibodies that might enhance entry of HIV into cells.** For example, enhancing antibodies are thought to be important in a few unusual viral infections such as dengue fever, Rift Valley fever, and yellow fever, in which the antibody binds to the virus and carries it into cells. **Thus, the more of a certain kind of antibody you have, the worse the infection can become** (see additional information below).

Sixth, Jon Cohen, writing for the journal *Science* (1994a) reported on a *Science* survey of an international sample of over 100 of the field's leading researchers, public health officials, and manufacturers. All told, 67 people from 18 countries on six continents reponded. And when it came to describing the obstacles that hinder vaccine development, the respondents—be they from Russia, Indonesia, Egypt, Europe, India, or Brazil—had remarkably similar views. **The scientific unknowns are the highest hurdles,** they said, but they also stressed that the field lacks the strong leadership and funding to speed progress.

Predictably, money—or rather, lack of it— was one of the most frequently mentioned obstacles. Even though vaccines are among the most cost-effective medical interventions ever devised, they are not big money-makers. **Drug companies are traditionally reluctant to invest in any form of vaccine development which carries high costs, low profits, and big risks of costly legal suits should accidents occur.** Their current analysis of the state of HIV/AIDS vac-

HIV VACCINE THERAPIES: PREVENTION AND THERAPY

A LOOK BACK AT THE FIRST VACCINE

The year 1996 marked the 200th anniversary of the first vaccine, which was developed against smallpox. As vaccine researchers launch a new century of challenging disease, they might find inspiration in the early beginnings of immunology, Edward Jenner's discovery.

According to lore, Jenner was a country doctor who heard a rumor that the cowpox virus could provide immunity to smallpox. Investigating the theory, Jenner endured the ridicule of his colleagues before proving his point.

In a now-famous 1796 experiment, Jenner scratched (inoculated) the arm of 8-year-old James Phipps infecting the boy with cowpox pus taken from a milkmaid carrying the virus. Two months later, he again inoculated James but this time he added some smallpox residue. The rest, as they say, is history: James remained healthy! A smallpox vaccine—and the field of vaccinology—was launched.

No viral epidemic has ever been conquered by drug therapy—prevention is the key, and primary prevention via vaccine inoculation is the cornerstone. But, there are enormous problems inherent in constructing an HIV vaccine. **First**, the virus has extraordinary diversity, leaving little chance that just a few subtypes could induce broadly protective immunity. **Second**, The attenuated (weakened) virus strategy that has been so successful for many infections, including smallpox, polio, and measles, will be very difficult if not impossible to implement for HIV. **Third**, HIV attacks the very immune cells that are essential in an immunization procedure, and the immune cell activation that accompanies any immunization will activate HIV replication.

With that said, immunologists are still driven to achieve a most difficult task, the production of an effective HIV-preventive vaccine. Since the first injections of an experimental HIV vaccine were given in the United States in 1987, more than 2,000 uninfected adults have received about 20 experimental vaccines; 17 people have become HIV-infected from the vaccines. Only a handful of HIV vaccines have made it to the second of the three stages of the trials that are needed before any vaccine can be marketed. As of mid-1996, no U. S. pharmaceutical company or University researched vaccine has reached the third stage, full-scale testing. Worldwide, through 1996, there are some 25 experimental vaccines in the first stage

of testing—to determine if the vaccine itself causes human illness.

DNA VACCINE

In March of 1996, the FDA approved the first human testing of a vaccine made with pure DNA. Apollon Inc. and the National Institutes of Health will test the experimental AIDS vaccine on 15 (13 men, 2 women) healthy people at the NIH hospital in Bethesda, Maryland in mid-1996. **Update 1997**–DNA vaccine experiments were not successful!

Potential AIDS vaccines have been given to healthy people before. But this marked the first time a healthy person has received the pure genetic material of any disease—causing agent.

Apollon made the vaccine from a gene responsible for forming one of the surface proteins of HIV.

Most vaccines against most diseases involve injecting someone with a protein of the disease-causing agent. The idea behind DNA-based vaccines is to use the body's own cells to make a portion of that protein, not enough to be infectious but enough that immune cells will recognize the protein if the disease-causing agent ever strikes.

Although scientists are mixing the old traditional ideas of vaccine production with the new, in general there remains the fear that the production of an effective HIV-preventive vaccine may not be possible. But, if it is, it won't be available before the year 2005 and even then it may only be 30% effective in preventing HIV infection! A successful AIDS vaccine will need to induce the formation of broad, cross-reactive neutralizing antibodies against an array of HIV antigens that encompass the majority of HIV strains active in the region of interest and at the same time confer some mucosal immunity. It should be mentioned that to date, there is only one vaccine available against a sexually transmitted disease (hepatitis B vaccine) and it does not stimulate mucosal immunity.

THERAPY

A full-scale test of a therapeutic AIDS vaccine made by San Diego's Immune Response Corporation (IRC) has gotten a go-ahead from the Food and Drug Administration for a 3-year, 2,500 person trial in the United States—the largest ever test of a vaccine, called **Remune**, in people already infected with HIV. This trial began in March 1996; IRC is using "killed" (inactivated) HIV that have had an cine research is particularly bleak. The National Institutes of Health (NIH) spends 8% of its AIDS budget—around $100 million a year—on vaccine work, but only about $5 million is being spent worldwide on preparing new candidate vaccines.

In 1990, AIDS researchers and stock analysts hailed Repligen Corp., a Massachusetts biotechnology firm, as a leader—many said **the** leader—in the race to develop a vaccine against HIV. Not only was Repligen collaborating with top AIDS researchers and publishing impressive scientific papers, the startup had won financial backing from pharmaceutical giant Merck & Co. A 1990 investors' guide from Shearson Lehman Hutton predicted that if human tests of the vaccine went well, Repligen and Merck might ask the U.S. Food and Drug Administration to license it as early as the end of 1994.

Fast forward to July 19, 1994. On that day, Repligen announced that, because of a "lack of available funding," it was stopping its HIV vaccine research and development program.

Seventh, economics clearly isn't the only factor that is discouraging companies from entering the search for an AIDS vaccine. Another is the fact that the science is very tough. Animal models used to test AIDS vaccines have severe limitations; the genetic diversity of HIV may require an effective vaccine to be based on many viral strains; and no researcher has successfully demonstrated which immune responses correlate with protection from HIV (Cohen, 1994b.)

Use of Whole Inactivated HIV: A Vaccine-Induced Enhancement of HIV Infection

Whole inactivated viruses are believed to be unsuitable for vaccine production because: (**1**)

one cannot be 100% certain that every HIV is inactivated, recall the Salk polio vaccine problem stated earlier and (**2**) the envelope surrounding HIV may prevent the production of suitable antibodies. The best reason not to use whole HIV, however, may be the possibility of **vaccine-induced enhancement** of disease. It has been shown by a number of investigators that

_____ **POINT OF INFORMATION 9.10** _____

PATHOLOGICAL UNIQUENESS OF HIV

There has been much written about the uniqueness of HIV. Perhaps the most singular feature is that it is lethal to humans. A national state of immunity has not yet been documented in humans. Once infected with HIV, there is a high probability of death within 10 to 15 years.

Most human pathological viruses, including HIV, behave in a somewhat similar fashion with one important exception. Other viruses, including all of the other sexually transmitted viruses, enter cells, cause cell lysis, and remain in the body. The body "learns" to live with viral infections, latent periods, and recurrent episodes. **But HIV is different: it infects and suppresses an immune system that holds other viral infections in check.** Perhaps it is because we survive these other viral infections that there has not been the urgency to learn more about host response to viruses: how viruses actually infect cells, become proviruses, and are activated to reproduce. There is not even a respectable spectrum of antiviral drugs available, mostly because we do not know enough about the viruses.

There are vaccines available for smallpox, polio, measles, mumps, yellow fever, rubella, rabies, and influenza; but, only one vaccine—hepatitis B is available for a sexually transmitted viral disease. And, only one vaccine has ever eradicated a human disease, the smallpox vaccine.

some HIV antibodies actually help HIV enter host cells, primarily monocyte cells (Koff, 1988). This phenomenon is called **antibody-enhanced infectivity**. Antibodies that enhance HIV infectivity have been identified in the serum of HIV-infected patients and in HIV-infected and immunized animals.

The viral antigens responsible for the enhancement phenomenon must be identified and removed before a vaccine is made; otherwise there would be an increased risk of HIV infection following vaccination (Homsy et al., 1989; Levy, 1989).

Testing HIV Vaccines

Whether a vaccine will stimulate antibody production and is **safe** can be easily determined. It will not require a long time nor will it require many volunteers. But to gauge a vaccine's **efficacy** (effectiveness) will require a large number of volunteers who are free of HIV but in danger of becoming infected with it (members of behavioral high risk groups). To determine a vaccine's efficacy, two large groups of subjects are selected, one that receives the vaccine and one that receives a placebo, to see whether the vaccinated group has a lower rate of HIV infection. In carrying out efficacy trials, the number of participants, the length of the follow-up period, the rate of HIV infection, and the presumed efficacy of the vaccine are related to each other. Because the rate of HIV infection is low, even in "high-risk" populations, researchers estimate they will need to study several thousand participants to determine whether an HIV vaccine is effective. The original polio vaccine trial was completed in a year but required nearly half a million children.

An important variable in determining the parameters of the trial is whether the vaccine is prophylactic (preventative) or therapeutic. If the vaccine actually prevents infection, the trial will measure the rate at which participants develop HIV antibodies. If, however, the vaccine allows infection but prevents or greatly retards disease progression, the trial will measure the rate at which disease develops and will therefore require many more years of follow-up.

Morality of Testing HIV Vaccines

Designers of the vaccine trials are thus confronted with a paradox unique to HIV/AIDS. If safer-sex and safe-needle practices are not taught, volunteers who believe they are protected by the unproven vaccine (which may actually be a placebo) could take more risks and increase their chances of becoming infected. **If such practices are taught**, and by ethical standards, they must be, volunteers could cut their risk so effectively that they are never exposed to HIV leaving the vaccine with nothing to fight. **In a way, the trial depends on the failure of education.** To get around this potential conflict of interest, phase III trials of an AIDS vaccine will have to rely on populations in which the number of infections remains high regardless of education, like young high-risk gay men and injection-drug users. **There is also the additional problem of creating vaccine HIV-positive persons who can not be distinguished from those who are HIV-infected.** They, too, will be subjected to adverse social, employment, and other discrimination following a positive antibody test.

Having to use volunteers from high behavioral risk groups, such as gay men, prostitutes, and injection drug users—assuming a sufficient number could be recruited—presents its own set of complications. It will be necessary for investigators to keep track of volunteers for as long as 5 years and to be informed of their drug and sexual practices during this time. This may be extremely difficult, considering that the same volunteers will be engaged in illegal activities.

Partners and spouses of AIDS-infected hemophiliacs are at high risk of acquiring infection and would be excellent as vaccine volunteers, but their limited numbers diminish the prospect of evaluating vaccines in this population. There is the possibility of testing an HIV vaccine overseas—particularly in Africa, which has a significant AIDS problem.

HIV Vaccine Costs

Perhaps the most difficult moral question is the cost of the vaccine. A successful vaccine that sells for a high price will be of little use to poor and uninsured Americans and most people of de-

———— BOX 9.10 ————

RETHINKING "STERILIZING IMMUNITY"

Since the AIDS virus was first isolated, HIV/AIDS immunologists have been searching for a vaccine that can completely prevent HIV infection. Vaccine researchers feared that if even a single HIV particle infected a cell, it might ultimately lead to AIDS. So the only safe course was to create a vaccine that blocked infection completely, producing so-called **"Sterilizing Immunity."** The usual means for developing such a vaccine has historically been monkey experiments using SIV, the simian cousin of HIV. But monkey studies with disappointing results forced researchers to rethink this all-or-nothing strategy. Immunologists now point to a phenomenon that, just a few years ago, seemed implausible: the immune system does have some capacity to contain infection with the AIDS virus. Therefore, even a vaccine that fails to deliver sterilizing immunity should still be able to delay or prevent disease. As a result of this new thinking, prevention of symptoms, rather than sterilizing immunity, is being considered as a hallmark of vaccine success.

Staging a trial with a disease as a clinical end point would probably require several years—and tens of thousands of people—to arrive at a statistically meaningful answer. And that makes it tough, since retaining people in a vaccine trial for more than a few years is difficult, and the costs of running multiyear tests is astronomical. A trial with infection as an end point might take as little as 3 years and require fewer than 3,500 people (Cohen, 1993).

THE USE OF THE TUBERCULOSIS VACCINE: IT IS NOT 100% EFFECTIVE

In spite of conflicting evidence of its ability to prevent infection, the tuberculosis (TB) vaccine is, surprisingly, the most widely used vaccine in the world. Its rise to prominence began in 1908, when Albert Calmette and Camille Guérin at the Pasteur Institute in Paris developed a weakened strain of a bacterium that causes TB in both cows and humans. They first tested this vaccine in people in 1921; since then, more than 3 billion people have received the BCG (bacille Calmette-Guérin) vaccine.

Although BCG is recommended by the World Health Organization's Expanded Program on Immunization, doubts about its effectiveness remain. Some clinical trials have shown it to protect 80% of those vaccinated; others have found it to offer no protection at all. Numerous theories have been proposed to explain these conflicting results, including the possibility of subtle differences in the BCG vaccines used.

The relatively low incidence of TB in the United States, coupled with uncertainties about the effectiveness of the BCG vaccine, has led the U.S. Public Health Service to recommend TB testing and drug therapy for those infected, rather than vaccination. But TB cases are on the rise, and the spread of the hard-to-treat multidrug-resistant tuberculosis (MDR TB) has encouraged the Centers for Disease Control and Prevention (CDC) to take another look at BCG.

The CDC sponsored a review of 14 prospective trials and 12 case-control studies of the BCG vaccine. After analyzing these studies, it was concluded that the vaccine protected just over half of those inoculated.

It's on the lower end of efficacy for a vaccine, but it still provides protection for some people. BCG is effective and should be considered for use in the United States (Christensen, 1994b).

It can be argued that regardless of whether BCG is 80% or less than 50% effective, it is a better treatment than treating drug-resistant TB with an ineffective drug.

---

veloping nations, who have no more than a few dollars a year to spend on health care. Ten years have passed since the discovery of a vaccine for hepatitis B, a viral disease that is also spread by sexual contact and the sharing of hypodermic needles. But the product has yet to reach many poor people in the United States and Third World countries largely because it costs more than $120 for a series of three injections. Polio and measles vaccines are relatively cheap but are still not in universal use and they have been available for decades!

HUMAN HIV VACCINE TRIALS

The goal in producing HIV vaccines is to destroy HIV or keep it in check so that it causes no further damage. The ideal vaccine will stop progressive immunodeficiency and restore the immune system. In order to determine if an HIV vaccine will meet these criteria it must ultimately be tested in human vaccine field trials.

The basic principle behind human vaccine trials has changed little since the 19th century. To test for an HIV/AIDS vaccine, several thousand people at high risk for the disease will be inoculated with the experimental agent, most likely an altered version of HIV or some portion of it. The vaccine should not be dangerous enough to cause the disease, but enough like HIV to confer immunity by triggering the production of antibodies and other virus-fighting components of the immune system. The subjects in the trial will be carefully monitored to see if they have a better rate of avoiding infection than others who were not vaccinated.

In 1994, there were at least 15 candidate HIV Prophylactic vaccines and 10 therapeutic vaccines in phase I or II clinical trials in Europe and North America (Lurie et al., 1994). As of early 1998, with the exception of the U. S. Army vaccine study, no vaccine has satisfactorily completed testing in a phase III trial.

In June of 1994 the National Institutes of Health (NIH) delayed human testing of two of its most promising vaccines until sometime in 1997 because of insufficient efficacy and safety data.

The two candidate vaccines had not been formally tested for efficacy. During phase I and II vaccine studies, 12 of 1,500 volunteers became HIV-positive before the complete immunization sequence was administered (WHO, 1995). Thus NIH concluded that the vaccine was unlikely to be effective enough to make the 4,500-person trial worthwhile. The phase III efficacy trial was to involve 9,000 people. Using this large number of people was to show whether the vaccines were more than 60% effective or less than 30% effective. A larger follow-up would be required if their effectiveness was between those levels. (Belshe et al., 1994; Macilwain, 1994). In November of 1995, Jean-Paul Levy, director of the French National Agency for AIDS Research, described phase III trials as an **absurdity** given the lack of basic knowledge. We are unsure if we will ever be able to get a vaccine for this virus, which is different to any virus for which

we have ever created a vaccine (Butler, 1995). Regardless of the United States decision of not to begin vaccine trials, the world Health Organization, in October, 1994, recommended large-scale trials of HIV vaccines moved forward. The first candidate countries for the vaccine experiments are Uganda and Thailand. These trials are set to begin sometime in 1996. Data from these trials will not be available for some 7 years. (HIV vaccines Get Green Light for Third World Trials, 1994; Weniger, 1994; Cohen, 1995; Science, 1996). In February 1996 the National Institutes of AIDS and Infectious Diseases announced a joint phase II vaccine with Pasteur-Meriuex of France and Biocine Inc. of California. Early in 1997, Pasteur Merieux tested one version of the vaccine in about 100 patients. It uses the canary-pox virus to carry HIV genes into the body, where the genes produce proteins that can trigger an immune system alarm. The vaccine and a follow-up booster shot generated antibodies in all 100, a sign the immune system kicked into gear. It also triggered the mobilization of killer T cells, the immune system's attack force, in 40% of the people. If the canary-pox prototype passes current safety tests, the company expects to begin an efficacy trial of 3,500 people in the United States in 1998 and smaller trials in Uganda and Thailand over the next few years. **The outcome is anybody's guess!**

In April of 1996, a 5-year vaccine field trial conducted under the auspices of the Walter Reed Army Institute of Research in Washington D.C. and the National Institute of Allergy and Infectious , followed 608 voluteers for 5 years, until December 1995, Half were given the gp160 vaccine and half a placebo. The results show that microgenesys vaccine did not affect the cause of HIV disease in HIV-infected volunteers (Nature, 1996). The vaccine was noneffective!

Liability Is a Major Hurdle in Vaccine Development

Jon Cohen (1992) states that some pharmaceutical and biotechnical companies are very concerned about potential damage suits by injured trial subjects. Some companies have stopped their HIV vaccine development work due to the fear of **liability**. Given our litigious society, concerns of product liability are slowing the progress in vaccine research.

In 1986, the National Childhood Vaccine Injury Compensation Act was passed by Congress. The act was made necessary because of the large number of liability cases that arose from the vaccines for polio, diphtheria-tetanus-pertussis, and swine flu. This act allowed for the reward of victims **without** punishing the vaccine manufacturers. HIV/AIDS vaccine manufacturers are **not** covered by this act because this **no fault** program was designed to include **only childhood vaccines**. Vaccine manufacturers are asking Congress for similar adult/adolescent vaccine liability protection. The World Health Organization, which planned to begin efficacy trials in four countries in 1997, is currently analyzing the liability issue and expects to find potential solutions by the beginning of 1998.

Vaccine Testing Confidentiality

Confidentiality must be maintained for the duration of the vaccine trials because people immunized with candidate AIDS vaccines who mount effective immune responses will appear positive for HIV antibody. They may be subject to the social stigma and discrimination associated with being truly HIV-positive.

Vaccine-induced seroconversion may lead to difficulties in donating blood, obtaining insurance, traveling internationally, or entering the military. Vaccine-induced antibodies may be long-lived, thus volunteers in AIDS vaccine trials must be given some form of documentation that certifies that their antibody status is due to vaccination and not HIV infection. The National Institute of Allergy and Infectious Disease has recently (1993) provided a tamper-proof identification card to help uninfected participants in vaccine trials. The seroconversion issue may play a major role in recruitment efforts and in the future welfare of vaccine trial participants (Koff, 1988). So the question for anyone is: **Should I enter an HIV vaccine trial when I know safeguards are limited?** I know why I ought to do it...but! (**Class discussion**)

Is an Effective Vaccine Enough to Stop HIV Disease/AIDS?

Data from the San Francisco Young Mens Health Study, which is an HIV transmission study of young gay men, suggests that it is very unlikely that effective vaccines alone will eradicate HIV in San Francisco. Sally Blower and colleagues (1994) suggest that an effective vaccine could cause a sharp **increase** in new HIV infections because of the false sense of security it may create causing people to take greater risks. Their work suggests that risk behavior change and mass vaccination would have to occur together.

Finally, the Question: Have AIDS Prevention Programs Produced Long-Term Behavior Change?

Kyung-Hee Choi and colleagues (1994) state unequivocally that current AIDS prevention programs have produced long-term behavior changes. In their study they critically review the scientific literature on AIDS prevention programs in an attempt to determine the extent to which behavioral intervention research has demonstrated the efficacy of methods for reducing risk behaviors. They focused on the three most critical questions in intervention research: (1) have AIDS prevention programs had long-term success in behavior change; (2) what recommendations can be made to program developers; and (3) where should HIV prevention research be heading. They reviewed published abstracts, journal articles, and other reports that formally evaluated intervention programs aimed at changing HIV risk behavior. They selected evaluation research on HIV testing and counseling since August 1991, because Higgins and colleagues (1991) provided critical evaluations of relevant materials presented or published up to July 1991. Intervention studies reviewed were divided by AIDS risk or intervention target groups (gay or bisexual men, IDU, heterosexuals, young adults, and adolescents) and treatment units (individual, group, organization, or community) or implementation settings (clinic, school). Each intervention was summarized in terms of its content, duration, intensity and impact, and was assessed according to methodologic strength (inclusion of comparison groups, subject self-selection, sample attrition, analysis of secular trend). The report by Choi and Coates is recommended reading for those wanting greater detail on the question of whether HIV/AIDS prevention programs are working and what else can be done.

SUMMARY

The key to stopping HIV transmission lies with the behavior of the individual. That behavior, if the experience of the past 16 years can be used as an indicator, has proven to be very difficult to change.

Changing sexual behavior and using a condom is referred to as **safer sex**. The latex condom is the only condom believed to stop the passage of HIV; and a spermicide should be used with the condom. Oil-based lubricants must not be used because they weaken the condom, allowing it to leak or break under stress. Water-based lubricants are available and should be used. There is at least one female condom, called a vaginal pouch, approved by the FDA. It is inserted like a diaphragm. It offers protection to both sexual partners.

Many cases of HIV infection have come from contaminated blood transfusions. A test developed in 1985 to screen all donated blood in the United States has reduced the risk of HIV transfusion infection. But blood bank screening has reduced the size of the blood donor pool. Many hospitals are encouraging people who know they might need an operation to donate their own blood for later use—autologous transfusion.

To date there is no FDA-approved vaccine for pre- or post-HIV infection. Scientists have ruled out the possibility of an attenuated HIV vaccine because HIV may mutate to a virulent form once injected into the body. Inactivated whole virus vaccines are also being held back because there is no 100% guarantee that all HIV used in the vaccine will be inactivated.

Even if a vaccine is developed, will it be effective against all of the HIV mutants in the HIV gene pool? Can the threat of vaccine-induced enhancement of HIV infection be overcome? Will an animal model be developed that will allow investigators to study each step of the HIV infection process so that a proper therapy can be designed? How are vaccine testing agencies going to handle the ethical question of vaccine seroconverting normal subjects to positive antibody status? The social repercussions will be devastating for those who, when tested, test HIV-positive even though they are HIV free.

There are some 5.3 million health care workers in the United States. It is crucial that they adhere to the Universal Protection Guidelines set down by the CDC, as a significant number of them are exposed to the AIDS virus annually. The risk of HIV infection after exposure to HIV-contaminated blood is about 1 in 200.

A few states have implemented HIV-partner notification; many other states are beginning to experiment with HIV-partner notification or contact tracing programs. It is too early to tell just how successful locating and testing high behavioral risk partners will be, or the cost-to-benefit ratio. One thing is certain; if these programs are to be successful, they will have to ensure confidentiality to those who are traced. Partner notification or contact tracing continues to work well for other sexually transmitted diseases.

REVIEW QUESTIONS

(*Answers to the Review Questions are on page 578.*)

1. Which is the better condom for protection from STDs, one made from lamb intestine or one made from latex rubber? Explain.

2. Which lubricant is best suited for condom use? Explain.

3. Briefly explain safer sex.

4. True or False: If a person has unprotected intercourse with an HIV-infected partner, he or she will become HIV-infected. Explain.

5. Yes or No: If injection drug users (IDUs) were given free equipment—no questions asked—would that stop the transmission of HIV among them? Explain.

6. What is the current risk of being transfused with HIV-contaminated blood in the United States?

7. What do you think should happen in cases where a person who knows he or she is HIV-

positive, lies at a donor interview, and donates blood?

8. Why do most scientists wish to avoid using an attenuated HIV vaccine or an inactivated HIV vaccine?

9. What is the advantage of using recombinant HIV subunits in making a vaccine?

10. Explain vaccine-induced enhancement. How does it occur?

11. Why is it necessary to practice strict confidentiality with respect to volunteers for AIDS vaccine tests?

12. What are universal precautions? Who formulated them?

13. True or False: Research continues to show that AIDS prevention messages are effective in causing teens to change their sexual behaviors.

14. True or False: Latex condoms eliminate the risk of HIV transmission.

15. True or False: Partner notification is usually performed by the infected individual or a trained and authorized health department official.

16. True or False: The Centers for Disease Control and Prevention estimates that as many as 1 in 100,000 units of blood in the blood supply may be contaminated with HIV.

17. True or False: The three types of vaccines that scientists are interested in developing are preventive, therapeutic, and perinatal vaccines.

18. True or False: Used disposable needles should be recapped by hand before disposal.

19. True or False: Prompt washing of a needle-stick injury with soap and water is sufficient to prevent HIV infection.

REFERENCES

AMORTEGUI, A.J., et al. (1984). The effects of chemical intravaginal contraceptives and betadine on *Ureaplasma urealyticum. Contraception*, 30: 35–40.

ANDERSON, FRANK W.J . (1993). Condoms: A technical guide. *Female Patient*, 18:21–26.

BARBER, HUGH R.K. (1990). Condoms (not diamonds) are a Girl's best friend. *Female Patient*, 15:14–16.

BAYER, RONALD et al. (1992). HIV Prevention and the two faces of partner notification. *Am. J. Public Health*, 82:1158–1164.

BAYER, RONALD, et al. (1993). AIDS and the limits of control: Public health orders, quarantine and recalcitrant behavior. *Am. J. Public Health*, 83:1471–1476.

BELSHE, ROBERT, et al.(1994). HIV infection in vaccinated volunteers. *JAMA*, 272:431.

BENOWITZ, STEVEN. (1997). Politics polarizing issues in needle-exchange study. *The Scientist*, 11:1,6–7.

BIRD, KRISTINA D. (1991). The use of spermicide nonoxynol-9 in the prevention of HIV infection. *AIDS*, 5:791–796.

BLOWER, SALLY M., et al. (1994). Prophylactic vaccines, risk behavior change, and the probability of eradicating HIV in San Francisco. *Science*, 265:1451–1454.

BOLCH, O.H., JR, et al. (1973). In vitro effects of Emko on *Neisseria gonorrhoeae* and *Trichomonas vaginalis. Am. J. Obstet. Gynecol.*, 115:1145–1148.

BURNETT, JOSEPH. (1995). Fundamental basic science of HIV. *Cutis*, 55:84.

BURRIS, SCOTT, et al. (1996). Legal strategies used in operating syringe-exchange programs in the United States. *Am. J. Public Health*, 86:1161–1166.

BUTLER, DECLAN. (1995). AIDS vaccine needs focused effort as drug firms back off research. *Nature*, 378:323–324.

CHRISTENSEN, DAMARIS. (1994a). A shot in time: The technology behind new vaccines. *Science News*, 145:344–345.

CHRISTENSEN, DAMARIS. (1994b) Another look at the TB vaccine. *Science News*, 145:393.

CHOI, KYUNG-HEE, et al. (1994). Prevention of HIV infection. *AIDS*, 8:1371–1389.

CLEMENT, MICHAEL J. (1993). HIV disease: Are we going anywhere? *Patient Care*, 27:13.

COHEN, JON. (1992). Is liability slowing AIDS vaccines? *Science*, 256:168–170.

COHEN, JON. (1993). A NEW GOAL: Preventing disease, not infection. *Science*, 262:1820–1821.

COHEN, JON. (1994a). Bumps on the vaccine road. *Science*, 265:1371–1372.

COHEN JON. (1994b) Are researchers racing toward success, or crawling? *Science*, 265:1373–1374.

COHEN, JON. (1995). Thailand weighs AIDS vaccine tests. *Science*, 270: 904–907.

CONNELL, ELIZABETH B.(1989). Barrier contraceptives—their time has returned. *Female Patient*, 14:66–75.

Consumer Reports. (1989). Can you rely on condoms? 54:135–141.

DES JARLAIS, DON, et al. (1995). Maintaining low HIV seroprevalence in populations of IDUs. *JAMA*, 274:1226–1231.

DE VINCENZI, ISABELLE. (1994). A longitudinal study of HIV transmission by heterosexual partners. *N. Engl. J. Med.*, 331:341–347.

DRUCKER, LURIE, et al. (1997). An opportunity lost: HIV infection associated with lack of a national needle-exchange program in the USA. *Lancet*, 349:604–608.

ETZIONI, AMITAI. (1993). HIV sufferers have a responsibility. *TIME*, 142:100.

EZZELL, CAROL. (1987). Hospital workers have AIDS virus. *Nature*, 227:261.

FARR, GASTON, et al. (1994). Contraceptive efficacy and acceptability of the female condom. *Am. J. Public Health*, 84:1960–1964.

FINDLAY, STEVEN. (1991). AIDS: The second decade. *U.S. News World Rep.*, 110:20–22.

FISHER, ALEXANDER A. (1991). Condom conundrums: Part 1. *Cutis*, 48:359–360.

FISHER, PETER. (1990). A report from the underground. *International Working Group on AIDS and IV Drug Use*, 5:15–17.

FRANCIS, DONALD P., et al. (1987). The prevention of acquired immunodeficiency syndrome in the United States. *JAMA*, 257:1357–1366.

GERBERDING, JULIE LOUISE. (1991). Reducing occupational risk of HIV infection. *Hosp. Pract.*, 26:103–118.

GLANTZ, LEONARD. (1996). Annotation: Needle exchange programs and the law—time for a change. *Am. J. Public Health*, 86:1077–1078.

GOSTIN, LAWRENCE, et al. (1997) Prevention of HIV/AIDS and other blood-born diseases among injection drug users. *JAMA*, 277:53–62.

GREEN, JOHN, et al. (1996). Bacterial infection following blood product transfussion: Some bad blood bugging you? *Primary Care Rev.*, 2:13–18.

GRIMES, DAVID A. (1992). Contraception and the STD epidemic: Contraceptive methods for disease prevention. *The Contraception Report: The Role of Contraceptives in the Prevention of Sexually Transmitted Diseases*, III:1–15.

GUTTMACHER, SALLY, et al. (1997). Condom availability in New York City public high schools: Relationships to condom use and sexual behavior. *Am. J. Public Health*, 87:1427–1433.

HAGEN, HOLLY. (1991). Studies support syringe exchange. *FOCUS*, 6:5–6.

HART, GRAHAM J., et al. (1991). Prevalence of HIV, hepatitis B, and associated risk behaviors in clients of a needle exchange in central London. *AIDS*, 5:543–547.

HEARST, NORMAN, et al. (1995). Collaborative AIDS prevention research in the developing world: the CAPS experience. *AIDS*, 9 (suppl 1):51–55.

HICKS, D.R., et al. (1985). Inactivation of HTLV/LAV-infected cultures of normal human lymphocytes by nonoxynol-9 in vitro. *Lancet*, 2:1422–1423.

HIGGINS, D.L., et al. (1991). Evidence for the effects of HIV-antibody counseling and testing on risk behaviors. *JAMA*, 266:2419–2429.

HIV vaccines get the green light for third world trials. (1994). *Nature*, 371:644.

HO, DAVID, et al. (1995). Rapid turnover of plasma virons and CD4 lymphocytes in HIV infection. *Nature*, 373:123-126.

HOMSY, JACQUES, et al. (1989). The Fe and not CD4 receptor mediates antibody enhancement of HIV infection in human cells. *Science*, 244:1357–1359.

HOOKER, TRACEY. (1996). HIV/AIDS: Facts to consider, 1996. *National Conference of State Legislature*. Denver, Co., February, pp. 1–64.

JUDSON, FRANKLYN N. (1989). Condoms and spermicides for the prevention of sexually transmitted diseases. *Sexually Transmitted Dis. Bull.*, 9:3–11.

KAPLAN, EDWARD, et al. (1993). Let the needles do the talking! Evaluating the New Haven needle exchange. *Interfaces*, 23:7–26.

KOFF, WAYNE C. (1988). Development and testing of AIDS vaccines. *Science*, 241:426–432.

LACKRITZ, EVE, et al. (1995). Estimated risk of transmission of HIV by screened blood in the United States. *N. Engl. J. Med.*, 333:1721–1725.

LEVY, JAY A. (1989). Human immunodeficiency viruses and the pathogenesis of AIDS. *JAMA*, 261:2997–3006.

LEWIS, DAVID. (1995). Resistance of microorganisms to disinfection in dental and medical devices *Nature Med.*, 1:956–958.

LICHTENSTEIN, BRONWEN. (1996). Needle exchange programs: New Zealand's experience. *Am. J. Public Health*, 86:1319.

LURIE, PETER, et al. (1994). Ethical behavioral and social aspects of HIV vaccine trials in developing countries. *JAMA*, 271:295–302.

MACILWAIN, COLIN. (1994). U.S. puts larger-scale AIDS vaccine trials on ice as premature. *Nature*, 369:593.

MANDELL, WALLACE, et al. (1994). Correlates of needle sharing among injection drug users. *Am. J. Public Health*, 84:920–923.

MARWICK, CHARLES. (1995). Released report says needle exchanges work. *Med., News Perspect.*, 273:980–981.

Morbidity and Mortality Weekly Report. (1988). Partner notification for preventing human immunodeficiency virus (HIV) infection—Colorado, Idaho, South Carolina, Virginia. 37:393–396; 401–402.

Morbidity and Mortality Weekly Report. (1989a). Guideline for prevention of transmission of HIV and hepatitis B virus to health care workers. 38:3–17.

Morbidity and Mortality Weekly Report. (1989b). AIDS and human immunodeficiency virus infection in the United States: 1988 Update. 38:1–33.

Morbidity and Mortality Weekly Report. (1992a). Childbearing and contraceptive-use plans among women at high-risk for HIV infection—selected U.S. sites, 1989–1991. 41:135–144.

Morbidity and Mortality Weekly Report. (1992b). Sexual behavior among high school students—United States, 1990. 40:885–888.

Morbidity and Mortality Weekly Report. (1993a). Update: Barrier protection against HIV infection and other sexually transmitted diseases. 42:589–591.

Morbidity and Mortality Weekly Report. (1993b). Impact of new legislation on needle and syringe purchases and possession—Connecticut 1992. 42:145–147.

Morbidity and Mortality Weekly Report. (1995). Notification of syringe-sharing and sex partners of HIV-infected persons—Pennsylvania, 1993–1994. 44:202–204.

Morbidity and Mortality Weekly Report. (1996). School-based HIV-prevention education-United States, 1994. 45:760–764.

Morbidity and Mortality Weekly Report. (1997). Update: Syringe-exchange programs—United States, 1996. 46:565–568.

NARA, PETER. (1989). AIDS viruses of animals and man: Non living parasites of the immune system. *Los Alamos Sci.* 18:54-84.

Nature. (1996). Controversial AIDS vaccine fails to delay disease. 380:662.

Office Nurse. (1995). Contraception: how today's options stack up. 8:13–14.

PARRAN, THOMAS P. (1937). *Shadow on the Land: Syphilis*. New York: Reynal and Hitchcock.

PERRONE, JANICE. (1989). U.S. cities launch new AIDS weapon. *Am. Med. News,* March:68–71.

PINES, MAYA. (1993). Blood: Bearer of life and death. *Howard Hughes Med. Inst.,* 6:17.

POTTS, MALCOLM. (1994). Urgent need for a vaginal microbicide in the prevention of HIV transmission. *Am. J. Public Health,* 84:890–891.

RAYMOND, CHRIS ANNE. (1988). U.S. cities struggle to implement needle exchanges despite apparent success in European cities. *JAMA,* 260:2620–2621.

ROPER, WILLIAM L., et al. (1993). Commentary: Condoms and HIV/STD prevention—clarifying the message. *Am. J. Public Health,* 83:501–503.

ROSENBERG, MICHAEL J., et al. (1992). Commentary: Methods women can use that may prevent STDs including HIV. *Am. J. Public Health,* 82:1473–1478.

ROTHENBERG, KAREN, et al. (1995). The risk of domestic violence and women with HIV infection: Implications for partner notification, public policy, and the law. *Am. J. Public Health,* 85: 1569–1576.

RUTHERFORD, GEORGE W. (1988). Contact tracing and the control of human immunodeficiency virus infection. *JAMA,* 259:3609–3670.

SATTAR, SYED A., et al. (1991). Survival and disinfectant inactivation of HIV: A critical review. *Rev. of Infect. Dis.,* 13:430–447.

Science. (1996). Uganda may host AIDS vaccine trial. 272:657.

SELLERS, DEBORAH, et al. (1994). Does the promotion and distribution of condoms increase teen sexual activity? Evidence from an HIV prevention program for Latino youth. *Am. J. Public Health,* 84:1952–1958.

SINGH, B., et al. (1982). Demonstration of a spirocheticidal effect by chemical contraceptives on *Treponema pallidum. Bull. Pan. Am. Health Organ.,* 16:59–64.

STIMSON, GERRY V., et al. (1989). Syringe exchange. *International Working Group on AIDS and IV Drug Use,* 4:15.

STOECKLE, MARK, et al. (1996). Infectious diseases. *JAMA,* 275:1816–1817

STONE, KATHERINE M., et al. (1986). Personal protection against sexually transmitted diseases. *Am. J. Obstet. Gynecol.,* 155:180–88.

STRAUS, STEPHEN, et al. (1994). Placebo-controlled trial of vaccination with recombinant glycoprotein D of herpes simplex virus type 2 for immunotherapy of genital herpes, *Lancet,* 343:1460.

STRATTON, P., et al. (1993). Prevention of sexually transmitted infections: Physical and Chemical barrier methods. *Infect. Dis. Clin. North Am.,* 7(4):841–859.

THOMPSON, DICK. (1992). Getting the point in New Haven. *Time,* 139:55–56.

TIERNO, PHILIP M. (1988). AIDS overview: New guidelines for handling specimens. *Am. J. Cont. Ed. Nurs.,* Special Issue:1–14.

Time. (1992). Closed: Needle Park. 139:53.

U.S. Public Health Service. (1994). Counseling to prevent unintended pregnancy. *Am. Fam. Phys.,* 50(5):971.

VOELKER, REBECCA. (1995a). Scientists zero in on new HIV microbicides. *JAMA,* 273:979–980.

VOELKER, REBECCA. (1995b). Lessons from cat virus. *JAMA,* 273:910.

WEI, XIPING, et al. (1995). Viral dynamics in HIV infection. *Nature,* 373:117–122.

WEINSTEIN, STEPHEN P., et al. (1990). AIDS and cocaine: A deadly combination facing the primary care physician. *J. Fam. Prac.,* 31:253–254.

WELLER, SUSAN. (1993). A meta-analysis of condom effectiveness in reducing sexually transmitted HIV. *Soc. Sci. Med.* 36:1635–1644.

WENIGER, BRUCE C. (1994). Experience from HIV incedence cohorts in Thailand: Implications for HIV vaccine efficacy trials. *AIDS,* 8:1007–1010.

WHITE, NICK, et al. (1988). Dangers of lubricants used with condoms. *Nature,* 335:19.

WITTKOWSKI, KNUT. (1995). The potential of nonoxynol–9 for the prevention of HIV infection reconsidered. AIDS, 9:310.

WODAK, ALEX. (1990). Australia smashes international needle and syringe exchange record. *International Working Group on AIDS and IV Drug Use,* 5:28–29.

World Health Organization. (1995). Scientific and public health rationals for HIV vaccine efficacy trials. *AIDS,* 9:1–3.

Incidence and Prevalence of HIV Infections, AIDS Cases, and Deaths Among Select Groups in the United States

CHAPTER CONCEPTS

♦ AIDS is a new plague.

♦ Men make up 80% of all AIDS cases; 20% are women.

♦ The majority of people with AIDS can be associated with certain lifestyle risks.

♦ AIDS can be associated with single or multiple exposures.

♦ AIDS cases can be separated by sex, age group, race, ethnicity, and sexual preference.

♦ Risk is strongly tied to social behavior.

♦ Behavioral risk groups include homosexual and bisexual men, injection drug users (IDUs), hemophiliacs, transfusion patients, and the sex partners of these people.

♦ IDU is strongly associated with HIV infection.

♦ All military personnel are tested for HIV.

♦ Two per 1,000 college students are HIV-infected.

♦ Thirty states report HIV-infected by name

♦ High rates of HIV infection have been found among prisoners.

♦ The greatest HIV threat to health care workers is needlestick (syringe) injuries.

♦ All 50 states and U.S. territories must report all AIDS cases.

♦ People do not always tell the truth when completing questionnaires, especially with regard to sexual behavior.

It is easy to be overwhelmed by statistics in reporting on HIV infections and AIDS cases and to lose track of the human faces of the epidemic. But certain numbers, like the **first half million documented AIDS cases reported in October 1995** and over 440,000 dead by the end of 1998, take on a compelling quality of their own. Therefore within this chapter there are many statistics presented on all facets of the

HIV/AIDS pandemic. After reading this chapter one will have gained a deeper insight into the spread of HIV and those who are affected by HIV: those who have it, and those who don't—those who will suffer and those who won't. But in reality we are all impacted by this disease in one way or the other!

The **prevalence** of a disease refers to the percentage of a population that is affected by it at a given time. For example, the total number of AIDS cases or number of HIV infections reported in the United States, by your state or city to the CDC, say for the year 1996. The **incidence** means the number of times an event occurs in a given time frame, for example, the number of new AIDS cases each month or new HIV infections each week (events that occur within a specified period of time). The two terms are similar. Much has been learned about the prevalence of HIV infection, HIV disease, and its terminal stage called AIDS since the 1981 CDC report that awakened the world to this new epidemic.

Although cases of AIDS appear retrospectively to have occurred in the United States as early as 1952, the **AIDS pandemic** is con-

sidered to have begun with the initial report early in 1981. Since then, there has been a rapid rise in reported AIDS cases (Table 10-1). The accelerated rise in AIDS cases means that there must be a reservoir of asymptomatic HIV-infected people who **with time** progress to AIDS.

If the accumulative world AIDS deaths had occurred in a single year, this pandemic would top the list of the worst natural disasters of the 20th century. Natural disasters are often analyzed in terms of global vulnerability to events with a rapid onset such as tropical storms, earthquakes, and volcanic eruptions. The slower onset of the AIDS pandemic, with about 440,000 deaths from early 1981 through the end of 1998, sets it apart from natural disasters; but in terms of cost and human suffering, it is no different. If only the 35,000 to 45,000 deaths per year from 1991 through 1998 are used as reference points, the yearly numbers are still greater than the number of deaths caused by most of the natural disasters recorded in this century. By the end of this century, AIDS will be the most common cause of death in the United States (HIV Guideline Panel, 1994).

Is it your impression that some of your friends and associates *still* regard HIV/AIDS as someone else's problem? HIV/AIDS has invaded *all* segments of society worldwide! It is EVERYONE'S problem!

The 1990s are the second decade of HIV disease/AIDS. The prevalence of HIV infection and new AIDS cases will continue to increase dramatically. More people have died in the United States of AIDS in any 2 years from 1988

TABLE 10-1 AIDS Cases a Percentage of Total Population: United States, 1982–1997

Year	Total Population[a]	Number of AIDS Cases[b]	Percent with AIDS
1982	231,534	1,500	<0.0005
1983	233,981	2,760	<0.001
1984	236,158	4,445	0.001
1985	238,740	8,249	0.003
1986	241,078	12,932	0.005
1987	243,400	21,070	0.009
1988	245,807	31,001	0.013
1989	248,239	33,722	0.014
1990	248,710	44,755	0.018
1991	252,177	53,176	0.020
1992	254,462	49,106	0.019
1993	257,301	106,618	0.041
1994	260,507	80,901	0.031
1995	262,605	74,180	0.028
1996[c]	265,513	69,151	0.026
1997[c]	266,473	61,300	0.023

[a]United States total resident population in thousands.

[b]Number of AIDS cases reported, by year, to the Centers for Disease Control and Prevention, Atlanta, Georgia, USA. **AIDS cases are underreported by 10% to 20%.**

[c]1997 data are estimated based on reports adapted from HIV/AIDS Surveillance Report, June 1997.

_____ BOX 10.2 _____

THE HIV/AIDS PANDEMIC HAS LIMITS

Epidemics or pandemics typically reach a point of saturation whereby incidence levels off under 100% of the population. This happens because some people either are naturally immune or avoid exposure to the disease. Thus AIDS will not wipe out entire populations, but the point of saturation for HIV (number of susceptible persons infected) probably varies substantially from population to population and cannot be predicted with any precision.

National Number of Persons Living With AIDS (1994)	Number of PLWA in Your City (1994)

$$\frac{170,000}{1,200,000} \times \frac{(e.g.,)\ 1,000}{x} = 170,000$$

(Estimated national number of HIV - infected persons)

$$x = 1,200,000,000$$

$$x = \frac{1,200,000,000}{170,000}$$

$$= 7,509$$

(About 7,509 persons in this sample city are HIV-infected.)

through 1998 than died during the 8 years of the Vietnam war. In the United States, for 1996, and 1997 about 178 people a day were diagnosed with AIDS and between 120 and 200 a day become HIV-infected. Worldwide, 9,000 become HIV-infected each day, 1,000 of these are children. Currently one person dies of AIDS in the United States about every 13 minutes; worldwide, at least two every minute.

OLD FORMULA FOR ESTIMATING HIV INFECTIONS

The estimated prevalence of HIV infection in the United States is an important measure of the extent of the nation's HIV disease/AIDS problem. Initial estimates on the number of HIV-infected people were based on the CDC formula: for every diagnosed case of AIDS, there are 50 to 100 people who are HIV-infected. The estimate was crude, but data essential for greater specificity were lacking. This was a new plague and no one was prepared for it. A workable definition for what constituted an AIDS patient had to be agreed upon. Surveillance networks also had to be set up to gather information on areas of highest incidence, who was being infected, and routes of transmission.

NEWER FORMULA FOR ESTIMATING HIV INFECTIONS

A newer formula proposed by the CDC for use in determining the number of HIV-infected persons is as follows:

Single or Multiple Exposure Categories

In Table 10-2, the number of AIDS cases through June 1997 are presented with respect to adult/adolescent, **single** or **multiple** exposure categories. For example, under **_Single Mode of Exposure_**, heterosexual contact accounts for 9% of all AIDS cases. Under **_Multiple Modes of Exposure_**, 5% of AIDS cases occurred among injection drug users who also had heterosexual contact. In other words, Table 10-2 lists the numbers and percentages of all reported AIDS cases broken down into seven categories of people who contracted HIV/AIDS from a single risk mode of exposure and 26 categories of people who contracted HIV/AIDS from multiple risk modes of exposure. Note that of the total number of adult/adolescent AIDS cases, 79% occurred from **single risk** modes of exposure. Of this 79%, 47% occurred among men who had sex with men and 21% among injection drug users.

A composite representation of all AIDS cases by exposure category reported through 1997 is shown in Figure 8-1.

BEHAVIORAL RISK GROUPS AND STATISTICAL EVALUATION

Behavioral Risk Groups and AIDS Cases

As the pool of AIDS patients grew in number during 1981–1983, individual case histories were separated into **behavioral risk groups**. The early case histories of AIDS patients

TABLE 10-2 Adult/Adolescent AIDS Cases by Single and Multiple Exposure Categories, Reported through June 1997, United States

Exposure Category	AIDS Cases No.	(%)
Single Mode of Exposure		
1. Men who have sex with men	286,661	(47)
2. Injection (IJ) drug use	124,684	(21)
3. Hemophilia/coagulation disorder	3,673	(1)
4. Heterosexual contact	53,119	(9)
5. Receipt of transfusion of blood, blood component, or tissue	8,063	(1)
6. Receipt of transplant of tissues/organs	12	(0)
7. Other/undetermined	95	(0)
Single Mode of Exposure Subtotal	476,257	(79)
Multiple Modes of Exposure		
1. Men who have sex with men; IJ drug use	33,600	(6)
2. Men who have sex with men; hemophilia	151	(0)
3. Men who have sex with men; heterosexual contact	8,366	(1)
4. Men who have sex with men; receipt of transfusion/transplant	3,260	(1)
5. IJ drug use; hemophilia	182	(0)
6. IJ drug use; heterosexual contact	27,251	(5)
7. IJ drug use; receipt of transfusion	1,541	(0)
8. Hemophilia; heterosexual contact	83	(0)
9. Hemophilia; receipt of transfusion/transplant	779	(0)
10. Heterosexual contact; receipt of transfusion/transplant	1,452	(0)
11. Men who have sex with men; IJ drug use; hemophilia	43	(0)
12. Men who have sex with men; IJ drug use; heterosexual contact	4,528	(1)
13. Men who have sex with men; IJ drug use; receipt of transfusion/transplant	573	(0)
14. Men who have sex with men; hemophilia; heterosexual contact	20	(0)
15. Men who have sex with men; hemophilia; receipt of transfusion/transplant	34	(0)
16. Men who have sex with men; heterosexual contact; receipt of transfusion/transplant	252	(0)
17. IJ drug use; hemophilia; heterosexual contact	60	(0)
18. IJ drug use; hemophilia; receipt of transfusion/transplant	36	(0)
19. IJ drug use; heterosexual contact; receipt of tranfusion/transplant	892	(0)
20. Hemophilia; heterosexual contact; receipt of transfusion/transplant	32	(0)
21. Men who have sex with men; IJ drug use; hemophilia; heterosexual contact	8	(0)
22. Men who have sex with men; IJ drug use; hemophilia; receipt of transfusion/transplant	13	(0)
23. Men who have sex with men; IJ drug use; heterosexual contact; receipt of transfusion/transplant	153	(0)
24. Men who have sex with men; hemophilia; heterosexual contact; receipt of transfusion/transplant	5	(0)
25. IJ drug use; hemophilia; heterosexual contact; receipt of transfusion/transplant	18	(0)
26. Men who have sex with men; IJ drug use; hemophilia; heterosexual contact; receipt of transfusion/transplant	5	(0)
Multiple Modes of Exposure for AIDS Cases	83,337	(14)
Risk Not Reported or Identified	44,582	(7)
Total AIDS Cases	604,176	(100)

(Source: For exposure categories. CDC HIV/AIDS Surveillance Report, through June 1997, 9:1–39)

clearly separated people according to their social behavior and medical needs. AIDS patients were placed into the following six risk behavior categories: (1) homosexual and bisexual men; (2) injection drug users; (3) hemophiliacs; (4) blood transfusion recipients; (5) heterosexuals; and (6) children whose parents are at risk. Each of these groups is considered to be at risk of HIV infection based on some common behavioral denominator. That is, those within these groups represented a higher rate of AIDS cases than people whose needs or behaviors excluded them from these groups. However, because there is some mixing between individuals in behavioral risk groups, HIV infection has gradually spread to lower-risk behavioral groups. Over time the behavioral risk groups have been aligned and defined according to age, exposure category, and sex (see Table 10-2).

A review of AIDS cases by sex/age at diagnosis, and race/ethnicity reported through December 1996 in the United States, shows that white, black, and Hispanic males between the ages of 20 and 44 make up 79% of all male AIDS cases. Between ages 20 and 59, they make up 96% of all male AIDS cases. Of the total number of male AIDS cases, 50% are white, 31% are black, and 17% are Hispanic. Figure 10-1 shows the distribution of **male** adult/adolescent AIDS cases reported for 1996 in the United States. Figure 10-2 shows the distribution of **male** adult/adolescent AIDS cases per 100,000 population in the United States.

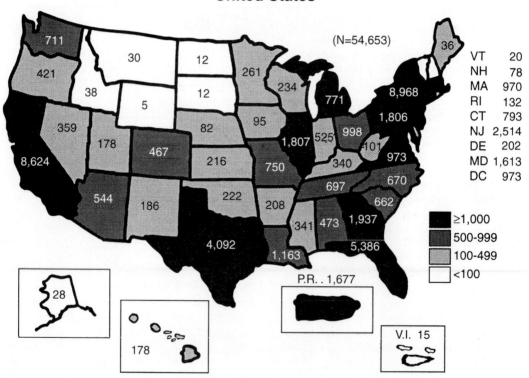

FIGURE 10-1   One Year of New AIDS Cases, Male Adults/Adolescents Across the United States, Reported for 1996. (Total AIDS cases for 1996, 69,151) (*Source: Courtesy of CDC, Atlanta*)

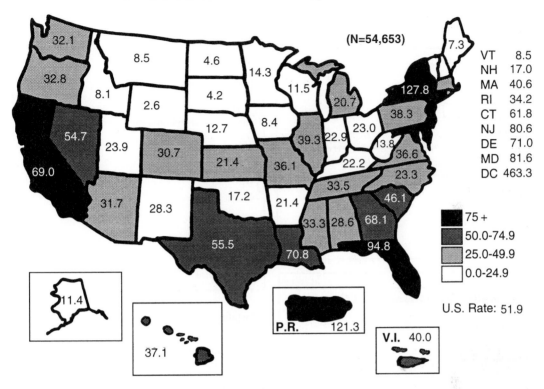

Adolescent/Adult Men AIDS Annual Rates per 100,000 Population United States — Cases Reported in 1996

(N=54,653)

VT	8.5
NH	17.0
MA	40.6
RI	34.2
CT	61.8
NJ	80.6
DE	71.0
MD	81.6
DC	463.3

75 +
50.0-74.9
25.0-49.9
0.0-24.9

U.S. Rate: 51.9

P.R.   121.3

V.I.   40.0

FIGURE 10-2   Rates of Reported AIDS Cases Per 100,000 Population Among Adolescent and Adult Men by State of Residence—United States, 1996. (*Source: Courtesy of CDC, Atlanta*)

Statistical Evaluation of Selected Risk Behavioral Group AIDS Cases

Adult/Adolescent AIDS Cases— October 31, 1995 is the time in history when the United States reached **a half million** (501,310) reported AIDS cases (*MMWR*, 1995a) (Figure 10-3). Through 1997, 650,000 AIDS cases and 403,000 AIDS-related deaths were reported to the CDC. Sixty-nine percent of all AIDS cases reported occurred between 1993 through 1997. Cumulative through 1996, 9% of AIDS cases have occurred among the heterosexual population, 26% occurred among injection drug users, and 56% occurred in the male homosexual/bisexual IDU population. For the first time (1996) since the United States AIDS pandemic began, more blacks were diagnosed with AIDS (41%) then whites (38%). Table 10–3 presents the total number of AIDS cases for 1996 and their distribution based on race, sex, and exposure group.

Figure 10-4 shows that the percentage of AIDS cases for ethnic related adult/adolescent groups are in striking contrast to the population percentages of each group. For example, in 1996 whites made up 74% of the population and represented 38% of adult/adolescent AIDS cases. Blacks made up 12% of the population but represented 41% of the adult/adolescent AIDS cases. Hispanics made up 10% of the population but represented 19% of the adult/adolescent AIDS cases.

FIGURE 10-3 A Profile of the First 650,000 AIDS Cases: June 1981 Through 1997—United States. Four hundred and three thousand people had died of AIDS to this point in time. Data may not add to 100% due to rounding off. (*Source: MMWR, 1995b, updated*)

Collectively, in 1996, blacks and Hispanics made up 22% of the population but make up 60% of adult/adolescent and 85% of pediatric AIDS cases **reported**. Thus, blacks and Hispanics contribute disproportionately high percentages to the total number of reported AIDS cases.

In 1995, 1 in 350 black men in the United States aged 25–44 years was diagnosed with AIDS, which is about **five times higher** than the annual incidence rate among white men (1 in 1,800). For black women in the same age group this rate was 1 in 1,100, for Hispanic women 1 in 2,500, whereas among white women this was 1 in 15,000 (Coutinho et al., 1996).

According to 1993 data analyzed by Philip Rosenberg (1995) of the National Cancer Institute, 1 in every 92 American men between **ages 27 and 39 may be HIV-infected**. The findings were especially dismal for African-American men, with 1 in 33 estimated to be HIV infected. The estimate was 1 in 60 for Hispanic men. And although women were more than four times **less likely** to be infected with HIV, the statistics were equally high for women of color. One in 98 African-American women and 1 in 222 Hispanic women are estimated to be infected with HIV. By comparison, the number of white women infected with HIV was 1 in 1,667. If the trends continue,

TABLE 10-3 Adult/Adolescent Behavioral Risk Groups, Race and Sex: Percent of Total AIDS Cases—United States, 1996

HIV/AIDS	No. of Cases[a]	% of Cases
Exposure Group		
Homosexual/bisexual male	27,389	40
Injection drug user (IDU)	17,027	25
Homosexual/bisexual IDU	2,967	4
Hemophiliac	318	1
Heterosexual contact	8,821	13
Transfusion related	551	1
None of the above	11,400	16
Total	68,473	100
Race/Ethnicity (all cases)		
White (non-Hispanic)	26,229	38
Black (non-Hispanic)	28,346	41
Hispanic	13,984	19
Other	1,718	2
Sex (adults only)		
Male	54,653	80
Female	13,820	20
Age Group (yrs)		
13–19	405	0.5
20–24	2,432	3.6
25–29	11,374	14.2
30–39	33,021	45.8
40–49	18,395	26.0
50–59	5,870	7.3
60 and above	2,201	2.6

[a]Total in each category = 68,473 adult/adolescent plus 678 pediatric = 69,151 = 100% of cases for 1996.

(Adapted from AIDS Surveillance Year End Report, 1996)

Rosenberg noted, HIV/AIDS in young people and minorities must be considered "endemic in the United States."

The Harvard AIDS Institute reported in October 1996 that by the year 2000, more than half of all AIDS cases in the United States will be among blacks. By the same year, a black person will be nine times more likely to be diagnosed with AIDS than someone who is not black. The Institute estimated that nearly 100 blacks and Hispanic Americans are diagnosed with AIDS every day (1 every 14 minutes) in the United States.

Figure 10-5 is a United States map of all AIDS cases reported to the CDC through the year 1997. Note that the highest incidence of AIDS cases occurs along the coastal regions.

Behavioral Risk Groups and Percentages of HIV-Infected People

Beginning 1998, investigators at the CDC found that HIV infection remained largely confined to the populations at recognized behavioral risks: homosexual men, injection drug users, heterosexual partners of injection drug users, hemophiliacs, and children of HIV-infected mothers. In the general population, rates for HIV infection include 0.04% for first-time blood donors, 0.14% for military applicants, 0.33% for Job Corps entrants, 0.19% to 0.87% for child-bearing women, and 0.30% for hospital patients. Data reported by the CDC in 1990 indicated that while the number of new AIDS cases increased by 5% in cities, it had increased by 37% in rural areas. This trend continues.

Comments on a Variety of Individual Behavioral Risk Groups

It must be kept in mind that because a group of people is at risk for HIV does not mean that these people are predestined to become infected. People are placed within these groups because of their social behavior, a behavior that has been associated with a high-, medium- or low-risk of becoming HIV-infected. Essentially there is no zero-risk group because a scenario can always be formulated to show that under certain circumstances one or more members of that group could become HIV-infected.

The point of placing people in behavioral risk groups is not to offend them but to provide a warning that certain behavior might make them more vulnerable to HIV infection. It is not the race or ethnic group that people belong to that places them at high or low risk for infection, it is their behavior.

The fact that AIDS was first identified in 1981 in seemingly well-defined behavioral groups (homosexual men, injection drug users, hemophiliacs, Haitian immigrants) probably contributed to a false sense of security among people who did not belong to any of these groups. However, as information about HIV and AIDS accumulated, it became

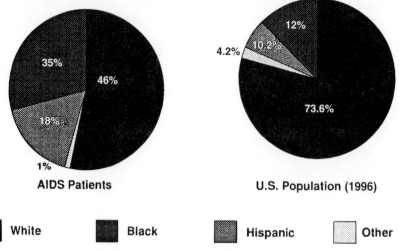

AIDS Patients

U.S. Population (1996)

■ White ▦ Black ▒ Hispanic □ Other

FIGURE 10-4 Racial and Ethnic AIDS Patient Classification. Adult AIDS cases show a disproportionate percentage among blacks and Hispanics. Fifty-four percent of reported AIDS cases occur among racial and ethnic minorities. The figures reflect higher rates of AIDS in blacks and Hispanic injection drug users and their sex partners. Percentages of the population are based on the numbers of AIDS cases in the United States estimated through 1997. U.S. population data (over 267,000,000).

clear that HIV was transmitted in body fluids. This had grave implications for all social groups. On reflection, the people in the original high-risk groups simply had the bad luck of being in the way of a newly emerging infectious agent as it first began to spread. It is highly probable that in the different behavioral risk groups there were lifestyle or medical history factors that increased the efficiency with which the virus was transmitted.

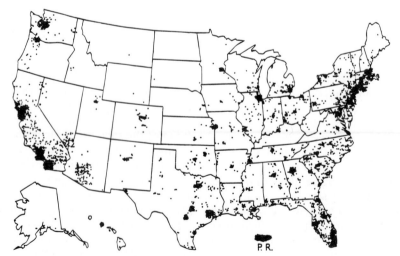

FIGURE 10-5 Surveillance Report Showing the Approximate Location of AIDS Cases that Occurred through the Year 1997.

Men Who Have Sex with Men (MSM)— In 1981, 100% of all AIDS cases reported to the CDC occurred in homosexual males. For 1993, 46% of the 106,618 new AIDS cases occurred in gay males; in 1995, 43%in 1996, 40% (*MMWR*, 1995a; HIV/AIDS surveillance report, 1996). It appears that in the 1990s, the number of gay male AIDS cases, as a percentage of all AIDS cases, is significantly decreasing. The *Morbidity and Mortality Weekly Report* (1995b) documents the disproportionate occurrence of AIDS among black and Hispanic MSM compared with white MSM from 1981 through 1995. This finding underscores the need for community planning groups to consider culturally appropriate prevention services when addressing the HIV-prevention needs of radical/ethnic minorities. There are indicators of a second wave in the HIV/AIDS epidemic among gay males.

In a survey by Robert Hays and colleagues (1990, 1992), of gay men aged 18 to 25, 42% reported having engaged in unprotected anal intercourse in the previous 6 months. In a study of 258 gay men aged 17 to 25 conducted at gay dance clubs in San Francisco, 12% were found to be infected with HIV (Lemp, 1991). Finally, studies show that a significant percentage of gay men who had originally adopted safer sex behaviors are "relapsing" to unsafe sex (Stall et al., 1990; Lemp et al., 1994).

As most people who have attempted to change behavior know, it is difficult to maintain new behavior patterns over a long period of time. Increasing attention and concern has been focused on the issue of relapse. High seroprevalence levels among homosexual men (estimated to be 50% in high incidence cities such as San Francisco) make relapse to risky behaviors a significant source of new infections and justify continued interventions to reinforce behavior change.

SIZE OF THE HOMOSEXUAL COMMUNITY. Estimating the size of the homosexual population continues to be a problem for the CDC. Because of the lack of available information on sexual practices, the CDC has relied on the 1948 Kinsey report, *Sexual Behavior in the Human Male*, for its estimate that 2.5 million (10%) American males are **exclusively** homo-

sexual, while another 2.5 to 7.5 million have **occasional** homosexual contacts. These numbers are refuted by some recent surveys like the 1992 National Opinion Research Center that reports that among males, 2.8% are exclusively gay, and among women, 2.5% are exclusively lesbian. Judith Reisman argues in her 1990 book, *Kinsey, Sex and Fraud*, that male homosexuals make up about 1% of the population. The group, Coloradans for Family Values and the Washington-based Family Research Institute believe about 3% of the male population is exclusively gay. In the late 1980s, Congress approved two national surveys of sexual behavior but this action was stopped in the United States Senate.

Using data collected from HIV testing conducted in 1986 and 1987, the CDC estimates that 20% of exclusively homosexual men are HIV-infected. This means (depending on whose numbers are used) that between 500,000 and 625,000 gay males are HIV-infected. For bisexuals and men with infrequent homosexual encounters, the CDC tabulates a prevalence rate of 5%, meaning that between 125,000 and 375,000 of this population are HIV-infected (Booth, 1988). Approximately 6% of all IDU-associated AIDS cases occur in the homosexual/bisexual male population. These cases may reflect HIV transmission either by contaminated syringes or sexual activity.

Injection Drug Users— According to the CDC, as many as 33% of the nation's 1.2 million injection drug users may be HIV-infected. This behavioral risk group contains the nation's second largest group of HIV-infected and AIDS patients. An association between injection drug use and AIDS was recognized in 1981, about 2 years before the virus was identified. AIDS in IDUs and hemophiliacs offered the first evidence that whatever caused AIDS was being carried in and transmitted by human blood. From the first reported IDU AIDS cases in 1981 through 1997, 27% of all adult/adolescent AIDS cases occurred in IDUs. Of IDUs, 74% listed IDU as their **only** risk factor for HIV infection; 26% were also homosexual/bisexual. The CDC estimates that through 1997 47% of women and 22% of men with AIDS were/are strictly IDUs.

IDUs have been reported in all 50 states and the District of Columbia. Fifty-two percent of the accumulated 160,000 IDU-only AIDS cases occurred in New York and New Jersey. Among the adult/adolescent heterosexual AIDS cases over half had sexual partners who are/were IDUs. Beginning 1998, of the estimated 650,000 AIDS cases, 234,000 (36%) were directly or indirectly associated with IDU (*MMWR*, 1996a).

Rates for IDU-associated AIDS varied widely by area: rates in Puerto Rico, New Jersey, New York, and the District of Columbia were greater than 10 per 100,000; in 22 states, rates were lower than 1 per 100,000 population.

About 55% of all IDU-associated cases were reported in the Northeast, which represents about 20% of the population of the United States and its territories. The South reported 20% of IDU-associated AIDS cases, 5% from the Midwest, and the West reported the remaining 20%.

The rate of IDU-associated AIDS continues to be higher for blacks and Hispanics than for whites. Except for the West, where rates for whites and Hispanics were similar, this difference by race/ethnicity was observed in all regions of the country and was greatest in the Northeast. J. Peterson and colleagues (1989) reported that among **heterosexual** men, injection drug use accounts for 83% of black, 87% of Hispanic, and 45% of white AIDS cases. Through 1997, overall IDU-associated **male** AIDS cases represented 9% of all AIDS cases in whites, 36% in blacks, 37% in Hispanics, 5% in Asians/Pacific Islanders, and 15% in American Indians/Alaskan Natives. For **women** it was; white, 43%; black.47%; hispanoc, 44%; 17% Asian/Pacific Islanders; and 44% American Indian/Alaskan Natives.

Heterosexuals— The spread of HIV in the general population is relatively slow, yet potentially it is the source of the greatest numbers of HIV/AIDS cases. The CDC estimates there are 142 million Americans **without** an identified at-risk behavior, the general population.

Data from the CDC beginning 1998 indicated that 9% of all the AIDS cases in the United States occurred through heterosexual contact. But this must be placed in perspective. Although 9% of anything may be a significant number, beginning 1998 it stood for about 58,500 adult/adolescent/pediatric AIDS cases out of the total 650,000. Most of these heterosexual AIDS cases occurred in persons or the sexual partners of individuals with an identified behavioral risk. Relative to the general adult population, the number of heterosexual AIDS cases is only a fraction of 1%. Of the 40,000 new HIV infections expected to occur each year beginning 1996 through the year 2000, only 2,000 or 5% are expected to occur in the heterosexual population.

In the United States, CDC data for 1994 and 1995 indicate that 5% of heterosexual men in each year contracted HIV from women. Worldwide, through 1998, **heterosexuals** will make up 75% of the 35 million HIV-infected people. Over half of these people live in Sub-Saharan Africa (about 24 million). North America (1.5 million), Latin America (2.3 million), South and Southeast Asia (6.3 million), and Africa account for 97% of global HIV infections (Figure 10-6).

Of the 35 million HIV-infected people worldwide, over 90% live in nonindustrial nations. It is estimated that through 1998, 10 million people will have AIDS worldwide, 77% of those cases will be in Africa, 7% in Asia, 6% in the United States, and 3% in Europe. The Joint United Nations program an HIV/AIDS (UNAIDS) estimate that 7.3 million (72.5%) of the 10 million will have died (UNAIDS, 1996 updated).

The World Health Organization (WHO) projected that by the year 2000, up to 90% of all HIV infections globally will be transmitted heterosexually. In 1996, the WHO estimated that there are about to a half a **billion** heterosexuals who are at moderate to high risk of exposure to HIV because of multiple sexual partners. In addition, there are about 10 million homosexuals and 5 million drug users who are also at moderate to high risk because of multiple sex partners or regular sharing of injection equipment. Most HIV infections in North America have been transmitted homosexually to men who practiced receptive anorectal intercourse, whereas most of those occurring in Africa and parts of the Caribbean have been transmitted heterosexually to both women and men during vaginal intercourse.

Heterosexual transmission accounts for a growing proportion of HIV/AIDS cases in Europe and Latin America, and is proliferating at explosive rates in parts of Thailand and India (Aral et al., 1991). Homosexual transmission still predominates in North America, but heterosexual transmission is increasing.

Hemophiliacs— There are about 16,000 to 20,000 hemophiliacs in the United States. At least half are HIV-positive and through 1997, 2,650 of them have died . Of those infected, over 98% received HIV in blood products that were essential to their survival. By mid-1985, an HIV blood screening test was put into effect nationally. From that point, the risk of HIV infection from the blood supply has been significantly lowered but a small risk still exists. Scandals in knowingly selling HIV-positive blood for transfusions and in production of the blood factor essential for hemophiliacs have surfaced in France, Germany, the United States, Canada, and Japan in the 1990s. (For discussion, see Chapter 8.)

From 1982 through 1997, 4,567 adult/adolescent, 400 sexual partners of hemophiliacs, and 255 hemophilic pediatric AIDS cases have been reported. Almost all of these cases are the result of HIV infections that occurred prior to 1985.

Military— The incidence of HIV infection can be measured best in groups that undergo routine serial testing. Because active duty military personnel and civilian applicants for the service are routinely tested for HIV antibody, there is a unique opportunity to measure the incidence of HIV infection in a large, demographically varied subset of the general population.

Since October 1985, all military personnel on active duty, as well as all civilian applicants for military service, have undergone mandatory testing for HIV antibody. Over the next 2 years, the armed forces screened 3.96 million people for exposure to HIV. Of the 3.96 million tested, 5,890 (0.15%) were HIV-positive. This total included active duty personnel, members of the National Guard, members of reserve units, and would-be recruits. The recruits who tested positive have been barred from entering the service. Those carrying HIV who are already in uniform are allowed to stay in the service as long as they remain asymptomatic. They are, however, ineligible for overseas duty and must undergo close health monitoring.

Through 1997, there were an estimated 1,049 HIV-positive persons in the military who became HIV-positive **while serving in the military**. The Navy has the highest incidence of HIV, with 2.5 per 1,000 people. The rate in the Army is 1.4 per 1,000; in the Marines, 1 per 1,000; and in the Air Force, 0.99 per 1,000. The higher rate in the Navy may reflect that Navy personnel are based primarily on the East and West Coasts, which have the highest number of AIDS cases.

Early in 1996, the U.S. Congress passed a defense bill that contained a provision dedicated to discharging all HIV-positive persons from the military. This decision is under appeal.

College Students— Between April 1988 and February 1989, the blood of 16,863 students enrolled at 16 large universities and three private colleges was tested for HIV antibodies. Thirty students, 28 males and 2 females, tested HIV-positive for an overall rate of 2 per 1,000 or 0.2%. With 12.5 million students enrolled in American colleges and universities, the rate of 2 in 1,000 means there are about 25,000 HIV-infected college students.

The study was conducted by the CDC with The American College Health Association (Gayle et al., 1988). Because the samples were not identified, students who tested positive could not be informed. All blood samples from 10 of the 19 campuses were HIV-negative. At five campuses the rate of HIV-positive blood ranged from four to nine samples per 1,000. In contrast, the rate of HIV in the general heterosexual population is about 0.02% and the rate for military personnel in about the same age group tested over a similar time period was 0.14%.

The important question is **why** college students have a rate of HIV infection 10 times higher than the general heterosexual population. Are college students less well informed than the general heterosexual population?

Surveys indicate that college students are well educated about HIV/AIDS. Why, then, the higher rate of infection? Perhaps it's the age-old dilemma of information versus behavior. **They know what to do—but they don't do it.**

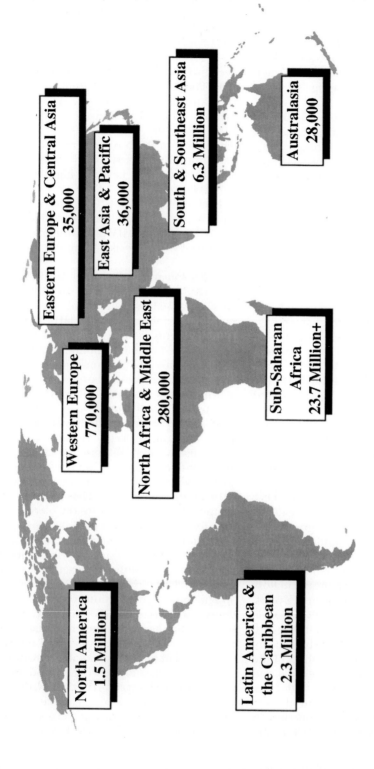

Global Total: 35 Million

FIGURE 10-6 Estimated Number of Global HIV Infections Projected by the World Health Organization through 1998. Of the 35 million HIV-infected persons, 26 million **are living** in some state of HIV/AIDS illness. Over 1 million of these are children of 209 countries reporting AIDS cases to the WHO and UNAIDS; 194 have reported AIDS cases. (*Source: Pan American Health Organization Quarterly Report, September 1996 updated*)

There is a difference between knowledge and action based on that knowledge. College students have always had information on drug use, alcoholism, pregnancies out of wedlock, and sexually transmitted diseases; but this knowledge has not appreciably reduced at-risk behaviors. STDs are at an all-time high in teenage and college students.

COLLEGE STUDENTS AND NATIONAL ISSUES. In April of 1994, the Roper College Track poll asked undergraduate students at 4-year colleges and universities, "What are the national issues you are most concerned about?" Their overwhelming response was AIDS. Of the top 10 issues listed most frequently, 50% of students listed AIDS as their main concern, followed by crime at 34%, drugs 21%, quality of education 20%, cost of health care 19%, moral values and race relations at 17% each, the budget deficit 16%, and environmental damage and poverty each at 15%.

Prisoners— Beginning 1997, the nation's prison population was at an all-time high of over 1,650,000 adults: contained in 1,300 state and 71 federal prisons.

According to the United States Bureau of Justice Statistics, 2.4% of these people or 39,600 are HIV-positive and of these, 17% have AIDS (Rubel et al., 1997). The total number of **prisoners**, **parolees**, and **probationers** in 1996 was 4,450,000 with an HIV-positive rate of 2.4% or 107,000 being HIV-positive (DeGroot et al., 1996). Beginning 1997, about 5,500 adult inmates in U.S. state and federal prisons and jails had died of AIDS. And, an additional 5,500 people with AIDS were still in prisons and jails (*MMWR*, 1996c). In 1995 through 1997, **four states**—New York, Florida, Texas, and California—had **more than half** the known cases of HIV in prison. Condoms are not available in prisons of these four states. In fact, only six prison systems in the United States distribute or sell condoms to male inmates (Hooker, 1996) and only two of the six distribute dental dams and condoms to female inmates. **No** United States correctional facility distributes bleach or syringes to inmates (Mahon, 1996).

Blood testing of inmates at 10 selected prisons indicated that 1 in every 24 prisoners is infected with HIV. This study also found that incarcerated women under age 25 had a higher HIV seroprevalence (5.2%) than incarcerated young men (2.3%). The rate was comparable among older women (5.3%) and older men (5.6%). Non-whites were almost twice as likely to be infected as whites. Rates varied widely among the 10 institutions from 2.1% to 7.6% for men, and 2.7% to 14.7% for women (Vlahov et al., 1991).

In general, prisoners diagnosed with AIDS were infected prior to their incarceration—most are IDUs (Francis, 1987). Infected inmates most often transmit the virus to others through homosexual and drug-related activities. For that reason 21 states segregated HIV-infected and AIDS patient prisoners from the other prisoners. In September of 1989, a court order in the state of Connecticut ended their prison segregation policy. Similar antisegregation lawsuits have been filed in Alabama and Oregon. Through 1997, 10 other states had laws that allow for isolation or segregation of HIV-infected inmates.

A number of state prisons have instituted either mass screening programs or large-scale blind serological surveys for HIV infection. The Federal Bureau of Prisons tests a 10% sample of federal prisoners. Other jurisdictions conduct screening or testing programs for selected groups of prisoners, such as known injection drug users and homosexuals.

The incidence of AIDS is about 14 times higher in state and federal correctional systems (202/100,000 prisoners) **than in the United States population** (15/100,000 population) (Gostin et al., 1994). Anne DeGroot and colleagues (1996) report a summary of HIV testing results of prisoners in 42 state prisons and report that the rate of HIV infection is **10-to 100-fold higher** than in the general population. In 1993, the WHO reported that AIDS is responsible for 30% of all deaths in United States prisons. It is the leading cause of death in the New York and Florida prison systems. In 1991, according to the *People with AIDS Coalition Newsline*, 66% of inmate deaths in New York and New Jersey resulted from AIDS. In Florida in 1994, 67% of all deaths in the state prisons were related to AIDS. Of these, 42% were due to tuberculosis or *Pneumocystis* pneumonia (24%), both are successfully treated complications of

HIV infection if diagnosed early enough (De Groot et al., 1996).

TURNOVER IN PRISON POPULATIONS CREATES AN HIV TRANSMISSION PROBLEM FOR THE GENERAL POPULATION. Large numbers of at-risk individuals cycle through prisons and jails every year. The turnover rate for some prisons is as high as 50% per year. Because the prevalence of HIV is so high among the prison population, on release from prison, they can spread HIV to others. For example, the *AIDS Quarterly Report* in May 1990 stated that in 1992, 15,000 HIV-infected prisoners left the New York prison system to join the general population, and because of confidentiality laws, no one will know who they are. At Riker's Island facility in New York, of 21,000-plus prisoners, one in four are reported to be HIV-infected (National Press Release, 1989). A blinded serosurvey performed by the New York City Department of Health in 1991 determined that 26% of women and 16% of men in New York City prisons were HIV-seropositive (De Groot et al., 1996).In Florida, 3.4% of its prison population of 65,000 is HIV-positive (2,210).

The Elderly— AIDS cases remain relatively low among people between the ages 65 and 90. Howard Fillit and colleagues (1989) reported that nationally 10% of the total AIDS cases occur in people over age 50. Beginning 1998, this represented over 60,000 people. Three percent of AIDS occurs in people over age 60 or over 19,000 people and 0.7% occurs in people over 70 or over 4,500 people. One AIDS patient was 90 years old when diagnosed. He became HIV-infected from a blood transfusion during surgery at age 85. He became symptomatic about 4 years later and died 1 year later of *Pneumocystis carinii* pneumonia.

In **Florida**, a state with a large retired population, the number of recorded AIDS cases among those over age 50 has risen from 6 in

─────── **POINT OF INFORMATION 10.1** ───────

WHERE OLDER PATIENTS WITH HIV DISEASE CAN GET HELP

The problem of AIDS in persons 50 and older has received little recognition. But a few organizations now provide literature or services aimed specifically at older patients and their physicians:

American Association of Retired Persons
601 E St. NW
Washington, D.C. 20049
(202) 434-2277

Publishes free fact sheet, "AIDS: A Multi-generational Crisis" (Stock No. D14942), that includes listings of referral services.

Senior Action in a Gay Environment (SAGE)
208 W. 13th St.
New York, NY 10011
(212) 741-2247

Provides a variety of services to gays in their 50s or older. Also offers training, education, counseling, and therapy and is a source of information for physicians and hospitals. Operates chiefly in the area surrounding New York City (NY, NJ, CT).

Healthcare Education Associates
70 Campton Pl.

Laguna Niguel, CA 92677
(714) 240-2179

Publishes a training manual for use in discussion groups: "AIDS and Aging: What People Over 50 Need to Know." "Leaders Guide" and "Participant's Workbook" are $13.95; workbook alone, $5.

HIV/AIDS in Aging Task Force
425 E. 25th St.
New York, NY 10010
(212) 481-7670

Arranges conferences and education seminars; participants include physicians. Provides support for establishing task forces and seminars throughout the country.

National Institute on Aging
Public Information Office
Federal Bldg. 31 (Room 5C27)
Bethesda, MD 20892
(301) 496-1752

Publishes fact sheet, "Age Page: AIDS and Older Adults," available as a FAX transmission by calling (800) 222-2225.

1984 to 1,341 in 1993 to over 7,500 through 1997, or nearly 12% of the state's cases.

In general, Americans over 50 are potentially at risk, sometimes without realizing it, when they begin dating following a divorce or the death of a spouse. Others are at risk because they are IDUs or continue to have multiple sex partners or have a sex partner who practices unsafe sex. Individuals who acquire HIV infection at older ages progress to AIDS more rapidly, on average, than individuals infected at younger ages (excluding pediatric cases).

The majority of AIDS cases in the elderly once occurred due to HIV-contaminated blood transfusions; now the new elderly cases of AIDS most often include IDU or sexual activities (El Sadr et al., 1995; Gordon et al., 1995). It is believed that with the growing number of elderly people in the United States and better therapy for those who are HIV-infected in their early and late 50s, there will be an increasing number of elderly HIV-infected and AIDS patients who must be cared for. The male-female ratio in the age 50 and over is about 9:1 (Ship et al., 1991).

Health Care Workers— Health care workers are defined by the CDC as people, including students and trainees, whose activities involve contact with patients or with blood or other body fluids from patients in a health care setting. They represent 7.7% of the United States labor force.

The risk of HIV transmission from health care worker to patient during an exposure-prone invasive procedure is remote. There is a greater and well-documented risk of transmission from an infected patient to a health care worker.

As the pandemic of HIV infections continues to increase, workers in every health care field will be involved in the detection, counseling, therapy, maintenance, quantity, and quality of life for the symptomatic HIV-infected and for those expressing AIDS. Although the largest number of HIV-infected people are asymptomatic, each day many of them begin to experience signs and symptoms of HIV disease; and each day new cases of AIDS are diagnosed. As the number of patients increases, additional health care workers are required to meet their needs. As this work force

enlarges to meet the demands of the estimated numbers of AIDS cases in the coming years, precautions must be practiced to prevent health care workers themselves from becoming HIV-infected.

Ruthanne Marcus and colleagues (1988) reported that, across the board, health care workers exposed to HIV-contaminated blood have about a 1 in 300 chance of becoming infected. Other more recent reports place the risk of HIV infection at 1 in 250.

Health Care Workers with HIV/AIDS

Beginning 1997, the CDC had received reports of 52 health care workers in the United States with **documented** occupationally acquired HIV infection and 111 with possible occupa-

--------- POINT OF INFORMATION 10.2 ---------

HEALTH CARE WORKERS AND HIV EXPOSURE

Prospective studies of health care workers (HCWs) who have sustained an exposure to HIV-infected blood or bloody body fluid are the most important studies to define the risk of occupational transmission. David Henderson and colleagues (1990) have reviewed these studies, which are summarized in Table 10-4.

It is notable that prospective studies have not documented a single case of HIV transmission after skin or mucous membrane exposure to HIV-infected blood or body fluid. These studies illustrate the low risk of non-needlestick exposure. However, there have been six cases of percutaneous (passage through unbroken skin) transmission documented, for a rate of 0.29% (approximately 1 in 300).

TABLE 10-4 Summary of Prospective Studies of Health Care Workers Exposed to HIV-Infected Blood or Bloody Body Fluid

Type of Exposure	# Exposures	# (%) Seroconversion
Skin	5,568	0 (%)
Mucous membrane	1,051	0 (0%)
Percutaneous	2,042	6 (0.29%)

(Source: University of Colorado Health Sciences Center, Denver, CO 80262. *AIDS NEWSLINK*, Spring 1996)

tionally acquired HIV infection (nurses account for the largest number of cases). Twenty-four of the documented cases have developed AIDS. Five had died by the end of 1997. These are small numbers when compared to some 7,000 hepatitis B transmissions to health care workers every year in the United States (Osborne, 1993 Aiken et al., 1997).

Through 1997, of the 111 possible occupationally acquired HIV-infected workers, 58 have developed AIDS (*MMWR*, 1992b; Bell, 1996). The number of persons with occupationally acquired HIV infection is probably greater than the totals presented here because not all health care workers are evaluated for HIV infection following exposures and not all persons with occupationally acquired infection are reported.

Of the estimated 650,000-plus adult/adolescent/pediatric AIDS cases entering 1998, about 22,750 (3.5%) are health care workers, including an estimated 2,600 (0.4%) physicians, 4,940 (0.76%) nurses, and 3,575 (0.55%) dentists (Toufexis, 1991, updated). Overall, by 1998, 75% of the health care workers with AIDS, including an estimated 1,300 physicians, 90 surgeons, 330 dental workers, 3,045 nurses, and 290 paramedics, have died. The Medical Expertise Retention Program (MERP) in San Francisco in November 1991 estimated that 7,000 to 10,000 physicians and 50,000 to 70,000 other HCWs in the United States are HIV-positive (Williams, 1991).

Like other adult AIDS patients, health care workers have a median age of 35 years. Males account for 91.6% of cases and 62% are white.

Ninety-five percent of the health care workers with AIDS were classified into known transmission categories. Health care workers with AIDS were significantly **less likely** to be injection drug users and **more likely** to be homosexual or bisexual men (*MMWR*, 1996b).

Needlestick Injuries— Health care workers are in a quandary about the possibility of becoming HIV-infected via needlesticks. Articles such as "Needlestick Risks Higher Than Reports Indicate" or "The Risk of HIV Transmission via Needlesticks Is Low" convey conflicting impressions.

The kinds of needlesticks most likely to occur in hospital or health care settings come from disposable syringes, IV line/needle assemblies, prefilled cartridge injection syringes, winged steel needle IV sets, vacuum tube phlebotomy assemblies, and IV catheters, in that order. Needlesticks and penetration of sharp objects account for about 80% of all health care workers' exposures to blood and blood products. An estimated 1,000,000 needlesticks occur in the United States each year (Lumsdon, 1992).

ESTIMATES OF HIV INFECTION AND FUTURE AIDS CASES

In 1987, Otis Bowen, then Secretary of Health and Human Services, said "AIDS would make black death pale by comparison."

As long as the number of newly infectious people each year exceeds the number who die, the pandemic will continue to build.

Reportability

The CDC considers a case of AIDS reportable when: (1) an otherwise healthy person is HIV-positive and has an unusual opportunistic infection (protozoal, fungal, bacterial, or viral) or a rare malignancy; or (2) an individual with a positive HIV antibody test has a T4 cell count of less than 200 per cubic millimeter of blood,

——————— BOX 10.3 ———————

HIV/AIDS DATA DEFICIENCIES

Neither the United States nor any other country has an **accurate count** of the number of people infected by HIV. Much of the testing to date comprises small samples of high-risk groups, such as prostitutes and drug addicts, and is therefore unrepresentative of entire populations. Within countries, infection rates vary widely from region to region, further complicating the problem of generalizing from a small sample. Counting the number of AIDS cases and AIDS-related deaths is also difficult, particularly since health care systems in many countries lack the required diagnostic ability. Some developing countries have AIDS rates 100 times higher than reported. Moreover, some governments suppress what information they have. Further **improvements in data collection may reveal a crisis of even greater magnitude than is portrayed in this text**.

which is about one-fifth the normal level; or (3) an individual with a positive HIV antibody test has been diagnosed with pulmonary tuberculosis, invasive cervical cancer, or recurrent pneumonia.

AIDS— AIDS is reportable in all 50 states, the District of Columbia, and United States territories. AIDS surveillance has been crucial in identifying people at risk for the disease and the modes of transmission. AIDS surveillance data together with HIV surveys are important components of public health programs directed toward controlling HIV infection, and assist in providing the most accurate picture of the HIV epidemic in the United States.

By the end of 1993, all 50 states, the District of Columbia, and four territories (Guam, Pacific Islands, Puerto Rico, and the Virgin Islands) reported adult/adolescent cases. The CDC also reported the numbers of adult/adolescent/pediatric AIDS cases per 100,000 population in metropolitan areas with a population of 500,000 or more. Of the 94 such cities, 14 had no reported pediatric AIDS cases in 1989. By December 1993, all have reported pediatric AIDS cases. The 10 leading metropolitan areas for AIDS through 1997 (1 through 10) were: New York City; Miami, FL; Jersey City, NJ; San Francisco, CA; Fort Lauderdale, FL; West Palm Beach, FL; Newark, NJ; San Juan, Puerto Rico; Baltimore, MD; and New Orleans, LA. Beginning 1998, the seven states and territories reporting the highest incidence of AIDS cases for adult/adolescents were, from highest to lowest: Washington, DC; Puerto Rico; New York; California; Florida; Texas; and New Jersey. **Fifty-eight percent of all United States AIDS cases occur in 5 states**, New York, California, Florida, Texas, and New Jersey, in highest to lowest order respectively. **Seventy percent of all AIDS cases occur in 9 states**(Ones previously cited plus Georgia, Illinois, Maryland, and Pennsylvania).

HIV— Through 1996, only two states, Maryland and Washington, require that HIV infection reports carry the name of persons who are symptomatic. Thirty states report the HIV-infected by name (Table 10-5).

How Many People in the United States Are HIV-Infected?

How many people in the United States are HIV-infected? And just how many cases of AIDS are expected to occur and when? Although projections have been made, the numbers are in question. **Why**? They come from surveys and incidence data that lack rigorous scientific documentation. For example, publications give information such as "researchers **believe** that the current number of HIV-infected people in the United States ranges from 1% to as high as 10%" (Slack, 1991). But even if this range is to be believed, the difference between 1 in every 100 versus 10 in every 100 is very significant. This range implies that the data are questionable, and that is what raises the spectrum of concern. How many people in the United States and worldwide have HIV disease and how many have AIDS? **How large a problem is the HIV pandemic**? The answers to such questions are crucial to the allocation of funds for research and medical programs and for medical preparedness of institutions that will be hit hard as the number of cases increases.

All health care institutions and personnel will be affected by the increase in AIDS cases as will allied health service and support occupations, insurance companies, the funeral industry, and the work force in general.

United States Estimates Lead to Confusion

AIDS is a global pandemic. About 35 million people are expected to be HIV-infected by the end of 1998 including about 9 million AIDS cases (Figure 10–6). During 1996 HIV/AIDS-associated illnesses killed 1.3 million people—300,000 were children under age 5. UNAIDS and the WHO estimate that beginning 1996 through each year of the 1990s there will be about 3.3 million new HIV infections or about 9,000 per day—8,000 adults and 1,000 children! The World Health Organization estimated that by the year 2000, most of the 1 to 1.5 million HIV-infected people in the United States will have AIDS. Worldwide, there will be 16

TABLE 10-5   Status of HIV Infection Reporting—United States, June 1997

	Confidential HIV Reporting Required		
Name[a]	Anonymous[b]	HIV Pediatric Reporting Only	HIV Reporting Not Required[c]
Alabama	Georgia	Connecticut	Alaska
Arizona	Iowa	Texas	California
Arkansas	Kansas		Delaware
Colorado	Kentucky		District of Columbia
Florida	Maine		Hawaii
Idaho	Montana		Massachusetts
Illinois	New Hampshire		New Mexico
Indiana	Rhode Island		New York
Louisiana			Pennsylvania
Maryland[d]			Vermont
Michigan[e]			
Minnesota			
Mississippi			
Missouri			
Nebraska			
Nevada			
New Jersey			
North Carolina			
North Dakota			
Ohio			
Oklahoma			
Oregon (for children <6			
South Carolina			
South Dakota			
Tennessee[d]			
Utah			
Virginia			
Washington[d]			
West Virginia			
Wisconsin			
Wyoming			

All states require reporting of AIDS cases by name at the local/state level. The 1998 session of Congress expects to pass the **HIV Prevention Act of 1997**. The HIV Prevention Act adds HIV to 52 other notifiable contagious diseases such as gonorrhea, hepatitis A, B, and C, syphilis, tuberculosis, and AIDS that must be reported to the Centers for Disease Control.

[a]Names of HIV-infected people are provided to local or state health departments.

[b]Individual reports of people with HIV infection are provided to local or state health departments. Reports may contain demographic and transmission category information but do not record identifiers.

[c]Some states receive HIV reports on a voluntary basis.

[d]Requires HIV reports with names for symptomatic HIV-infected persons only.

[e]Names are reported to the local health department only.

(Source: HIV/AIDS Surveillance Report, June, 1997, 9:1–39)

times that number of AIDS cases (Figure 10-7) and 40 million cases of HIV infection. However, J. Chin and colleagues (1990), averaging the data of 14 experts, suggest that, by the year 2000, there will be about 18.3 million HIV-infected and 6.1 million AIDS cases. In 1992, a Harvard research group of 40 HIV/AIDS experts estimated that by the year 2000 there would be between 38 and 110 million HIV-infected adult/adolescents and 10 million children. By then, there will also be 24 million adult and several million pediatric AIDS cases. The estimates of HIV infections by the Harvard group is over twice that of the World Health Organization. Regardless of whose figures are more accurate, it is clear that the HIV/AIDS pandemic of the 1990s will be much worse than for the 1980s.

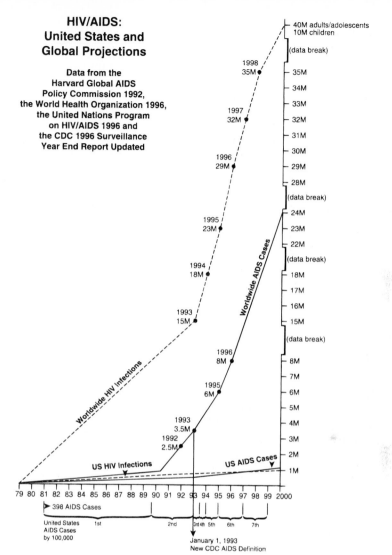

HIV/AIDS:
United States and
Global Projections

Data from the
Harvard Global AIDS
Policy Commission 1992,
the World Health Organization 1996,
the United Nations Program
on HIV/AIDS 1996 and
the CDC 1996 Surveillance
Year End Report Updated

40M adults/adolescents
10M children

(data break)

1998
35M — 35M
— 34M
1997
32M — 33M
— 32M
— 31M
— 30M
1996
29M — 29M
— 28M
(data break)
— 24M
1995
23M — 23M
— 22M
(data break)
1994
18M — 18M
— 17M
— 16M
1993
15M — 15M
(data break)
1996
8M — 8M
— 7M
1995
6M — 6M
— 5M
1993
3.5M — 4M
1992
2.5M — 3M
— 2M
US HIV Infections   US AIDS Cases
— 1M

Worldwide AIDS Cases

Worldwide HIV Infections

79 80 81 82 83 84 85 86 87 88 89 90 91 92 93 94 95 96 97 98 99 2000

▶ 398 AIDS Cases

United States   1st   2nd   3rd 4th 5th   6th   7th
AIDS Cases
by 100,000

January 1, 1993
New CDC AIDS Definition

FIGURE 10-7   United States and Global Projections for Total Number of
HIV and AIDS Cases. Beginning 1998, about 650,000 United States AIDS
cases were reported to the CDC. Most of these cases were diagnosed
according to the 1987 CDC AIDS definition guidelines. On January 1, 1993,
the CDC changed the definition of AIDS to include all persons with a T4
cell count of **less than 200**. The new definition raised the number of AIDS
cases in the United States from 1992 to 1993 by about 111%. The expected
number of adult/adolescent cases for 1993, 49,100, became 106,618. The
new definition has raised the number of persons living with diagnosed and
reported AIDS in the United States through 1996 to about 250,000. By the
year 2000, the United States is projected to have about 1.5 million AIDS
cases—worldwide, the number of AIDS cases is expected to be about 24
million. By the year 2000, 10% of all HIV infections and 12.5% of total
AIDS cases will be in the United States. William Hazeltine, AIDS
researcher formerly at the Dana Farber Institute, and now with Human
Genome Sciences Inc., said that if prevention does not work or a cure is

TABLE 10-6   Estimated[a] Prevalence of HIV-Infected People in the United States

	Estimated Number in U.S.	Proportion Infected with AIDS Virus	Estimated Number Infected
Homosexual men	2.5 million	20–25%	500,000–625,000
Bisexual men and men with highly infrequent homosexual contacts	2.5–7.5 million	5%	125,000–375,000
Regular injection drug users (at least weekly)	900,000	25%	225,000
Occasional injection drug users	200,000	5%	10,000
Hemophilia A patients	12,400	70%	8,700
Hemophilia B patients	3,100	35%	1,100
Heterosexuals without specific identified risks	142 million	0.021%	30,000
Others, including heterosexual partners of people at high-risk, heterosexuals born in Haiti and Central Africa, transfusion recipients	N.A.	N.A	45,000–127,000
Total			945,000–1.4 million

[a]Public Health Service in 1986 and the CDC in 1987 made the above *rough estimates.*

(Source: CDC; Figures projected in 1986 remained unchanged through mid-1995. **In March 1995, CDC announced 50% to 59% reduction of HIV people in the United States—from 1,200,000 to between 600,000 and 700,000.**)

WHOSE FIGURES ARE CORRECT?: ISSUES OF CREDIBILITY

The Public Health Service (PHS) in 1986 estimated that 1.5 million Americans were HIV-infected (Table 10-6). The PHS and the CDC (1987) estimated that by 1991 there would be 270,000 cases of AIDS and 179,000 people with AIDS would have died since 1981; by 1992, 365,000 Americans would demonstrate AIDS and 263,000 would have died of AIDS. These are ominous figures about the future of AIDS in the United States, **but were they responsible figures?** In fact, by 1992 there were 206,559 reported AIDS cases and 140,282 deaths—the estimates were off by 44% and 47%, respectively.

In mid-1988, New York City's Health Commissioner, who had relied on the CDC's methodology for calculating the number of future HIV-infected AIDS cases, cut the estimated number of HIV-infected gay and bisexual men from 250,000 to 50,000—an 80% reduction.

The Commissioner also reduced the total estimated number of HIV-infected New Yorkers from 400,000 to 200,000—a 50% reduction. The reason for these reductions was that the numbers of AIDS cases expected from a pool of 400,000 infected people were not happening.

A number of insurance companies, pharmaceutical manufacturers, and other industrial companies wanted more reliable prevalence figures. The demand for reliable data resulted in hiring research firms that specialize in population surveys. One such company, the Hudson Institute, reported that in 1989, 1.9 million to 3 million Americans were HIV-infected. The 3 million estimate is double the 1986 PHS and the 1987 CDC estimates.

Allan M. Salzberg, Chief of Medicine at the Veterans Center in Miles City, Montana, devised a computer model of the AIDS epidemic. It forecasts a future with 3 million American AIDS cases and 10 million infected by the year 2000 (Thomas, 1988). In mid-1989, the General

FIGURE 10-7   (*continued*)
not found, some **1 billion** people could be HIV-positive by the year 2025. Global population on through 1998 was about 6 billion. For the year 2000, it is projected to be about 6.2 billion people. (*Source: Harvard Global AIDS Policy Commission 1992 and World Health Organization 1993, 1994, National Census Bureau 1997 and projected data*)

Accounting Office (GAO) of the U.S. Congress reported that it analyzed 13 forecasts of the number of AIDS cases to occur by the end of 1991 and found that the range of predictions was so large—from 84,000 to 750,000—that they could not be used as a meaningful guide to health services planning. The GAO concluded that a range of 300,000 to 485,000 AIDS cases by the end of 1991 was more realistic than the PHS's and CDC's estimates of 270,000. (Recall only 206,000 were reported.)

James Curran of the CDC reported that blind HIV testing of Job Corps applicants revealed a rate of HIV infection 2.5 times higher than that found in military personnel. Job Corps data extrapolated to the general population would mean that there are 900,000 cases of HIV infection in the United States.

Scott Holmberg (1996) estimated the prevalence and incidence of HIV in 96 United States, metropolitan areas (MSAs) with populations greater than 500,000. From his data, he estimates that there are 1.5 million injection drug users, 1.7 million gay and bisexual men, and 2.1 million at-risk heterosexuals, and, among them, an estimated 565,000 HIV infections with 38,000 new infections occurring each year. This means there are about 700,000 total HIV-infected people in the United States with 40,000 new HIV infections occurring yearly. He states that roughly **half of all estimated new infections are occurring among injection drug users**, most of them in northeastern cities, Miami, and San Juan, Puerto Rico. Gay and bisexual men still represent most HIV infections, although the incidence of new infections, (25%), is much lower now than it was a decade ago. Heterosexual cases makeup the remaining 25% (Katz et al., 1997).

John Karon and colleagues (1996), **based on data from three different sources and methods of calculation, estimate there are between 650,000 and 900,000 (0.3% of the population) HIV-infected people in the United States**.

According to the CDC projections in Figure 10-8, about 35,500 AIDS cases should have occurred in 1988—34,261 (98%) were reported. In 1989, 46,000 were expected; 40,530 (88%) were reported. In 1990, 56,000 were expected and 44,757 (80%) cases were reported. In

1991, 65,000 were expected and 53,176 (82%) were reported; and in 1992, 80,000 AIDS cases were expected and 49,106 (61%) were reported. If one adds in the CDC's estimate of 15% to 20% of unreported AIDS cases, the projected and reported numbers through 1992 become more closely aligned. For 1993, before the implementation of the new AIDS definition, 65,211 cases were projected. Due to the 1993 change in the definition of AIDS, a total of 106,618 adult/adolescent cases were reported, a 37% increase over the expected and a 111% increase over the number of cases reported in 1992. The number of AIDS cases projected for 1994, 1995 and 1996 occurred. After the backlog of AIDS cases based on the new definition is reported, the increase in new AIDS cases per year is expected to stabilize at a 3% to 5% increase for each year through the 1990s. Table 10-7 presents data on the time it took for the first, second, third, fourth, fifth, and sixth 100,000 AIDS cases to occur in the United States and the estimated time for the seventh 100,000 AIDS cases.

Rise in HIV/AIDS Cases Among Heterosexuals

In 1989, while the number of new AIDS cases rose by 11% among gay males, it increased by 36% or more among heterosexuals and

---POINT OF INFORMATION 10.3---

UNITED STATES: 650,000 AIDS CASES BEGINNING 1998

It took 7 years (1981–1987) for the first 50,000 AIDS cases to be **reported** in the United States (50,352). Over the next 5 years an additional 152,865 AIDS cases were reported (a total of 203,217 or 31% of the 650,000 AIDS cases to be reported by the beginning of 1998). During the next 5 years, between the end of 1992 and the beginning of 1998, an additional 446,783 AIDS cases or 69% of all AIDS cases will have been reported.

The data in Table 10-7 show that it took 8 years (1981 to 1989) to accumulate the first 100,000 AIDS cases. In a little over half that time (1989 to mid-1993), 4.6 years, 300,000 new AIDS cases occurred.

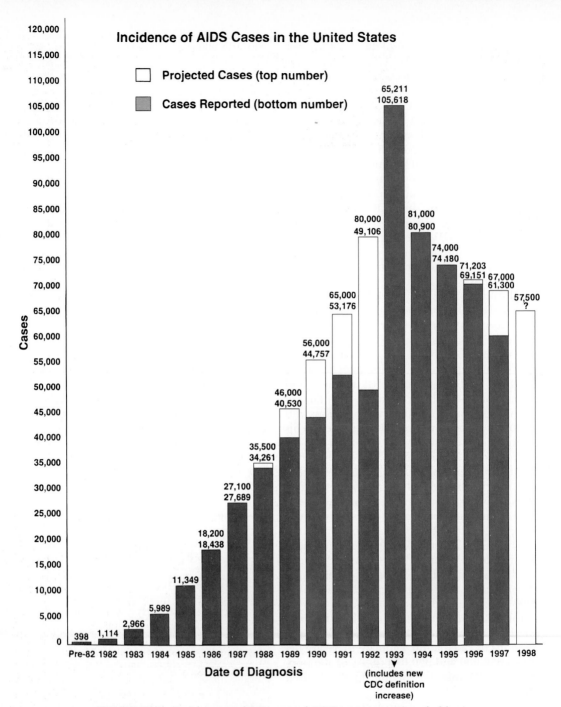

FIGURE 10-8 Incidence and Estimates of AIDS in persons 13 and older by Year of Diagnosis—United States, pre-1982 through 1998. The total for 1995 reflects an 9% reduction in AIDS cases from 1994 due to a drop in the backlog of persons to be identified as AIDS cases according to the 1993 definition of AIDS. Estimates for 1997 and 1998 reflect a 3% and 8% reduction respectfully from 1996.

TABLE 10-7   AIDS Cases Comparison—50,000 vs. 100,000

Dates in Years	Time in Months[a]	AIDS Cases by 50,000	AIDS Cases by 100,000
1987	84	First	—
Jun. 89	17	Second	First (8 years)
Nov. 90	17	Third	—
Nov. 91	12	Fourth	Second (29 months)
Nov. 92	12	Fifth	—
Mar. 93	5	Sixth	Third (17 months)[b]
Jul. 93	5	Seventh	—
Dec. 93	5	Eighth	Fourth (10 months)[b]
Oct. 94	10	Ninth	—
Oct. 95	12	Tenth	Fifth (22 months)[b]
Jul. 96	9	Eleventh	—
Apl. 97	9	Twelfth	Sixth (24 months)[b]
Jan. 98	9	Thirteenth	—
Oct. 98	9	Fourteenth	Seventh (18 months)[b]

[a]Reported AIDS cases beginning 1981 through 1996. Estimated for 1997, 1998.
[b]Rapid increase in AIDS cases due to new January 1, 1993 CDC AIDS definition.

newborns. In 1993, due to the new AIDS definition, **heterosexual contact** AIDS cases increased 130% over 1992, from 4,045 to 9,288. This number increased by 8,585 in 1994 by 8,093 in 1995. and by 8,821 in 1996. AIDS cases attributed to gay males or bisexual males increased 54% from 25,864 cases in 1992 to 48,266 in 1993. There were 35,524 new cases in 1994, 30,671 in 1995, and 27,316 in 1996.

The groups most affected by the expanded 1993 definition were women, blacks, heterosexual injection drug users, and hemophiliacs. The increase was greater among women (151%) than among men (105%), and greater among blacks and Hispanics than whites. Young adults ages 13 to 29 accounted for 27% of the heterosexual contact cases. On average, women accounted for about 35% of the heterosexual contact cases from 1993 through 1997.

James Chin (1990), an epidemiologist in charge of AIDS surveillance at the WHO, predicts that by the year 2000, heterosexual transmission will predominate in most industrialized countries. The growth of the epidemic may have been slower among heterosexuals than it has been among gays or injection drug users, but it will continue to increase because HIV infection is a sexually transmitted disease and most people in society are heterosexual.

Conclusion

There is one thing on which all prognosticators agree: There is no reliable baseline from which to organize and analyze the data. There is no standard curve available to indicate the number of people from each behavioral risk group who will either become HIV-infected or develop AIDS.

There are no reliable means of obtaining data on human sexual behavior. Over the years, a constant theme has emerged from groups working on HIV/AIDS data: That is (1) extracting sensitive behavior risk information from HIV-infected or AIDS patients is difficult for even the most experienced interviewer; and (2) as HIV infection spreads beyond initially identified behavioral risk groups, assessing risk by sexual history becomes even less reliable. People do not always tell the truth when answering questions about their sexual preferences and sexual habits.

**SHAPE OF THE HIV PANDEMIC:
UNITED STATES**

Based on the HIV presentation of HIV infections in Figure 10-9 during the years 1981 through 1983, HIV infections reached their peak and then rapidly declined. In 1988, the number of **new** HIV infections appears to have leveled off

Shape of the HIV Epidemic, United States

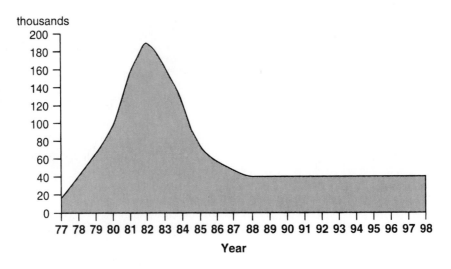

FIGURE 10-9   Rate of HIV Infection 1997 through 1998: United States.
(*Source: Dr. Don C. Des Jarlais, Beth Israel Medical Center, updated*)

at about 40,000 a year through 1998. Unless a preventive vaccine is found, the rate of new HIV infections in the United States is expected to remain at 40,000 annually. This may mean the new prevention campaigns **will not** significantly reduce new infections. Society has, in a sense, reduced new HIV infections to its lower limit.

Class Discussion: Is the last statement plausible—have we reached a point at which further expenditures will not significantly reduce the rate of infection—that all society can do now is wait on a preventive vaccine? **What** would be **your solution** given that we have actually reached this point and **no** vaccine is forthcoming?

ESTIMATES OF DEATHS AND YEARS OF POTENTIAL LIFE LOST DUE TO AIDS IN THE UNITED STATES

Deaths Due to AIDS

Each year in the United States there are about 2,300,000 deaths. AIDS has, since 1992, caused on average 40,000 of these deaths each year. AIDS now accounts for about 1.8% of deaths

each year. That is, two people of each 100 who die, die of AIDS.

Former Surgeon General C. Everett Koop has said on a number of occasions that "AIDS is virtually 100% fatal." Looking back over the number of AIDS cases diagnosed and comparing them to the number of AIDS patients who have died would indicate that a diagnosis of AIDS is a death sentence. Figure 10-10 presents a sobering look at the numbers of AIDS patients who have died since those first CDC reported cases in 1981. People with HIV disease/AIDS are now dying at the rate of about 3,000 a month. About 95% of those diagnosed with AIDS in 1981 have now died. And about 60% of AIDS cases diagnosed up through 1996 have died. In New York City, 17 people a day died from AIDS from about 1989 through 1995. **BUT**, AIDS deaths dropped in New York by 30% in 1996, from 7,046 in 1995 to 4,944 in 1996, and the number is expected to fall again in 1997. **Nationwide**, AIDS deaths fell 23% in 1996. Deaths for men fell 22%. The drop was 28% among whites, 16% among Hispanics, and 10% among black men. Deaths in women dropped 7%, reflecting rising female case loads.

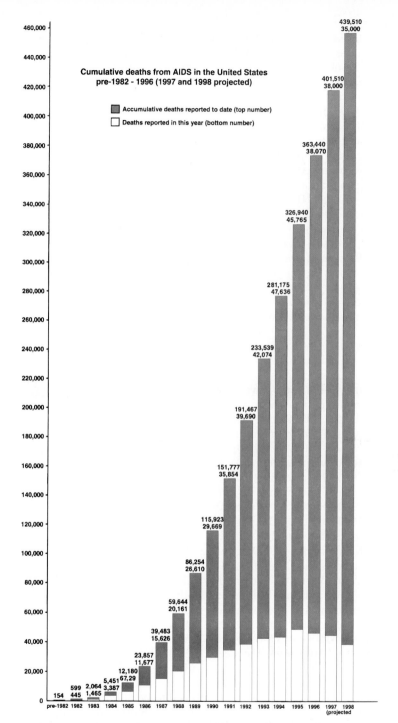

FIGURE 10-10 Cumulative Deaths from AIDS in the United States pre-1982–1996 (1997 and 1998 projected). By the end of 1988, there were 60,000 deaths due to AIDS. Beginning 1997 there were about 363,500 AIDS deaths. About 440,000 will have died by the end of 1998.

Many of the deaths that would have occurred in 1996 and 1997 are being **POSTPONED** through the use of combination cocktail drug therapy and in particular the use of at least **one protease inhibitor** within the drug cocktail.

The majority of AIDS deaths have occurred among homosexual/bisexual men (59%) and among women and heterosexual men who were injection drug users (21%). Most (75%) of AIDS deaths have occurred among people 25 to 44 years of age and about 24% occurred in those over age 45. In 1992, HIV disease/AIDS became the number one cause of death among black and Hispanic men ages 25 to 44 and second among black women ages 25 to 44 (*MMWR*, 1994b). **Between January 1993 and December 1995 AIDS was the leading cause of death in all Americans aged 25 to 44** (*MMWR*, 1995a). For 1996 it dropped to second. AIDS is the **eighth** leading cause of death overall in the United States.

According to the CDC (1993), deaths from HIV disease/AIDS are **underreported by 25% to 33%**. Although most deaths occurred among whites, proportional rates have been highest for blacks and Hispanics. During 1994, the number of deaths per 100,000 population, aged 25 to 44 years, was 178 for black men and 47 for white men. It was 9 times as high for black women (51) as for white women (6). In proportion, since 1985, the rate of death was higher for women than for men (*MMWR*, 1996d). By the year 1990, 86,254 AIDS patients died. By the end of 1997, 402,000 AIDS patients had died. To place the death rate due to AIDS in perspective, each day about 140,000 people die from assorted causes while about 95 to 100 die each day from AIDS. Worldwide, through 1998, of an estimated 35 million HIV-infected persons, about 26 million will be alive with HIV disease. About 40% are women. Although the **rate of increase in new AIDS cases has slowed**, the number of new cases continues to exceed the number who die of AIDS.

Prevalence and Impact of HIV/AIDS

However the impact of the disease is measured—by deaths, AIDS cases, or monetary losses—it is just beginning. The worldwide impact during the 1990s will be 5 to 10 times that of the 1980s. As this process unfolds, the United States will find itself progressively more involved with prevention programs and with the political changes that HIV/AIDS will bring about in countries with a high incidence of HIV/AIDS.

LIFE EXPECTANCY

In 1995, the Metropolitan Life Insurance Company published data that shows that life expectancy reached its peak in the United States in 1992 at 75.8 years. For the years 1993 and 1994 it dropped to 75.5 years. The forecast is that continued loss due to AIDS will further erode life expectancy.

A mortality analysis of homosexual males indicates that gay men in Vancouver, British Columbia, have a life expectancy 8 to 20 years shorter than non-gay men in the same area (Hog et al., 1997). The researchers note that if the trend continues, "we estimate that nearly half of gay and bisexual men currently aged 20 years will not reach their 65th birthday." The study collected vital statistics from 1987 to 1992 and assessed mortality rates based on 3%, 6%, and 9% prevalence rates of homosexual and bisexual men. "Under even the most liberal assumptions, gay and bisexual men in this urban center are now experiencing a life expectancy similar to that experienced by all men in Canada in the year 1871."

SUMMARY

In 1981, the CDC reported the first case of AIDS in the United States, and, from that time onward, has constantly tracked the prevalence of AIDS cases in different geographical areas and within different behavioral "risk" groups. In all behavioral risk groups, the common denominator is the exchange of body fluids, in particular blood or semen. The heterosexual population at large is considered to be at low risk for HIV infection in the United States. By 1993, all states and the District of Columbia, Puerto Rico, and the Virgin Islands have reported AIDS cases in people who have had heterosexual contact with an at-risk partner.

A major problem exists in attempting to determine the number of HIV-infected people. Several different approaches have been used by the CDC to estimate the total number of HIV infections. These estimates can be evaluated by examining their compatibility with available prevalence data.

With respect to race and ethnicity, the cumulative incidence of AIDS cases is disproportionately higher in blacks and Hispanics than in whites. The ratio of black to white case incidence is 3.2:1 and the Hispanic to white ratio 2.8:1. This racial/ethnic disproportion is also observed in HIV-positive blood donors and in applicants for military service. Even among homosexual and bisexual men and IDUs, where race/ethnicity-specific data are available, blacks appear to have higher seroprevalence rates than whites.

With regard to prostitution, in a large multicenter study of female prostitutes, black and Hispanic prostitutes had a higher rate of HIV infection than white and other prostitutes. This disproportion existed for both prostitutes who used injection drugs and for those who did not acknowledge injection drug use.

The risk of new HIV infections in hemophiliacs and in people who receive blood transfusions has declined dramatically from 1985 because of the screening of donated blood and heat treatment of clotting factor concentrates. Evidence also indicates an appreciable decline in the incidence of new infections in homosexual men. However, the risk of new infections appears to remain high in IDUs and in their heterosexual partners. In several metropolitan cities, the prevalence of HIV infection in IDUs has been increasing.

Studies conducted by the CDC along with the American College Health Association revealed that in 1989, two college students per 1,000 were HIV-infected.

There are some 5.3 million health care workers in the United States. Even though they are supposed to adhere to Universal Protection Guidelines set down by the CDC for their protection, a significant number are exposed to the AIDS virus annually. A relatively small number of those infected have progressed to AIDS.

Estimating the number of HIV-infected people in the United States continues to be a numbers game. Various agencies and private industries have, for different reasons, attempted to determine the number of HIV-infected people. The numbers from the different groups vary widely. However, the 1986 CDC estimated numbers of 1 to 1.5 million HIV-infected people may be too high. However, the number of new AIDS cases occurring each year are within 10% to 20% of the CDC estimated figures.

Beginning 1998, with some 700,000 to 900,000 people HIV-infected in the United States and with 40,000 new infections occurring each year through the year 2000, the face of AIDS in America is changing. **It's a younger face than it used to be. It's more likely to be a face of color than it used to be.** And more people with HIV disease and AIDS are from areas outside of major cities. Overall, the number of new AIDS cases appears to be leveling. But the HIV epidemic should be viewed as many different epidemics in different stages that vary according to age, race, gender, and locality. Although gay and bisexual men continue to make up the largest portion of AIDS cases, the epidemic is increasing more rapidly among people who become infected though heterosexual contact and through sharing syringes to inject drugs. Every year women are composing a larger portion of AIDS cases, many who did not realize they were at risk. (See Chapter 11 for specifics on HIV/AIDS in women, children, and teenagers.)

REVIEW QUESTIONS

(Answers to the Review Questions are on page 578.)

1. How did the CDC estimate the numbers of HIV-infected people in the United States? In what year was this done? In retrospect, how accurate are their estimates?

2. Why are people placed in potential HIV risk groups?

3. True or False: The time it takes for HIV-infected people to become AIDS patients is different for each ethnic group, risk group, and exposure route. Explain.

4. What percentage of all U.S. HIV-infected IDUs are in the New York–New Jersey region?

5. What percentage of newborns from HIV-infected mothers are HIV-infected?

6. Eventually, what percentage of HIV-infected children will result solely from HIV-infected mothers?

7. What is the rate of college students currently HIV-infected? Is this more or less than the rate for military personnel? Explain.

8. Compare the college student rate of HIV infection with the rate of HIV infection for the general U.S. population.

9. What is the risk of a health care worker converting to seropositivity after exposure to HIV-contaminated blood?

10. What single job-related event causes the greatest risk of HIV infection among health care workers?

11. What percentage of the total number of AIDS cases in the United States represents health care workers?

12. Are health care workers more apt to become infected with the hepatitis B virus or the AIDS virus?

13. In May of 1989, four states had no reported pediatric cases. Name these four states. What might this imply about HIV infection in these states?

14. In mid-1989, the government's General Accounting Office said _____ cases of AIDS will have occurred in the United States by the end of 1991. How many did the CDC predict?

15. Do you think people of the United States openly and truthfully discuss their sexual habits with survey personnel? What does the text say?

16. How many AIDS patients are estimated to die by the end of 1998?

17. Data on AIDS deaths indicated that of AIDS patients diagnosed between 1981 through 1997, _____% had died.

REFERENCES

AIKEN, LINDA, et al. (1997). Hospital nurses' occupational exposure to blood: prospective, retrospecture and institutional reports. *AM. J. Public Health*, 87:103–107.

ARAL, SEVGI O., et al. (1991). Sexually transmitted diseases in the AIDS era. *Sci. Am.*, 264:62–69.

BELL, DAVID. (1996). Occupational risk of HIV infection in health care workers. *Improv. Manage. HIV Dise.*, 4:7–9.

BOOTH, WILLIAM. (1988). CDC paints a picture of HIV infection in U.S. *Science*, 242:53.

BOOTH, WILLIAM. (1989). Asking America about its sex life. *Science*, 243:304.

CHIN, J., et al. (1990). Projections of HIV infections and AIDS cases to the year 2000. *Bull. WHO*, 68:1–11.

COUTINHO, ROEL, et al. (1996), Summary of Track C: Epidemiology and public health. *AIDS* 10 (suppl. 3):S115–S121.

DE GROOT, ANNE, et al. (1996). Barriers to care of HIV-infected inmates: a public health concern. *AIDS Reader*, 6:78–87.

DOLAN, KATE, et al. (1995). AIDS behind bars: Preventing HIV spread among incarcerated drug infections. *AIDS*, 9:825–832.

EL-SADR, WAFFA, et al. (1994). *Managing Early HIV Infection: Quick Reference Guide for Clinicians.* Agency for Health Care Policy and Research. Publication #94-0573, Rockville, MD.

EL-SADR, WAFFA, et al. (1995). Unrecognized human HIV infection in the elderly. *Arch. Intern. Med.*, 155:184–186.

FAY, ROBERT E., et al. (1989). Prevalence and patterns of same-gender sexual contact among men. *Science*, 243:338–348.

FELDMAN, MITCHELL, et al. (1994). The growing risk of AIDS in older patients. *Patient Care*, 28:61–72.

FILLIT, HOWARD, et al. (1989). AIDS in the elderly: A case and its implications. *Geriatrics*, 44:65–70.

FRANCIS, DONALD P. (1987). The prevention of acquired immunodeficiency syndrome in the United States. *JAMA*, 257:1357–1366.

GAYLE, HELENE. (1988). Demographic and sexual transmission differences between adolescent and adult AIDS patients, U.S.A. *Fourth International Conference on AIDS.*

GORDON, STEVEN, et al. (1995). The changing epidemiology of HIV infection in older persons. *J. Am. Geriatr. Soc.*, 43:7–9.

GOSTIN, LAWRENCE, et al. (1994). HIV testing, counseling and prophylaxis after sexual assault. *JAMA*, 271:1436–1444.

HAYS, ROBERT B., et al. (1990). High HIV risk-taking among young gay men. *AIDS*, 4:901.

HAYS, ROBERT B. (1992). AIDS and gays: Look for a second wave. *Med. Asp. Human Sexuality*, 26:61.

HENDERSON, DAVID, et al. (1990). Risk for occupational transmission of human immunodeficiency virus type 1 (HIV-1) associated with clinical exposures. *Ann. Intern. Med.*. 113:740.

HIRSCHHORN, LISA. (1995). HIV infection in women: Is it different? *AIDS Reader*, 5:99–105.

HIV Guideline Panel. (1994). Managing early HIV infection. *Am. Fam. Phys.,* 49:801–814.

HIV/AIDS Surveillance Report. (December 1996). 8:1–36.

HIV Surveillance Report. (June 1997). 9:1–39.

HOGG, ROBERT, et al. (1997). HIV disease shortens life expectancy of gay men by up to 20 years. *Inter.J. Epidemiol.*26:657–661.

HOLMBERG, SCOTT. (1996). The estimated prevalence and incidence of HIV in 96 large U.S. metropolitan areas. *Am J. Public Health,* 86:642–654.

HOOKER, TRACEY. (1996). HIV/AIDS: Facts to consider—1996. National Conference of State Legislatures, Denver, CO, pp. 1–64.

KARON, JOHN, et al. (1996). Prevalence of HIV infection in the United States, 1984 to 1992. *JAMA,* 276:126–130.

KATZ, MITCHELL, et al. (1997). Postexposure treatment of people exposed to HIV through sexual contact or IDLL. *N. Eng. J. Med.,* 336:1097–1100.

LEMP, GEORGE. (1991). The young men's survey: Principal findings and results. A presentation to the San Francisco Health Commission, June 4.

LEMP, GEORGE, et al. (1994). Seroprevalence of HIV and risk behaviors among young homosexual and bisexual men. *JAMA,* 272:449–454.

LUMSDON, KEVIN. (1992). HIV-positive health care workers pose legal, safety challenges for hospitals. *Hospitals,* 66:24–32.

MAHON, NANCY. (1996). New York inmates' HIV risk behaviors: the implications for prevention policy and programs. *Am. J. Public Health,* 86:1211–1215.

MARCUS, R., et al. (1988). AIDS: Health care workers exposed to it seldom contract it. *N. Engl. J. Med.,* 319:1118–1123.

MARTORELL, REYNALDO, et al. (1995). Vitamin A supplementation and morbidity in children born to HIV-infected women. *Am. J. Public Health,* 85:1049–1050.

MICHAELS, DAVID, et al. (1992). Estimates of the number of motherless youth orphaned by AIDS in the United States. *JAMA,* 268:3456–3461.

Morbidity and Mortality Weekly Report. (1990). HIV prevalence, projected AIDS case estimates. Workshop, Oct. 31–Nov. 1, 1989. 39:110–119.

Morbidity and Mortality Weekly Report. (1991). The HIV/AIDS epidemic: The first 10 years. 40:357–368.

Morbidity and Mortality Weekly Report. (1992a). HIV prevention in the U.S. correctional system, 1991. 41:389–391, 397.

Morbidity and Mortality Weekly Report. (1992b). Surveillance for occupationally acquired HIV infection—United States, 1981–1992. 41:823–824.

Morbidity and Mortality Weekly Report. (1993). Update: Mortality attributable to HIV infection among persons aged 25–44 years—United States, 1991 and 1992. 42:869–873.

Morbidity and Mortality Weekly Report. (1994a). Heterosexually acquired AIDS-United States, 1993. 43:155–160.

Morbidity and Mortality Weekly Report. (1995a). Update: Trends in AIDS among men who have sex with men—United States, 1989–1994. 44:401–404.

Morbidity and Mortality Weekly Report. (1995b). First 500,000 AIDS cases—United States, 1995. 44:849–853.

Morbidity and Mortality Weekly Report. (1996a). AIDS Associated with Injection Drug Use—United States, 1995. 45:392–398.

Morbidity and Mortality Weekly Report. (1996b). Case central study of HIV seroconversion in health-care workers after percutaneous exposure to HIV-infected blood—France, United Kingdom, and United States, January 1988–August 1994. 44:929–933.

Morbidity and Mortality Weekly Report. (1996c). HIV/AIDS education and prevention programs for adults in prisons and jails and juveniles in confinement facilities—United States, 1994. 45:268–271.

Morbidity and Mortality Weekly Report. (1996d). Update: Mortality Attributable to HIV Infection among persons aged 25–44 years—United States, 1994. 45:121–125.

Nations Health Report. (1995). Women learn of progress, share deep concerns on HIV/AIDS issues. XXV:10.

OSBORNE, JUNE E. (1993). AIDS policy advisor foresees a new age of activism. *Fam. Prac. News,* 23:1, 45.

PETERSON, J.L., et al. (1989). AIDS and IV drug use among ethnic minorities. *J. Drug Issues,* 19:27–37.

REISMAN, JUDITH. (1990). *Kinsey, Sex and Fraud: The Indoctrination of a People.* Lafayette, LA: Huntington House Press.

ROSENBERG, PHILIP. (1995). Scope of the AIDS epidemic in the United States. *Science,* 270: 1372–1376.

RUBEL, JOHN, et al. (1997). HIV-related mental health in correctional settings. *FOCUS,* 12:1–4.

RYDER, ROBERT, et al. (1994). AIDS orphans in Kinshasa, Zaire: Incidence and socioeconomic consequences. *AIDS,* 8:673–679.

SHIP, J.A., et al. (1991). Epidemiology of AIDS in persons aged 50 years or older. *J. Acquired Immune Deficiency Syndrome,* 4(1):84–88.

SLACK, JAMES D. (1991). *AIDS and the Public Workforce: Local Government Preparedness in Managing the Epidemic.* Tuscaloosa: The University of Alabama Press.

STALL, R., et al. (1990). Relapse from safer sex: The next challenge for AIDS prevention efforts. *J. Acquired Immune Deficiency Syndrome,* 3:1181.

THOMAS, PATRICIA. (1988). Official estimates of epidemic's scope are grist for political mill. *Med. World News*, 29:12–13.

TOUFEXIS, ANASTASIA. (1991). When the doctor gets infected. *Time*, 137:57.

UNAIDS. (1996). The HIV/AIDS situation in mid 1996: Global and regional highlights, Geneva 27, Switzerland, pp. 1–14.

VLAHOV, D., et al. (1991). Prevalence of antibody to HIV-1 among entrants to U.S. correctional facilities. *JAMA*, 265:1129.

WEISFUSE, ISAAC C., et al. (1991). HIV-1 infection among New York City inmates. *AIDS*, 5:1133–1138.

WILLIAMS, PATRICIA. (1991). Job fears may impede care for seropositives. *Med. World News*, 32:39.

WILSON, J., et al. (1990). Keeping your cool in a time of fear. *Emergency Medical Services*, 19:30–32.

CHAPTER

11

Prevalence of HIV Infection and AIDS Cases Among Women, Children, and Teenagers in the United States

CHAPTER CONCEPTS

♦ A global estimate of HIV-positive women is presented.

♦ In proportion there are significantly more black women with AIDS than white women.

♦ Injection drug use is the major route of HIV infection for women.

♦ From 1994 through 1997 at least 38% of women in the United States contracted HIV from men through sex.

♦ Injection drug use and prostitution are strongly associated with HIV infection.

♦ AIDS is the leading cause of death for women ages 25 to 34.

♦ First 100,000 AIDS cases in women in the United States are documented in January 1998.

♦ Women make up 40% of worldwide AIDS cases.

♦ "Pediatric" means **under** age 13 in the United States and **under** age 15 in Canada.

♦ About 95% of pediatric AIDS cases receive the virus from their HIV-infected mothers.

♦ In proportion there are significantly more black and Hispanic pediatric AIDS cases than for whites.

♦ Perinatal HIV infection without drug intervention is about 30%; with drug intervention it is about 8%.

♦ Not all newborns that test HIV-positive are HIV-infected.

♦ Seven of 10 people are sexually active by age 19.

♦ Eighty-six percent of all sexually transmitted diseases occur in the 15 to 29 age group.

♦ The total number of HIV-infected teenagers is unknown.

♦ Black and Hispanic teenagers account for a disproportionate number of AIDS cases compared to whites.

♦ Teenagers are being exposed to quality HIV prevention but they choose to ignore it.

Just 10 years ago, women, children, and teenagers seemed to be on the periphery of the HIV/AIDS pandemic. **Now . . . they are at the center of this pandemic. The fear of becoming infected and an inability to ensure that they remain uninfected are common to virtually all women**.

Worldwide beginning 1998, there were an estimated 9 million AIDS cases of 32 million people infected with HIV. About 3,700,000 (40%) of these AIDS cases are women. Of the HIV-infected, 17,280,000 are men and 14,720,000 are women (Figure 11-1). Beginning 1997, about 50% of all new HIV infections occurred in women.

In sub-Saharan Africa, the ratio of women to men infected with HIV/AIDS is currently 6:5 and rising. In Rakai and Masaka, rural districts of Uganda, a 1994 national report indicated that of 1,300 young women aged 15 to 25, 70% were HIV-infected. When compared with HIV-infected young men of the same villages and age group, there was a female-to-male ratio of 6:1. In Rwanda and Tanzania, young women under age 25 accounted for 20% of female AIDS cases and men under 25 for less than 9% of male cases. The male-to-female ratio of AIDS cases among Ethiopian teenagers is 1:3; in Zimbabwe, it is 1:5. In Brazil, the ratio of male-to-female infection in Sao Paulo has changed from 42:1 in 1985 to 2:1 in 1995. In Northern Thailand, HIV prevalence among women coming to prenatal clinics reached 8% in 1993. And 72% of sex workers are HIV-infected. In the United States, women as a percentage of HIV/AIDS cases rose 8% from 1981 to 1987, but 19% from 1993 to 1995 and 20% in 1996. Through 1997, seventy-five percent of HIV transmission worldwide was associated with heterosexual (vaginal) inter-

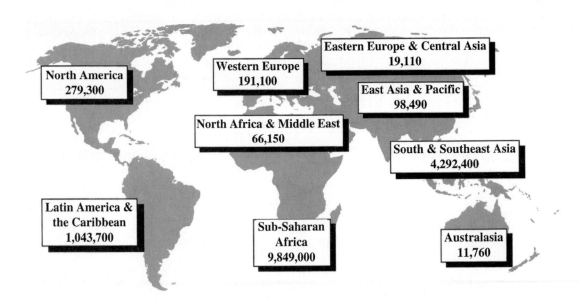

Global Total: 14.7 Million HIV Positive Women

FIGURE 11-1 Estimate of HIV-Positive Women Worldwide Beginning 1998. For comparison, beginning 1993 there were **5 million** HIV-positive women worldwide; by the end of 1993, women made up an estimated **8 million** HIV cases. Through 1997 there were **14.7 million** HIV-positive women, or about 47% of all HIV-positives worldwide were women! There will be about 16.4 million HIV-positive women globally by the end of 1998.

course. Women are biologically more vulnerable to HIV infection than men because HIV in semen is in higher concentration than in vaginal and cervical secretions and because the vaginal area has a much larger mucosal area for exposure to HIV than the penis.

Transmission of HIV from male to female is 2 to 10 times more effective than from female to male (*World Health Organization*, 1994). Paradoxically, since time immemorial women have been blamed for the spread of sexually transmitted diseases. Among certain peoples in Thailand and Uganda, STDs are known as "**women's diseases**." And in Swahili, the language of much of east Africa, the word for STD means, literally, "**disease of woman**." Also, it is not coincidental that the countries in which HIV is now spreading fastest heterosexually are generally those in which women's status is low.

Every minute of every day, every day of the year, two women worldwide become infected by HIV, and every 2 minutes a woman dies from AIDS (525,600 AIDS deaths/year). The WHO estimated that by the year 2000, over 18 million women will have been infected with HIV, 7 million of whom will already have progressed to AIDS. Prevalence rates of other sexually transmitted diseases have always been higher among females than among males in those under age 29 (Mongella, 1995; United Nations, 1995).

WOMEN: HIV-POSITIVE AND AIDS CASES—UNITED STATES

In rural America, HIV/AIDS due to heterosexual transmission is increasing faster than in any other part of the country. Women most at risk are ethnic minorities and the economically disadvantaged. Among sexually active teenagers, college students, and health care workers nationwide, nearly 60% of the heterosexual spread of HIV is among women (Pfeiffer, 1991).

In 1982, it was thought that all female AIDS cases were associated with injection drug usage. It soon became apparent that some of these women had become infected through heterosexual contact with HIV-infected males. Additional AIDS cases from heterosexual transmission appeared in 1983, and the percentage of female cases in the heterosexual category has continued to increase. The trend in heterosexual vaginal transmission may serve as a marker for future trends in HIV transmission.

HIV/AIDS in women is a national tragedy, but in addition women are the major source of infection in infants. From 1993 through 1997, about 96% of HIV-infected children, aged 0 to 4 years, got the virus from their mothers.

At the end of 1988, women made up 6,964 or 9% of the total adult AIDS cases in the United States. By the end of 1996, women accounted for an estimated 15% of total AIDS cases (Table 11-1). Sixty-eight percent of all female AIDS cases have been reported in the four years between 1993 and the beginning of 1997. And they have been reported from all 50 states and territories. About 75% of these females are between the ages of 13 and 39 and 25% are over age 40 (Guinan, 1993). Between 1989 and the beginning of 1998, female AIDS cases were and continue to be twice as frequent among black women than among white, and almost three times higher in black women than in Hispanic women (Figure 11-2). The number of reported female AIDS cases across the United States for 1996 is seen in Figure 11-3. The number of all female AIDS cases for 1996 is shown in Figure 11-4.

Among the most alarming HIV/AIDS statistics to emerge is that of HIV transmission through heterosexual contact. Of the total reported cases acquired through heterosexual contact in the United States, 66% are women. Of AIDS cases that occur in women ages 13 to 24, 49% are due to heterosexual contact.

Figure 11-5 presents the cumulative source of United States female AIDS cases in 1996. In 1996, of the 68,473 persons aged ≥ 13 years reported with AIDS, 13,820 (20%) occurred among women—nearly threefold greater than the proportion (534 [7%] of 8,153) reported in 1985. The proportion of cases among women has increased steadily since 1981 (Table 11-1). The median age of women reported with AIDS in 1996 was 35 years, and women aged 15 to 44 years accounted for 84% of female AIDS cases. Through 1997, women aged 50 years and older accounted for 9% of all female AIDS cases. And most of these women became infected through heterosexual

sexual activities (Schable et al., 1996, updated). More than three fourths (76%) of AIDS cases among women occurred among blacks and Hispanics.

In 1996, the Northeast region accounted for the largest percentage of AIDS cases reported among women (44%), followed by the South (36%), West (9%), Midwest (7%), and Puerto Rico and U.S. territories (4%). In the Northeast, 1.4% of women with AIDS resided outside metropolitan areas compared with 10.2% of women who resided outside metropolitan areas in the South. Of all AIDS cases among women, 61% were reported from five states: New York (26%), Florida (13%), New Jersey (10%), California (7%), and Texas (5%).

Of all women with AIDS who were initially reported without risk but who were later reclassified, most had heterosexual contact with an at-risk partner (66%) or a history of injection drug use (27%). In 1996, of the 40% of women reported with AIDS attributed to heterosexual contact (as opposed to 6% heterosexual contact AIDS cases for men), 35% reported contact with a male partner who was an injection drug user; 5%, a bisexual male; 2%, a partner who had hemophilia or had received HIV-contaminated blood or blood products; and 58%, a partner who had documented HIV infection or AIDS but whose risk was unspecified (*HIV/AIDS Surveillance Report*, 1996).

TABLE 11-1   Reported AIDS Cases for Women, United States

Year	Number	% Increase	Total
1981 (From June)	6		
1982	47		
1983	144		
1984	285		
1985	534		
1986	980		
1987	1,701		
1988	3,263		
1989	3,639		
1990	4,890		
1991	5,732	1992–1994 151[b]	Through 1994 (58,995)
1992	6,571		
1993	16,824[a]		Through 1995 (73,095)
1994	14,379		Through 1996 (estimated) (86,915)
1995	14,100		Through 1997 (estimated) 99,915
1996	13,820		
1997	(projected) 13,000		
Men	402,800 (1981–1996)		
Total:	581,429 (1996)[c]		
Estimated	646,429 (1997)		

[a]The large increase in women's AIDS cases for 1993 over previous years was due to the January 1, 1993 implementation of the new definition of AIDS. Fifty-two percent of cases are associated with IDU. Most of the remaining cases occurred in women who are sexual partners of IDUs.

[b]Reported male AIDS cases for 1993 were up 113%, in women, 128% (Hirschhorn, 1995).

[c]Total AIDS cases include 7,629 pediatric.

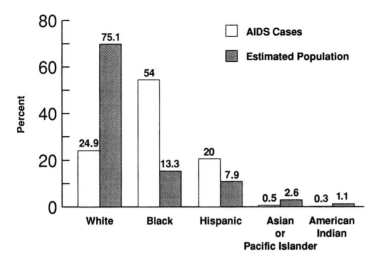

FIGURE 11-2 Incidence of AIDS Cases Among Women of Different Ethnic Groups, United States. Worldwide, every minute, two women become HIV-infected, and every 2 minutes, a woman dies of AIDS. (*Source: Courtesy of CDC, Atlanta, 1993, updated*)

[An excellent resource on HIV/AIDS in women can be obtained from the CDC National AIDS Clearinghouse 1-800-458-5231 and the Women's Information Service and Exchange (WISE), 125 Fifth St., N.E., Alanta, Georgia 30308, (800) 326-3861.]

In 1994 and 1995, 60% of all new female HIV infections in the United States occurred in women by age 20 (Cotton, 1994). To identify women at risk accurately, physicians need to be aware of the known demographic, epidemiological, and transmission risk factors related to HIV in women.

Figure 11-6 shows the risk factors of the sexual partners of 5,522 women who contracted their infection through heterosexual contact in 1996. Many women may not be aware that their partners are in these behavioral risk categories, but those who are should be given the opportunity to discuss the risks and should be counseled to undergo testing. These data illustrate the importance of obtaining as much information as possible concerning a person's sexual partners.

As the frequency of HIV/AIDS increases in women, the question of whether AIDS will ex-

Adolescent/Adult Women AIDS Annual Rates per 100,000 Population
United States — Cases Reported in 1996

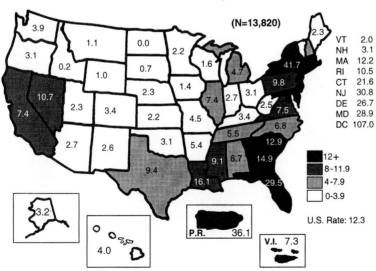

FIGURE 11-3 Rates of Reported AIDS Cases per 100,000 Population Among Adolescent and Adult Women by State of Residence—United States, 1996. (*Source: Courtesy of CDC, Atlanta*)

Chap. 11 *Prevalence of HIV Infection and AIDS Cases Among Women, Children, and Teenagers* **335**

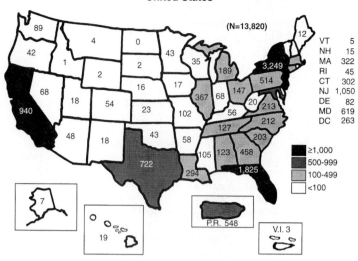

Adolescent/Adult Women AIDS Cases Reported in 1996
United States

(N=13,820)

VT	5
NH	15
MA	322
RI	45
CT	302
NJ	1,050
DE	82
MD	619
DC	263

≥1,000
500-999
100-499
<100

FIGURE 11-4 One Year of New Women AIDS Cases Across the United States, Reported for 1996. (Total AIDS cases for 1996, 69,151) (*Source: Courtesy of CDC, Atlanta*)

plode in the heterosexual community of the United States becomes more a question of **when will the number of female AIDS cases equal male cases**. Worldwide, women accounted for 25% of all HIV-infected adults in 1990. Beginning 1998 that percentage had risen to about 50%. The World Health Organization predicts that by the year 2000, women will constitute the majority of HIV-infected adults.

FIGURE 11-5 Cumulative Major Sources of HIV Infections in United States Women. (*Source: U.S. Centers for Disease Control and Prevention, Year End Surveillance Report 1996*)

Transmission Categories

Injection drug use (IDU) has, since 1981, been the major route of HIV transmission for women. Beginning in the 1990s, however, female AIDS cases through heterosexual contact is increasing rapidly and may equal IDU by the turn of the century. Blood transfusions and use of blood products make up 4% of female AIDS cases and in 12% of cases the cause is undetermined.

HIV infection has occurred in a substantial number of women exposed to semen from a single HIV-infected male. In one case, 10 out of 17 women became HIV-infected through vaginal intercourse with one HIV-infected man (Allen et al., 1988). In another case, a male is accused

————— **ANECDOTE** —————

I was referred to an eye doctor who is a specialist in retinal detachment in HIV/AIDS patients. After looking at my chart, the first thing he said to me was "Sex or drugs?" I knew he was trying to pigeonhole me. But I said, "Excuse me," and he repeated, "Sex or drugs?" I told him, "I don't do drugs anymore and sex with you, I don't think so!"

Commentary: Women with HIV/AIDS have to deal with a lot of attitude from people, including health care providers.

HIV INFECTION AMONG WOMEN

Alarming News for Women (*World News Tonight* ABC, September 7, 1993). Until now, AIDS has been perceived to be a disease primarily afflicting homosexual men and injection drug users. **In nine U.S. cities, AIDS has become the leading cause of death in women of childbearing age. For the first time, in 1992, the number of women infected with AIDS through heterosexual transmission approximated those women infected via virus-contaminated needles.** In 1993, the number of women infected via heterosexual transmission surpassed those infected via injection drug use.

There are 6 million women ages 18 to 40 in the United States who are unmarried and having sexual relationships. Those most at risk for HIV infection are: (**1**) those who have multiple sexual partners (defined as having more than four different partners/year), and (**2**) those women who **do not** insist on the use of a condom.

The nation's top five cities with a female population of 100,000 or more that have the highest incidence of AIDS among women are as follows:

Rate/100,000 Women (1993)

City	White	Black (non-Hispanic)
(1) New York, NY	41.5	90.9
(2) West Palm Beach, FL	38.1	295.4
(3) Ft. Lauderdale, FL	34.1	199.5
(4) Newark, NJ	29.6	105.5
(5) Miami, FL	29.1	125.2

Clearly, in all five cities, HIV disease and AIDS affects black, non-Hispanic women disproportionately.

Three of the nation's cities with the highest incidence of AIDS in women are located in Florida within a 70-mile radius of each other (West Palm Beach, Ft. Lauderdale, and Miami). This area is an epicenter of HIV infection for Florida women. Florida has 10% of the nation's AIDS cases. The other areas of highest incidence of AIDS in women are Puerto Rico, followed by New Jersey, New York, the District of Columbia, Florida, Connecticut, Maryland, Delaware, Massachusetts, Rhode Island, Georgia, and South Carolina (Guinan, 1993). Nationally, through 1997, 15% of female AIDS cases are in women. In Florida's Palm Beach County the rate is 24%; in Broward and Dade Counties, 18%. The epidemiologist for the state of Florida stated that what is happening in Florida is happening in the inner cities nationwide. What may distinguish the AIDS epidemic in women is that it hinges on the low self-esteem and lack of personal power experienced by women in many walks of life.

Most of Florida's women with AIDS are poor and receive their medical care through the public health system. Among women in South Florida, HIV transmission is associated with crack cocaine. Pam Whittington, Director of the Boynton Community Life Center, a family support facility in southern Palm Beach County, said, "If you have 10 women on crack, probably eight of them are HIV-infected."

Crack cocaine is cheap and readily available. Its use contributes to anonymous, high-risk sex with multiple partners. Those who cannot afford crack exchange sex for it. In isolated communities of crack users, there is a high degree of sharing sex partners, many of whom are HIV-positive.

of HIV-infecting between 30 and 50 women. Ending 1997, authorities are still searching for him. To date there are six cases of transmission through artificial insemination **reported** in the United States, and six other cases are known to have occurred (Joseph, 1993). Four of eight Australian women who received semen from a single infected donor became infected. HIV-contaminated semen had been injected into the uterus through a catheter.

Prostitutes

The term **prostitute** is used in preference to the more recently coined "**sex worker.**" No single term can adequately encompass the range of sex for money/drugs/friendship/accommodation transactions that undoubtedly occurs worldwide. However, the term prostitute is at least relatively clear in referring to those who are directly involved in trading sex for

WOMEN + SEXUAL PARTNERS + DECEPTION = AIDS

Across the world, women in support groups or with a close friend have been telling their stories of **trusting** their sexual partners and ending up with AIDS. Their trust was violated—their lives forfeited. Here are but a few examples of the thousands of similar cases worldwide.

1. She is 48 years old with curly red hair and bags beneath her eyes. She slouches slightly in the office chair, stretching out her feet. From her eye shadow to her sneakers, everything is blue. Married to one husband for 28 years, she has children and grandchildren. She also has AIDS. She did not use drugs or have multiple sexual partners. **She did have sex with her husband without a condom!**

2. One 23-year-old had a boyfriend with hemophilia; he never used condoms and never mentioned HIV, even though he had already infected another woman.

3. A divorced man with two children did not tell his 46-year-old girlfriend he had AIDS, even when he was hospitalized with an AIDS-related infection.

4. A 7-year live-in partner of a woman denied infecting her, even though he tested positive for HIV; she did not know he was having sex outside their relationship.

5. Because she had **only two boyfriends,** because "we were perfectly ordinary," they did not use condoms.

6. This woman with a baby did not know "my man was shooting up drugs and sharing needles." Not until he died of AIDS.

7. She **never** dreamed her partner had used a needle. When the doctor said she had AIDS, she replied, **"You have made a mistake.** I cannot have AIDS. How could I have that?"

All these women discovered their HIV status only after they became seriously ill with infections that they **should not** have had. Heterosexual transmission is rising dramatically. A seldom mentioned fact is: a large percentage of the infected women are married or in committed relationships.

---

money or drugs. In the United States, prostitutes represent a diverse group of people with various lifestyles. About 31% of female IDUs admit to engaging in prostitution. They need money to support their drug habit, pay rent, and eat. Cities with large numbers of IDUs subsequently have large numbers of prostitutes. Evidence is overwhelming—IDU, prostitution, and HIV infection are strongly associated.

In a multi-city study, HIV antibody was detected in 13% of 1,378 female prostitutes; **80% of the infected prostitutes reported using injection drugs** (Darrow et al., 1989). For prostitutes **without** histories of injection drug use, HIV seroprevalence was 5%; HIV infection in this group was greater among blacks and Hispanics and among those who had had more than 200 paying sex partners. The point is that **non-injection-drug-using prostitutes in the United States play a small role in HIV transmission**. This is believed to be because of the low incidence of HIV infection among their male clients and on the insistence by many prostitutes that their clients use condoms (Felman,

1990). In Africa and Asia, however, prostitution plays a major role in HIV transmission.

Women Who Have Sex with Women (Lesbians)

Research on female-to-female transmission remains inconclusive. But the large numbers of HIV-positive women and women with AIDS should alert women who have sex with women that they cannot assume their partners are uninfected because they are lesbians. Daron Ferris and colleagues (1966) report that 80% of lesbian women have had sex with men during their lifetime. Also, certain sexual behaviors common among lesbians probably put them at risk for transmitting and receiving HIV through vaginal fluid, menstrual blood, sex toys, and cuts in the vagina, mouth, and on the hands.

The evidence is clear: HIV infection is present among lesbians, and lesbians engage in behaviors that put them at risk for HIV infection, in some cases, at higher risk than most others in society. Whether or not lesbians put

1% Transfusion recipient

35% Injection drug users

58% Risk not specified

6% Bisexual male

<1% Hemophilia

FIGURE 11-6 Risk Category of Sexual Partners of Women with Heterosexually Acquired AIDS, for 1996, United States. Thirty-five percent of women who contracted AIDS through heterosexual contact had partners who were injection drug users. Fifty-eight percent acquired HIV from partners with other risk factors. (*HIV/AIDS Surveillance Report, 1996*)

their female sexual partners at risk is less clear. In fact, there is a great deal of controversy about this question. Some HIV/AIDS investigators believe the risk of sexual transmission increases as the number of HIV-positive lesbians increases. Others believe that lesbians are not getting infected through lesbian sex, but only through unsafe behaviors like IDU. Female-to-female transmission has been reported in one case and suggested in another (Curran et al., 1988).

Susan Chu and colleagues (1994) reported the findings of a special surveillance project, Female-to-Female Sexual Contact and HIV Transmission, conducted by nine states (Arizona, Colorado, Connecticut, Delaware, Florida,

Georgia, Michigan, New Mexico, and South Carolina) and two local health departments (Los Angeles and Washington). They interviewed 1,122 women reported with HIV/AIDS between January 1990 and September 1993.

Only 10 of these women reported sexual contact **only with other women** in the past 5 years. Of these 10, eight (80%) reported injection drug use, one had received a blood transfusion before March 1985, and one had an undetermined mode of exposure. She reported one instance of sexual intercourse with a man in 1981. In addition, she has had two female sex partners who had HIV disease; one, a bisexual woman, was reported to have died of "pneumonia," the other informed her she

—————— POINT OF INFORMATION 11.2 ——————

SPECIAL PROBLEMS FOR HETEROSEXUAL WOMEN

Heterosexual women are at far greater risk of contracting AIDS during heterosexual intercourse than heterosexual men for several reasons.

1. During vaginal contact, women are exposed to semen carrying significant quantities of lymphocytes. Conversely, men are exposed to small amounts of potentially infected vaginal fluids and cervical secretions (fewer lymphocytes).

2. The mucosal surface area available for HIV penetration is significantly smaller in men than in women. The entire vagina and cervix are of a mucosal nature. In men, the urethra is the only mucosal surface area exposed to female secretions.

3. During the act of sexual intercourse, the vaginal mucosa often suffers microscopic abrasions, drawing lymphocytes to the area. This makes vaginal tissue more susceptible to HIV-positive semen. Abrasions do not normally occur within the male urethra.

4. There are more HIV-infected men than women. In Western Europe, Australia, and North America, the ratio of HIV-infected men to HIV-infected women is about 6:1 (Aggleton et al., 1994). Because of the greater number of infected men, the sexually active woman is at increased risk. This is particularly true if the woman has multiple partners and lives in an area with a large population of HIV-infected men.

had been diagnosed with AIDS. The woman described herein could have been infected from female-to-female sexual contact, especially considering the risk behavior and clinical status of some of her female partners.

George Lemp and colleagues (1995) reported on HIV infection in 498 lesbian and bisexual women. Six were HIV-positive but, there was **NO** evidence of women-to-women transmission! The Women's AIDS Network (1988) of San Francisco states in their publication *Lesbians and AIDS* that if there is a possibility that either woman is carrying the virus, she should not allow her menstrual blood, vaginal secretions, urine, feces, or breast milk to enter her partner's body through the mouth, rectum, vagina, or broken skin.

Special Concerns of HIV/AIDS Women

First, HIV/AIDS has a profound impact on women, both as an illness and as a social and economic challenge. Women play a crucial role in preventing infection by insisting on safer sexual practices and caring for people with HIV disease and people with AIDS. The stigma attached to HIV/AIDS can subject women to discrimination, social rejection, and other violations of their rights.

Women need to know that they can protect themselves against HIV infection. Women have a traditionally passive role in sexual decision making in many countries. They need knowl-

TABLE 11-2 Barriers to Medical Care for HIV-Infected Women

Poverty
Lack of health insurance
Primary care provider for children and family
Competing health needs
Injection drug use
Inconvenient location and times of clinic
Transportation
Fear of disclosure
Domestic violence
Undocumented immigration status
Competing health needs of family members (children, partner, etc.)
Culturally based fears or mistrust of the health care system
Denial
Lack of education about risk for HIV infection

Adapted from Hirschhorn, 1995.

edge about HIV and AIDS, self-confidence, the skills necessary to insist partners use safer sex methods, and good medical care (Table 11-2).

Efforts to influence women to practice safer sex must also be joined by efforts to address men and their responsibility in practicing safer sex.

Second, women get pregnant. Women who are ill and discover they are pregnant need information about both the potential impact of pregnancy on their own health and maternal–fetal HIV transmission.

Third, women have the role of mothering. From this role come two important consequences. First, when a woman becomes ill with HIV disease or AIDS, her role as caretaker of the child or children or other adults in the household is immediately affected. The family is severely disrupted and each family member has to make adjustments. Second, the mother must cope with her own life-threatening illness while she also deals with the impact of the disease on her family. Demographic studies show that many HIV-infected or AIDS women have young children; and these women are often the sole support of these children.

Fourth, a woman's illness may be complicated further by incarceration and the threat of foster care proceedings. If the mother is healthy enough to care for her child, she must still cope with the complex issues of medical and home care, school access, friends, and family stress.

Fifth, worldwide, women make up over 40% of AIDS cases and 80% of these (40%) women are mothers of children. An estimated 3 million women will have died of AIDS ending the 1990s, and over 18 million will have become HIV-infected. Yet little is known about how HIV infection occurs in women and what is the appropriate standard for their clinical care. Initially, what became known about HIV disease was derived from studies on men, who for the most part differ from women in race, income, and risk behavior. And what female-derived information there is on HIV disease in women came mostly from studies on pregnant women which have focused primarily on perinatal issues. In 1986, only 3% of participants of federally funded HIV/AIDS clinical trials were women. By 1996, this figure rose to 26%.

To date, little is known about the pharmacokinetics of HIV/AIDS drugs in women, nor is it

AN AIDS CLINICAL DRUG TRIAL—BY DEFINITION

A clinical drug trial is a government funded and organized study of an experimental or unproven drug to determine the drug's safety and efficacy (whether or not it works). Drug trials for HIV/AIDS, sponsored by the FDA, are organized into the AIDS Clinical Trials Group (ACTG). Guidelines are set to determine how the ACTGs may be run and who is eligible to participate. Taking part in a trial may entitle persons to receive medical examinations and checkups and to have their overall health monitored. For many people with AIDS, the ACTGs are the only means of access to certain potentially life-saving drugs, and the only form of health care they may ever receive.

Historically, FDA policy on admitting women into clinical trials has been confusing and dis-

criminatory at best. Until recently, the FDA has had an outright ban on all women of childbearing potential from participation in early stages of drug trials. In March of 1994, the Food and Drug Administration (FDA) took two important steps to ensure that new drugs are properly evaluated in women. **First,** it provided formal guidance to drug developers to emphasize its expectations that women would be appropriately represented in clinical studies and that new drug applications would include analyses capable of identifying potential differences in drug actions and value between the sexes. **Second,** the agency altered its 1977 policy to include most women with childbearing potential in the earliest phases of clinical trials (Merratz et al., 1993).

clear whether gender influences specific illnesses. For example, does HIV infection increase cervical and vaginal disease and pelvic inflammatory disease? Why are certain opportunistic diseases more aggressive and damaging to females? And how are the drugs used to treat opportunistic infections metabolized in women?

1995 Update— According to Arlene Bardeguez (1995) and other similar reports (Cohen, 1995; Garcia, 1995), gender does not influence the prevalence of AIDS-defining illnesses, with the exception of invasive carcinoma of the cervix and possibly Kaposi's

sarcoma. Access to HIV-related care and therapies is the dominant factor influencing the prevalence of AIDS-defining illnesses among women (Table 11-3). Injection drug use in HIV-seropositive women leads to a higher incidence of certain diseases, particularly esophageal candidiasis, herpes simplex virus, and cytomegalovirus. Once an initial diagnosis of AIDS has been made, several major AIDS-defining illnesses appear more frequently in women: toxoplasmosis, herpes genital ulcerations, and esophageal candidiasis.

The currently proposed female-specific markers of **HIV disease** include **cervical dys-**

ONE WOMAN'S COMMENTS ON HER HIV DISEASE TREATMENTS

"I was fired from my job when they found out I was HIV-positive. The boss said, 'You have a modern problem—and this is an old-fashioned business.' "

This woman, in 1995, was 29 years of age and HIV-positive since age 22. When her T4 cell count dropped to 250, her M.D. put her on zidovudine (ZDV, also called AZT). She was not given any literature or verbal explanation of how this drug would affect her. In 12 months she became anemic; she could not sleep or hold down food, and her menstrual cycle became erratic. Without explanation, she next received two other HIV repli-

cation inhibitors, ddI and ddC. The side effects were very bad: consistent premenstrual symptoms; mood swings; increased cravings for certain foods, alcohol, or drugs; breast tenderness; and bloating. But, there was no literature for her to read and her M.D. said, "I knew how the drugs affected men, but I knew nothing of what to expect when I gave these drugs to women." "I stopped taking these drugs—they were killing me faster than the virus! I have severe yeast infections, shingles, sinus infections, and a host of other infections. My M.D. is dealing with me like I'm some kind of experiment."

TABLE 11-3 Frequency of AIDS-Defining Illnesses in HIV-Positive Women and Men

	Women (%)	Men (%)
Pneumocystis carinii pneumonia	43	48
Wasting syndrome	21	20
Esophageal candidiasis	26	19
HIV-associated encephalophaty	6	6
Herpes simplex infection	6	4
Toxoplasmosis of the brain	6	4
Mycobacterium-avium intracellulare complex	6	6
Extrapulmonary cryptococcosis	4	4
Cytomegalovirus infection	3	4
Cytomegalovirus retinitis	3	4
Extrapulmonary tuberculosis	2	3
Cryptosporidosis	2	2
Lymphoma	2	4
Kaposi's sarcoma	2	20

From CDC, AIDS Public Information Data Set—updated through 1997.

plasia and **neoplasia** (tumor), **vulvovaginal candidiasis**, and **pelvic inflammatory disease** (PID). HIV-infected women have been found to have a higher incidence of cervical abnormalities on routine screening.

The 14 most common AIDS-defining illnesses in HIV-seropositive women are listed in Table 11-3. No gender-related differences in survival of HIV-positive persons have been documented when access to medical care is considered. The shorter observed survival of women in some studies is thought to occur because of the lack of access to physicians who are knowledgeable about HIV-related care and therapies (Table 11-2).

Female HIV/AIDS Deaths

Women's deaths in the United States, rose from 18 cases in 1981 to 55,952 beginning 1998. That is, 56% of all women with AIDS have died. AIDS is now the leading cause of death for all women between the ages of 25 and 34, the third leading cause of death for all women between the ages of 25 and 44, and the fifth leading cause of death in white women. It is the leading cause of death for black women between the ages of 25 and 44 (*MMWR*, 1996c).

Through 1994, in the United States, **48% of women who died of AIDS were diagnosed after their deaths, at autopsy**. They died without knowing they had AIDS. Eleven percent of women with AIDS died within 30 days after the diagnosis.

Identifying and Preventing HIV Infection

Identification of HIV-Positive Women— At age 26, a woman and her physicians were baffled when she began suffering from a variety of strange medical conditions: fevers, throat sores, unexplained vaginal bleeding, and fatigue. **It took a variety of doctors and 7 years to find out what was wrong. She tested HIV-positive!**

This woman's difficulty in getting diagnosed points out the extent to which women still are invisible when it comes to AIDS. After more than 17 years into the epidemic, the message still hasn't reached primary care physicians: Their female patients may be at risk. This young woman said, "I went into doctors' offices and all they saw was a white, middle-class woman, not someone at risk for HIV."

Early identification of women with HIV infection is a pressing problem. Risk-based screening at a Johns Hopkins perinatal clinic showed that 43% of HIV-positive women were not identified as at-risk on the basis of such screening, with infection being found in 20 (9.5%) of 211 women admitting to risk behaviors and in 15 (1.6%) of 949 who were not at risk according to their response to screening questions (Garcia, 1995). Recent epidemiologic data indicate that the most common AIDS-indicator illnesses among both men and women are esophageal candidiasis and

PROPORTION OF WOMEN TAKING HIV TEST

From 1991 to 1993, the proportion of women aged 18–44 years who have ever been tested for HIV increased 60% (from 18.8% to 31.8%). Increases were similar across all sociodemographic groups (*MMWR*, 1996b). As in 1991, in the 1993 survey, higher percentages of black and Hispanic women (46.1% and 39.7%, respectively) compared with white women (27.9%) reported having been tested for HIV. Similarly, a higher proportion of women with <12 years of education reported having been tested for HIV (36.9%) compared with high school graduates (31.5%) or those with college education (30.4%). In addition, more women living in poverty reported having been tested for HIV (40.2%) than did women living at or above the poverty level (30.3%). HIV testing trends among women aged 18–44 years were similar to those in 1991 with respect to marital status, risk perception, and region of residence; however, the proportions of women tested in all three groups increased during 1991–1993. During 1991–1993, **the proportion of women tested who had higher perceived risk for HIV did not increase; however, the proportion tested with low or no perceived risk nearly doubled.** (Data about HIV testing and other AIDS-related knowledge and attitudes were collected in 1994 and 1995.)

Class Discussion: A. How can one explain the higher level of HIV test taking among the **poor** and **less educated** than in those economically advantaged and better educated? **B.** Give several reasons why the percentage of those with higher perceived risk for HIV **did not increase** while the percentage taking an HIV test among low risk individuals **doubled!**

Pneumocystis carinii pneumonia, with women having a somewhat greater frequency of the former and a somewhat reduced frequency of the latter (Table 11-3).

Prevention— To prevent HIV infection, women have been told to reduce their number of partners, to be monogamous, and to protect themselves by using condoms. But these goals, generally speaking, do not fit the realities of women's lives or they may not be under their control.

Women do not wear the condom. For women to protect themselves from HIV infection, they must not only rely on their own skills, attitudes, and behaviors regarding condom use, but also on their ability to convince their partner to use a condom. Gender, culture, and power may be barriers to maintaining safer sex practices.

Women who have more than one partner in their lifetime often practice serial monogamy, remaining with one partner at a time. People living as couples reduce the number of their sexual partners. Still, in many phases of life, sex is practiced with new partners in new relationships. American women, on average, are single for many years before their first marriage; they might be single again after a divorce; they might marry again; and, in later phases especially, they might be widowed. For some women, multiple partners throughout life are an economic necessity, urging them to reduce the number of partners is meaningless unless the economic situation for these women is improved (Ehrhardt, 1992). In addition, public health strategies not necessarily targeted to women can also play an important role for women. Syringe exchange and drug treatment are important strategies because almost half of all HIV infections in women are due to injection drug use. Because women are now more likely to be infected by men through heterosexual contact, programs that specifically target men, especially IDUs, will have a beneficial impact on women's programs.

Childbearing Women

Without therapy the perinatal incidence of 30% for HIV infection is second only to that for gay men. Beginning 1998, there were an estimated 90,000 HIV-infected women of childbearing age in the United States; perhaps 30% know that they are infected. Women, in general, have two children before they find out they are infected (Thomas, 1989). The birth of an infected child may serve as a **miner's ca-**

nary—the first indication of HIV infection in the mother. In New York, in 1993, 25% of HIV-infected babies were born to mothers who did not know they were HIV-infected. In the United States, 0.17% of childbearing women are HIV-positive (Luzu-riaga et al., 1996). Some 5,800 infants were born to HIV-infected mothers each year from 1988 through 1992 and 6,500 to 7,000 such births occurred each year from 1993 through 1997. Seven thousand infants with a 30% HIV infection rate means about 2,100 HIV-infected infants/year.

Pregnancy and HIV Disease— (See Chapter 7 for more information of HIV transmission and zidovudine therapy for the newborn.) Early findings in pregnant women indicated that those with T4 cell counts of less than **300/μL** of blood were more likely to experience HIV-associated illness during pregnancy. Pregnant HIV-infected women exhibit a greater T4 cell count decline during pregnancy than do women without HIV infection. T4 cell counts in the HIV-infected do not return to prepregnancy levels. However, the overall declines in HIV-infected women likely represent declines that would have occurred in the absence of pregnancy and suggest that pregnancy does not accelerate disease progression.

Over the last 6 years, HIV-positive pregnant women have been attracting more attention from the medical establishment, **first**, because there are better medications for the HIV-positive mother and fetus, and **second**, because of the relatively high incidence of HIV births.

Class Discussion: Nationwide, approximately 1.7 of 1,000 pregnant women are HIV-infected, an incidence much higher than that of **fetal neural tube** defects, for which pregnant women are screened routinely. **Should less be done for HIV pregnancies?**

Reproductive Rights— These are central to a woman's right to control her body. The choice of becoming pregnant or terminating the pregnancy are continually disputed.

However, as more women become HIV-infected and give birth to HIV-infected children, childbearing may come under the surveillance of the state. Women of childbearing age may be among the first groups to undergo mandatory testing as part of an attempt to control the birth of HIV-infected newborns.

Reproductive rights take on new meaning with HIV-infected pregnancies. The state has traditionally expressed an interest in protecting the rights of the fetus. This interest was transcended in the 1973 *Roe v. Wade* decision when the Supreme Court recognized a woman's right to choose an abortion. The court ruled that a woman's right to privacy must prevail against the state's interest in protecting

--------- **BOX 11.2** ---------

HIV-INFECTED WOMEN: DIFFICULT CHOICES DURING PREGNANCY

She was 19 years old, a nursing student, pregnant, and HIV-positive. She spent 4 1/2 months of pregnancy in constant fear for herself and for her baby. She waited, her health began to falter, then she decided to have an abortion.

Several studies have reported that HIV-positive women who perceived their risk of infecting their fetus to be greater than 50% were more likely to abort than those who perceived a lower risk. HIV-positive women who chose to continue their pregnancy cited the desire to have a child, strong religious beliefs, and family pressure (Selwyn et al., 1989).

For women who are HIV-positive, pregnancy poses difficult choices. First, pregnancy may mask the presence of HIV disease symptoms and having a child poses other questions such as: Can the mother cope with a normal or infected child? and Who will care for the child if the mother becomes too ill or dies? Such questions bring up a moral issue for **Class Discussion: Do couples have a right to have children when one of the partners is known to be HIV-positive? If the woman is HIV-positive? If both are HIV-positive? Is there any stage of HIV disease/AIDS when you think a women should lose the right to become pregnant? (See Chapter 7 for the four stages of HIV disease).**

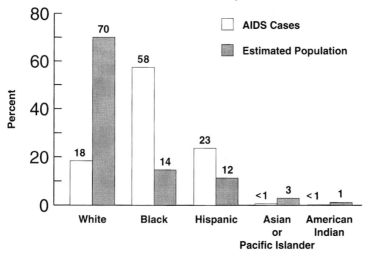

AIDS Cases: Children, United States

Percent

80
70
60
58
40
23
20 18
14
12
0 <1 3 <1 1

White | Black | Hispanic | Asian or Pacific Islander | American Indian

☐ AIDS Cases

▨ Estimated Population

FIGURE 11-7 Pediatric AIDS Cases—United States through 1996. The number of pediatric AIDS cases in proportion to the ethnic pediatric population is presented in percent. Due to rounding, numbers may not add up to 100%. (*Source: CDC, Atlanta, GA, 1996*)

the future life of the fetus. The state's interest in fetal survival tends to diminish, however, when the mother is infected with HIV (Franke, 1988). (See Chapter 7 for recent information on preventing HIV infection of the fetus.)

PEDIATRIC HIV-POSITIVE AND AIDS CASES—UNITED STATES

Pediatric AIDS in the United States affects two age groups: (1) infants and young children who became infected through perinatal (vertical)

─────── SIDEBAR 11.1 ───────

NATURAL CONCEPTION IN HIV-NEGATIVE WOMEN WITH HIV-INFECTED PARTNERS

An increasing number of couples in which the man is HIV-positive and the woman HIV-negative want children. Insemination with sperm from *seronegative donors* is the only safe option, yet most couples wish to have a child who is biologically theirs.

Between 1986 and 1996, Laurent Mandelbrot and colleagues (1997) followed 104 consecutive pregnancies in 92 HIV-negative women with HIV-positive partners. All were single pregnancies, conceived without the use of assisted reproduction techniques. Most couples had received nondirective preconceptual counseling on the risks of heterosexual HIV transmission. Prior to pregnancy, most of the men were symptom-free, 14 (13%) had HIV-related symptoms, and one died of AIDS during the pregnancy. Twenty-one men were receiving antiretroviral therapy at the time of conception. One-third of partners reported inconsistent or no condom use; **in 68 pregnancies conception resulted from unprotected intercourse during ovulation, only after one episode of intercourse in 17 of these cases.** After conception, couples were advised to use condoms, and women were tested monthly for HIV infection. Follow-up was 3 months in all cases and more than 6 months in 95 cases. There were 92 deliveries, four abortions, six miscarriages, and two lost to follow-up in the second trimester. No seroconversions occurred within the first 3 months following conception. Seroconversion was observed in two women at 7 months of pregnancy and in two others postpartum; all such cases arose in couples reporting inconsistent condom use. The investigators suggest that their data show that male-to-female HIV transmission is infrequent during natural conception.

transmission, and (2) school-age children, the majority of whom acquired HIV through blood transfusions (mostly hemophiliacs).

Beginning 1998, over 8,000 pediatric AIDS cases were **reported** and about 4,500 (55%) have died from AIDS. Pediatric AIDS cases represent about 1.3% of the total number of AIDS cases to date. It is estimated that for each pediatric AIDS case **reported** there are three to four other HIV-infected children. Thus an estimated 20,000 to 28,000 children in the United States have HIV (Luzuriaga et al., 1996; Rodriguez et al., 1996). Of the pediatric AIDS cases, 3% were/are hemophilic children who received HIV-contaminated blood transfusions or blood products (pooled and concentrated blood factor VIII injections). About 5% of pediatric AIDS cases occurred in nonhemophilic children who were transfused with HIV-contaminated blood. Ninety percent of pediatric AIDS cases received the virus from HIV-infected mothers who transmitted it to them either during the fetal stage (perinatal), during labor or as the newborn passed through the birthing canal, or from breast milk soon after birth. From 1994 through 1997, 95% of HIV-infected newborns contracted HIV before or during the birthing process. In 2% of pediatric AIDS cases, the route of HIV infection cannot be determined. The Pediatric AIDS Foundation reported in April of 1995 that hospital costs for each HIV-infected newborn were $35,000 per year (*Nations Health Report*, 1995). In a study from Childrens Hospital of Wisconsin, the cost of care for children with HIV was estimated at $418,863 per patient (*AIDS Clinical Care,*

1996:8, 23). Based on the data of Susan Davis (1995), there are an ending 1997, estimated 15,300 children living with HIV disease.

Beginning 1997, 27 states (no territories) reported on **HIV-infected children.** They reported a total of 1,390 HIV-positive children. Of the 27 reporting states, only two **with the highest incidence of pediatric HIV, New Jersey and Texas, were on the list of the 27 reporting states.** Nine states, New York (25%), Florida (16%), New Jersey (9%), California (7%), Texas (4%), Pennsylvania (3%), Maryland (3%), Illinois (3%), and Georgia (2%) have 72% of **all reported** pediatric AIDS cases. AIDS infection is now the **sixth** leading cause of death in children between the ages of 1 and 14.

Ethnic Prevalence of Pediatric AIDS Cases

Children of color make up 14% of all children in the United States but account for 57% of pediatric AIDS cases. Whites make up 70% of children and account for 18% of pediatric AIDS cases. Hispanics make up 12% of children and account for 23% of pediatric AIDS cases (Figure 11-7).

The 1990s: Decade of the Orphans

The increasing death rate for women affects the care of their children: the estimated 90,000 HIV-infected women of childbearing age in the United States, who were alive in 1992, will leave approximately 125,000 to 150,000 children when they die during the 1990s. Worldwide, the former World Health Organization estimated that by the year 2000, 5 to 10 million

--- **POINT OF INFORMATION 11.5** ---

CHILDREN ORPHANED BY AIDS

By the end of 1995 an estimated 24,600 children, 21,000 adolescents, and 35,100 young adults in the United States had been orphaned by the HIV/AIDS epidemic. An estimated 13% of children and 9% of adolescents whose mothers died in 1991 lost their mothers to AIDS. More youths now lose their mothers to AIDS than to motor vehicle injuries. Unless the course of the epidemic changes drastically, by the year 2000, the cumulative number of U.S. children, teens, and young adults left motherless due to AIDS will exceed 144,000. Worldwide, one in every three children orphaned by HIV/AIDS is younger than 5 years old. Since the beginning of the global epidemic about 10 million children under the age of 15 have lost their mothers to HIV/AIDS. Of these maternal orphans, 90% have been in sub-Saharan Africa.

——— BOX 11.3 ———

ORPHANED CHILDREN DUE TO AIDS AND HIV INFECTION

AIDS orphans present a chilling illustration of the far reaching effects of the AIDS pandemic.

His mother was young, single, and HIV-positive. When she went to the hospital to give birth, she checked in under a false name and address and then slipped out of the hospital leaving her baby who was only a few hours old. Today the boy is 2 years old. No one has yet to offer him a home.

An increasing number of HIV-infected children are being left in hospitals because their HIV-infected mothers and fathers are unable to care for them and no one else wants them. The hospital becomes their home. James Hegarty and colleagues (1988) reported that for 37 children at Harlem Hospital Center, one third of the total in-patient days and over 20% of the cost was for social rather than medical services. By the end of 1994, there were an estimated 24,000 AIDS-related orphan children in the state of New York.

As HIV continues to spread across the nation and HIV-infected women continue to become pregnant, the question is: What will happen to their HIV-infected babies? For one young woman who passed the AIDS virus to her baby 2 years ago, the decision has been made. The baby has AIDS and is in foster care. The mother is very ill. The courts are now deciding whether her six other children should also be put in foster care.

David Michaels and Carol Levine (1994) indicate that by the end of 1995, an estimated 24,600 children, 21,000 adolescents, and 35,100 young adults in the United States will have been orphaned by the HIV/AIDS epidemic. An estimated 13% of children and 9% of adolescents whose mothers died in 1991 lost their mothers to AIDS. More youths now lose their mothers to AIDS than to motor vehicle injuries. Unless the course of the epidemic changes drastically, by the year 2000, the cumulative number of U.S. children, teens, and young adults left motherless due to AIDS will exceed 144,000. The great majority of these children, uninfected by the virus—will begin to affect already burdened social services in major American cities. Things will get immediately worse in such places, where children already spend years going from foster home to foster home and caseworkers are overwhelmed by long lists of families needing everything from housing to medical care. Using the same projections, as many as 98,000 young people 18 and older will become motherless and in some cases be called upon to care for younger family members.

Orphans are often referred to as the **silent legacy** of AIDS. It is expected that about a third of the children orphaned will be from New York City, which has the nation's largest number of AIDS cases. Other cities expected to be hit hard are Miami, Los Angeles, Washington, Newark, and San Juan, Puerto Rico. Most of these orphans will be the children of poor black or Hispanic women whose families are already dealing with stresses like drug addiction, inadequate housing, and health care. Relatives who might in other circumstances be called upon to care for the children often shun them because of the stigma attached to AIDS.

HIV-infected women who abandon their babies are often already sick themselves and face an early death. Few can bear the thought of watching their children struggle through a short life should they have passed the virus during pregnancy. Though the majority of infected mothers do not abandon their offspring, such babies are becoming an increasingly common feature of the AIDS pandemic almost everywhere. And they are part of a larger problem that is turning out to be one of the most serious social consequences of the pandemic—THE PHENOMENON OF AIDS ORPHANS.

The vast majority of the children orphaned by the AIDS pandemic, up to the end of this century, will be in sub-Saharan Africa, where formerly the extended family could always be relied upon to take on the dependents of those who died. But today the continent's age-old, traditional social security system—which has proved itself resilient to so many social changes—is buckling under due to the unprecedented strain caused by the increasing number of AIDS cases.

———— **BOX 11.3** (*continued*) ————

children under age 10 will be orphaned because of HIV/AIDS (*MMWR*, 1996).

Vertical HIV Transmission

Vertical transmission means that HIV passes directly from the infected mother into the fetus or infant. The exact time of HIV transmission to the fetus during pregnancy is unknown. It has been shown to occur as early as the 15th week of gestation. Perinatal (at or near the time of delivery) infection occurs as

does 10% to 15% of HIV transmission through breast-feeding. The European Collaborative Study [1994] reported the HIV transmission rate during cesarean delivery from an HIV-disease mother to be 12% versus 18% for vaginal delivery.

Breast-feeding by mothers with HIV infection established **before** pregnancy increases the risk of vertical transmission by 14%. When a mother develops primary HIV infection **while** breast-feeding, the risk of transmission rises to 29%. Some studies have reported transmission

———— **POINT OF INFORMATION 11.6** ————

WORLDWIDE: CHILDREN WITH HIV/AIDS

Basing its HIV/AIDS estimations and projections on assumptions very similar but not identical to those applied by UNAIDS and WHO, the François-Xavier Bagnoud Center for Health and Human Rights of the Harvard University School of Public Health estimates through 1997, worldwide, about 3,700,000 children have acquired HIV infection through mother-to-child transmission since the beginning of the global epidemic. Because of the rapid progression of pediatric HIV infection to the onset of AIDS and the short survival once pediatric AIDS has set in, most of these children have already died. About one quarter of all AIDS-related deaths thus far have been in children who were infected vertically.

To date, over 85% of all children infected through mother-to-child transmission have been in sub-Saharan Africa. During 1995 through 1997, each year approximately 500,000 children were born with HIV infection (about 1,400 per day); of these children, 67% were in sub-Saharan Africa, 30% in South-East Asia, 2% in Latin America, and 1% in the Caribbean.

Beginning 1998, about 1.5 million children are living with HIV/AIDS, of whom 65% are in sub-Saharan Africa. HIV incidence among children in sub-Saharan Africa, South-East Asia, and the Caribbean is higher than HIV incidence among adults in all other regions of the world. HIV/AIDS prevalence among children is almost 35 times higher in the developing world than in the industrialized world.

rates to be higher during vaginal delivery than cesarean section. But the increased risk of transmission is not enough to offset the general risks associated with cesarean sections, and surgery is not performed unless other indications exist. (This issue remains under investigation, however.) In general it is believed that 50% of HIV-positive babies are infected during the last 2 months of pregnancy and 50% are infected during the birthing process or through breast-feeding.

A working definition of the timing of maternal HIV transmission has been established to differentiate infants infected in utero (in the uterus) from those infected near the time of or during delivery (perinatally). In utero infection occurs in approximately 20% of HIV-infected infants. Children who are infected in utero have a more rapid progression to AIDS and generally become symptomatic during the first year of life. Those infected perinatally have no detectable HIV at birth but demonstrate HIV in the blood by 4 to 6 months of age. These children constitute the majority of HIV-infected infants and have a slower progression to AIDS, about 8% per year (Diaz et al., 1996).

Rate of Transmission— The worldwide rate of HIV transmission from mother to child varies geographically. In Africa, maternal transmission is as high as 50%, while in parts of Europe, transmission is 15%. In the United States, the overall rate is 25% to 30%. The Public Health Service and 16 other national health organizations have recommended that HIV testing be offered to all women at risk prior to or at the time of pregnancy. (Pre- and post-counseling of at-risk females who want to become pregnant or have become pregnant is covered in Chapter 13.)

Because newborns who test HIV-positive **may not be HIV-infected**, infected mothers in developed nations (mothers in underdeveloped nations have been advised to breast-feed because of the lack of available health care and nutrition), are advised not to breast-feed their children. The reason a newborn can test positive and not be infected is because the mother's HIV antibodies can enter the fetus during pregnancy (gestation). Because of the presence of maternal HIV antibody, the newborn may ap-

pear to be infected but is not. The HIV antibody will be lost with time and the child will revert to **seronegativity** (no HIV antibody in the serum).

Perinatal Transmission— Many factors that influence perinatal HIV transmission are not known; but, influencing factors do exist because one mother gave birth to an HIV-infected child followed by an uninfected child who was followed by an infected child (Dickinson, 1988)!

There are multiple factors involved in HIV transmission risk, including maternal immunity and viral load, placental conditions, route of delivery, duration of membrane rupture, and fetal factors (birth order, gestational age). This knowledge has led to trials of various interventions, such as drug therapy to reduce viral load (the number of HIV RNA strands present in the mother at the time of birth) and cesarean section to reduce HIV exposure during delivery.

Viral RNA Load Associated with Perinatal HIV Transmission— Although the close association between stage of HIV infection in a pregnant woman and likelihood of perinatal transmission has been established, there are no precise numerical criteria for pregnancies at **high** and **low** risk of transmission. Viral load measurements are now helping to quantitate this risk.

As explained in Chapters 4 and 7, **viral RNA load refers to the number of copies of HIV RNA in the blood**. Separate studies in 1996 and 1997 on pregnancy and viral loads showed that in one study of 30 HIV-infected women giving birth, 20 of the 22 mothers who did not transmit HIV to their children had a low plasma HIV RNA level (less than 30,000 copies/mL) while 8 of 8 transmitting mothers had plasma HIV RNA levels above 30,000 copies/mL. In a second study (Dickover et al., 1996), 20 of 97 newborns were born HIV-positive. The 20 transmitting mothers each had over 50,000 copies of plasma HIV RNA per milliliter at delivery. An RNA copy number of **50,000** has scientists calling it a **breakpoint for defining a high-risk pregnancy for HIV transmission.** None of 63 women with less than 20,000 HIV RNA copies per milliliter produced truly HIV-positive babies. These studies are supported by the work of Donald Thea and colleagues (1997).

ECONOMIC COSTS FOR HIV TESTING AND ZIDOVUDINE TREATMENT OF HIV-POSITIVE WOMEN AND THEIR NEWBORNS

Testing: The **yearly cost for testing 4 million pregnant women** in the United States is estimated **at $120 million** based on a $30 cost of an HIV test.

Treatment: Currently, each year in the United States approximately 7,000 HIV-positive women become pregnant and approximately 1,000 to 2,000 of their newborns will be HIV-positive. Assuming transmission rates are reduced from 25.5% to 8.3% as found in the ACTG 076 trial, treatment costs of $104,502 for 100 HIV-positive pregnant women and their newborns are offset by the reduction of $1,701,333 associated with fewer cases of pediatric HIV infection for a net savings of $1,596,831.

Update 1977: At San Francisco General and the University of California–San Francisco medical centers—the two main hospitals in San Francisco where HIV-positive mothers are treated—there have been no cases of HIV transmission to newborns since April 1995. And, city health records for 1995 through 1997 show no new pediatric AIDS cases from birth to age 12.

Outcomes of Treating 100 Human Immunodeficiency Virus (HIV)-Positive Pregnant Women and Their Infants With Zidovudine

Outcome Categories	Zidovudine Treatment for 100 Woman–Infant Pairs	No Antiretroviral Treatment for 100 Woman–Infant Pairs
Zidovudine costs		
Prenatal, mothers	$83,440	$0
Intrapartum, mothers	$3,542	$0
Postpartum, infants	$2,520	$0
Total zidovudine costs	$89,502	$0
Other costs associated with zidovudine treatment	$15,000	$0
Total treatment costs	$104,502	$0
No of HIV-positive infants	8.3	25.5
Pediatric HIV treatment costs	$820,992	$2,522,325
Total medical care costs	$925,494	$2,522,825
Total cost savings attributable to treatment with zidovudine per 100 woman–infant pairs	$1,597,331	

Source: Mauskopf et al., 1996.

Nucleoside Reverse Transcriptase Inhibitor Monotherapy that Appears to Reduce HIV Transmission During Pregnancy— For many HIV investigators, the hard search for drugs to combat HIV replication has paid off. The use of zidovudine, in all AIDS Clinical Trials Groups (ACTG) of pregnant women to date, has lowered the incidence of HIV-infected newborns from HIV-infected mothers.

Summary of Results of ACTG Protocol 076— On February 21, 1994, the National Institute of Allergy and Infectious Diseases and the National Institute of Child Health and Human Development announced the interim results of a randomized, multicenter, double-blind, placebo-controlled clinical trial, ACTG Protocol 076. Eligible participants were HIV-infected pregnant women at 14 to 34 weeks of gestation who had received no antiretroviral therapy during their current pregnancy, had no clinical antiretroviral therapy, and had T lymphocyte counts $\geq 200/\mu L$ at the time of entry into the study.

Enrolled women were assigned randomly to receive a regimen of either ZDV or placebo. The ZDV regimen included oral ZDV initiated at 14 to 34 weeks of gestation and continued throughout the pregnancy, followed by intravenous ZDV during labor and oral administration of

ZDV to the infant for 6 weeks after delivery. The placebo regimen was administered identically. Blood specimens were obtained for HIV culture from all infants at birth and at 12, 24, and 78 weeks of age. A positive viral culture was considered indicative of HIV infection. Sera from the infants at 15 and 18 months of age were also tested for HIV antibody.

The estimated transmission rate was 25.5% among the 184 children in the placebo group compared with 8.3% among the 180 children in the ZDV group. This was a 60% reduction of HIV transmission into newborns within the ZDV group! This use of ZDV has the potential to reduce the rate of perinatal transmission substantially, which would reduce overall child mortality. Based on what has been recently learned about perinatal transmission and viral load, ZDV may be reducing HIV transmission by reducing viral load. ZDV did not appear to delay the diagnosis of HIV infection.

Toxicity

Observed toxicity specifically attributable to ZDV was minimal among the women in this study (*MMWR*, 1994; Goldschmidt et al., 1995).

Zidovudine appeared to have minimal toxicity for infants; although anemia was observed, it was mild, temporary, and completely reversible, with no transfusion or administration of other blood products being required (long-term effects of ZDV on exposed children are unknown). In short, **the use of ZDV is known to reduce perinatal HIV transmission.** But it is not 100%, because 8% of ZDV pregnancies will still deliver HIV-infected infants. And that is if therapy is given to all HIV-positive pregnant women!

The full lessons of ACTG 076 have yet to be learned. For example, How does zidovudine work? Would a different drug regimen have been even more effective? The most pressing questions, however, relate to the developing world, where up to 98% of the nearly 15 million women infected with HIV and where almost all of the 3 million perinatally infected infants live. Are there differences, for example, in maternal nutrition, metabolism, health status, or birthing practices that might affect drug

safety and efficacy in these settings? HIV subtype B predominates in North America and Europe, but will zidovudine be as effective for the other HIV subtypes that prevail in Africa and Asia? (See Chapter 3 for discussion of HIV subtypes.)

Economic disparities are also of concern. The cost of medication alone for ACTG 076 was about US$600 per mother-and-child pair which is a prohibitive cost for most developing economies. The year 2000, over 90% of the 5 to 10 million HIV-infected children will live in developing countries.

Pediatric HIV Transmission Goal by Year 2000

The goal is to reduce perinatal HIV transmission to 2% by the year 2000. There is an excellent chance this will occur. Using the drug zidovudine in **combination** with other nucleoside or non-nucleoside reverse transcriptase enzyme inhibitors and one or more of the protease inhibitors offers the **realistic potential** of reaching this goal. It may not be possible to reduce vertical transmission to less than 2% because in studies through 1997, HIV transmission has occurred even with **very low levels of HIV RNA in some patients.** It is not certain, therefore, that more complete viral suppression will result in the absence of vertical transmission. As with the use of zidovudine, questions remain on the safety of the fetus/newborn when exposed to these drugs (Bryson, 1996).

States and Territories Most Affected by Pediatric Cases

The incidence of reported AIDS cases in the United States bears a striking similarity to the incidence of cancer in children. But unlike cancer or the other major causes of death in children whose contributions to childhood mortality have remained stable over the years, the impact of HIV infection is increasing. For infants and young children (ages 1 through 4), AIDS is already among the seven leading causes of death, surpassing all other infections, and is likely to be among the five leading causes of death within the next several years.

There is evidence that HIV was present in female IDUs as early as 1977 because their babies developed AIDS (Thomas, 1988). As the number of HIV-infected women of childbearing age rises, so does the number of HIV-infected babies.

Pediatric AIDS, in the United States is most widespread among blacks, Hispanics, and **the poor of the inner cities** (Figure 11-7). Beginning 1998, New York had the highest incidence of pediatric AIDS cases followed by Florida, New Jersey, California, Puerto Rico, and Texas. Combined, these cases accounted for 66% of all AIDS cases reported among children.

Risk exposures for HIV infection among the mothers of children with perinatally acquired AIDS included injecting drug use (41%), sexual contact with a partner with or at risk for HIV/AIDS (34%), and receipt of contaminated blood or blood products (2%). No risk was specified for 13% of cases. Ten metropolitan areas account for more than 50% of all Pediatric AIDS cases: New York, Miami, Newark, Los Angeles, San Juan, Washington, DC, West Palm Beach, Philadelphia, Nassau/Suffolk, and Jersey City. New York City, Newark, New Jersey, and Miami report the largest numbers. The epidemic is also spreading into smaller communities. Through 1997, pediatric AIDS cases have been reported in 48 of 50 states (North Dakota, Wyoming, Gaum and the Pacific Island, have not yet reported a pediatric AIDS case).

Incidence of HIV Infection in Newborns—United States

Susan Davis and co-workers' (1995) estimated that 14,920 HIV-infected infants were born in the United States between 1978 and 1993. Approximately two thirds of these infants were born between 1988 and 1993, the years for which estimates could be based on data from a recent survey of childbearing women.

An estimated 12,240 of these children were living with vertically acquired HIV at the beginning of 1994. Over half (56%) were born since 1988 and thus are less than age 5. Of these, an estimated 3,180 (26%) were younger than 2 years, 4,240 (35%) were aged 2 to 4 years, and 4,820 (39%) were aged 5 years or older.

AIDS Cases Among Children Declining

The findings reported in "AIDS Among Children–United States, 1996" present a documented decline in the incidence of perinatally acquired AIDS. From 1992 through 1995, the estimated annual number of perinatally acquired AIDS cases declined 27%, from 905 to 663. During this time, the estimated annual number of cases declined 39% among non-Hispanic white, 26% among non-Hispanic black, and 25% among Hispanic children. The proportionate decrease in the number of children with perinatally acquired AIDS from the six areas reporting in the highest number of cases was greater than the decrease for all remaining areas and for all areas combined (*MMWR*, 1996a).

There are many reasons to believe that, with continued HIV counseling of HIV-positive pregnant women and use of AIDS drug cocktails that lower viral loads, fewer children will become infected and this will translate into a continued decrease in children with AIDS (Figure 11-8).

TEENAGERS: HIV-POSITIVE AND AIDS CASES—UNITED STATES

Teenagers often say, **"I KNOW HOW TO BE SAFE,"** but the statistics on teenage pregnancy, smoking, drinking of alcohol, drug use and, in particular, injection drug use, sexual behavior, and the use of contraceptives indicates otherwise. Studies on teenage risk-taking continue to show that about half of teens are **NOT WORRIED ABOUT BECOMING INFECTED WITH HIV AND THAT RELATIVELY FEW TEENAGERS HAVE CHANGED THEIR SEXUAL BEHAVIORS BECAUSE OF THEIR CONCERNS ABOUT THE HIV PANDEMIC.**

Teenagers/Young Women at Greatest Risk

Sixty percent of all new HIV infections globally occur among young women ages 15 to 24, with twice as many young women infected as young men in this age group. In the United States, 25% of all new HIV infections are estimated to occur in young people between the ages of 13 and 20.

FIGURE 11-8 An HIV-Infected Orphan. This 4-year-old child lies in her hospital bed. She was left to society as her mother died of AIDS and no one has come forth to claim her. (*Photograph courtesy of Archive Photos*)

While more research needs to be done on this topic, several factors associated with teenagers and young women are clear: **(1)** they tend to be partnered with **older men** who have had more sexual partners and have a greater chance of being infected with HIV and other sexually transmitted diseases (STDs); **(2)** their risk of HIV infection is greater because of their immature cervix and relatively low vaginal mucous production presents less of a barrier to HIV.and **(3)** many lack the education, social status, economic resources, and power in sexual partner relationships to make informed choices.

Safer Sex

There was a time when safer sex meant not getting caught by your parents. With time, sexually transmitted diseases and in particular HIV/AIDS have changed the meaning of safer sex. Today, over half of teenagers (aged 13 to 19) in the United States have had sex by the time they reach 16, and 7 in 10 are sexually active by 19. Many enter the sexual arena unprepared for the responsibility of their actions (Table 11-4). About 1 million teenage women become pregnant, outside of marriage, each year.

Whether or not society openly discusses it, teens clearly are having sex. Many women—and most men—have their first sexual relations prior to marriage, usually during their teens, and most often those first encounters are unprotected. Research in family planning has revealed that the quality of reproductive health information is generally low among adolescents. This is a reflection in part of the lack of social acceptance of providing sex education and contraceptive services to teens in many countries. In the developing world, contraceptive services are often available only to married women, and in some situations, only to women who have already borne one or more children.

The guiding philosophy in dealing with sexuality in many cultures is "**if you don't talk about sex they won't do it.**" This logic, however, is critically flawed. Teenagers are sexual beings at varying stages of self-awareness and understanding. Many teenagers continue to engage in sexual intercourse despite lack of access to any accurate information about sex and, in most cases, engage in "unsafe sex." **Safer sex** requires an ability to distinguish between risky and nonrisky sexual activities **and** an ability to choose safer sex.

———— **POINT OF VIEW 11.2** ————

PERILS OF UNSAFE SEX

As one teenager put it, "When you're a teenager, your hormones are raging and you think you're indestructible. But sex is how I got AIDS."

TABLE 11-4 Sexually Active Teenagers by High School Year and Age (%)

High School Year	Age Group	Female	Male	Combined
9th Grade	14–15	31.9	48.7	40.3
10th Grade	15–16	42.9	52.5	47.7
11th Grade	16–17	52.7	62.6	57.7
12th Grade	17–19	66.6	76.3	71.5

Source: CDC HIV/AIDS Surveillance Report, November 1991:1–18.

In a 1990 nationwide survey, 19% of high school students have had four or more sex partners by their junior year and 29% had four or more by their senior year (*MMWR*, 1992). Teenagers are experiencing skyrocketing rates of sexually transmitted diseases (STDs). **Every 10 seconds a teenager somewhere in the United States is infected with an STD.** (That's equal to 3 million teenagers aged 13 to 19 years.) People under age 25 account for 66% of all new STDs every year. One in four teens will contract an STD before finishing high school. In California, for example, 15- to 19-year-olds have the highest rates of gonorrhea and chlamydia of any age group in the state. Experts fear that if these diseases are being transmitted, then HIV is too (California Department of Health Services, 1995).

In April of 1992, the *MacNeil/Lehrer Report* estimated that 40,000 to 80,000 teenagers will become HIV-infected during the 1990s. Yet AIDS cases are relatively rare among 13- to 19-year-olds. This is because of the 9- to 15-year time average from HIV infection to AIDS diagnosis. In 1981, there was **one** reported teenage AIDS case, by 1991 there were **789** reported cases. Beginning 1998, there were **4,550** (0.7% of the total AIDS cases). Between 1990 and 1992 the number of AIDS cases in 13- to 24-year-olds increased by 77% (House Select Committee, 1992). It is projected that after 1994 the number of teenage AIDS cases will double annually (Black et al., 1990; Burkhart, 1991).

HIV/AIDS Won't Affect Us!

In 1996, it was estimated that at least two teenagers per hour are becoming HIV-infected (8,760 per year) and this is expected to increase markedly through and beyond the year 2000. (Office of National AIDS Policy 1996). This means that regardless of available information on prevention, and, according to several large-scale studies, **teenagers do know** how HIV is transmitted, there has been a continuing increase in HIV infections within the preteen and early teen population! They continue to engage in sexual intercourse **without condoms!**

How Large Is the Teenage and Young Adult Population?

There are about 28 million teenagers between the ages of 13 and 19. This number is expected to increase to 43 million over the next 24 years (Sells et al., 1996). There are 18 million people ages 20 to 24, and about 22 million between the ages of 25 and 29. That's 68 million people between the ages of 13 and 29. Eighty-six percent of all STDs occur in the age group of 15 to 29. It has been estimated that 34% of all heterosexual adults with AIDS were infected with HIV as teenagers.

Estimate of HIV-Infected and AIDS Cases Among Teenagers and Young Adults

The total number of HIV-infected teenagers is unknown. But it is known that 56% of teenagers who were tested for HIV infection through 1994 did **not** return for their results!

Federal health agencies estimate that teenagers make up about 20% of the HIV-infected population. They are a silent pool for eventual cases of AIDS. About 20% of the total number of AIDS cases in the United States, or 1 in 5 occur in people ages 20 to 29 (about 130,000 through 1997). Most of these people, given the 9- to 15-year period before being diagnosed with AIDS, were infected as teenagers! About 50% of HIV-infected teenagers come from six locations: New York, New Jersey, Texas,

California, Florida, and Puerto Rico. The overall male-to-female ratio of AIDS cases in the United States is now about 7:1, but among 13- to 19-year-olds, the ratio is less than 3:1.

In New York City, teenagers account for 29% of all New York AIDS cases. AIDS is the sixth leading cause of death among persons aged 15 to 24 and fourth among women aged 25 to 44 years (*MMWR*, 1995a,b). Sixty percent of new HIV infections in women now occur during their adolescent years. About 500,000 people in the United States under the age of 29 are HIV-positive.

Teenagers and Incidence of AIDS Cases by Gender and Color

Teenagers of color account for 59% of reported teen AIDS cases. Among males, white teenagers account for 47% of reported teen AIDS cases, followed by blacks (30%) and Hispanics (21%). Among females, black teenagers account for 56%, white for 27%, and Hispanic for 17%. Teenage females, unlike their adult counterparts, are more likely to become infected with HIV through sexual exposure than through injection drug use. A program that followed a large group of HIV-infected adolescents found that although 85% of females contracted HIV infection through heterosexual intercourse, very few were aware that their male partners had HIV infection at the time of their exposure (Futterman et al., 1992).

Teenage HIV Infections Worldwide: At-Risk Behavior Is Universal

Worldwide, Faustin Yao (1992) reports that 20% to 25% of all new HIV infections are occurring among teenagers. Of the 30 million HIV-positive people worldwide early 1997, 10 million became HIV-infected between the ages of 15 and 24.

Teenage Women at Greatest Risk

Teenage women are leading the next wave of the HIV epidemic worldwide. In Asia, Africa, and North America, HIV infections are increasing at an alarming rate among young women, with the highest rates now being found in the 15- to 19-year age group. Many more young women than young men are being HIV-infected worldwide.

Helene Gayle (1988) states that the proportion of teen females in the United States with AIDS is greater than for adult females; and the proportion of teen females infected via heterosexual contact is greater than for adult females. A 1993 study at Montefiore Medical Centre, New York, found that of HIV-positive teenage girls, 85% had contracted the virus through sex with males; 26% reported having **anal sex** either for contraceptive purposes or to retain vaginal virginity. One new face of the epidemic in the United States may be reflected in the behavior of teenage women.

Categories of Teenage HIV Infection

For 1993 and 1994, the current breakdown for HIV infection among teenagers was as follows: males who have sex with males account for 29%, patients with hemophilia and other coagulation disorders account for 31%, heterosexual contact represents 14%, intravenous drug use 17%, and nonhemophilia-related transfusions and organ donations 9%.

David Rogers, vice chairman of the National Commission on AIDS (which dissolved in 1993), said, "We have let issues of taste and

---
BOX 11.4

HIV SPREADING RAPIDLY AMONG TEENAGE GAY MALES

Results of the first national survey of young gay and bisexual men (teens and early twenties) showed that 7% in the survey were HIV-infected (HEALTH, 1996). Researchers interviewed 1,781 men ages 15 to 22 in six urban counties: Miami's Dade County, Dallas County and Los Angeles, San Francisco, and Santa Clara and Alameda counties in California. Results of the interviews demonstrated that 5% of the young men ages 15 to 19 and 9% of those ages 20 to 22 were HIV-infected. Four percent of whites, 7% of Hispanics, and 11% of blacks were infected. And, 38% reported unprotected anal sex within the previous 6 months. These 1994/1995 data, when compared to those data of a similar 1992/1993 survey, were about the same! Education and prevention control measures do not appear to be changing teenage gay sexual behaviors with regard to preventing HIV infection.

THOUGHTS AND COMMENTS FROM A GENERATION AT RISK

"If you're going to educate kids about AIDS, you have to educate them about drugs as well. If you're a youth, you're going to experiment with drugs, especially if you live in a metropolitan area. Even though you get stupid with drugs, you still think about things you don't want to do, but you do it anyhow."—**16-year-old HIV-positive youth from San Francisco**

"We grow up hating ourselves like society teaches us to. If someone had been 'out' about their sexuality. If the teachers hadn't been afraid to stop the 'fag' and 'dyke' jokes. If my human sexuality class had even mentioned homosexuality. If the school counselors would have been open to a discussion of gay and lesbian issues. If any of those possibilities had existed, perhaps I would not have grown up hating what I was. And, just perhaps, I wouldn't have attempted suicide."—**Kyallee, 19**

"People say HIV is this or that group's problem, not mine. But for HIV, it's a matter of risk behaviors, not risk groups. Because if you say it's a risk group thing, I don't identify with that group, so I'm not at risk. That makes people feel invincible to HIV."—**HIV-positive youth**

"I was infected with HIV by my first partner when I was 16 years old. Now at 20 I have this virus that's taking my life because everything I heard when I was younger was sugar-coated. We need more complete information than what we are being given. Even the pamphlets concerning HIV/AIDS prevention are too basic and bland. We need to know real stuff."—**Ryan, age 20**

"We, the young people of this country, need a place where we can go to ask our questions, where we won't be teased or ridiculed. We need a place where we can ask about our mixed up feelings, about sex, and about AIDS."—**15-year-old high school student from Concord, NH**

"If I could talk to the President, or a Senator, or anyone in the Federal Government who can make a difference, I'd tell them to take a look, learn a lesson from the youth that are currently dealing with the disease. Listen to them, hear their stories and then see that they have a future. If they don't have that future, then we don't have an America."—**Allan, San Francisco**

(Adapted from a *Report to the President*, March 1996)

morality interfere with the delivery of potentially life-saving information to young people."

Do you think he is correct? What is the down side of his statement? (Class Discussion)

Runaway Teenagers

Each year since 1993, an estimated 3 million adolescents dropped out of high school. Youth drop-outs have higher frequencies of behaviors that put them at risk for HIV/STDs, and are less accessible to prevention efforts. Many teenagers choose to run away from home.

The Homeless

An estimated 1 to 2 million runaway teenagers are homeless each year. These youth may engage in behaviors such as ID use, having multiple sexual partners, exchange of sex for money or drugs, and unprotected sexual intercourse that place them at risk for HIV infection. HIV seroprevalence studies among homeless youth have shown rates that are higher than adolescents in other settings (Rotheram-Borus et al., 1991).

David Allen and co-workers (1994) report that in general HIV infection rates among the homeless youth populations were comparable with persons attending STD clinics. In nine of 16 sites, HIV seroprevalence rates among homeless youth were higher than the median rates of youth attending STD clinics within the same city. These studies can only hint at how far HIV has infiltrated specific groups of teenagers.

Teenagers, the Health Profession, and HIV Transmission

In 1993, 7,500 ninth graders, in 39 Philadelphia schools, over a 10-month period were surveyed regarding what teens most wanted in a health care provider (their physician's office). Their number one concern was contracting HIV from their health care person (physician/nurse). Other top concerns were: wanting to see the medical staff wash their hands, and removing instruments from sterile packaging. When asked how many of the 1.5 million HIV-infected people in the United States occurred as a result of a health care visit, the answers ranged from 100,000 to 1,000,000 (a hundred thousand to a million). To date, only six cases of HIV transmission are believed to have occurred from a dentist to his patients (see Chapter 8, for an in-depth discussion of this case). Clearly there is room for improving quality information among the teenagers of the United States.

If you are a teenager or know of one who needs help or has HIV/AIDS questions, call: **NATIONAL TEENAGERS AIDS HOTLINE** 1-800-234-8336.

SUMMARY

AIDS surveillance and HIV seroprevalence studies indicate that a significant proportion of HIV infection among women in the United States is acquired through heterosexual contact. Because more men than women are HIV carriers, a woman is more likely than a man to have an infected heterosexual partner. The predominance of heterosexually acquired HIV infection in women of reproductive age has important implications for vertical HIV transmission to their offspring: nearly 30% of children with AIDS were infected by mothers who acquired infection through heterosexual contact. One of the greatest tragedies of the AIDS pandemic is orphaned children. They are left in hospitals because (**1**) their parents have died of AIDS or cannot care for them, or (**2**) no one wants them. AIDS at present is relatively rare among 13- to 19-year-olds, but 20% of AIDS cases, due to a 9- to 15-year period before AIDS diagnosis, had to begin with HIV-infected teenagers.

REVIEW QUESTIONS

(Answers to the Review Questions are on page 579.)

1. By the end of 1998, how many women are expected to be HIV-positive worldwide?

2. Globally, what percent of new HIV infections occur in women?

3. What are the major routes of HIV transmission into women?

4. What is the most likely way a female prostitute in the United States becomes HIV-infected?

5. By the year 2000, how many women worldwide will have become HIV-positive and how many will have died from AIDS?

6. AIDS is now the _____ cause of death for all women between ages _____ and _____. It is the _____ leading cause of death in _____ women between the ages of _____ and _____ and the _____ cause of death for black women ages _____ to _____.

7. Beginning 1998, in the United States how many HIV-infected women are of childbearing age?

8. Beginning 1998, only two states have **not** reported a pediatric AIDS case. Which states are these?

9. Since 1994, what percentage/year of HIV-infected newborns received HIV from their mothers?

10. List three major factors that are associated with perinatal HIV transmission.

11. Where do most of the orphaned AIDS children come from? Why are they called AIDS orphans?

12. What percentage of teenagers have had sexual intercourse by the age of 16?

13. Currently, _____ teens/hour are being HIV-infected in the United States?

14. How many teenagers are there between the ages of 13/19 in the United States?

15. What percentage of HIV infections are occurring globally among women ages 15 to 24?

16. What percentage of all new HIV infections in the United States occur between ages 13 and 20?

17. About how many people in the United States under the age of 29 are estimated to be HIV-positive?

18. What is the National Teenagers AIDS Hotline telephone number?

REFERENCES

AGGLETON, PETER, et al. (1994). Risking everything? Risk behavior, behavior change, and AIDS. *Science*, 265:341–345.

ALLEN, DAVID, et al. (1994). HIV infection among homeless adults and runaway youth, United States, 1989–1992. *AIDS*, 8:1593–1598.

ALLEN, J. R., , et al. (1988). Prevention of AIDS and HIV infection: Needs and priorities for epidemiologic research. *Am. J. Public Health,* 78:381–386.

BARDEGUEZ, ARLENE. (1995). Managing HIV infection in women. *AIDS Reader, Suppl.,* Nov/Dec, pp. 2–3.

BLACK, STANTON B., et al. (1990). HIV risk behaviors in young black people: Can we benefit from 30 years of research experience? *AIDS Public Policy J.,* 5:17–23.

BRYSON, YVONNE. (1966). Perinatal HIV transmission: recent advances and therapeutic interventions. *AIDS,* 10(Suppl. 3):S33-S42.

BURKHART, DYMPNA. (1991). Who said the sexual revolution is over? *Med. Asp. Human Sexuality,* 25:9.

BUTLER, DECLAN. (1993). Who side is focus of AIDS research? *Nature,* 366:293.

California Department of Health Services, STD Control Branch. (1995). Sexually transmitted diseases in California. *Surveillance Report.*

CHU, SUSAN, et al. (1994). Female-to-female sexual contact and HIV transmission. *JAMA,* 272:433.

COHEN, JON. (1995). Women: Absent term in the AIDS research equation. *Science,* 269:777–780.

COTTON, PAUL. (1994). U.S. sticks head in sand on AIDS prevention. *JAMA,* 272:756–757.

CURRAN, JAMES W., et al. (1988). Epidemiology of HIV infection and AIDS in the United States. *Science,* 239:610–616.

DARROW, W.W., et al. (1989). HIV antibody in 640 U.S. prostitutes with no evidence of intravenous (IV) drug abuse. *Fourth International Conference on AIDS.* Bio-Data Publishers: Washington, DC.

DAVIS, SUSAN, et al. (1995). Prevalence and incidence of vertically acquired HIV infection in the United States. *JAMA,* 274:952–955.

DIAZ, LESLIE, et al. (1996). Factors influencing mother-child transmission of HIV. *J. Fla. Med. Assoc.,* 83:244–248.

DICKINSON, GORDON M. (1988). Epidemiology of AIDS. *Int. Ped.,* 3:30–32.

DICKOVER, RUTH, et al. (1996). Identification of levels of maternal HIV-RNA associated risk of perinatal transmission: Effect of maternal Zidovudine treatment on viral load. *JAMA,* 275:599–610.

EHRHARDT, ANKE A. (1992). Trends in sexual behavior and the HIV pandemic. *Am. J. Public Health,* 82:1459–1464.

European Collaborative Study. Cesarean section and risk of vertical transmission on HIV infection. (1994). *Lancet,* 343:1464–1467.

FELMAN, YEHUDI M. (1990). Recent developments in sexually transmitted diseases: Is heterosexual transmission of HIV a major epidemiologic in the spread of AIDS? III: AIDS in Sub-Saharan Africa. *Cutis,* 46:204–206.

FERRIS, DARON, et al. (1966). A neglected lesbian health concern: Cervical neoplasia. *J. Fam. Pract.,* 43:581–584.

FRANKE, K. (1988). Turning issues upside down. In: *AIDS: The Women,* I. Rieder and P. Ruppelt, eds., San Francisco: Cleis Press.

FUTTERMAN, DONNA, et al. (1992). Medical care of HIV-infected adolescents. *AIDS Clin. Care,* 4:95–98.

GAYLE, HELENE, et al. (1988). Prevalence of HIV among university students. *N. Engl. J. Med.,* 323:1538–1541.

GOLDSCHMIDT, RONALD, et al. (1995). Zidovudine and prevention of perinatal HIV transmission. *Am. Fam. Physician,* 52:745–749.

GUINAN, MARY S. (1993). AIDS: Your patients are at risk. *Menopause Manage.,* 11:10–18.

GWINN, MARTA, et al. (1991). Prevalence of HIV infection in childbearing women in the U.S.: Surveillance using newborn blood samples. *JAMA,* 265:1704–1708.

HEALTH. (1966). AIDS still spreading rapidly among young gay men. *Am. Med. News,* 39:30 (March issue).

HIRSCHHORN, LISA. (1995). HIV infection in women: Is it different? *AIDS Reader,* 5:99–105.

HIV/AIDS Surveillance Report. (1995). Year end 7:1–36.

HIV/AIDS Surveillance Report. (1996). Year end, 8:1–39.

House Select Committee on Children, Youth and Families. (1992). A decade of denial: Teens and AIDS in America. Washington, D.C., May.

JOHNSON, TIMOTHY, et al. (1995). Current issues in the primary care of women with HIV. *Female Patient,* 20:51–58.

JOSEPH, STEPHEN C. (1993). The once and future AIDS epidemic. *Med. Doctor,* 37:92–104.

LEMP, GEORGE, et al. (1995). HIV seroprevalence and risk behaviors among lesbians and bisexual women in San Francisco and Berkley, California. *Am. J. Public Health,* 85:1549–1552.

LUZURIAGA, KATHERINE, et al. (1996). DNA polymorase chain reaction for diagnoses of vertical HIV infection. *JAMA,* 275:1360–1361.

MANDELBROT, LAURENT, et al. (1997). Natural conception in HIV-negative women with HIV-infected partners. *Lancet,* 349:850–851.

MAUSKOPF, JOSEPHINE. (1996). Economic impact of treatment of HIV-positive women and their newborns with zidovudine: implications for HIV screening. *JAMA*, 276:132–137.

MERRATZ, RUTH, et al. (1993). Women in clinical trials of new drugs. *N. Engl. J. Med.*, 329:292–296.

MONGELLA, GERTRUDE. (1995). Global approaches to the promotion of women's health. *Science*, 269:789–790.

Morbidity and Mortality Weekly Report. (1992). Selected behaviors that increase risk for HIV infection among high school students–United States, 1990. 41:236–240.

Morbidity and Mortality Weekly Report. (1993). Update: Acquired immunodeficiency syndrome–United States, 1992. 42:547–557.

Morbidity and Mortality Weekly Report. (1994). Update: Impact of the expanded AIDS surveillance case definition for adolescents/adults on case reporting–United States, 1993. 43:160–170.

Morbidity and Mortality Weekly Report. (1995a). Update: AIDS–United States, 1994. 44:64–67.

Morbidity and Mortality Weekly Report. (1995b). Update: AIDS among women–United States, 1994. 44:81–84.

Morbidity and Mortality Weekly Report. (1996a). AIDS among children–United States, 1996. 45:1005–1010.

Morbidity and Mortality Weekly Report. (1996b). HIV testing among women aged 18–44years–United States, 1991 and 1993. 46:733–736.

Morbidity and Mortality Weekly Report. (1996c). Update: Mortality attributable to HIV infection among persons aged 25–44 years–United States, 1994. 45:121–125.

Office of National AIDS Policy. (1996). Youth and HIV/AIDS: An American agenda. *Report to the President*, pp. 1–14.

PFEIFFER, NAOMI. (1991). AIDS risk high for women; care is poor. *Infect. Dis. News*, 4:1, 18.

RODRIGUEZ, ZOE, et al. (1996). Medical care and management of infants born to women infected with HIV. *J. Fla. Med. Assoc.*, 83:255–261.

ROTHERAM-BORUS, M., et al. (1991). Sexual risk behaviors, AIDS knowledge, and beliefs about AIDS among runaways. *Am. J. Public Health*, 81:208–210.

SCHABLE, BARBARA, et al. (1996). Characteristics of women 50 years of age or older with heterosexually aquired AIDS. *Am. J. Public Health*, 86:1616–1618.

SELLS, WAYNE, et al. (1996). Morbidity and mortality among US adolescents: an overview of data and trends. *Am. J. Public Health*, 86:513–519.

SELWYN, PETER A., et al. (1989). Knowledge of HIV antibody status and decisions to continue or terminate pregnancy among intravenous drug users. *JAMA*, 261:3567–3571.

THEA, DONALD, et al. (1977). The effect of maternal viral load on the risk of perinatal transmission of HIV. *AIDS*, 11:437–444.

THOMAS, PATRICIA. (1988). Official estimates of epidemic's scope are grist for political mill. *Med. World News*, 29:12–13.

THOMAS, PATRICIA. (1989). The epidemic. *Med. World News*, 30:41–49.

United Nations Economic and Social Council. (1995). *Second Review of the Niarobi Forward-Looking Strategies*, p. 11.

Women's AIDS Network. (1988). Lesbians and AIDS: What's the connection? *San Francisco AIDS Foundation*, 333 Valencia St., 4th Floor, P.O. Box 6182, San Francisco, CA 94101-6182.

World Health Organization, Geneva. (1994). *Women's Health*, p. 18.

YAO, FAUSTIN K. (1992). Youth and AIDS: A priority for prevention education. *AIDS Health Promotion Exchange No. 2*, Royal Tropical Institute, The Netherlands: 1–3.

Prevalence of HIV Infection, AIDS Cases, and Deaths Outside the United States

CHAPTER CONCEPTS

♦ Worldwide, about 9,000 persons a day become HIV-infected.

♦ The majority of all HIV infections worldwide occur in people ages 15–24.

♦ Worldwide, over 1 million people die of AIDS each year.

♦ Over 90% of all AIDS-associated deaths occur in people under age 50.

♦ The number of HIV infections worldwide has tripled since 1990!

♦ In Africa and India, HIV is mainly transmitted heterosexually.

♦ Prostitution is a major route of HIV transmission in Africa and India.

♦ It is estimated that there will be a 20% decline in population in East Africa by the year 2001 due to AIDS.

♦ In Europe, France and Italy have the two highest rates of AIDS cases, respectively.

♦ Mexico ranks eighth in the number of AIDS cases in the world.

♦ Cuba mandates national screening for HIV-infected people.

♦ The former Soviet Union reported its first AIDS case in 1987.

♦ China reported its first AIDS case in 1988.

♦ Asia will surpass Africa in numbers of HIV infections and AIDS cases by the year 2000.

♦ AIDS cases are being reported from 209 countries to the World Health Organization.

There are enormous disparities in the quality of life for people born in different parts of the world. The Third World contains three fourths of the Earth's population. There, 87% of all births and 98% of all infant and childhood deaths occur. One in 10 people suffers from a tropical disease, 190 million children are undernourished, and 10 million people die of acute respiratory and diarrheal infections each year.

With regard to HIV disease/AIDS, data from the World Health Organization (WHO) suggests that Americans are in a relatively enviable position. People in the United States have lived through 17 years of HIV transmission, with the current rate of new infections in the United States appearing to be stabilized (World Health Organization, 1992 updated). The current rate of new HIV infections in the United States has stabilized at 40,000 per year, down from 100,000 new infections per year through the 1980s. This is not true for persons living in many countries in the developing world where the HIV epidemic progresses unchecked. Since 1990, the number of HIV infections **worldwide** has more than **tripled** (1990, 10 million; 1998, 35 million).

About 94% of the world's estimated 35 million (through 1998) HIV-infected persons now live in developing countries. And the majority of the HIV-infected worldwide are between the ages of 15 and 24. Worldwide, according to Peter Piot (Figure I-4), director of UNAIDS, about 9,000 new HIV infections are occurring daily. That is about 1 HIV infection every 10 seconds, 24 hours a day! About 88% of the world's total HIV-infected people live in sub-Saharan Africa and in South and Southeast Asia (Friedland, 1996 updated). The global epidemic has intensified despite a massive prevention effort. In many countries with high infection rates, education campaigns have spread the news about HIV, but this has not led as yet to a decrease in the frequency of high-risk sexual behavior adequate to affect the epidemic.

Because HIV infection occurs disproportionately in certain behavioral high-risk groups, seroprevalence may differ markedly between neighboring countries, urban and rural areas within a country, or social strata within an urban population.

GLOBAL PREVALENCE OF HIV INFECTION AND AIDS

Various sources, including the WHO's global program on AIDS, estimated that, by the end of 1994, there were about 5 million AIDS cases worldwide. In late 1992, the Harvard Global AIDS Policy Coalition estimated that, from 1981 to 1992, the number of HIV-infected people worldwide increased from 100,000 to 12.9 million: 7.1 million men, 4.7 million women, and 1.1 million children. Using current **UN-AIDS, WHO,** and **CDC** figures on numbers of HIV and AIDS cases, by the end of 1997 there will be 32 million HIV-infected, 9 million of whom will have AIDS, and of these 9 million, 8 million will have died. By the end of 1998, 35 million will be HIV-positive, of whom 10 million will have AIDS and 9 million will have died (Figure 12-1). And in 1999, 38.5 million will be HIV-positive, of which 11 million will have AIDS and over 10 million will have died. Projection to the year 2000 indicates 42 million HIV-positive, of which between 12 and 13 million will have AIDS and 11 to 12 million will have died. To appreciate the effect the AIDS death toll will have on countries with the higher incidence of AIDS deaths, see Figure 12-2.

The history of HIV infection suggests that about 90% to 95% of those infected will, on average, become AIDS patients within 9 to 15 years. Beginning 1997, there were 209 countries

——— BOX 12.1 ———

THE GLOBAL COURSE OF THE HIV PANDEMIC, 1998–1999

Through 1998, an estimated 35 million adults and children worldwide have been HIV-infected. Of these, 26 million people are living with HIV disease, 10 million of these have AIDS, and 9 million have died. An additional million people plus will die each year of the pandemic through the year 2000. Children will make up about 23% of those deaths, adults about 77%. Of the 24.8 million HIV-infected children, 94% live in developing nations. Over 26 million live in sub-Saharan Africa and in South and Southeast Asia. These data stand in stark contrast to the estimated 750,000 to 800,000 HIV-infected persons living in the United States and the estimated 35,000 to 40,000 HIV-infected people living in Canada.

OTHER POINTS OF INFORMATION

♦ Of the cumulative 35 million HIV-infected people worldwide through 1998, about 31.5 million are adults and about 3.5 million are children.

♦ Of the 35 million infected, over 30 million infections will have occurred in sub-Saharan Africa and in South and Southeast Asia. These data are in stark contrast to the estimated 1.5 million HIV infections in the United States and the estimated 50,000+ in Canada.

♦ Over 90% of all AIDS-associated deaths occur in people under age 50.

♦ The majority of newly infected adolescent/adults are between the ages of 15 and 24.

♦ Through 1998, 9 million people will have died of AIDS. By the year 2001, about 2 million will die each year of AIDS. Children now make up about 23% of these deaths; adolescents/adults make up about 7%.

♦ Overall, of the 24.8 million adolescents/adults living with HIV disease ending 1998, about 45% are women and that proportion is increasing.

♦ Worldwide, about 85% of HIV infections have been transmitted through unprotected sexual intercourse (condoms were not used). Ending 1998, heterosexual intercourse will account for 80% of all adult HIV infections, homosexual intercourse for 10%, injection drug use for 5% to 10%, and breast-feeding and blood transfusion for about 3%.

♦ The average of several published reports on the number of new HIV infections occurring daily, worldwide, is 9,000, over 3 million per year.

♦ Worldwide, about 1,500 children per day are born HIV-infected. Of these children, 67% are born in sub-Saharan Africa, 30% are born in Southeast Asia, 2% in Latin America, and 1% in the Caribbean.

♦ Worldwide, through 1998, about 10 million children under the age of 15 have lost their mother to AIDS.

reporting to the WHO on AIDS. One hundred and ninety-four countries on the seven continents have reported AIDS cases to the WHO. Figure 12-3 presents a global overview of the number of HIV-infected people through 1998.

Figure 12-4 presents the global distribution of the estimated 10 million AIDS cases beginning 1999.

Table 12-1 offers the **estimated** cumulative number of: HIV infections, AIDS cases, AIDS-associated deaths, and the total number of people living with HIV disease and AIDS worldwide, ending 1998.

THE ECONOMICS OF PREVENTING HIV INFECTION IN DEVELOPING COUNTRIES

According to the World Bank's *World Development Report 1993: Investigations in Health,* the cumulative annual spending in developing countries for the prevention of HIV infection is less than $200 million. In sub-Saharan Africa, the total amount spent is about $90 million. That translates into less than 20 cents per person for the region with the greatest burden of HIV/AIDS in the world. National health bud-

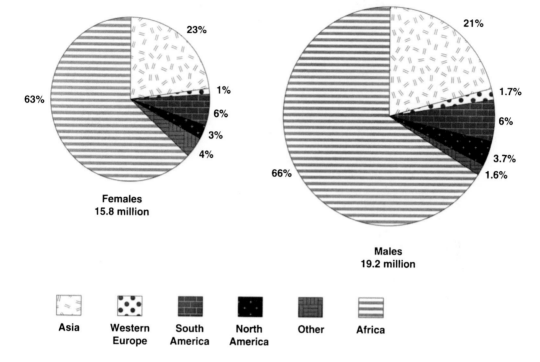

FIGURE 12-1   Cumulative Global Distribution of HIV-Infected Children and Adults. Ending 1998, there will be about 35 million children and adults HIV-infected worldwide. About 10 million will have died. By the end of 1999, there will be about 38 million persons who have been HIV-infected. The large increase in new HIV infections over the past years and in future years is and will continue to be attributed to the marked increase in HIV infections in Africa and Asia.

gets are already strained, and any additional money to be allocated to medical care for AIDS patients must come from developed countries.

The reality is that the resources, whether from in-country budgets or donor sources, are already far too small to undertake the prevention effort. At the Ninth International AIDS Conference (June 1993), Michael Merston, head of the World Health Organization's Global Program on AIDS, estimated that a 10-fold increase (to $2 billion) of funds spent on preventing the spread of HIV and other sexually transmitted diseases would avert 10 million new HIV infections by the year 2000 (Biggar, 1993).

Clearly the expensive drug therapies available in the developed nations cannot be afforded in the developing nations. And, even if they were made available, the problems of drug maintenance, distribution, and people compliance (i.e., taking each separate drug on time, perhaps 20 to 30 pills each and every day) poses very difficult problems. Many hundreds of thousands of HIV-infected people do not live in areas where the drugs can be kept and patients monitored.

SPREAD OF AIDS OUTSIDE THE UNITED STATES

The AIDS pandemic has demonstrated unprecedented speed in its diffusion. Whereas the great cholera pandemics took nearly 20 years to sweep across Europe, HIV/AIDS has reached most of the world within 7 years. The question now is whether research, behavior modification, and education—all of which require international cooperation—will be able to meet the AIDS challenge.

Population in Millions for the Year 2020

No AIDS Cases
Subtracting AIDS Deaths
Current Population

Difference
between forecast
without AIDS and
forecast with AIDS ▼

millions

U.S. — 323.1 / 321.4 / 260.7	-0.5%
Brazil — 210.5 / 197.5 / 158.7	-6.6%
Zaire — 101.7 / 92.9 / 42.7	-9.5%
Thailand — 76.6 / 62.9 / 59.5	-21.8%
Uganda — 49.8 / 34.1 / 19.8	-46.0%
Zambia — 23.2 / 15.8 / 9.2	-46.8%
Haiti — 11.3 / 9.5 / 6.5	-18.9%

FIGURE 12-2 Projecting Future AIDS Mortality. Each country's population forecast with and without AIDS. (*Source: Center for International Research, U.S. Census Bureau.*)

Through 1998, 93% of the estimated 35 million people who have been HIV-infected belonged to developing countries. Over two-thirds of these people are/were from sub-Saharan African nations such as Zambia, Zimbabwe, Kenya, and Uganda. The life expectancy in sub-Saharan Africa was up to age 70 before HIV/AIDS. Now in many places it is under age 40. Children make up 25% of AIDS deaths in Africa.

A brief summary concerning the number of AIDS cases in **Africa, the Americas, Europe,** and **Asia** is presented.

AFRICA

By the end of 1994, the United Nations Health Agency estimated that sub-Saharan Africa had over 3 million AIDS cases and that over 2 million Africans had already died from AIDS. Africa, with about 12% of the world's population, is now **reporting** about 25% of the world's AIDS cases. It is estimated to have over 65% of the total number of HIV-infected adults and 90% of the world's HIV-infected children (DeCock et al., 1993). Sixty percent of HIV infections occur in the 15- to 24-year-old age group. About 6,000 Africans become HIV-infected each day; that is 250 per hour or four per minute. The highest number of cases have been reported from urban areas in central, eastern, and southern Africa (Figure 12-5). About half of all reported AIDS cases in Africa originate from East Africa—Uganda, Kenya, Tanzania, Rwanda, and Burundi (Barongo et al., 1992).

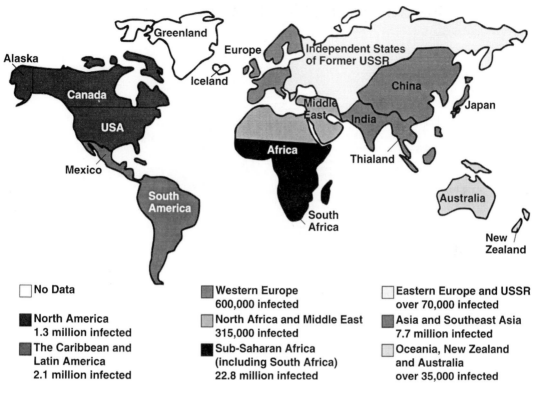

No Data

North America
1.3 million infected

The Caribbean and Latin America
2.1 million infected

Western Europe
600,000 infected

North Africa and Middle East
315,000 infected

Sub-Saharan Africa (including South Africa)
22.8 million infected

Eastern Europe and USSR
over 70,000 infected

Asia and Southeast Asia
7.7 million infected

Oceania, New Zealand and Australia
over 35,000 infected

FIGURE 12-3 Estimated Global HIV Infections through 1998. This map shows the global proliferation of the AIDS virus. Although sub-Saharan Africa has the greatest number of HIV-infected people, other regions are catching up. (*Adapted from Palca, 1991 and updated*)

Through 1998, the WHO and UNAIDS estimate that there will be about 20 million HIV-infected adults and 1.5 million infected children in Africa. The WHO estimates by the year 2000 there may be 40 million HIV-infected adults and as many as 10 million orphans in the 197 reporting countries worldwide.

Major routes of HIV transmission in Africa are heterosexual, mother-to-child, and transfusions with unscreened blood. The latter is being reduced as blood for transfusion is now being screened in most major urban areas.

Between 20% and 30% of sexually active adults between the ages of 20 and 40 are believed to be infected with HIV in some urban areas of sub-Saharan Africa. The HIV seroprevalence in rural areas, where the majority of the population lives, remains much lower but is increasing.

First AIDS Case in Africa?

There was a report in 1960 of a young white patient who was treated in 1959 for Kaposi's sarcoma. The investigator stated that this may have been the first case of AIDS in Africa (Sonnerfeld, 1990).

AIDS in Africa was officially recognized among the indigenous African population soon after it was recognized in the United States. Some investigators contend that AIDS was present in Africa in the 1970s. It was reported that a Danish surgeon contracted AIDS in Zaire in 1976; and Vandepitte and colleagues (1983) diagnosed the disease in a

Estimated: 10 Million AIDS Cases Worldwide

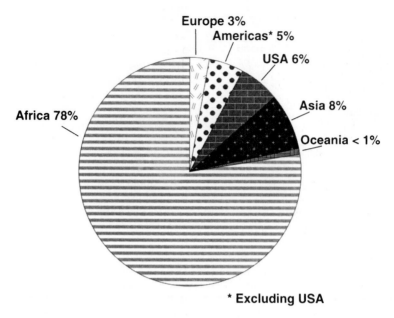

FIGURE 12-4   Global Distribution of 10 Million AIDS Cases, January 1999.

Zairean visitor to Europe in 1976. Saxinger and colleagues (1985) found HIV antibodies in samples collected in the West Nile region of Uganda between 1972 and 1973. There is also a report of a husband and wife in Uganda having AIDS in 1976. These are believed to be the first **reported** AIDS cases in Uganda.

In 1986, for a variety of political and economic reasons, such as possible international discrimination and fear of loss of tourist trade and foreign investments, only nine of Africa's 51 countries reported that they had AIDS patients. Yet, in 1987, Jonathan Mann stated "No area in the world is more affected by HIV than Africa." The WHO estimates that one in three of the 40 million people in Southern Africa will be HIV-infected by the year 2010.

Reduction of African Population Due to AIDS

In July of 1996, the Washington-based **World Population Reference Bureau** reported that sub-Saharan Africa will have 1.25 billion in-

habitants by 2025– 100 million less than without the effects of AIDS.

In the past, demographers assumed that the impact of AIDS would be relatively modest and would not significantly affect the continent's population growth. The report states that "it now seems likely that AIDS will alter the demographic prospects of some 20 to 30 countries. In Africa, Botswana, Kenya, Malawi, Uganda, Zambia, and Zimbabwe will be among the worst-affected countries. Kenya, often projected to pass the 60 million mark within 30 years, may see its potential future population reduced by half." (See Figure 12-2.)

Northern Africa: Egypt

In Egypt, entering 1998, HIV/AIDS carries such a stigma that it is practically unmentionable. The government insists that every person carrying HIV was infected either through blood transfusions while working in the Gulf or through sexual contact in Europe.

TABLE 12-1 Global Estimates of HIV Infections, AIDS Cases, and Deaths Associated with AIDS, Through 1998

Cumulative HIV infections	
Adults	31.5 million
Male	18.3 million
Female	13.2 million
Children	3.5 million
Total	**35.0 million**
Cumulative AIDS cases	
Adults	8.0 million
Male	4.6 million
Female	3.4 million
Children	2.0 million
Total	**10.0 million**
Cumulative HIV/AIDS deaths	
Adults	7.2 million
Male	4.2 million
Female	3.0 million
Children	1.8 million
Total	**9.0 million**
People living with HIV/AIDS	
Adults	24.8 million
Male	14.4 million
Female	10.4 million
Children	1.2 million
Total	**26 million**

Data updated from publications from the joint United Nations Programs on HIV/AIDS, the WHO, and the CDC.

A decade has passed since the first AIDS case was **reported,** yet the country still has no reliable figures on the epidemic. In 1986, 513 HIV infections and 88 cases of AIDS were **reported** to the World Health Organization. The real figures **now** could be anywhere between 5,000 and 20,000 HIV-positive and 1,000 AIDS cases, which is still low for a population of close to 60 million people.

One explanation for the low rate could be that cultural, social, and religious norms discourage promiscuity. But these taboos also put women at risk and make it very difficult for them to protect themselves. Islam has laid down principles for appropriate sexual behavior, but sex education is forbidden. This taboo is being reinforced by a new breed of **fundamentalist women,** who believe that AIDS is a plague of immoral Western society.

They are ignoring the fact that many men practice unsafe sex before—and often during—marriage. Many women, even those with infected husbands, believe that condoms are immoral and that "God curses the woman who refuses to sleep with her husband when he wants to."

AIDS Program—On paper, Egypt has a model AIDS program, though officials admit there has been some delay in its implementation of the proposed activities. The program is run by the ministry of health with the cooperation of the WHO and directed by a committee of medical experts and government officials. Local offices have been set up in Greater Cairo, the Delta, and Upper Egypt. The only action to be recommended is a campaign for widespread sex education, in order to prevent the spread of AIDS.

By the end of 1994, all hospitals in Cairo and some of those in rural areas were equipped to test for HIV.

Surveillance systems have also been put in place. So far only high-risk groups—including drug addicts and people with sexually transmitted diseases (STDs) and blood disorders—have been tested. One million blood samples from STD clinics and family planning and rehabilitation centers were tested, of which 15 carried the virus—one in every 100,000.

Testing—The government's testing policy is not so enlightened. Testing of foreigners is mandatory and any found positive must leave the country within 10 days. Prisoners, women arrested for prostitution, homosexuals, and blood donors are all tested randomly and **without consent.**

HIV tests are available in many labs and private clinics, but they are not confidential. Often, positive results are reported to the authorities **before they are reported to the patient.**

Counseling services are widely available, but there is insufficient social and economic support for people living with AIDS or for their families. Each province has only one team of social workers, psychologists, nurses, and doctors who provide moral support, counseling, and sometimes financial help, but people are very reluctant to come forward. There is a telephone hotline which offers advice to patients or relatives and to suspected carriers (*Nazz Ki Pukaar,* 1996)

——— BOX 12.2 ———

THE BEGINNING: JULIANA'S DISEASE
(Adapted from Laurie Garrett's, *The Coming Plague*)

It was first noticed in the village of Lukunya, on the Ugandan border, sometime in early 1983.

The Ugandan trader came through selling cloth for women's **kangas** (skirt-like cloth) patterned with the name **Juliana.** A poor village girl traded sex for a **kanga.**

Some months later the girl became sick; she had no appetite, could not hold down food, and had constant diarrhea. In a few weeks she had to be carried everywhere. Before she died, two other women, who also traded sex for Juliana's cloth, came down with the disease.

The people of Lukunya decided that the Ugandan was a witch, and that Juliana's cloth had evil powers.

Within a year the curse had spread to four neighboring villages. By 1984 Juliana's disease cases were appearing at Kidenya's hospital in the Kagera District's capital at Bukoba, and the Ndolage Missionary Hospital on the **other side** of the district. The Bukoba doctors were convinced the disease was something new. No treatment could save those affected. Rumors of widespread witchcraft were spreading throughout the Kagera region; the Juliana mystery had to be solved.

In September 1984, a village paramedic brought nearly two dozen patients to Bukoba in a single day; blood and stool samples were taken from all. Studies of the samples with microscopes and special stains revealed nothing. The patients all told a similar tale of a young barmaid in their town who gave Juliana's disease to the men, who in turn gave it to their wives.

The three doctors pooled their meager resources and financed a trip for one to the capi-

tal for Nyamuryekunge. Carrying blood samples and all available information on the patients, the doctor traveled southeastward for days by boat, truck, bus, and car, finally reaching Muhimbili Medical School, where his former professors studied the samples, read the reports, and debated the nature of Juliana's disease. In the end they agreed only on one thing: nobody could find a microorganism that could be causing the illness. That meant it must be something new.

Visiting the medical library, a surgeon found Gottlieb's description of *Pneumocystic carinii* pneumonia cases among Los Angeles men in the United States, the CDC's reports on acquired immune deficiency syndrome in Haiti, the list of symptoms in the *New England Journal of Medicine,* and evidence in *Science* of a new retrovirus discovery in laboratories in the United States and France. He carefully compared the Kagera patients' symptoms and the Muhimbili laboratory findings from their samples with the observations in the American medical journals.

It was a perfect match, except for the types of patients involved: Kagera had no homosexuals, drug users, or hemophiliacs on blood factor VIII. But they now knew that Juliana's disease was AIDS. One doctor later remembered that the news was a death sentence for his people.

"I thought surely this will be the greatest war we have ever fought. Surely many will die. And surely we will be frustrated, unable to help. But also **I thought the Americans will find a treatment soon. This will not be forever."**
IT WAS JANUARY 1985!

HIV Transmission in Africa

The WHO estimates by the end of 1998, 67% of the world's 35 million plus HIV-infected people will live in Africa. That is over 23 million HIV-infected people. Likewise, Africa has 67% of the total AIDS cases or about 6.7 million cases. Currently, about 19 million HIV-infected adults live in sub-Saharan Africa. Available evidence suggests that it is unlikely that the spread of HIV will be brought under

control in the near future (DeCock et al., 1994). **About 66% of HIV infections occur in those under age 25.**

Injection drug use has traditionally been a rarity in sub-Saharan Africa. However, there are indications that the practice may be catching on, particularly in port areas and among educated and affluent city-dwellers.

Other areas hard hit by the epidemic are those of central and east Africa. These areas account for one-sixth of the region's popula-

FIGURE 12-5 Map of Africa. AIDS began to appear in Central Africa at about the same time it was being recognized in the United States. Increasing numbers of cases have been reported in urban centers in Zaire, Zambia, Rwanda, Uganda, Tanzania, and Burundi. HIV infection among prostitutes in these countries is high (see text for details).

Legend (Percent HIV Positive):
- No Data
- 0.1 or less
- 0.2 to 1.0
- 1.1 to 5.0
- 5.1 to 10.0
- Over 10

tion, but between one-half and two-thirds of its infections. Here, in several towns and cities, about one-third of all men and women aged 15 to 49 are estimated to be HIV-positive.

Heterosexual Contacts—Data from AIDS studies in Zaire and Rwanda show about an equal number of men and women with AIDS. The major risk factor in HIV transmission appears to be related to the number of **heterosexual partners**, engaging in sexual inter-

course with prostitutes, and not treating the large variety of STDs that are continually being transmitted unchecked. In Rwanda, one in four women of childbearing age is HIV-positive (Commenges et al., 1992). In some cities 30% of pregnant women are HIV-infected (DeCock et al., 1994).

Studies by John and Pat Caldwell (1996) have ruled out other known methods of transmission in most of Africa. For instance, they found that because **anal intercourse** is considered abhorrent for a variety of reasons, in-

——— BOX 12.3 ———

IMPACT OF HIV/AIDS ON LIFE EXPECTANCY

Demographers now estimate that by the **year 2010** the mean national **life expectancy will fall** from 67 to 33 years in Zambia, from 67 to 40 in Zimbabwe, and from 59 to 31 in Uganda; all courtesy of HIV and tuberculosis.

Zimbabwe, formerly Rhodesia, is surrounded by South Africa, Zambia, Botswana, and Mozambique in southern Africa; the country's population totals 10 million people. With 30,000 reported AIDS cases, Zimbabwe ranks ninth in the world for AIDS incidence. This figure only includes those people who have been tested. People often die before they can be tested; in addition, some clinicians do not formally test patients but simply diagnose them on the basis of clinical symptoms. Thus, the number may be as much as 10 times higher. Likewise, reporting from other countries may be inaccurate.

Ninety percent of all hospital deaths in Zimbabwe are HIV-related. The ratio of men to women with AIDS is 1:1. In Africa, where the mother is the primary caregiver, orphans are defined as children who have lost their mothers. By the year 2001, Zimbabwe will be home to half a million orphans. The health budget for Zimbabwe from 1994 to 1995 was $250 million. This amounts to approximately 30 cents per person (McCarty, 1996).

cluding its connection with witchcraft, the practice is almost completely suppressed in much of sub-Saharan Africa. Also, intravenous drugs are seldom used there: marijuana is widely consumed, but **injected opiates** are too expensive for these impoverished societies.

Contraception: Use of Condoms by Rwandans—It is the interaction and passage of fluids, particularly beer and milk, in the form of social exchange or gift, which constitutes for Rwandans the essential social bond. Blockage of the flow through the individual body or between bodies was traditionally considered to be pathological. The practice of **kunyaza**, a form of wet sex, in which the female is aroused to secrete copiously before penetration, is closely linked to fundamental Rwandan notions of self in relation to other. Sex follows the mode of flow, blockage, and the ideal of reciprocity. Children are built in utero, over time, through repeated intercourse and mixing of fluids. A condom would block this essential flow of fluids, thus contradicting a most basic cultural notion (Taylor, 1990).

In Kigali, Rwanda, 30% of adults are HIV-infected. In Uganda, there is one doctor for every 23,000 people and one hospital for every 200,000 people.

Uganda

In late 1993, one in every eight Ugandans was HIV-infected—that is about 2 million of 17 million Ugandans. And 300,000 have AIDS. In some districts in Uganda, over half of all deaths are due to AIDS and 9 out of 10 of those deaths occur in people under age 35. In countries like Uganda, where a mother often has to walk 20 miles to get an aspirin for her sick child, the practical problems of getting a constant supply of condoms and learning to use them properly may never be resolved. As one young Ugandan said to the Health Minister, "You tell me that AIDS can make me ill in 10 years, but 25 people died here the past weekend. My father died young of TB . . . and my brother, out of school for 3 years, still has no job. Can AIDS really make life worse?"

Prostitution—The major route of HIV transmission in Africa is prostitution. Unofficial estimates by mission doctors in Kampala, Uganda, put the prevalence of HIV infection among the city's prostitutes at 70%, and at 20% in other adults (Culotta, 1991).

A research team from the University of Nairobi, Kenya, the University of Manitoba, Canada, and the Institute of Tropical Medicine in Belgium tested 535 Nairobi prostitutes in January 1985 and found that 348, or 65% of

COMPLEXITIES OF HIV PREVENTION IN DEVELOPING COUNTRIES: OBSTACLES TO OVERCOME

At the 11th International Conference on AIDS (Vancouver, July 7–12, 1996) several speakers described the obstacles to preventing HIV infection in their countries. Two of those speakers remarks are highlighted here to emphasize the vast differences that exist in health care between the West and the developing world.

SPEAKER ONE: a 24-year-old HIV-positive mother of two from Zambia who works as an AIDS educator. Ostracized after having tested HIV-positive at age 20, she went on to have two children despite being perceived by her colleagues as irresponsible and "a bad example to hold up as an educator." She did this, she explained, because "it is very difficult to come to terms with not having children, especially in Zambia, a place where childless women are outcasts." She went on to explain the paradoxical effect of AIDS awareness. An older man she described as a "sugar daddy" takes schoolgirls to fancy hotels *because he thinks they are free of HIV.* "The girls—and often their parents—see the sugar daddy as a way of relieving their poverty." As a result, almost one in five urban girls are HIV-positive by age 20. Lack of resources is a problem in AIDS control, but wasteful spending is another problem, she noted, citing an assistance program that spent the majority of its funds, not in Zambia, but in universities in donor countries.

SPEAKER TWO: a medical doctor who provided a less personalized but still sobering analysis of the realities of AIDS and economic development. He punctured the simplistic notion that epidemic disease is inevitably linked to the lack of development, citing historical examples such as the demise of feudalism and the triggering of European economic dominance in the wake of the Black Death. He said, **"Makers of coffins may contribute as much to an economy as makers of cradles."** With AIDS, economic and social factors are inevitably linked to medical ones in a complex web. As an example, he pointed to the Akosombo Dam on the Volta River in Ghana, which displaced people from agriculture and left many women, who were the principal farmers, without income. When construction ended, they migrated to urban areas to continue **sex work,** which produced a great deal of capital that was reinvested in their original region. It also produced a high rate of HIV infection, and many of these women are returning home to consume their assets and die. On a purely economic scale, the AIDS epidemic in this population might be viewed as just one of the costs of economic development, but this narrow view would fail to address the enormous social and political damage, not to mention the economic effects, yet to come.

Reports such as the two presented here, while sobering, are also encouraging: The complex reality of AIDS in its broadest social context is at least being acknowledged, a prerequisite for any effective response (Dobkin, 1996).

them, were HIV-positive. Of the remaining 185, by 2 years later 120 of them had become HIV-positive. Thus, of the original 535 prostitutes in 1985, 504 or 94%, were HIV-positive by 1987 (Niftrik, 1988). According to surveys, each Nairobi prostitute averages 1,000 male sexual partners per year, most of whom are truck drivers going inland from the port of Mombasa.

One of the highest concentrations of HIV/AIDS cases in Africa is found along the route from Uganda to Zaire. Reports indicate 27% to 60% of prostitutes in Kinshasa, Zaire, are HIV-positive; and 88% of prostitutes in Rwanda are infected (Quinn, 1988). Thirty-

seven percent of prostitutes in Kinshasa age 20 and older were HIV-infected; only 8% female nonprostitutes of the same age were infected. There is little reason to believe that similar situations do not exist in other equatorial African capitals. According to *Inside South Africa,* 60% of prostitutes in Entebbe and Kampala in Uganda tested in a combined study were found to be HIV-positive.

Condom use among prostitutes is infrequent. Only 23% of prostitutes say they have ever used condoms. Prostitutes say that customors refuse to use condoms or refuse to pay if made to wear a condom; "We die either way—of starvation or of AIDS." Condoms in Zaire

———— BOX 12.4 ————

AIDS IN AFRICA

CBS: Interviewer (CBS:I): "They don't often say it, but a lot of scientists around the world have been watching the spread of AIDS in central Africa with a mixture of horror and fascination. Horror because of the sheer numbers of infected; fascination because the region is a kind of human laboratory for studying heterosexual transmissions. The fact is, among African heterosexuals, the disease is spreading much more rapidly than heterosexuals in the West. At the same time, central African countries like Uganda look back at the West with embarrassment and anger. They're embarrassed by talk of African promiscuity. And they are angry when outspoken scientists, like Dr. Robert Gall of the National Center Institute, say that while no one can prove where AIDS began, and isolated cases do appear early in the West, all scientific signposts still lead to an origin in Africa."

Response from Head of AIDS Education for Uganda (AFT): "We don't have homosexuals and drug addicts. We don't have them. So this disease must be foreign. If anyone's to blame, it's Western homosexuals and drug addicts."

CBS: I: "And then there was this man, who was too sick even to give us his name. This scene may well be a dark vision of the future for all of Uganda. It was just a few years ago that the disease was first noticed in this province. 'Slim disease,' they called it, the disease that makes you thin. And at first, everyone thought that it would stay here. But the disease didn't stop in the provinces. It traveled this road toward the capital city because this is the highway used by the truck drivers. John Nsambo is bringing coffee back from the region around the lake, the neighboring countries of Zaire and Burundi [Figure 12-5]. The AIDS virus may well be part of his cargo, and his trip up the highway tells a lot about the way the disease began to spread. As he heads toward the city, he stops at four or five truck stops along the way. At every truck stop, the women are waiting. By now, as many as 76% of them are infected with the virus. Some of them are ordinary prostitutes, one-night stands. Others are what Ugandans call temporary wives, a woman supported by several regular customers who drop by before heading home to the principal wife. Here and in the rest of Africa, AIDS is a completely heterosexual disease."

CBS: I: "Whatever the reason, it took only two years for AIDS to make its way up the highway

from Lake Victoria into the capital city, Kampala. It moved with lightning speed through the suburbs, the workers, the housewives, still affecting men and women equally, moving straight on to the city's educated professionals, what Ugandans call their "Mercedes Benz set." Some studies show that in parts of the city, 20% of the young people are already infected, and at the current rate, all of them will be infected in just 10 years.

What does that mean to the future of Uganda if this disease is concentrating among the professional people?"

AFT: "Well, it is a disaster. It will mean that young people from the age of about 18 to 40, the bread-winners, the well-to-do, will—will die off."

CBS:I "So you could lose an entire generation?"

AFT: "We could, yes. We could lose the entire generation unless something drastically is done about it."

CBS:I: "While American hospitals worry about the thousands, the millions of dollars they'll spend treating AIDS, here at Mulago they worry about enough money to buy rubber gloves for the health workers or a few disposable needles. Here, when they give a man or woman a blood test for AIDS at $1.75, they've just spent the entire per capita health budget for the year. (In the United States, $500 per year are spent on each citizen's health care.)

A Sister at the N'Sambya St. Francis Hospital has one of Uganda's five machines for screening blood to be used in transfusions; just a fraction of the number of machines in New York City alone. The day we were there, she tested blood samples from donors, and the results were 28% positive. But when the donors who tested positive came to get their results, *if they looked healthy, they weren't told they were carrying the virus*. The doctors said there was no point in giving someone a possible death sentence when you have no counselors to help them deal with the news. Even if it means they spread the disease to others, the doctors say, one cruelty doesn't justify another. One woman who tested positive saw 10 doctors; no one told her the truth."

CBS:I: "This male worries too. He's from Rakai, and he's been ill for months. It was an 8-hour ride to get to the doctor. But the doctor he is going to see is the witch doctor who will charge him 5 months of his wages for just one treatment. The doctor and his associate, who is called the professor, begin the treatment with a magical X-ray. They toss some coins and keys and produce an instant diagnosis. They say they can tell from the demons in the dark if the patient has AIDS, or slim disease, and that they'll adjust the pre-

scription accordingly; though when we were there, it was always the same concoction of herbs and roots."

cost less than one penny each but the demand for them is so low, health care workers can not even give them away.

Some blacks in South Africa see HIV as a threat, as a plot by whites to preserve apartheid by persuading blacks to use condoms, thus reducing the blacks' pregnancy rate.

In **Tanzania** (East Africa), the mean of Dar es Salaam have a unique phrase for AIDS: *"Acha Iniue Dogedego Siachi,"* a Kiswahili translation of "Let it kill me as I will never abandon the young ladies." Women as well as public health officials are understandably concerned. One young prostitute said, "Even if I

take precautions, how can I be completely safe while I have no control over so many things—including my own husband?" (Earickson, 1990).

In **Ghana** (Northwest Africa) about all Ghanaian prostitutes in Cote d'Ivoire are HIV-positive. Many are returning home sick and destitute—to use up the little money they saved and then die (Decosas, 1996).

Socioeconomic Issues

The frequency of AIDS cases is highest among the upper class and the revenue-producing

---

POINT OF INFORMATION 12.3

TESTIMONY FROM THREE HIV-POSITIVE WOMEN IN NORTHWEST AFRICA, MOROCCO

Case I: She was HIV-positive and widowed at age 25. Her 48-year-old husband died of AIDS 17 days **after** their wedding. She found it hard to understand what the doctor was saying when he explained that she was the carrier of an invisible virus that is spread mainly through sexual intercourse. She was born in a rural area and never went to school. Of course, she had heard of AIDS, but she didn't know what it was. She was a virgin when she married. Her husband, who knew he was ill, demanded a certificate of **virginity.** Marrying a virgin is supposed to have purifying virtues. But that marriage will kill this woman.

Case II: She is a 33-year-old housewife, entirely dependent on her husband, and so she has little chance of negotiating with him about limiting the number of pregnancies or preventing STDs and AIDS. She said, "I can't stand the pill, but my husband refuses to use a condom. He says it's a piece of rubber that reduces his pleasure. And we had six children! But there's nothing I can do. If I nag him about it he'll find another

wife and I'll be out in the street. Of course I'm afraid of AIDS, but I'm even more afraid of being kicked out. So . . ."

Case III: She is a 35-year-old widow with three daughters. "When my husband died, he left me a small house, but my in-laws sold it, and I found myself in the street overnight. What else could I do? I started 'going out' to feed my children. I had no choice." This woman has been selling sex for 10 years in a small Casablanca street. No one knows about it in her family, who live some 50 kilometers away and think she works in a factory. She only uses condoms when a customer asks her to because a lot of men don't like condoms. Also she states, "There's so much competition. All these high school students. If I refuse to do it, there are a hundred girls ready to, without condoms or anything." She has such a low image of herself, her body, and her status. She feels she has nothing to lose. If she contracts AIDS or anything else, so what? (Himmich, 1996).

AIDS CAUSES BUSINESS FAILURE

In Kasheni, a Tanzanian village bordering Lake Victoria, a village chairman turns the pages of a worn personal file in which he keeps photographs of villagers who have died. Among the snapshots of family groups is a photo of fit and smiling young men who made up the local football team. More than half have died of AIDS. He recalls a market in nearby Rukunyo, where Tanzanian and Ugandan traders did brisk business in second-hand clothing, bicycles, and other goods. Then people began to fall ill. It was discovered that the illness was AIDS, traders drifted away, the market died, and the surrounding bars and hotels closed their doors.

population. These are male and female Africans 20 to 40 years old—the bread-winners, the food-producers, the backbone of the African labor force. In Luska, Zambia, 33% of blood donors between age 30 and 35 were HIV-positive; 68% of skilled Zambian copper-

belt workers were HIV-positive. In Nairobi, Kenya, 2% of all medical personnel tested positive.

Deaths due to AIDS are occurring so rapidly that African funerals which normally last up to a week are in jeopardy of being shortened. One of the reasons is that, as the labor force decreases, fewer relatives of the deceased can be spared time off for the lengthy traditional funeral. It has been estimated that there could be a 20% decline in population in East Africa by the year 2001.

Obstacles to fighting AIDS in Africa were set out forcefully by N'Galy Bosenge, director of the National AIDS Program in Zaire, as he addressed the Fifth International Conference on AIDS (1989).

First among the obstacles is poverty. "We lack resources not only for AIDS, but for health in general . . ., The situation in Europe and North America—where homosexuals and [injection] drug users are well-defined risk groups—makes it easy to target prevention and control programs. But apart from prosti-

BOX 12.5

ANGOLA: AN EXAMPLE OF THE IMPACT OF HIV/AIDS ON ITS SOLDIERS AND ITS CIVILIANS

"Combat killed 500,000 Angolans; the first years of peace may kill 1 million. . . . Angola is not prepared psychologically, physically or economically for a disease that will hit with epidemic force."—Eben Moussi of the World Health Organization, 1996.

Experts estimate at least 10% of Angola's 10 million population harbors HIV. The country has been divided by war for 20 years. Laboratories are in ruins. Health care workers are unable to do any HIV testing.

Boys as young as 13 were drafted by the thousands into the armies. They received their sex education from platoon mates on the march.

Sexual myths specific to Angola have also helped spread HIV. For example, legend has it that sexual relations with a virgin girl can cure a man with a sexually transmitted disease, condoms cause impotence, girls can't get AIDS, and a smelly root paste will cure it.

Young Angolan girls are now five times as likely to be infected as boys of the same age.

THE MILITARY ISSUE

HIV infection is so high among African soldiers that they run a far greater risk of dying from AIDS than they do from warfare.

Studies found at least 65% of army hospital beds in Uganda and Zaire were filled by soldiers with AIDS. More than half of Zimbabwe's soldiers are infected with HIV. And at least 100,000 Angolan government and rebel troops, half the fighting force, are HIV-positive. They are marching home to civilians who are war-weakened and vulnerable to HIV infection.

When people are warned about AIDS, they shrug. Danger to them is mines, bandits, and starvation. AIDS does not make the list.

Also at risk for HIV infection are the more than 7,000 international troops and tens of thousands of aid workers from around the world who are deployed across Angola under a U.N. reconstruction plan.

——— BOX 12.6 ———

EXAMPLE OF TRIBAL TRADITION, LUSKA, ZAMBIA

Throughout Africa, polygamy has been culturally tolerated for centuries. The custom is still practiced in many black African states.

Sanford Mweupe looks back on the days when he had only two wives to worry about. So do the two wives. Domestic life has been strained since events led to what was delicately referred to as "the confusion."

In 1988, after his brother died, Mweupe was chosen by the family's elders to perform a ceremony called **"ritual cleansing."** According to tribal tradition, the brother's two widows had to be purged of their husband's spirit by having sex with a member of his family.

Mweupe's brother had died of AIDS, and the widows may also have been infected. Mweupe's wives pleaded with him not to keep the tradition but the elders insisted he cleanse the widows and then take them as his wives. He was warned by modern doctors, but a traditional healer assured him it would be safe.

Mary Mweupe was pregnant with her third child—her husband's 18th—when Mweupe's brother died.

Mweupe took some precautions. He took his brother's widows to a traditional healer who gave them injections and said they were free of AIDS. He also brought some condoms over to his brother's house on the day the families gathered for the ceremony.

He said "I wanted to use them, but the grandmother of one of the widows saw them and she said this would not be according to the tradition. She said the widows would not be cleansed. I was afraid she would tell other people and make me a laughingstock, so I did not use them."

After the families drank beer in his brother's yard, Mweupe and the two widows retired inside. He stayed with them for a week. He agreed to go beyond his cleansing duties and take them as his wives, assuming responsibility for their five children, as well as a sixth who was born 7 months after the ceremony.

When Mweupe went home at week's end to the first and second Mrs. Mweupe, the reunion was less than warm. Mweupe told his wives that he should not sleep with them because of the possibility of infection. But after a time they insisted. They said he was their only husband—who else could they sleep with?

The consequences are still unclear, because Mweupe and the two sisters have not been tested for the HIV virus.

(Adapted from John Tierney, The New York Times, Sept. 17, 1990)

---

tutes, there really are no risk groups in Africa: 90% of cases are from the general population."

Will Africa's Experience Be Repeated Elsewhere?

Conditions in Africa that contributed to the AIDS disaster included sexual behavior patterns conducive to the spread of HIV infection, high incidence of STDs, nonuse of condoms, government inattention to the problem in its early years, and contaminated blood supplies in some places. Whenever such conditions prevail, the African experience is likely to be repeated. In certain Latin American and Asian countries, conditions resemble those of Africa. The number of new AIDS cases in Asia is expected to pass those occurring in Africa by 2001.

THE AMERICAS (NORTH, SOUTH, AND CENTRAL)

By the end of 1998, about 988,000 AIDS cases and 462,000 deaths will have been **reported** by 47 countries and territories in the Americas. The Americas represent 47% of worldwide AIDS cases **REPORTED** but only 34% of the **estimated** AIDS cases, worldwide, through 1998. The Americas will contribute about 6% to 7% of the 9 million **estimated deaths** due to AIDS, worldwide, through 1998. The number of **reported** cumulative AIDS cases and deaths due to AIDS in the Americas by REGION (with subregions and countries listed) through early September 1996 are found in Table 12-2. Approximately 73% of the AIDS cases in the Americas have been **reported** by the United States.

In North America and many urban areas of Latin America, most AIDS cases occur among

HIV/AIDS IN UGANDA

In Uganda, AIDS is known as **"grandmother's disease"** because the grandmother is often the only family member left to raise children—the mother and father have died of AIDS and the grandfather was killed years ago during civil war.

One in four young adults is **HIV-infected in Uganda's cities.** In Roki, a district in Southern Uganda, where the first AIDS cases were diagnosed, over 50% of adults are HIV-positive. Every family in Roki has lost someone—a mother, father, or child. There are over 400,000 orphaned children in Roki due to AIDS (Figure 12-6). Ebraphim Samba, head of the WHO regional office for Africa, said, **"You go to parts of Uganda now and see orphaned children and elderly people, and in between there's nothing. It doesn't take a genius to see that's a disaster for the economy and for society."**

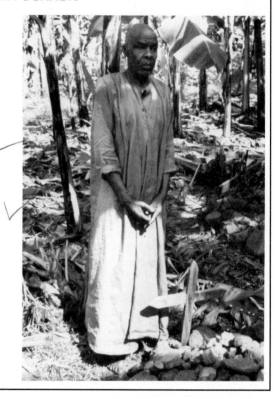

FIGURE 12-6 Grieving for Lost Children. A sole Ugandan parent grieves at the graveside. He mourns the loss of seven children and grandchildren who have died of AIDS. (*Photograph by E. Hooper, World Health Organization, Geneva*)

homosexual or bisexual men between the ages of 20 and 49 and among injection drug users. Over 50% of homosexual men in some urban areas have been infected. The proportion of cases involving heterosexual contact in these areas is estimated at about 5%. In some areas of Latin America, especially in the Caribbean, there is an increasing trend towards heterosexual transmission which now accounts for the majority of new HIV infections in some places (*PAACNOTES*, 1990). To better understand the distribution of AIDS cases by **AGE** and **SEX** in subregions of the Americas, see Figure 12-7. To review the annual incidence of AIDS cases for the three major regions of the Americas, see Figure 12-8.

BOGUS HIV CERTIFICATES IN KENYA

Nairobi—Kenyatta Hospital is selling HIV-negative certificates, according to the Dutch gay publication *De Gay Krant*. The certificates, supplied within 15 minutes, are going for the rough equivalent of $40, and no medical tests are done. The report states that the certificates are valuable to people who wish to become foreign laborers or visit the United States, where HIV-seropositive immigrants and visitors are not permitted to enter the country.

TABLE 12-2   Number of Reported Cumulative Cases of AIDS in the Americas per Year and Deaths, by Region, through 1996

Subregion and Country or Territory	Cumulative Total	Total Deaths
Regional total	742,273	443,407
(Adults, 729,154; Pediatric, 13,119)		
Latin America	169,489	77,885
Andean Area	18,435	8,950
Bolivia		
Columbia		
Ecuador		
Peru		
Venezuela		
Southern Cone	11,595	4,404
Argentina		
Chile		
Paraguay		
Uruguay		
Brazil	88,099	43,744
Central American Isthmus	11,142	3,114
Belize		
Costa Rica		
El Salvador		
Guatemala		
Honduras		
Nicaragua		
Panama		
Mexico	31,293	16,332
Latin Caribbean	8,925	1,341
Cuba		
Dominican Republic		
Haiti		
Puerto Rico		
Caribbean	10,165	6,046
Anguilla		
Antigua and Barbuda		
Aruba		
Bahamas		
Barbados		
Cayman Islands		
Dominica		
French Guiana		
Grenada		
Guadeloupe		
Guyana		
Jamaica		
Martinique		
Montserrat		
Netherlands Antilles		
Saint Kitts and Nevis		
Saint Lucia		
St. Vincent and the Grenadines		
Suriname		
Trinidad and Tobago		
Turks and Caicos Islands		
Virgin Islands (UK)		
North America	595,571	372,332
Bermuda		
Canada		
United States of America		

Source: *AIDS Surveillance in the Americas*, Quarterly Report, December 1996.

Canada

The first reported case of HIV/AIDS in Canada was diagnosed in 1979. In July of 1993, Canada changed their definition of AIDS to follow CDC's January 1, 1993 definition with the exception that Canada does not include T4 counts to **diagnose** AIDS cases (*Canadian Quarterly Surveillance Update*, July 1994). Through April 1997, the Federal Centre for AIDS received reports on 14,836 AIDS cases, 13,822 males and 1,013 females. These included 14,677 adults/adolescents and 159 children (Figure 12-9). A total of 10,837 have died (73%). AIDS is the **second** leading cause of death among persons aged 25 to 44 years. Adult cases in Canada are defined as ages 15 to 65; pediatric, less than age 15. About 17% of AIDS cases occur in males and 27% in females between ages 15 to 29. With a 9- to 15-year delay in the onset of AIDS, one in five people with AIDS were infected as teenagers. As in the United States, the largest number of AIDS cases occur in the 30- to 39-year age group, 45% of males and 36% of females. There are about 3,000 **new** HIV infections each year.

Michael Chretian, the chairman of a 1988 report entitled "AIDS: A Perspective for Canadians," said that Canada lags behind the United States in incidence of AIDS cases by 2 or 3 years. About 70% of AIDS cases occur in three cities: Montreal, Toronto, and Vancouver. Twenty-five percent of Canadians live in Montreal and Toronto.

About 69% of AIDS cases are among homosexual and bisexual males. About 10% of AIDS cases involve heterosexual contact and about 8.5% are injection drug users. Seven and one-half percent of AIDS cases in Canada are women. About one in four women with AIDS was/is an injection drug user. Two-thirds of all AIDS cases in Canada were diagnosed after 1990. The report on AIDS issued by the Royal Society of Canada opposes mandatory testing for HIV infection, and supports antidiscrimination legislation, education on condom use, and dispensing clean needles to drug addicts.

Canada experienced about a 20% drop in deaths due to AIDS for 1996 when compared to 1995 data (*AIDS in Canada*, 1997).

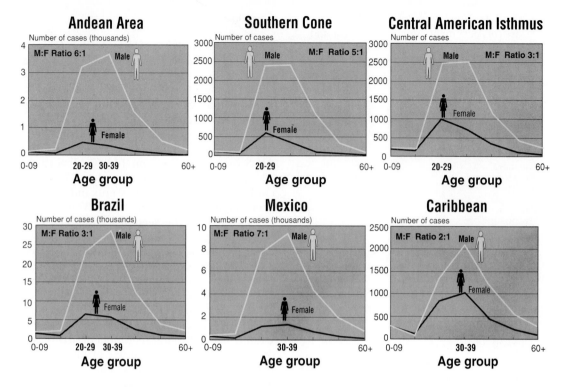

FIGURE 12-7   The Incidence of AIDS Cases by Age Group in Each Subregion of the Americas. In the Southern Cone and Central America, the age of the highest infection is the group between 20 and 29 years old for both sexes and for females in Brazil. In the Andean Area, Mexico, and the Caribbean, the age of infection is between 30 and 39 years old for males and females, as well as for males in Brazil (see Table 12-2).

Mexico

The first **reported** woman to be diagnosed with AIDS in Mexico in 1985 was a 52-year-old housewife living in Mexico City; her only known behavioral risk was having unprotected sexual intercourse with her husband. The majority of Mexican women with HIV infection and AIDS are between the ages of 20 and 45. The primary reason for their infection is the lack of knowledge due to the lack of HIV prevention programs.

In 1988, Mexico ranked eighth in total number of AIDS cases reported to the WHO. By June of 1996, Mexico had reported a total of 29,954 AIDS cases. Thirty-four percent of AIDS cases are in Mexico City, 64% are in provincial towns and cities, and 2% are in the outlying areas. Most affected are middle- and upper-class Mexicans. Mexico now ranks second to Brazil for AIDS cases in Latin America (United States Department of State, 1992; Pan American Health Organization, 1994).

As elsewhere in the world, most AIDS cases occur in the 25- to 45-year age group. Through January 1997, about 47% of the female AIDS patients became HIV-infected via blood transfusions and 53% from heterosexual contacts (Uribe-Salas et al., 1997). Of men with AIDS, 93% became infected through sexual activities. Of these, 56% are homosexuals, 27% are bisexuals, and 10% are heterosexuals. Injection drug users (IDUs) account for less than 1%, apparently because of the high cost of injection drugs (Sternberg, 1989).

Rate per Million Population

* 1997 data are incomplete due to delayed reporting.

FIGURE 12-8   Annual Incidence Rates of AIDS in the Americas (per Million), Three Major Regions, 1982–1997.

Latin America and the Caribbean

Latin America and the Caribbean region are heterogeneous and diverse, with a total of 44 countries and territories, an estimated population of over 470 million people with a variety of ethnic backgrounds, and four main languages (English, Spanish, French, and Portuguese). The rate of spread of HIV/AIDS has been slower than in other developing regions of the world, but the pandemic is well established and there is a wide variation in the level of HIV infection and the speed of the many epidemics among subregions and countries.

By the end of 1988, over 10,000 AIDS cases from Latin America and the Caribbean had been reported to the WHO. Beginning 1997, over 193,000 cases were reported (26% of re-

ported AIDS cases in the Americas). Still, it is estimated that 30% to 50% of cases are not reported. Jonathan Mann believes they are underreported by about 60% (Mann et al., 1988). The concentration of AIDS cases here, as elsewhere, is largely in urban areas. Through 1986, most AIDS cases occurred among homosexual males and IDUs. The primary modes of HIV transmission in the subregions are homo/bisexual (Andean Area, Southern Cone, Brazil, and Mexico; see Table 12-2) and **heterosexual** (Central American Isthmus and the Caribbean). HIV transmission attributed to injection drug use is common in the Southern Cone and Brazil with 29.7% and 26.5%, respectively (*AIDS Surveillance in the Americas,* 1996). Nearly all Caribbean islands have reported at least one case of AIDS. Rates range

Number of cases reported

	15	15-19	20-29	30-39	40-49	50+	TOTAL
Males	83	41	2350	6220	3732	1396	13822
Females	81	4	284	360	137	147	1013

Age Group (Years)

Women (n = 1,013)   %

Heterosexual Contact	58.8
Injection Drug Use	16
Blood Recipient	11
Perinatal	6.7
Clotting Factor	1.1
Occupational Exposure	0.1
No Identified Risk	6.3

Pediatric (n = 159)   %

Perinatal Transmission	78
Blood Recipient	7.6
Clotting Factor	6.3
No Identified Risk	8.1

- Range of age at AIDS diagnosis: newborn to 85 years
- Mean age at AIDS diagnosis: 37.6 years
- 25% of AIDS cases with age at diagnosis less than or equal to 31 years
- 50% of AIDS cases with age at diagnosis less than or equal to 36 years
- 75% of AIDS cases with age at diagnosis less than or equal to 43 years

FIGURE 12-9   Total Reported AIDS Cases in Canada by Age Group and Sex Canada (*N=14,836: reported deaths 10,837*). Data reported to April 15, 1997. *(Source: Division of HIV/AIDS Epidemiology, BCDE, Laboratory Centre for Disease Control, Health Canada)*

from a low of 2.3 per 100,000 people in Cuba to a high of 556 per 100,000 in the Bahamas (Caribbean Epidemiology Centre, 1994). Six islands—Bahamas, Barbados, Bermuda, Jamaica, Trinidad, and Tobago—account for 90% of all AIDS cases in the Caribbean. Early cases of AIDS in the Caribbean were reported in Haiti in 1979 and in Trinidad in 1983. In Haiti, one recent study found one in 10 pregnant *nonprostitutes* to be HIV-infected (Palaca, 1991).

Transmission—Modes of HIV transmission in the Caribbean are similar to those in the United States and also to those in Africa. Initial cases tended to be among homosexual and bisexual men. But, as the pandemic has progressed, the mode of HIV transmission has become increasingly heterosexual and it is now (1997) the dominant mode. About 9% of

AIDS cases reported are among children under age 5.

The majority of AIDS cases in Bermuda are associated with IDUs, which are not a problem in most of the other Caribbean islands. On several islands, female prostitutes are HIV-infected; in Jamaica they constitute 12% of all AIDS cases. Some migrant farm workers, who work in the United States for 3 to 6 months each year, have become HIV-infected through heterosexual contact while abroad and have developed AIDS. They represent 14% of all AIDS cases in Jamaica.

Virtually all Caribbean islands now have HIV control programs which include screening of blood donors, public education, and counseling. Cuba has been unique in undertaking national screening and, in the past, isolating HIV-infected people in a sanatorium.

Cuba

As of early 1994, Cuba stopped its quarantine of people who test HIV-positive. Reasons for Cuba's reversal of policy on testing everyone for HIV is not known. Prior to this change in policy, everyone old enough to have sex was tested—*no exceptions.* By December of 1993, over 90% of 11 million people had been tested. Of these, 710 men and 297 women tested positive and were being confined in 13 sanatoriums. The government paid every sanatorium resident the salary he or she received prior to confinement. Almost all send money home to their families.

Except for cigarettes, everything was free—pots and pans, coffee makers, phone calls, detergent, rice, beans, zidovudine, antibiotics, and condoms. Within the sanatorium, no one taught abstinence; no one expected people to give up sex.

Beginning 1996, at least 248 of the 1,159 HIV-positive Cubans had died of AIDS. Cuba's experience has shown that there are effective, albeit draconian, public health measures for controlling the spread of HIV/AIDS.

Argentina

In Argentina, the first cases of AIDS in men occurred in 1983, and in women in 1987. Although the actual number of cases among women is low in comparison to that in other countries, the number has increased in recent years. From 1994 through 1997, among men with AIDS, the most common risk factor was the use of injection drugs, while among women with AIDS, the most common risk factor was heterosexual contact.

The increase in AIDS cases is occurring mainly in persons aged 20 to 34 years, who accounted for nearly 65% of all of the 9,000 reported AIDS cases in Argentina through 1996. Argentina reported the second highest incidence rate of AIDS cases (41 per million) in South America during 1993 (the most recent year with complete reporting for the Region of the Americas), preceded only by Brazil (80 per million). Underreporting is officially estimated to be 30% (Betts et al., 1996). A recent study by the World Health Organization estimated that 30% of inmates in Argentina's federal prison system are infected with HIV.

Brazil

> Equating AIDS with death can blunt a campaign's effectiveness. If you say "AIDS kills," street kids say, "It's just another thing that kills us. The police kill us too." Killing is not serious to them.
>
> *Ana Filgueiras*

With the exception of Haiti, Brazil ranks highest in Latin America for HIV infections. At the Fourth International Conference on AIDS (1988), Brazilian Health Minister Borges da Silveira said that Brazil had 4,946 cases of AIDS. Beginning 1997, Brazil had over 83,000 AIDS cases. It is now estimated that 1 million out of a population of 157 million Brazilians are HIV-infected. Two-thirds of all families live below the poverty level of $900 a year. Private insurers throughout Brazil **do not** pay for AIDS treatment. In 1985, 3% of AIDS cases were women; for 1993 it was over 20%. In 1988, heterosexual contact was considered responsible for 1% of men and 12% of women reported to have AIDS; for AIDS cases diagnosed in 1993, these figures had risen to 17% and 51%, respectively (Lurie et al., 1995).

In Brazil, surveys show that men are aware of the AIDS threat, but are reluctant to use condoms. In Rocinha, Rio's largest slum, 77% of sexually active male respondents to a survey said they never used condoms.

In addition to objections on grounds of pleasure, Brazilian men fault condoms for their high price and their poor quality. Priced out of reach of Brazil's poor majority, a pack of three condoms cost the equivalent of 1 kilogram (2.2 pounds) of rice or 2 kilograms of black beans. Brazil, with a population of 157 million, has **seven** free clinics for HIV testing.

About 70% of AIDS patients live in Sao Paulo or Rio de Janeiro, but AIDS is spreading into the rural areas. Blood banks are contaminated and 74% of the hemophiliacs in Rio de Janeiro are HIV-infected. Government figures show that in Rio de Janeiro, 34% of professional blood donors are HIV-infected.

TABLE 12-3 The Incidence of AIDS in Europe

Country	Cumulative through March 31, 1990	Cumulative through 1996
Albania	0	10
Austria	415	1,547
Belarus	0	16
Belgium	651	2,130
Bulgaria	7	40
Croatia	1	100
Czechoslovakia	23	76
Denmark	573	1,870
Estonia	0	9
Finland	58	232
France	9,718	43,904
Germany	4,672	15,771
Greece	295	1,380
Hungary	34	228
Iceland	13	44
Ireland	142	517
Italy	6,068	33,984
Latvia	0	12
Lithuania	0	9
Luxembourg	26	109
Malta	14	38
Moldova	0	6
Monaco	2	38
Netherlands	1,189	4,028
Norway	153	532
Poland	35	440
Portugal	410	3,256
Romania	478	3,970
Russian Federation	26	222
San Marino	1	2
Slovak Republic	0	14
Slovenia	0	56
Spain	5,295	38,939
Sweden	406	1,396
Switzerland	1,255	5,130
Ukraine	0	81
United Kingdom	3,157	12,714
Yugoslavia	120	570
Total	35,236	173,415

Cumulative AIDS cases reported by **38 countries**—World Health Organization (WHO) European Region, through March 31, 1990 and November 30, 1996. (Sources: WHO Surveillance Program, Geneva)

EUROPE

In 1993, most European countries expanded their AIDS case definition to that used in the United States. In Spain, the new definition was introduced on January 1, 1994. By the end of 1996, over 173,000 cases of AIDS, representing about 3% of the world's total, were reported from 38 countries in Europe (Table 12-3). This number represents an increase of about 80% over the 1990 number of AIDS cases. Over 60% of AIDS persons have died. The number of cases reported in central and eastern Europe remains low. The two countries with the largest number of AIDS cases are France and Italy (Figure 12-10).

About 85% of AIDS cases in Europe occur in homosexual males and IDUs. Women account for about 14% of total AIDS cases. And, over half of the women who have AIDS are IDUs (Smith et al., 1994). Regional differences in Europe are similar to those in the United States. The prevalence of AIDS cases in Europe is strikingly different from north to south and east to west. In Denmark, Sweden, and the United Kingdom, 70% to 90% of the total number of AIDS cases occur in the homosexual male population. At the beginning of 1992 in Southern Europe, in Italy 66% and in Spain over 50% of AIDS cases occurred in IDUs.

AIDS cases were first reported in France in 1978 (Coles, 1988). In 1997, the greater Paris area still had the largest number of AIDS patients. Of these, 70% were homosexual males and 7% were IDUs. However, as in the United States, homosexual AIDS cases have declined. In France, they went from 78% in the early 1980s to 53% in 1987. IDUs, on the other hand, increased from 6% in the early 1980s to 17% in 1987.

Jean-Baptiste Brunet, of Claude Bernard Hospital in Paris, reported that the incidence of AIDS cases among IDUs in Spain, France, and Italy is increasing at an annual rate of 16%. In 1985, 7% of Europe's AIDS cases were IDUs. In 1996, about 30% of AIDS cases were IDUs. It is estimated that over 1 million people in 38 European countries (Table 12-2) are HIV-infected and there are about 40,000 new HIV infections occurring each year. AIDS has killed about 22,830 people in France and about 16,992 in Italy through 1996. In Paris, over 40% of AIDS deaths occur in males between ages 25 to 44. In France, 120,000 are estimated to be HIV-positive; in England and Wales, 28,000 are HIV-positive (Bajors et al., 1995).

FIGURE 12-10 AIDS Cases in Western Europe Through 1997. The number of new AIDS cases in Western European countries increased 19- to 30-fold over the number diagnosed in 1986. The numbers under each Western European country represent diagnosed AIDS cases in 1986 and in 1997. AIDS cases in these countries are mostly in metropolitan areas.

EASTERN EUROPE:
THE FORMER SOVIET UNION

The former Soviet Union has only recently been alarmed by an increasing number of AIDS patients. The first case of AIDS was reported in 1987. Until 1990, Soviet officials still regarded AIDS as a Western problem. Foreign Ministry spokesman Gennady I. Gerasimov called AIDS "a scourge of God for the down-fallen morals in our world." In November 1988, the Soviet Union reported its first AIDS-associated death, a 29-year-old woman. But by the end of 1992, 600 AIDS cases had been re-

———— BOX 12.9 ————

POLAND'S HIV/AIDS EPIDEMIC

The rapid spread of HIV disease/AIDS in Poland is directly linked to a form of homemade heroin called **campuk**. It is easily and cheaply made in the kitchens of Polish homes. Campuk consists of poppy straw, acetone, ammonia, and water. After boiling to reduce the broth, the left-over residue consists of 25% heroin, 50% morphine, and 25% codeine—**it is highly addictive**. The problem is compounded because injection needles are scarce and so those addicted share needles. There are between 300,000 and 600,000 injection drug users in Poland. Few treatment facilities are available with even fewer medical supplies and too few medical staff to make a difference. Over 10,000 physicians left Poland in 1990. A single day clinic in Warsaw treats 25,000 addicts a year; 75% are HIV-positive. Because drugs are in limited supply, only the fatally ill receive Zidovudine. It is not unusual to have people die of AIDS within 2 years of diagnosis. The only hospital in Warsaw has a ward with 20 beds for AIDS patients, but only eight can be accommodated because of staff shortages.

PROSTITUTION (COMMERCIAL SEX WORKERS)

From January to October 1990, 500,000 Polish women lost their jobs and turned to the streets. Officially, 10,000 are registered prostitutes; however, the figure is probably much higher. Some of the women do not tell their clients they are HIV-infected or have AIDS.

One of these women said that in 2 or 3 hours she could make 3 months' salary. This woman bragged of having clients from New York, Sweden, and Finland. Warsaw is becoming the prostitution capital of Eastern Europe.

(Source: *AIDS Quarterly: The Crisis in Poland,* WGBH Educational Foundation)

———— BOX 12.10 ————

ONE MAN STARTS THE RUSSIAN AIDS EPIDEMIC

In 1981 the engineer returned from Africa to Elista carrying HIV. He married. The virus spread to his wife. She had a child. The child was infected, became sick, and in 1988 was sent to the hospital. Doctors did not know the child carried the virus.

In the hospital, the child received drug injections. The same drug was given to other children by doctors and nurses who used the **same syringe** because they thought children are sterile.

Some of these HIV-infected children were transferred to larger hospitals. At each of those hospitals, the pattern was repeated. New cases appeared 300 miles away in hospitals in Volgograd, Rostov-on-Don, and Stavropol. A total of 260 children and several of their mothers became HIV-infected before this chain of events was stopped.

Russian medical authorities realized there had not been a single case of AIDS infection in the area before this outbreak of HIV infections. When authorities recognized the disease, they began exhaustive medical detective work to track the epidemic to its source.

In 1989, more than 140,000 people were tested for HIV. The investigation led to the Russian engineer.

One aspect of this epidemic in Russian children remains puzzling. The investigation revealed that 21 mothers were infected. It seems they must have been infected by their children, but how?

The head of the AIDS laboratory of the Central Scientific Research Institute of Epidemiology in Moscow speculated the children may have had **bleeding mouth sores. Blood** from the sores may have entered the mothers' bloodstream during breast-feeding. But, American health authorities said that was unlikely.

ported. The most common route of HIV-transmission is IDU.

In March 1989, the Soviet Health Minister said that AIDS was a threat similar to that posed by nuclear weapons. In February 1989, Gerasimov cautioned the world that the Soviet Union would now require foreigners who planned to stay there for more than 3 months to show certificates proving they were HIV-free. In late 1994, the Russian Parliament approved compulsory HIV screening of foreigners (Butler, 1994). In April 1995, President Boris Yeltsin signed the AIDS law that imposes mandatory HIV testing on **almost** all **foreigners** who **plan** to spend 3 months or more in Russia. With a national population exceeding 150 million, the incidence of HIV infection and AIDS cases is negligible compared with that of the United States. Beginning 1997, Russia had registered 2,316 HIV-positive people and 1,000 cases of AIDS. But Russian health experts estimate the true numbers are 10 times higher.

Soviets receive prison sentences of up to 8 years for transmitting the virus and 5 years for exposing someone else to the virus in cases where transmission does not occur. Soviet law empowers authorities to test anyone suspected of carrying the AIDS virus.

ASIA

This region includes Bangladesh, Bhutan, Brunei Darussalam, Cambodia, China, India, Indonesia, Hong Kong, Japan, DPR Korea, Republic of Korea, Laos, Malaysia, the Maldives, Mongolia, Myanmar, Nepal, the Philippines, Singapore, Sri Lanka, Thailand, and Vietnam. It is home to **over 60% of the world's adult population, hence what happens in the region will have a major impact on the global AIDS pandemic**. By the year 2001, 42% of the estimated 40+ million HIV-infected people will live in Asia where the main route of HIV transmission is heterosexual (Wolffers, 1997).

Many of the first cases of HIV infection in Asia were discovered among homosexual men. However, the rapid spread of the virus in Asia has generally been among injection drug users followed by female commercial sex workers (CSW) and their clients (Ford et al., 1995).

South Asia's AIDS Pandemic

Southern Asia is made up of **14 countries** in South Central Asia and **10 countries** of Southeast Asia. Various international bodies, such as the World Health Organization and Harvard AIDS Institute, have now stated that within the next few years, South Asia will have more people living with HIV/AIDS than the rest of the world put together. It has been estimated that India (South Central Asia) alone will have approximately 12 million HIV/positive people by the year 2000 and 20 to 40 million people living with HIV by 2020.

The South Asian HIV epidemic has been defined as heterosexual, but there are doubts regarding the use of heterosexual versus homosexual terminology in this part of the world because of different cultural definitions of the two terms. All that can be stated for certain is that approximately 70% of HIV transmis-sion is through sexual intercourse. Needle use and infected blood supplies make up the remainder.

Through mid-1985, 44 countries in Asia had reported 250,000 AIDS cases. The WHO estimated that by the end of 1995, over 4 million Asians were HIV-infected. By the year 2000, an estimated 10 million Asians will be HIV-infected. By the year 2000, it is estimated that between 4 million and 8 million Asian children will have been orphaned by the disease. Many of the initial AIDS cases were linked to people who had been to areas where HIV disease and AIDS were more prevalent. HIV is believed to have entered Asia in the mid-1980s. Thus far, relatively few AIDS cases have been reported to the WHO from Asian nations. However, the WHO'S Global Program on AIDS (GPA) states that the rate of new HIV infection is rising dramatically—so fast, in fact, that, even though the disease was virtually unknown only a few years ago, by the end of this decade more Asians than Africans are expected to become infected each year (Palaca, 1991).

SOUTH CENTRAL ASIA

Pakistan

This is a land of 128 million people. In mid-1989, Health Minister Amir Haider Kazmi announced

——— BOX 12.11 ———

KARACHI, PAKISTAN: A WELL-GUARDED SECRET

Most people only know the name AIDS but nothing about prevention and how the disease spreads. There are deep-seated religious taboos against sex and the use of condoms. Social attitudes toward HIV infection and AIDS is one of **total rejection**. It is no wonder then that a man and wife, both HIV-positive, carried a vial of poison with them when they took their 2-year-old child in for an HIV test. If **positive**, they were going to **kill her** (they did not realize test results took several weeks). The results came back **negative**. The child lives, but the father was **deported** from the sheikdom and recently died of AIDS.

that HIV-antibody tests would be given to all foreigners living in Pakistan and to citizens who had lived abroad. By December 1993, 26 cases of AIDS had been reported to the WHO. Pakistan borrowed about $17 million to purchase the necessary testing equipment.

Beginning 1997, the official figure of 1,050 HIV-infected and 65 AIDS cases in Pakistan included only those which had been **reported** to various health centers. Sources in the World Health Organization (WHO) estimated there are over 40,000 HIV-infected and over 2,000 AIDS cases. By the year 2000, there may be over 4,000 AIDS cases and 80,000 HIV-infected in Pakistan.

India

India has a population of over 900 million people. India has more people than the continents of Africa, Australia, and Latin America combined. Through 1997, the Indian Health Organization estimated that there were over 3 million HIV-infected people in India and over 100,000 AIDS cases. The most common mode of HIV transmission is **heterosexual**. The first HIV-positive person was found in 1986. Through 1993, 500 AIDS cases had been reported. Estimates on HIV infection rates in India are difficult to make, but there are signs that an epidemic is at hand. In Bombay, the WHO estimates there are about 500,000 HIV-infected people. There are an estimated

200,000 women working as prostitutes; 57% are believed to be HIV-infected. It is estimated that each prostitute has about 6 clients in a 24-hour period! (Bhave et al., 1995).

Ishwar Gilada, India's current Secretary-General of India's Health Organization and a renowned HIV/AIDS expert, stated in 1996 that **Bombay may become the AIDS capital of the world**. In the city of Pune, located just south of Bombay, population 2.5 million, about 15% of married women, with no sexual contact outside of marriage, are HIV-positive.

The new data show that HIV has spread to over 1 million people in India, far beyond the port cities of Bombay and Madras where it first entered, and is beginning to threaten rural populations, which are virtually defenseless because of a lack of information and condoms. Vulimiri Ramalingaswami of the All India Institute of Medical Sciences in New Delhi said that India is "sitting on top of a volcano" (Dickman, 1991). S. Snood (1990) reported that some Indian hospitals have banned AIDS patients and some doctors hesitate to treat them. In Delhi, nearly all physicians refuse to treat AIDS patients. V. Sharma, of the Malaria Research Center, Delhi, India (1994) reports that by the year 2000 India could have 1 million AIDS patients and 5 million HIV-infected (*Harvard AIDS Review*, 1995).

SOUTHEAST ASIA

Thailand

The only country in Southeast Asia never to have been colonized, Thailand, or *Muang Thai* ("land of the free"), is bordered by Laos, Cambodia, Myanmar (Burma), and Malaysia (Figure 12-11). About 80% of the population of 58 million live in rural areas. About 6 million people live in the capital, Bangkok, but no other city in Thailand has a population of over 300,000.

According to the WHO, Thailand is the most AIDS-prone country in **Southeast Asia** mainly because of widespread prostitution and injection drug use. The first case of AIDS was **reported** in December 1984. By the end of 1997, Thailand health officials believe that about 1.5 million people were HIV-infected

————— BOX 12.12 —————

INDIA: THE EMERGING FACE OF AIDS

The transmission of HIV is mapping a deadly course throughout India. The passage of HIV from one human into another, one person at a time, occurs mainly through heterosexual transmission involving **sex workers** and **truck drivers** and through **blood transfusions**, the use of **injection drugs**, the practice of **ancient traditions**, and through **gay men**.

SEX WORKERS

From the cage girls of Bombay to the dancers in Calcutta's pleasure houses, from the tribal women along Rajasthan's highways to the call girls of New Delhi, India's sex industry is extraordinarily varied. "Want some high-risk entertainment for the evening?" asks a manager of an HIV intervention program in Calcutta's red light district. "Step out into the street, take your pick: **female prostitutes, male prostitutes, child sex workers, housewives, college students, starlets, virgins, fresh Nepali girls**."

In Bombay—a city that has nearly twice as many inhabitants as New York, yet almost 20 times as many sex workers—the narrow lanes of the Falkland Road area serve as viewing galleries. In the gloom, girls peer mutely from between the bars of 5-foot-high cages.

When a client selects a cage girl, her pimp collects the payment, then escorts them to a private room. After sex, the pimp quickly returns the girl to her cage. She receives no pay, and there is no discussion of safe sex; condoms are used only if the client requests one. Most cage girls in Bombay are infected with HIV. The inability to negotiate safe sex and the necessity to sell sex to survive have rendered sex workers throughout Bombay vulnerable to HIV: their seroprevalence rate shot up from less than 2% in 1988 to 57% in 1995.

Farther south in India, festivals and even monsoons can regulate the **sex industry**—and therefore the ebb and flow of HIV. During festival months in the town of **Palani**, women earn their living by selling food, flowers, and amulets to the religious pilgrims. When the festivals end, the stream of pilgrims dwindles and the women are forced to **sell sex** to support themselves.

On the outskirts of Palani, in the sugar cane fields, many people earn their living by working the crops. Their income is assured during the wet season. When the wet season ends, sources of income dry up. The men then migrate to the neigh-boring state of Kerala, where there is work. Separated from their wives, they spend a large part of their wages on local sex workers. At home, wives sell sexual favors to support themselves and their children.

Throughout India, whether in temple towns like Palani or cities such as Bombay, the rise of HIV seroprevalence among female sex workers has been mirrored by increased rates of infection among their clients. HIV infection among these men is detected when they seek treatment for other sexually transmitted diseases (STDs) (*Harvard AIDS Review*, 1995).

TRUCK DRIVERS

As dusk falls and laughter erupts from the tin-roofed cinema hall, village women in Tamil Nadu signal their availability to passing truck drivers by draping **saris** on the trees that line the highway. Millions of truckers drive India's highways daily, transporting nearly half of the country's goods from the southern ports to the plains of the Ganges, from the Himalayan foothills to the markets of Bombay. The truck drivers often stop at roadside tea stalls for a dish of curry. They also stop for sex.

The truckers' practice of hiring sex workers en route stems not only from the extended periods of separation from their wives, but also from the prevalent myth that spending long hours behind the truck's engine **heats up the body. Many truckers believe they can rid themselves of this harmful heat by having frequent sex**.

Studies show that India's long-distance truckers average 200 sexual encounters each year; at any given time, 70% of them have STDs. Preliminary surveys estimate that **nearly one-third of them are infected with HIV**. With India's network of roadways—the largest in the world—penetrating the country's remotest corners, the truckers act as efficient couriers of HIV as they drive from town to town. In truckers in Madras who requested testing because they have STDs and are concerned about their high-risk behaviors, HIV seroprevalence rates rose from about **60%** in 1993 to **91%** in 1995 (*Harvard AIDS Review*, 1995).

BLOOD TRANSFUSIONS

When asked why he does not screen blood for HIV, the owner of a major blood bank in the Indian state of Bihar replied, "There need be no fear of AIDS in Bihar. This is, after all, the birth-place of the Buddha." The blood bank owner speaks for millions of Indians when he dismisses the presence of HIV in his country. But at the same time India struggles to cope with the epidemic through denial, ignorance, fear, and stigmatization, it faces the fastest growing HIV epidemic in the world.

It is estimated that 12% of the country's HIV infections have been acquired through blood transfusion. A highly placed government official in Madras says, "How many have contracted HIV through blood transfusion is anyone's guess." Each year India's more than 1,000 blood banks transfuse approximately 2 million units of blood. Throughout the country, the demand for blood outstrips supply, due in part to the fear of contracting HIV through blood donation, which is coupled with a superstition that losing blood leads to impotence. Half of India's blood supply therefore comes from people who sell their blood for a living. Their desperation has opened the door to HIV infection. **A Bombay study found that 86% of commercial blood donors screened in 1992 were seropositive.** Some commercial blood donors engage in unprotected sex to earn income; others may have been infected through unsterile plasma-pheresis equipment (*Harvard AIDS Review*, 1995).

INJECTION DRUG USERS

In northeastern India, against a backdrop of political and ethnic turmoil, injection drug users (IDUs) are at the center of a raging HIV epidemic. For years, the region's hill tribes had smoked opium for medicinal and recreational purposes, but by late 1989, heroin of injectable quality had flooded the state of Manipur from the nearby Golden Triangle of Myanmar, Thailand, and Laos. Manipuri youth switched from smoking opium to injecting heroin—with disastrous consequences. Within 6 months of the initial detection of HIV in Manipur in 1989, seroprevalence among IDUs increased to 54%. The government responded by **banning the sale of hypodermic** syringes, so the IDUs began **sharing ink droppers instead of syringes**. To avoid wasting a single drop of the drug, the IDUs inject themselves with heroin from the droppers, draw out their blood, and reinject the mixture several times before passing the paraphernalia to the next user. By the time this process is complete, they have exchanged considerable amounts of blood. The as-

sistant director of the AIDS Unit in Manipur reports HIV seroprevalence rates in northeastern India of up to 90% among IDUs, 6% among spouses of IDUs, and 1% among prenatal women (*Harvard AIDS Review*, 1995).

ANCIENT TRADITIONS

Koovagam resembles many or most villages scattered across India. No telephones, no concrete—just a temple and the thatched huts of a small farming community. This southern village is mostly forgotten until the **Chittirai-Pournami festival**, when thousands of devotees from as far away as New Delhi and Bombay pour into Koovagam to offer prayers to the presiding deity. What sets this festival apart from hundreds of others in India is that many of the participants are considered **neither male nor female**, but belong to what is loosely defined as a **third gender**—the **hijras**. Dressed in saris, with sprigs of fresh jasmine in their plaited hair, **the hijras are eunuchs and transsexuals who sell sex for a living**. Also in attendance are the **dungas**, men who **become women** for the duration of the festival. The rest of the year, the dangas are husbands or single men who appear to be strictly heterosexual. But during the Chittirai-Pournami festival, they don saris, elaborate wigs, and bright plastic jewelry. They also flirt, saunter, and sell sex to other men attending the festival. In addition to the hijras and the dangas are the **panthis**. The majority of panthis are single or married men who attend the festival to have sex with the hijras and dangas and pay up to 10 rupees—approximately 50 cents—per sexual encounter. Then there are the **husbands** of the hijras, who are both sexual partners and bodyguards.

Those selling sex do not insist that their clients use condoms, as most of them do not worry about HIV, which remains an abstract concept to many Indians. There are few reliable studies on seroprevalence among hijras, who, according to one estimate, may number 10,000 in New Delhi alone. Surveys by the director of New Delhi's AIDS Control Cell suggest that one in three hijras there is infected with HIV.

The Chittirai-Pournami festival is but one example of how participation in ancient traditions facilitates the present-day spread of HIV through India. Another tradition with deep roots in Hinduism is the initiation of poor, low-caste girls into the **devadasi sect**. Dedicated to the goddess

Yellamma when they are young, devadasis historically served priests, assisted in religious ceremonies, and cleaned temples. With the decline of temples as power structures, however, their role was stripped of much of its religious import and they found themselves selling sex to survive. According to the Indian Health Organization, devadasis compose nearly 15% of India's approximately 10 million sex workers. The number of devadasis is the highest in the states of Karnataka and Maharashtra, where they constitute 80% of all sex workers. By 1994, it had become clear that adherence to the tradition had exacted a deadly toll: in Pune, more than half the devadasis had become HIV-infected.

THE PRACTICE OF MATA

In the neighboring state of Andhra Pradesh, some villagers continue the practice of **mata,** yet another ancient tradition that fuels the spread of HIV through the population. A beautiful harijan, or low-caste child, who attracts the attention of the village landlords is chosen to become a mata or **sacred mother.** She is then dedicated to a life of meeting her patrons' sexual needs: she is bathed ceremoniously in the temple pond, paraded through the village, then sent to a seasoned, senior mata who tutors the girl in her new role. When she reaches puberty, the mata is publicly auctioned. Men outbid one another to become her first sexual partner, **often in the belief that sex with a virgin will cure them of sexually transmitted diseases.** Afterward, the mata moves from home to home, where wives make way for her to share their beds with their husbands. The HIV

prevalence in these villages is unknown, but with Andhra Pradesh reporting an HIV infection rate of 1 in every 200 people, it is clear that the mata tradition is providing yet another deadly channel for the virus. Traditions such as those of the hijras, devadasis, and matas—rooted in ancient beliefs and passed down through generations—have left legacies of vulnerability. To combat HIV, India must first reconsider practices that now carry lethal consequences (*Harvard AIDS Review*, 1995).

GAY MALES:
THE UNDERGROUND CULTURE

In India, the illegal status of homosexuality has created an underground culture where HIV and STDs are rampant. While few studies exist on HIV seroprevalence rates among men who have sex with men, one 1995 study found that, among a sample of this group in the Sangali district of Maharashtra, half were infected. Every evening, hundreds of gay men gather along the shores of the Marina beach in Madras, a popular meeting place for men seeking sex with men. "When I want to send out a signal that I'm looking for a partner, I generally roll up a newspaper and carry it under one arm," said one gay male, a college student who cruises the beach and local parks in search of the **perfect man.** He knows about HIV and uses condoms; he belongs to a small, educated group of volunteers who conduct AIDS awareness programs. For most of Madras's 3,000 homosexual men retaining their anonymity takes precedence over seeking lifesaving information, counseling, and condoms.

with 6% of these people developing AIDS each year. At this rate, the country's 90,000 hospital beds are insufficient to cope with the pandemic. Over 50,000 people have died from AIDS for each of the years 1995, 1996, and 1997. Over 6,500 children are born HIV-infected each year. This number is expected to increase to over 7,000 per year by the year 2000.

HIV Transmission—Eighty-seven percent of all cases of HIV infection and AIDS occurred among men and women ages 15 to 49. Through 1997, **heterosexual transmission** accounted for 76% of the total number of cases, 10% are IDUs, and 1.2% are gay and bisexual

men. HIV infections have occurred via **heterosexual intercourse** due largely to HIV transmission through female commercial sex workers (CSW). This has led to HIV transmission from men to their noncommercial female partners and a subsequent increase in mother–infant transmission. A substantial number of HIV infections have occurred among men who have sex with men and a small number of infections is thought to have resulted from blood transfusions.

The ratio of HIV-infected men to women is about 6:1, with increasing numbers of women being infected by their husbands who became infected via commercial sex workers. Thai re-

FIGURE 12-11 Thailand and Its Bordering Countries. Buddhism is the national religion of Thailand, although 4% of the population are Muslims and 1% are Christians.

searchers estimate that if education and prevention programs fail, up to 4.5 million people may be HIV-infected by the year 2000, with 650,000 cases of AIDS and 500,000 AIDS deaths. AIDS will then be the leading cause of death in Thailand. Indirect economic costs will be, in US dollars, about $8.5 billion.

Thai Government's Response: Prevention—In 1991, the Thai National AIDS Committee adopted an official policy, the **100% condoms program,** to enforce condom use in the sex industry (Surasing Visrutaratna et al., 1995). Its purpose was to promote the use of condoms by CSW and their clients **without exception.** If a customer **refused** to use a condom, the CSW was to withhold service and refund the customer's money. The **"100% con-**

dom program"** is the centerpiece of their prevention campaign. This government-enforced program requires that all sex workers in brothels demand that clients use condoms, distributed by the government. Brothels are a particularly important site of AIDS transmission in Thailand, because the vast majority of men patronize them. Thailand's sophisticated network of clinics that treat and track sexually transmitted diseases determine if brothels comply; violators are shut down. The campaign is reinforced by aggressive education about condom use in schools, military bases, workplaces, and on television and radio. The question to be asked is, can this program be effectively administered? According to Wiwat Rojanapithayakorn (1995) who reviewed the 100% condom program, the results through 1994 were very impressive. Before 1989, the percentage of sex acts with CSW protected by condoms had been approximately 14%. By December 1994, it had risen to over 90%. During the same time, the numbers of men presenting at government clinics with major STDs (syphilis, lymphogranuloma venereum, nongonococcal urethritis, gonorrhea, chancroid) declined from around 199,000 to 28,000. This was the first indication that the incidence of HIV transmitted through commercial sex might have declined. Subsequent evidence confirmed the decline. These data suggest that the Thai HIV/AIDS Prevention and Control Program is one of the few programs in the world that has demonstrated success at a national level.

In some areas of Thailand, 23% of pregnant women and 10% to 15% of military draftees have tested HIV-positive (Dickman, 1991).

EAST ASIA

China

In 1985, four Chinese hemophiliac patients who underwent treatment with blood factor VIII supplied by a U.S. pharmaceutical company tested positive for HIV. A few months earlier, a naturalized U.S. citizen originally from Argentina became the first person in China with a **documented** case of AIDS. In 1986, a Chinese chef from New York City, also a natu-

ralized U.S. citizen visiting China to seek medical care, became the first Chinese person to
be diagnosed with AIDS. At this point, none of
the 31 previous AIDS cases had originated in
China, all supposedly were imported AIDS in
foreigners. China **reported** its first AIDS case
in 1988.

The Chinese government adopted an AIDS
policy in collaboration with the World Health
Organization and tested subpopulations
deemed most likely to have elevated risks of exposure to HIV: drug users, Chinese persons returning from abroad, hotel service personnel,
prostitutes in detention centers, consumers of
imported blood products, contacts of persons
who are HIV-positive, and blood donors. HIV
tests were also made of sera from selected clinics along the country's southern border (Yu et
al., 1996).

By August 1990, the national newspaper reported that China, with a population of about
1.2 billion people, had a total of 305 cases of
AIDS. Through 1997, government estimates
were that China had about 4,555 HIV-infected
people, of whom 160 had AIDS. However,
China's doctors estimate the number of HIV-
infected people to be over 100,000. Most
(67%) of the HIV/AIDS cases are due to IDU
involving heroin addicts in southwest Yunnan
Province (Zheng et al., 1994, 1995). But scattered reports of HIV/AIDS have come in from
23 of China's 31 provinces.

Beijing has the next largest number of
HIV/AIDS cases in China. In order to halt further cases of HIV infection, the Beijing officials asked the people to determine if their
words and deeds conformed to the standards
of the People's Republic and whether they
knew what to do and what not to do when making contact with foreigners to avoid HIV infection.

Chinese officials dismiss the idea that the
use of condoms might be able to control HIV
infection.

There are now over 50 laboratories in 29
provinces conducting HIV-antibody testing on
prostitutes, injection drug users, and other
high-risk groups. In addition to beginning a
national education campaign, China is also
concerned about sterilizing techniques in
some hospitals. Hospitals in major cities have
just started to use disposable needles, but many
still do not. Health care workers are now urged
to follow strict guidelines in sterilizing syringes
and needles.

Japan

There are over 125 million people in Japan.
The majority have a deep-seated fear of becoming HIV-infected, not just because of their
possible premature death, but because of the
shame it brings to the individual and to their
family and ancestors. The stigma of HIV infection is so bad, that thousands of Japanese
are taking advantage of an unusual program,
funded by the Japanese Ministry of Health and
Welfare, which has established an HIV-testing
clinic outside of Japan for its citizens. Those
who fly to Honolulu feel that taking a 4,000-
mile trip is a small price to pay for a **guarantee of anonymity**, which they are not assured
of at home, since someone there might recognize them and spread gossip. They know
that if a verdict of HIV-positive leaked out,
they would face the equivalent of a death sentence in Japanese society, even in the absence
of any symptoms. Stan Sesser (1995) writes
that "if you're Japanese and HIV-positive, your
family rejects you, and you can't even tell your
best friends. Sometimes people who are HIV-
positive say to us that they want to stay in
Hawaii to die."

In Japan, any physical disability can be a
stigma and a source of shame, and many
Japanese look down on people who cannot be
fully productive. But AIDS is the worst afflic-
tion of all, because it is perceived as a foreigners' disease in a country that is intensely
xenophobic (fearful of foreigners), and as a
gay disease in a nation where homosexuality is
still not discussed.

Questionable AIDS Data—The intense
shame about AIDS and the resulting secrecy
make it futile to try and determine how many
Japanese are infected with HIV. The official
government statistics show that by the end of
June 1994, Japan had a cumulative total of
764 AIDS cases, of whom 441 had died. The
total of 3,075 were HIV-positive. However,
the deputy director of the Office of

Infectious Disease Control, at the Ministry of Health and Welfare, and one of the government's top AIDS officials, conceded that this count was far from accurate. "Our HIV-positive cases are maybe fifteen to twenty thousand. That's a reasonable estimate." Such data would suggest that through 1997, there may be 26,000 or more with HIV disease and perhaps 6,500 cases of AIDS, of which 3,770 may have died.

Oceania

Oceania is made up of 12 countries and the Federated States of Micronesia. Total population is over 28 million. The number of HIV-infected people and AIDS cases is relatively low compared to the other countries of the world, but the **incidence** of AIDS cases is about equal to that of other countries. For example, in New Zealand there are about 21 new AIDS cases each year. Through 1997, there were an estimated 546 AIDS cases in a population of 3.6 million people. Of these cases, 89% occurred in gay men, 6% were among heterosexuals, and 3% among IDUs. The most affected age group are those between the ages of 19 and 49. In both New Zealand and Australia, the AIDS epidemic appears to have reached a plateau. However, the incidence of AIDS cases will remain steady for another decade before declining. In several other Oceania countries, plateaus or declines in AIDS incidence have also been observed in some subgroups. In the state of Victoria in Australia, the total number diagnosed with AIDS appears to have begun to decline around 1991 (Sharples, 1996).

SUMMARY

The United States now accounts for about 40% of reported AIDS cases worldwide. But many countries, for political and economic reasons, underreport their AIDS cases. Thus the total number worldwide is an estimate and the real number remains unknown. The WHO estimated that there were between 5 and 10 million HIV-infected persons worldwide in 1992. But, the Harvard Global AIDS Policy Coalition estimated the number of HIV-infected persons

worldwide to be 12.9 million. It is estimated that by the end of 1998, there will be 35 million HIV-infected persons, 10 million with AIDS, and 9 million who have died from AIDS.

AIDS cases have been reported from all seven continents and from 197 countries. Africa has been reporting increasing numbers of AIDS cases from about 1985. HIV transmission in Africa is primarily between heterosexuals and from infected mothers to offspring. Injection drug use and homosexual activities are considered rare in Africa. There are some reports of blood transfusion cases of HIV infection in Africa, but they are relatively few.

The number of HIV infections and AIDS cases have been increasing at an alarming rate in Asia, primarily in South Central (India) and Southeast (Thailand) Asia. It is believed that Asia will surpass Africa in number of HIV-infected people and people with AIDS by the turn of the century.

The point is that HIV infections continue to increase in all nations reporting to the CDC or the WHO. The largest number of AIDS cases have yet to appear. Will the separate nations be prepared to handle the many medical, economic, social, and political problems that will accompany the tremendous drain on national resources?

REVIEW QUESTIONS

(Answers to the Review Questions are on page 579.)

1. Worldwide, what is the estimated rate of HIV infection?

2. What is the primary route of HIV transmission in Africa? In India?

3. Name the two countries in Europe with the highest number of AIDS cases.

4. What is the incidence of new AIDS cases in Europe?

5. What route of HIV exposure is becoming the most prevalent throughout the United States and Europe?

6. Of the countries presented, which appears to have the largest rate of HIV transmission by bisexual males? Which country is isolating HIV-infected people in sanatoriums? Which countries mandate that foreigners must have certificates proving they are **not** infected with HIV?

7. Name the two European countries in which over 50% of AIDS cases occur in IDUs.

REFERENCES

AIDS in Canada. (1997). Quarterly Surveillance Update. Bureau of HIV/AIDS and STD Laboratory Center for Disease Control, Heath Canada.

AIDS Surveillance in the Americas. (1996). Quarterly Report, September. PAHO/HCA/96.008.

ANDERSON, JOHN, et al. (1992). HIV antibody testing and post-test counseling in the United States: data from the 1989 National Health Interview Study. *Am. J. Public Health,* 82:1533–1535.

BAJOS, NATHALIE, et al. (1995). Sexual behavior and HIV epidemiology in France and Britain. *AIDS,* 9:735–743.

BARONGO, LONGIN R., et al. (1992). The epidemiology of HIV infection in urban areas, roadside settlements and rural villages in Mwanza region, Tanzania. *AIDS,* 6:1521–1528.

BAYER, RONALD, et al. (1995). Testing for HIV infection at home (Sounding Board). *N. Engl. J. Med.,* 332:1296–1299.

BETTS, CLAUDE, et al. (1996). The changing face of AIDS in Argentina. *JAMA,* 276:94–95.

BHAVE, GEETA, et al. (1995). Impact of an intervention on HIV, STDs, and condom use among sex workers in Bombay, India. *AIDS,* 9(Suppl. 1):S21–S30.

BIGGAR, ROBERT. (1993). Editorial: When ideals meet reality—the global challenge of HIV/AIDS. *Am. J. Public Health,* 83:1383–1384.

BUTLER, DELAN. (1994). HOPES AND DOUBTS MIRED PARIS AIDS SUMMIT. *NATURE,* 372–308.

CALDWELL, JOHN, et al. (1996). The African AIDS epidemic. *Sci. Am.,* 274:62–68.

CARIBBEAN EPIDEMIOLOGY CENTRE. (1994). *1993 Surveillance Report of HIV/AIDS/STD in English-Speaking Caribbean Countries and Surinam.* Port of Spain: CAREC; August 1–27.

COLES, PETER. (1988). French government recognizes need for AIDS health campaign. *Nature,* 335:2.

COMMENGES, DANIEL, et al. (1992). Estimating the incubation period of pediatric AIDS in Rwanda. *AIDS,* 6:1515–1520.

CULOTTA, ELIZABETH. (1991). Forecasting the global AIDS epidemic. *Science,* 253:852–853.

DECOCK, KEVIN, et al. (1993). Clinical research, prophylaxis, therapy and care for HIV disease in Africa. *Am. J. Public Health,* 83:1385–1388.

DECOCK, KEVIN, et al. (1994). The public health implications of AIDS research in Africa. *JAMA,* 272:481–486.

DECOSAS, JOSEF. (1996). HIV and development. *AIDS,* 10(Suppl. 3):569–574.

DICKMAN, STEVEN. (1991). AIDS threatens Asia. *Nature,* 351:682.

DOBKIN, JAY. (1996). More notes from Vancouver. *Infect. Med.,* 13:744.

EARICKSON, ROBERT J. (1990). International behavioral responses to a health hazard: AIDS. *Soc. Sci. Med.,* 31:951–952.

FORD, KATHLEEN, et al. (1995). AIDS knowledge, risk behaviors and factors related to condom use among male CSWs and male tourist clients in Bali, Indonesia. *AIDS,* 9:751–759.

FRIEDLAND, GERALD. (1996). Freeze frame: a picture of the pandemic in 1996. *AIDS Clin. Care,* 8:82, 85.

GALLO, DANA, et al. (1997b). Evaluation of a system using oral mucosal transudate for HIV antibody screening and confirmatory testing. *JAMA,* 277:254–258.

Harvard AIDS Review. (1995). Special report: AIDS in India. Fall: 1–21.

HIMMICH, HAKIMA. (1996). The Maghreb: women in the front line. *Naz Ki Pukaar,* April 13:18, 20.

Lancet. (1993). Heterosexual AIDS: pessimism, pandemics and plain hard facts. 341:863–864.

LURIE, PETER, et al. (1995). Socioeconomic status and risk of HIV, syphilis and hepatitis B infection among sex workers in Sao Paulo State, Brazil. *AIDS,* 9:S31–S37.

MANN, JONATHAN, et al. (1988). The international epidemiology of AIDS. *Sci. Am.,* 259:82–89.

McCARTY, KATHY. (1996). AIDS care in rural Zimbabwe. *AIDS Reader,* 5:130–133.

Naz Ki Pukaar. (1996). Egypt's fundamentalists say condoms immoral. *News:* July 14:11.

NIFTRIK, JACK VAN. (1988). AIDS in Africa. *Med. Interface,* 1:12–17.

PALACA, JOSEPH. (1991). WHO AIDS program: moving on a new track. *Science,* 254:511–512.

PAN AMERICAN HEALTH ORGANIZATION. (1994). *AIDS Surveillance in the Americas.* June 10:94,015.

PHILLIPS, KATHRYN, et al. (1995a). Potential use of home HIV testing. *N. Engl. J. Med.,* 332: 1308–1310.

PHILLIPS, KATHRYN, et al. (1995b). Who plans to be tested for HIV or would get tested if no one could find out the results? *Am. J. Prevent. Med.,* 11(3): 156.

Physicians Association for AIDS Care. (1990). WHO Projects 6,500,000 HIV Cases Worldwide. July/Aug.:177, 211.

Quarterly Surveillance Update. AIDS in Canada. January 1994:1–30.

QUINN, THOMAS C. (1988). Epidemiology of HIV-1 and HIV-2 in Africa. *Excerpta Medica,* Sept.:42–48.

ROJANAPITHAYAKORN, WIWAT, et al. (1995). The 100% condom program in Thailand. *AIDS* 10:1–7.

SAXINGER, W.C., et al. (1985). Evidence for exposure to HTLV III in Uganda before 1973. *Science*, 227:1036–1038.

SESSER, STAN. (1995). Hidden death. *New Yorker Magazine*, V:LXX #37:62–91, Nov.

SHARMA, V.P. (1994). Malaria and AIDS. *Nature*, 369:700.

SHARPLES, KATRINA, et al. (1996). HIV/AIDS in New Zealand: an epidemic in decline? *AIDS*, 10:1273–1278.

SMITH, ELOE, et al. (1994). The AIDS epidemic among Scandinavian women, 1980–1990. *AIDS*, 8:689–692.

SNOOD, S. (1990). AIDS patients are safe to treat. *Nat. Med. J. India*, 3:149.

SONNERFELD, E.D. (1990). First AIDS case in South Africa? *South African Med. J.*, 78:4.

STERNBERG, RACHEL. (1989). Fighting taboos, fighting AIDS. *Am. Med. News*, Feb.:3, 25–28.

SURASING VISRUTARATNA, CHRISTINA, et al. (1995). Superstar and model brothel: developing and evaluating a condom promotion program for sex establishments in Chiang Mai, Thailand. *AIDS*, 9(Suppl. 1):S69–S75.

TAYLOR, C. C. (1990). Condoms and cosmology: the fractal person and sexual risk in Rwanda. *Soc. Sci. Med.*, 31:1023–1028.

UNITED STATES DEPARTMENT OF STATE. (1992). *Global AIDS disaster: implications for the 1990s.* Publication No. 9955.

URIBE-SALAS, FELIPE, et al. (1997). Low prevalence of HIV infection and STD among female commercial sex workers in Mexico City. *Am. J. Public Health*, 87:1012–1015.

VANDEPITTE, J., et al. (1983). AIDS and cryptococosis. *Lancet*, 1:925–926.

WOLFFERS, IVAN. (1997). Culture, media and HIV/AIDS in Asia. *Lancet*, 349:52–54.

World Development Report 1993: Investing in Health. Washington, D.C.: World Bank, April 1993. World Bank Report 11778.

WORLD HEALTH ORGANIZATION GLOBAL PROGRAMME ON AIDS. (1992). *Current and Future Dimensions of the HIV/AIDS Pandemic: A Capsule Summary, January 1992.* Geneva, Switzerland: World Health Organization. Publication WHO/GPA/RES/SFI/92.1.

YU, ELENA, et al. (1996). HIV infection and AIDS in China, 1985 through 1994. *Am. J. Public Health*, 86:1116–1122.

ZHENG, XIWEN, et al. (1994). Injecting drug use and HIV infection in Southwest China. *AIDS*, 8:1141–1147.

ZHENG, XIWEN, et al. (1995). HIV risk behaviors but absence of infection among drug users in detoxification centers outside Yunnan province, China, 1993. *AIDS*, 9:959–963.

Testing for HIV: Diagnosis of AIDS and Human Implications

CHAPTER CONCEPTS

- ELISA means enzyme linked immunosorbent assay; it is a screening test for HIV infection.
- Western blot is a confirmatory HIV test.
- The ELISA test has been used to screen all blood supplies in the United States since March 1985.
- HIV screening tests can produce both false positives and false negatives.
- A positive ELISA test only predicts that a confirmatory test will also be positive.
- False-positive readings result from a test's lack of specificity.
- There is a relationship between the incidence of HIV in the population being tested and the number of false positives reported. The higher the incidence, the fewer the false positives.
- Levels of test sensitivity and specificity must be determined.

- Several new screening and confirmatory HIV tests are now available.
- Improved screening of nation's blood supply.
- National HIV testing day proclaimed.
- Saliva and urine HIV test are FDA approved.
- The polymerase chain reaction test is the most sensitive HIV RNA test currently available.
- Other HIV RNA tests available are Amplicar and the branched-DNA test.
- AIDS cases have been reported in all 50 states.
- Competency and informed consent are necessary for most HIV testing.
- Mandatory HIV testing does not mean people can be forced to undergo testing.
- HIV testing for the most part is on a voluntary basis.
- Compulsory HIV testing is used in the military, prisons, and in certain federal agencies.

———— BOX 13.1 ————

♦ U.S Public Health Service guidelines for annual prenatal HIV counseling and voluntary HIV testing of all pregnant American women.

♦ FDA approves two home HIV Test Kits.

♦ New York is first state to legislate mandatory HIV testing and disclosure of newborn HIV status to mother and physicians.

♦ American Medical Association endorses mandatory HIV testing of all pregnant women and newborns.

DETERMINING THE PRESENCE OF ANTIBODY PRODUCED WHEN HIV IS PRESENT

HIV-antibody testing is the most readily available, inexpensive, reliable, and accurate method to identify whether a person is infected with HIV. HIV antibodies are found in the blood or in saliva. When properly performed, HIV-antibody testing is highly sensitive and specific.

——————— BOX 13.2 ———————

PRE-TEST PATIENT INFORMATION

It is important that you read and understand the following information before having the HIV-antibody test.

The HIV-antibody test is a blood test. It was first used in 1985 to screen donated blood. **This test is not a test for AIDS. But a positive result does mean that there is a high probability an HIV-infected person will eventually develop AIDS**.

Only anonymous test results remain absolutely confidential.

What Does the Test Reveal?

The test reveals whether a person has been exposed to HIV. The test detects the presence of HIV antibodies, an indication that infection has occurred. It does not detect the virus itself nor does it indicate the level of viral infection, only that one has been infected.

It is important to find out whether you are HIV-positive or negative so that you can prevent spreading the virus to others and seek early medical intervention.

What Tests Will Be Done?

Wherever the test is done, the procedures are similar. A blood sample is taken from the arm and analyzed in a laboratory using a test called *ELISA* (*enzyme linked immunosorbent assay*). If the first ELISA test is positive, the laboratory will run a second ELISA test on the same blood sample. If positive, another test, called Western blot, is run on the same blood sample to confirm the ELISA result.

What Do the Test Results Mean?

See Table 13-1.

Positive Result: A positive result suggests that a person has HIV antibodies and may have been infected with the virus at some time. People with

TABLE 13-1 The Meaning of Antibody Test Results

A Positive Results	B Negative Results
If you test positive, it does mean:	If you test negative, it does mean:
1. Your blood sample has been tested more than once and the tests indicate that it contained antibodies to HIV. 2. You have been infected with HIV and your body has produced antibodies.	1. No antibodies to HIV have been found in your serum at the time of the test.
If you test positive, it does *not* mean:	Two possible explanations for a negative test result exist:
1. That you have AIDS. 2. That you necessarily will get AIDS, but the probability is high. You can reduce your chance of progressing to AIDS by avoiding further contact with the virus and living a healthy lifestyle. 3. That you are immune to the virus.	1. You have not been infected with HIV. 2. You have been infected with HIV but have not yet produced antibodies. Research indicates the most people will produce antibodies within 6 to 18 weeks after infection. Some people will not produce antibodies for at least 3 years. A very small number of people may never produce antibodies.
Therefore, if you test positive, you should do the following:	If you test negative, it does *not* mean:
1. Protect yourself from any further infection. 2. Protect others from the virus by following AIDS precautions in sex, drug use, and general hygiene. 3. Consider seeing a physician for a complete evaluation and advice on health maintenance. 4. Avoid drugs and heavy alcohol use, maintain good nutrition, and avoid fatigue and stress. Such action may improve your chances of staying healthy.	1. That you have nothing to worry about. You may become infected, be careful. 2. That you are immune to HIV. It has not yet been shown that anyone is immune to HIV infection. 3. That you have not been infected with the virus. You may have been infected and not yet produced antibodies.

(Adapted from the San Francisco AIDS Foundation)

———— BOX 13.2 *(continued)* ————

a positive result should assume that they have the virus and could therefore transmit it:

♦ by sex (anal, vaginal, or oral) where body fluids, especially semen or blood, get inside the partner's body;

♦ by sharing injection drug "works" (needles, syringes, etc.);

♦ by donating blood, sperm, or body organs; or

♦ to an unborn baby during pregnancy or to a newborn by breast feeding.

Negative Result: If it has been 4 to 6 months since the last possible exposure to HIV, then a negative result suggests that a person is probably not infected with the virus. However, **false negatives** can occur. For example, if the test was too soon after HIV exposure, the body may not have had time to produce HIV antibodies. **Collectively, studies show that 50% of HIV-infected persons seroconvert (demonstrate measurable HIV antibodies) by 3 months after HIV infection and 90% seroconvert by 6 months. A small percentage seroconverted at 1 year or later. Most important, a negative result does not mean that you are protected from getting the virus in the future—your future depends on your behavior.**

Inconclusive Result: A small percentage of results are inconclusive. This means that the result is neither positive nor negative. This may be due to a number of factors that have nothing to do with HIV infection, or it can occur early in an infection when there are not enough HIV antibodies present to give a positive result. If this happens, another blood sample will be taken at a later time for a retest.

How Accurate Is the Test Result?

The result is accurate. However, as with any laboratory test, there can be false positives and false negatives.

False Positive: A small percentage of all people tested may be told they have the HIV antibody when, in fact, they do not. This can be due to laboratory error or certain medical conditions which have nothing to do with HIV infection.

False Negative: Some people are told that they are not HIV-infected when, in fact, they are. This can happen when the test is taken too soon after being infected—the body has not had time to produce HIV antibodies. This is called the **window period**.

Should the Test Be Performed?

Whether to have the test done is a personal decision. However, knowing your antibody status can help you address some very difficult questions. For example, if the test is negative, what lifestyle changes should be made to minimize risk of HIV infection? If the test is positive, how can others be protected from infection? What can be done to improve your chances of staying healthy?

(Source: Roche Biomedical Laboratories, Inc.)

REQUESTS FOR HIV TESTING

Public HIV/AIDS clinics in the United States are becoming overwhelmed with requests for HIV testing. Most of the requests are repeats. About half of the CDC-estimated 650,000 to 900,000 living HIV-infected persons in the United States have never been tested. They have not been tested because of fear, lack of access, or lack of education. In January 1988, 6% of people, when asked if they had ever been HIV-tested said yes; in December 1996, 38% said yes.

REASONS FOR HIV TESTING IN THE UNITED STATES

HIV testing in the United States is done to monitor the pandemic; to determine how many people are infected, how many are being infected in a given time period (incidence), and their location; to determine the impact of prevention efforts to slow the spread of HIV; to prompt behavior change, to provide entry into clinical care, if necessary, to provide a starting point for partner notification and education, and to protect the nation's blood supply. There is an immediate need to change our perception about being HIV-positive so that people feel good about taking the test to protect themselves and others, rather than the discrimination that now exists against those who have taken the test.

AIDS is diagnosed by evaluating the results of clinical findings during a physical examination, and by laboratory analysis of blood samples for the presence of antibodies to HIV. Until early 1983, the causative agent of AIDS was unknown. Up to that time, infection could only be determined after the person began to express the signs and symptoms associated with AIDS. Once the virus was identified, a means of detecting viral exposure was developed. There is no single diagnostic test for AIDS. To date all **screening** tests, in the United States, measure the absence or presence of antibodies against **HIV subtype B**, a strain of HIV found primarily in North America and Europe (Hu et al., 1996). HIV counseling and testing are important components of HIV prevention programs.

IMMUNODIAGNOSTIC TECHNIQUES FOR DETECTING ANTIBODIES TO HIV

Refinements in the field of immunological testing, serology, and the study of antigen– antibody reactions have produced test names that reflect the component parts of the test being used. In most cases, tests are based on the detection of antibodies present in the serum, in this case antibodies to HIV. One immunological test uses antibodies, which if present in the person's serum, form a complex with a given antigen. An enzyme is then connected to the antibody. The presence of the antibody can be determined by adding a reagent that will form a colored solution if antibody to HIV is present. This is called the **enzyme linked immunosorbent assay** (ELISA, el-i-sa). The ELISA test was first used in 1983 to detect antibodies against HIV subtype B.

Recently, a technique has been developed that uses fluorescently labeled antibodies against HIV-specific antigens. This technique, called the fluorescent antibody technique, and others are described.

ELISA HIV-ANTIBODY TEST

The initial application of the ELISA test outside the research laboratory, was used primarily in large-scale screening of the nation's blood supply. ELISA testing of the existing blood supply and all newly donated blood began in the United States in March 1985. The ELISA test is used as a screening test because of its low cost, standardized procedures, high reproducibility, and rapid results.

The ELISA test is now semi-automated. It uses an antigen derived from HIV cultivated in human cell lines. One such line is the human leukemia cell line **H9**. Whole viruses isolated from H9 **are disrupted** into subunit antigens for use. The subunits of HIV are then bound to a solid support system.

Two solid support systems are used in the seven ELISA screening test kits licensed in the United States. Some attach the antigens onto small glass beads (Figure 13-1A), while others fix the antigens onto the sides and bottoms of small wells (micro wells) in a glass or plastic microtiter plate (Figure 13-1B). The serum to be tested is separated from the blood and is diluted and applied to the HIV-coated solid support systems (Figure 13-2). The ELISA test takes from 3.5 to 4 hours to perform (Carlson et al., 1989) and costs between about $7 in state sponsored virology laboratories and about $60 to $75 in private laboratories.

In accordance with FDA recommendations, effective June 1992, blood collection centers in the United States began HIV-2 testing on all donated blood and blood components. The CDC does not recommend routine testing for HIV-2 other than at blood collection centers (*MMWR*, 1992).

———— **POINT OF INFORMATION 13.1** ————

HIV TESTING OF TEENAGERS

Laws regarding the counseling and testing of persons younger than 18 years of age generally give minors the ability to be tested without parental consent or knowledge. Through 1996, at least 16 states had laws specific to HIV, and all states give minors the ability to be treated for sexually transmissible diseases without parental consent.

Solid Supports

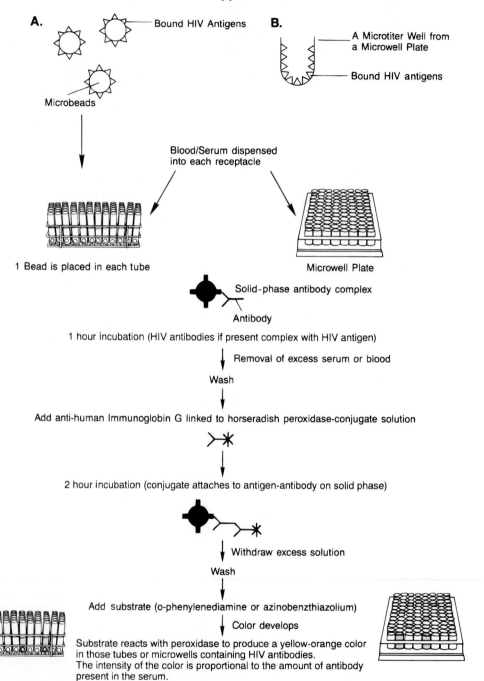

FIGURE 13-1 The ELISA Test. **A**, Microbeads with attached antigen in test tubes. **B**, Antigens bound to walls and bottom of microtiter wells.

C

D

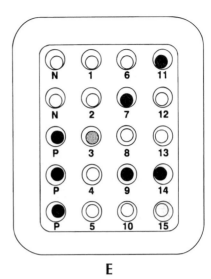

E

FIGURE 13-1 *(continued)* **C**, Microbeads are 7 mm in diameter. The test takes between 2.5 and 4 hours to perform. **D**, Microwell plates showing positive (yellow) and negative (clear) test results. The microtiter dispenser handles eight microwells at a time. **E**, Specimens positive for HIV antibody have a deeper color in this microwell tray. Serum specimens from 15 patients were tested for antibodies to HIV. Two negative and three positive control specimens are provided in the first column. In wells 7, 9, 11, and 14, the dark yellow color change, matching the color in the three positive control wells, indicates that the specimens are positive. Well 3 shows a weakly reactive result. The remaining specimens showed no color change and were interpreted as negative for HIV antibodies. (Adapted from Fang et al., 1989) (**C** and **D** *Courtesy of Roche Biomedical Laboratories, AIDS Testing Brochure*)

Understanding the ELISA Test

The ELISA test determines if a person's serum contains antibodies to one or more HIV antigens. Although there are some minor differences among the FDA licensed kits, test procedures are similar.

Problems with the ELISA Test

Any HIV screening test must be able to distinguish those individuals who are infected from those who are not. The underlying assumption of an ELISA test is that all HIV-infected people will produce detectable HIV antibodies. However, the HIV-infected population in general does not produce detectable antibodies for 6 weeks to 1 or more years after HIV infection, the **window period**. Most often, HIV antibody is present within 6 to 18 weeks. Thus, HIV-infected people can test HIV-negative. **This is a false negative result**. In some HIV-infected persons, as their disease progresses, the virus ties up the available antibody. Testing at this time would also produce false negative re-

IMPROVED ELISA TESTING, SCREENING FOR p24 ANTIGEN, AND BLOOD DONOR INTERVIEWS LOWER HIV IN NATION'S BLOOD SUPPLY

The increased sensitivity of current HIV-antibody ELISA tests, improved donor interviewing about behaviors associated with risk for HIV infection, and deferral of donors who test positive for HIV, hepatitis, human T-cell leukemia virus type 1 (HTLV-1), or syphilis have considerably improved the safety of the U.S. blood supply. In 1993, approximately six per 100,000 blood donations collected by the American Red Cross tested positive for HIV antibody. In addition, an estimated one in 450,000 to one in 660,000 donations per year (i.e., 18–27 donations) were infectious for HIV but were not detected by current screening tests.

Screening for p24 Antigen—In August 1995, the FDA recommended that all blood and plasma donations be screened for p24 antigen. FDA rec-

ommended p24 screening as an additional safety measure because 1) recent studies indicated that p24 screening reduces the infectious window period, 2) implementation of p24-antigen testing had become logistically feasible for mass screening, and 3) such testing would reduce the risk for HIV infection for persons who receive donated blood or blood products. Among the 12 million-plus annual blood donations in the United States, p24-antigen screening is expected to detect four to six infectious donations that would not be identified by other screening tests. FDA regards donor screening for p24 antigen as an interim measure pending the availability of technology that would further reduce the risk for HIV transmission from blood donated during the infectious window period (*MMWR*, 1996).

sults. Other reasons for false negative results are: immunosuppressive therapy, blood transfusions, some forms of cancer, B-cell dysfunction, bone marrow transplantation, and starch powder from laboratory gloves (Cordes et al., 1995).

False-positive reactions may also occur. This means that the person's serum does not contain antibodies to HIV but the test results indicate that it does.

Purpose of the ELISA Test

Because the original purpose of the ELISA test was to screen blood, the sensitivity (ability to detect low-level color formation; see Figure 13-1) of the test was purposely set high. It was reasoned that it was better to have some false positives and throw away good blood rather than to take in any HIV contaminated blood. Thus the ELISA test is a **positive predictive value** test. It only predicts that the serum tested will continue to test positive when a test with greater specificity, called a **confirmatory test**, is done.

In 1985, during the first month of donor screening, 1% of all blood tested HIV-antibody-positive. On ELISA retesting of these samples, only 0.17% (17/10,000) were HIV-antibody-positive. On subjecting these samples to a con-

firmatory test, only 0.038% (4/10,000) were actually HIV-positive. These early tests produced about 24 false positives for every true positive result. The main reason for such a high false positive rate or **lack of specificity** was that something other than HIV produced an antibody or other substance that reacted with HIV antigen causing the HIV test to appear positive.

People may test **false positive** who have an underlying liver disease, have received a blood transfusion or gamma globulin within 6 weeks of the test, have had several children, have had rheumatological diseases, malaria, alcoholic hepatitis, autoimmune disorders, various cancers, or DNA viral infections; are injection drug users; or have received vaccines for influenza or hepatitis B (Fang et al., 1989; MacKenzie et al., 1992). In each case, the person may have antibodies that will cross-react with the HIV antigens giving a false-positive reaction. Other reasons for false positives are laboratory errors and mistakes made in reagent preparations for use in the test kits.

Although high sensitivity tests eliminate HIV-contaminated blood from the blood supply, there is a downside to high sensitivity testing when proper procedure is **not** used. People told that they have tested positive have become emotionally distraught. Former Senator Lawton Chiles of Florida, at an AIDS conference in

A

D

B

C

E

FIGURE 13-2 (see page 404 for caption)

1987, told of a tragic example from the early days of blood screening in Florida. Of 22 blood donors who were told they were HIV-positive by the ELISA test, seven committed suicide.

There continue to be false positive reactions among blood donors and low-level risk populations because of a **low prevalence** of HIV infection in such populations. The American Red Cross Blood Services laboratories report that using current ELISA methodology, a specificity of 99.8% can be achieved (*MMWR*, 1988a).

Positive Predictive Value — The positive predictive value of the ELISA test indicates the percentage of true positives among total positives in a given population. To determine a positive predictive value:

Number of true positives ÷ Number of positives or true positives + false positives × 100%

There is also a negative predictive test. A negative predictive value refers to the percentage of individuals who test truly negative; they **do not** have HIV. It is determined by:

Number of true negatives ÷ Number of true negatives + false negatives × 100%

To safeguard against false-positive tests, the CDC recommends that serum that tests positive be retested twice (in duplicate). If both tests are negative, the serum is considered HIV-antibody-negative and further tests will only be done should signs or symptoms of HIV infection occur (Figures 13-3A and 13-3B). If one or both of the tests is positive, the serum is subjected to a confirmatory test, usually a Western blot (WB) (Figure 13-4). At blood banks, if the initial ELISA test is positive, the blood is discarded. If an individual's serum subjected to a confirmatory test is positive, the person is considered to be HIV-infected.

Although confirmatory tests can be used to determine true-positive results, they are too labor intensive and expensive to be used in screening a large population. Thus the positive predictive value of an ELISA test is an important first step in large-scale screening. Recall, however, that the predictive value depends on the prevalence of HIV infection in the population tested. The higher the prevalence of HIV infection in a given population, the more likely a positive ELISA test is to be a true positive; and conversely, the lower the prevalence of infection, the less likely a positive ELISA test is to be a true positive.

Levels of Sensitivity and Specificity in Testing for HIV — A test's **sensitivity** is its capacity to identify **all** specimens that **have** HIV antibodies in them. A test's **specificity** is its capacity to identify **all** specimens that **do not have** HIV antibodies in them.

Sensitivity is determined as follows:

Number of true positives ÷ Number of true positives + the false negatives × 100%

If 100 persons are actually HIV-infected and the test identifies only 90 of them as such, then we can say that the test has 90% sensitivity.

Specificity is determined as follows:

Number of true negatives ÷ Number of true negatives + false positives × 100%

FIGURE 13-2 (*see page 403*) Semi-Automated ELISA Test. **A,** Serum samples are individually machine diluted 1 to 400. This includes the dilution of positive serum negative samples supplied with the test kit. Beads containing the HIV antigens are placed into the individual sample holders. Antibodies, if present in the individual sera, attach to the HIV antigens. **B,** Excess serum is withdrawn from each sample and the beads are washed. **C,** The antihuman immunoglobulin-horseradish enzyme conjugate is added to each prepared sample. **D,** The samples are incubated. **E,** Each sample receives the chromogen or substrate (o-phenylenediamine or azinobenzthiazolium). A yellow-orange color appears in samples that contain antibodies to HIV. (*Courtesy of Florida Health and Rehabilitative Services, Office of Laboratory AIDS Unit, Jacksonville*)

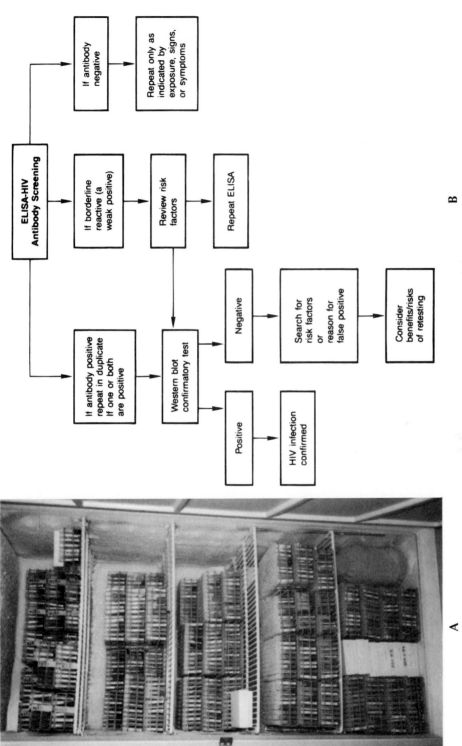

FIGURE 13-3 ELISA-INV Screen Flow Diagram. **A,** Frozen serum samples. The 7,500 samples in this freezer are part of the 13,000 samples collected statewide each month in Florida. From 1992 through 1997 an average of 245,150 tests each year were HIV-positive (3.5%/year). **B,** Either blood or serum can be screened for antibodies to HIV. If the ELISA test is positive, it is repeated in duplicate (left side of diagram). If duplicate tests are positive, a Western blot (WB) test is performed. Borderline reactions indicate that antibodies to HIV may be present but in small numbers (low titer) or that other antibodies present in the serum are cross-reacting with the HIV antigens. To determine the situation, the more specific WB test is required. For information on antibody screening procedures, see *MMWR,* 1988a. (**A,** *Courtesy of Florida Health and Rehabilitative Services, Office of Laboratory AIDS Unit, Jacksonville*)

405

Assume that, in a group of 500 people being tested for HIV antibodies, 100 individuals are actually not infected. If test results show that only 90, out of the 100, are identified as not having the virus, then the test has 90% specificity.

WESTERN BLOT ASSAY

The gold standard for determining a true-positive HIV-antibody test is still the **Western blot** (WB). This test is a method in which individual HIV proteins are used to react with HIV antibody in a person's serum. It should be understood that the WB test is not a **true** gold standard because it is not 100% certain, but it can come close to 100% if properly used.

Human cells in which HIV is being cultured are lysed or broken open, and the mixture of cell components and HIV components (proteins) are separated from each other. The viral proteins are placed on a polyacrylamide gel which then gets an electrical charge. The electrical current separates the viral proteins within the gel. This is called **gel electrophoresis**. The smallest HIV proteins will move quickly through the gel, separating from the next larger size, and so on.

Each different protein will arrive at a separate position on the gel. After proteins of similar molecular weight collect at a given site, they form a band; and these bands are identified based on the distance they have run in the gel. Because each band is a protein produced as a product of a different HIV gene, the gel band patterns give a picture of the HIV genes that were functioning and the location of each gene's products on the gel (Figure 13-4 and Table 13-2). The protein or antigen bands within the gel are "blotted," that is, transferred directly, band for band and position for position, onto strips of nitrocellulose paper (Figure 13-4).

FIGURE 13-4 Western Blot Strips. Each WB strip contains nine separate antigenic proteins of HIV. Human serum or blood can be applied directly to the strips. See text for details on reactions. Because false positives can sometimes occur with the ELISA test, additional testing is needed to evaluate specimens which are repeatedly reactive by ELISA. The Western blot is more specific but less sensitive than the ELISA and is recommended for blood banks and organ donor centers. Its clinical usefulness in trials to aid in evaluating specimens which are questionably positive by other methods has been proven. It is not a screening test because it lacks a high level of sensitivity. (*Courtesy of Roche Biomedical Laboratories, AIDS Testing Brochure*)

TABLE 13-2 Description of Major Gene Products of HIV and Capable of Inducing Antibody Response

Gene Product[a]	Description
p17/18[b]	GAG[c] protein
p24/25	GAG protein
p31/32	Endonuclease component of POL[d] translate
gp41	Transmembrane ENV[e] glycoprotein
p51/52/53	Reverse transcriptase component of POL translate
p55	Precursor of GAG proteins cleaved to p18 and p24
p64/65 p66	Reverse transcriptase component of POL translate
gp110/120 gp120	Outer ENV glycoprotein
gp160	Precursor of ENV glycoprotein

[a]Number refers to molecular weight of the protein in kilodaltons; measurement of molecular weight may vary slightly in different laboratories.

[b]Where two bands on acrylamide gel are too close for easy identification, they are presented as such, p51/53, etc.

[c]GAG = core.

[d]POL = polymerase.

[4]ENV = envelope.

(Adapted from *MMWR*, 1988a)

——————— BOX 13.3 ———————

THE PERFORMANCE RATE FOR THE COMBINED ELISA AND WESTERN BLOT HIV TEST—IS 99% ACCURACY GOOD ENOUGH? THE ANSWER: NO!

The Centers for Disease Control and Prevention (CDC) states that the two tests used to identify HIV— the ELISA and the Western blot (WB)—used in combination, have a better than 99% overall accuracy rate, but only if they are performed repeatedly. (The exact rate is unknown and the CDC states that it has no data on just how many false positives versus false negatives occur!) This **rate** is the percentage of correct test results in all specimens tested. With a 99% rate, if a population of 10,000 were tested, 9,900 would receive correct results, but 100 would receive erroneous results—either false positives or false negatives—including indeterminates.

If 99% accuracy is used as an example, then false positives would have to be less than 6/10ths (0.6%) of the erroneous results, because the CDC estimates that 0.6% of Americans are HIV-positive. That is, if false positives accounted for fully 0.6% of the errors, then the 0.6% of people who are HIV-positive would all be false positives, and that is not the case. However, if one assumes that only 0.2% are false positives, this leaves 0.8% as false negatives. So, of those same 100 people with erroneous results, 20% would be false positives and 80% would be false negatives. False-negative people are an unwitting threat to sex partners. But there is still another ramification: using the CDC estimate that 0.6% of Americans are HIV-positive, in a population of 10,000, 60 Americans that would test positive! This 60 must include all the false positives, 30, leaving only 30 people actually infected. This leads to the following conclusion: using a 99% accuracy, one finds as many false positives as true positives.

Even if the results of both AIDS tests, the ELISA and WB, are positive, the chances are only 50-50 that the individual is infected. This is why people with HIV-positive results must be tested repeatedly over the following 6 months to 1 year. The error rate at 99% accuracy is high with only two tests. (The CDC's *Morbidity and Mortality Weekly Report* shows an overall performance rate of only 98.4% on the Western blot alone—a lower accuracy than that used in this example. Even with repeated HIV-positive tests, the rare person may just be a false-positive tester.

The implications resulting from a false-positive test are broad for people tested at random. For example, a person was recently HIV-tested for a routine insurance examination. Because he or she had no behavioral risk factors and was in excellent health there was no concern about testing HIV-positive. The major concern was testing falsely positive— that risk, with a 99% accuracy testing procedure, is 30 out of 10,000 (0.3%). This may appear to be a low risk, but it isn't if you are one of the 30—after all, some 30 people out of 10,000 will be false positive. The results can destroy one's personal and professional life; other people believe your test results even if they are later found to be in error. It's like the newspaper scenario: retractions are found in small print on the back page — somewhere.

There is also the danger that false-positive people will not feel the need to avoid sex with truly infected people — a good route to infection.

But there is also room for optimism in these statistics. An individual who is a random false positive can find hope in them. This does not mean that he or she can take chances with other people's lives, of course, so each person must behave as though he or she is actually infected. But, inwardly, the random false HIV-positive individual can be cautiously optimistic.

The occurrence of even a small number of false-positive HIV tests can have profound implications. This is especially true when testing blood donors, since false-positive results waste resources in discarded blood units and require verification of positive results using more expensive tests. A false negative result, indicating that an individual is not infected, can have serious consequences for the blood recipient. Therefore, attempts to improve tests are a continuous challenge.

Once the antigen bands have been formed, serum that is believed to carry HIV antibodies is placed directly on them. That is, a test serum is added directly to antigen bands located on the nitrocellulose strip. If antibodies are present in the serum, they will form an antigen–antibody complex directly on the antigen band areas. After the strip is washed, the HIV antibody–antigen bands are visualized by adding enzyme-conjugated antihuman immunoglobulin G to the strip. Then the substrate or color agent is added. If antibody has complexed with any of the banded HIV proteins on the nitrocellulose strip, a color reaction will occur at the band site(s) (Figure 13-4). Positive test strips are then compared to two control test strips, one that has been reacted with known positive serum and one that has been reacted with known negative serum.

In contrast to the ELISA test, which indicates only the presence or absence of HIV antibodies, the WB strip qualitatively identifies which of the HIV antigens the antibodies are directed against. The greatest disadvantage of the WB test is that reagents, testing methods, and test-interpretation criteria are not standardized. The National Institutes of Health (NIH), the American Red Cross, DuPont company, the Association of State and Territorial Health Officers (ASTHO), and the Department of Defense (DoD) each define a positive WB differently.

It can be concluded from the criteria set up by different organizations to define a positive result that although the WB may be the gold standard of confirmatory testing, there is **no** agreement on what constitutes a positive WB test (Miike, 1987).

The WB procedure is labor-intensive, takes longer to run (12 to 24 hours), and is therefore more costly than the ELISA test. The WB is **less sensitive** than the ELISA **but more specific**.

Because the WB lacks the sensitivity of the ELISA test, it is not used as a screening test. Despite the high specificity of the WB, false positives do occur, but they occur less frequently than with ELISA tests because the WB is only run on serum or blood already suspected of containing HIV antibodies.

Relative Costs of ELISA and Western Blot Tests

The cost incurred to identify each true-positive HIV individual in a population with a 10% prevalence for HIV infection is presented in Table 13-3. Cost estimates are for tests performed on a contractual basis, that is, for screening large numbers of people versus testing of individuals. Note that the difference is quite significant.

OTHER SCREENING AND CONFIRMATORY TESTS

There are a variety of HIV-antibody and HIV-antigen detection tests now on the market and others are on their way. A few of these tests have been singled out because they are currently in use or because of their potential to make a contribution in the field of HIV antibody–antigen testing methodology.

Immunofluorescent Antibody Assay

The **immunofluorescent antibody assay** uses a known preparation of antibodies labeled with a fluorescent dye such as fluorescein isothiocyanate (FITC) to detect antigen or antibody. In the direct fluorescent antibody test, fluorescent antibodies detect specific antigens in cultures or smears. In the indirect fluorescent

TABLE 13-3 Incurred Costs to Identify True-Positive HIV-Antibody-Containing Sera in a Population with a 10% Prevalence of HIV-Antibody-Infected People

Price of testing under negotiated contracts:
Low estimate: $4.41 per specimen tested
High estimate: $7 for each ELISA, $60 for each Western blot
Price for individual testing: $47.50 for each ELISA, $121 for each Western blot
Best case:
Number of true positives: 9,920
Number of ELISAs performed: 100,000
Number of Western blots performed: 9,960 + 900 = 10,860
Low estimate: $4.41 × 100,000 divided by 9,920 = $44
High estimate: $7 × 100,000 plus $60 × 10,860 divided by 9,920 = $136.25
Individual testing: $47.50 × 100,000 plus $121 × 10,860 divided by 9,920 = $611.30

(Adapted from Miike, 1987; adjustment reflects charges through 1997)

SOME RELATIVE DRAWBACKS TO THE CURRENT HIV SCREENING TEST— ELISA/WESTERN BLOT

Regardless of the high sensitivity and high specificity or overall test performance, there are a few test-related problems. For example, although only 24 hours are required to complete the ELISA/Western blot testing procedures, most labs batch specimens for processing, causing a 1- to 2-week wait for definitive results. One study has shown that 40% of those tested never returned for their test results. Perhaps because of concern about maintaining anonymity or other factors, many individuals with HIV are not tested until they develop symptoms. Up to one-third of patients receive their HIV diagnosis within 2 months of an AIDS diagnosis.

Cost and time investment of the two-step process (pre- and post-test counseling) have also impeded testing. Even when tested without charge at a publicly funded clinic, clients must take time out of work or caring for children for waiting time, counseling, or travel. The true cost of this process has been estimated at $41 per test. And, individuals tested in private offices may incur not only the cost of the test by commercial or hospital labs, but also the physician's office fee (Sax et al., 1997).

ficity of the IFA test are similar to the Western blot, this method has been proposed as an alternative confirmatory test for positive ELISA results. The IFA method is relatively simple and is one of the quickest tests available.

In late 1992, the FDA approved Fluorognost for marketing, the first assay for HIV-IFA confirmation and screening.

The assay allows doctors to do in-office tests for antibodies to HIV in human serum or plasma. As opposed to the Western blot test, the current standard confirmation test, Fluorognost posts almost no indeterminate test results. In addition, the test takes only 90 minutes to complete, while the Western blot takes from 12 to 24 hours to process. This FDA-approved test allows smaller health care facilities, emergency rooms, and doctors' offices to conduct in-office HIV screening and confirmation with accuracy, ease, and low overhead.

Recombigen HIV-1 Latex Agglutination Test

Recombigen, a 5-minute HIV-antibody test that requires no special equipment, was FDA approved in December 1988. The test is designed for use with serum, plasma, or whole blood. Patient samples are placed on a card along with positive and negative controls that come with the kit. Each serum sample is combined with a suspension of latex microspheres (beads) coated with CBre3, a recombinant protein containing the most immunogenic segments of the HIV envelope glycoprotein gp120 and the transmembrane protein gp41. The ingredients are then mixed for 3 minutes either by tilting the card manually or by carefully mixing the solution on the card. If antibodies to HIV are present in a sample, they will form complexes with the protein-coated beads causing a visible agglutination reaction.

Positive readings should be confirmed with a Western blot assay. The accuracy of the test is thought to be comparable to that of other conventional screening assays.

Polymerase Chain Reaction

Interactions between HIV and its host cell extend across a wide spectrum, from latent to productive infection. The virus can persist in

antibody test, specific antibody from serum is bound to antigen on a glass slide.

The indirect procedure is modified for use in detecting antibodies to HIV. Cells that are HIV-infected will have HIV antigens on their cell membranes and will later fluoresce when the antihuman fluorescent conjugate is added.

A diluted sample of a person's serum is placed on a slide prepared with HIV antigens and incubated to allow antibody–antigen reaction if there are HIV antibodies in the serum. The slides are then rinsed to get rid of excess serum and other materials. Fluorescent antihuman antibody is then placed on the slide and incubation allows antihuman HIV antibody complexing to occur. The slide is again rinsed and dried. Fluorescence, if any, is observed using a special fluorescence microscope. The indirect fluorescent antibody (IFA) test is now used in many laboratories as a screening procedure. In as much as the sensitivity and specicells as unintegrated DNA, as integrated DNA with alternative states of viral gene expression, or as a defective DNA molecule. Determining the fraction of cells in the blood that are latently or productively infected is important for the understanding of viral pathogenesis and in the design and testing of effective therapies. Determining the number of infected cells in a heterogeneous cell population and the proportion of those cells that are carrying the virus but not producing new viruses requires the identification of the proviral DNA and viral mRNA in single cells.

The **polymerase chain reaction (PCR)** is a technique by which any DNA fragment from a single cell can be exponentially multiplied to an amount large enough to be measured. This technique indirectly measures **viral load** and thus enables an assessment of viral load and viral expression in different parts of the body of HIV-infected patients. Thus PCR could be an ideal diagnostic test for HIV infection, since it directly amplifies proviral HIV DNA and does not require antibody formation by the host. It is already used in settings where antibody production is unpredictable or difficult to interpret, such as in acute HIV infection or in the perinatal/postnatal period. For HIV testing, the technique used is to copy a segment of proviral DNA found in cells such as T4 lymphocytes and macrophages that carry the virus. The PCR is so sensitive that it can detect and amplify as few as six molecules of proviral DNA in 150,000 cells or one molecule of viral DNA in 10 μl of blood. This level of sensitivity is unparalleled by any other technology.

Finding these few molecules of DNA to copy and amplify is, as the saying goes, like finding a needle in a haystack. The needle in this case is the proviral DNA molecule. It is only a miniscule fraction of the total DNA content of a given cell and far less when mixed in with the DNA of over one million cells as used in some HIV PCRs.

One of the first uses of the PCR in HIV/AIDS research was to show that HIV was present in people who were suspected of being infected but did not produce HIV antibodies. The HIV provirus was detectable in their cells. The PCR's most recent use has been in the detection of HIV provirus in newborns of HIV-infected mothers (Rogers et al., 1989).

In 1993, researchers reported that, in HIV-infected persons, 4% to 15% of peripheral blood lymphocytes were infected with HIV. The percentage of these cells that contained HIV mRNA, an indicator of viral replication, ranged from less than 1% to 8%. The data indicate that, in HIV-positive individuals, a significant proportion of peripheral blood lymphocytes are infected with HIV, but that the virus is in a latent state in the majority of these cells.

Now that there are some good therapies available to treat opportunistic disease which help slow the onset of AIDS, the diagnosis of individuals who carry the provirus is critical because they may benefit from early treatment. The PCR test will become even more important with the advent of an HIV vaccine. Vaccinated people will become HIV-antibody-positive. The PCR test will be used to identify those who are truly HIV-infected.

How PCR Works— The PCR (Figure 13-5) was developed by Kary Mullis and colleagues at Cetus Corporation (Mullis et al., 1987; Keller et al., 1988). The procedure requires the synthesis of **oligomer primers** (short 16 to 25 nucleotide sequences of DNA) that will hybridize or bind to the segment of DNA to be copied. The primer is required because the polymerase enzyme used to copy the desired DNA sequence needs an initial DNA sequence of nucleotides to add on to.

In the case of the HIV provirus, the primers need to hybridize to a DNA sequence adjacent to the gene area to be copied—for example, the GAG gene DNA sequence that produces the p24 protein. Because DNA is double-stranded, a primer molecule is attached to each strand (Figure 13-5). After primer attachment, a polymerase enzyme (usually Taq 1) is added. The polymerase enzymes, using the primers as starting points, add one nucleotide at a time as they copy their single DNA strands.

After each strand of the DNA segment has been copied at a temperature of 70°C, the reaction is heated to 93°C to **separate** the newly synthesized strands from the original DNA strands. This is called **denaturation**. The temperature is then cooled to 37°C to permit the additional primer molecules to attach (anneal) to the newly synthesized DNA sequences and the original DNA sequences (Figure 13-5). After **primer attachment**, the temperature is raised to 70°C and the polymerase enzyme molecules, starting at the primer sites, **copy** each strand of DNA. At the end of this second cycle there are four copies of each of the original DNA single strand sequences. By repeating the cycles of **denaturation**, **annealing**, and **synthesis**, the original DNA sequence can be amplified exponentially according to the formula 2^n where n is the number of cycles.

Single-Use Diagnostic Test

In late 1992, the FDA approved a rapid (10-minute) screening test for detecting HIV antibodies. This test is a single-use diagnostic system (**SUDS**). According to the manufacturer, in clinical trials the test had a sensitivity of 99.9% and a specificity of 99.6%, which is comparable to other approved HIV tests used by clinical laboratories. This test can be used in a physician's office, and requires no special equipment and only minimal staff training. The process involves taking a small quantity of serum or plasma and mixing it with an antibody capture reagent. It is then poured into a test cartridge with HIV antigens, followed by a wash step and the addition of enzyme–antibody and a chromogen. Results are available in approximately 10 minutes. Positive results, indicated by a blue-colored window, should be confirmed with other assays.

List price in 1997 was $9 per test, but the control must be purchased separately.

Saliva and Urine Tests

By the end of 1994, there were at least nine **serum** HIV-antibody **screening** tests and four confirmatory tests available in the marketplace. Because HIV antibodies are present in body fluids other than blood (e.g., urine and saliva), HIV-antibody assays have been developed for their use. Collecting samples of urine and saliva is noninvasive, easier, less dangerous, and less expensive. Such tests are particularly useful in developing nations where there is a shortage of refrigeration and sterile equipment (Constantine, 1993); Frerichs et al., 1994).

At least one HIV saliva test, **OraSure** (Figure 13–6), had received FDA approval for use in the United States in late 1994. But the FDA withheld permission to market OraSure until June of 1996. Previously, people whose OraSure pad tested positive had to give a blood sample to confirm the results. Now both the initial and confirming (Western blot) tests can be performed with the OraSure pad. OraSure is comparable to blood tests in cost and speed. But the FDA says it is slightly less accurate than blood tests. Although the OraSure kit performs well, at this point its niche in the clinical lab is not entirely clear. The manufacturer suggests it may be useful

---

POINT OF INFORMATION 13.3

SALIVA HIV TEST: IS IT AS GOOD AS THE ELISA?

According to Wesley Emmons and co-workers (1995), a blinded study to determine the accuracy of detecting HIV antibody in human saliva was performed at the United States National Naval Medical Center. Naval medical center personnel tested commercially available (OraSure) saliva test kits. Test kit performance was as follows:

An absorbent pad, mounted on a lollipop-like plastic stick, was placed between the lower cheek and gum, rubbed along the tooth-gum margin 20 times, and held there for 2 minutes; the collected fluid was then centrifuged. A 1:4 dilution of saliva was used for ELISA tests (1:400 is usual for serum testing) and 200-μL samples

for Western blot confirmation (as compared with 20 μL for serum testing).

All 195 HIV-seropositive adults were positive for HIV antibodies on ELISA tests of saliva samples, and 190 of them (97.4%) had strongly positive Western blot results (the other five blots were indeterminate). Saliva samples from all 198 HIV-seronegative controls were negative on ELISA (del Rio et el., 1996).

Oral disease, mouth sores, and tobacco use did not seem to affect its accuracy. The OraSure test is the first saliva test to received FDA approval in December of 1994. The OraSure kit is only available to professional health care workers.

Polymerase Chain Reaction

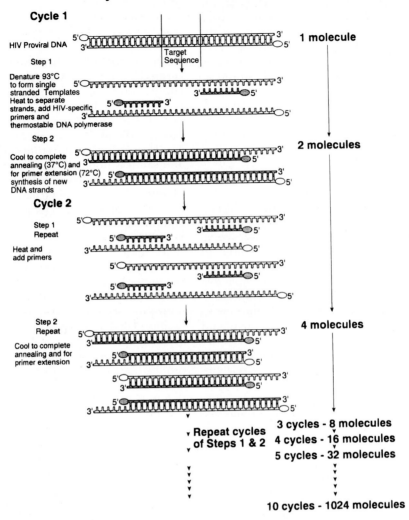

Cycle 1

HIV Proviral DNA

Step 1

Denature 93°C
to form single
stranded Templates
Heat to separate
strands, add HIV-specific
primers and
thermostable DNA polymerase

Step 2

Cool to complete
annealing (37°C) and
for primer extension (72°C)
synthesis of new
DNA strands

Cycle 2

Step 1
Repeat

Heat and
add primers

Step 2
Repeat

Cool to complete
annealing and for
primer extension

Target
Sequence

1 molecule

2 molecules

4 molecules

Repeat cycles
of Steps 1 & 2

3 cycles - 8 molecules
4 cycles - 16 molecules
5 cycles - 32 molecules

10 cycles - 1024 molecules

FIGURE 13-5 Polymerase Chain Reaction. A source of DNA containing
the sequence to be amplified is mixed with two primers, nucleotide
triphosphates and the DNA polymerase Taq 1 (Taq 1 is a DNA polymerase derived from the bacterium *Thermus aquaticus*). The primers are
synthetic oligonucleotides of *known sequence*. Therefore, the boundaries
of the DNA sequence to be copied are already known. *Cycle 1:* Primers
are added in excess (1 million-fold). Using DNA polymerase, the primers
are extended by DNA synthesis. The first cycle takes about 5 minutes.
Cycle 2: The product from cycle 1 is denatured, reannealed, and primer
extension occurs once again. This cycle takes place as many as 50 times
so that the primer-extended sequence increases thousands of times. The
original DNA sequence can be amplified exponentially according to the

(continued on next page)

HIV Gene Probes

Gene probes or genetic probes are an idea borrowed from methodologies used in recombinant DNA research. The idea is to isolate a DNA segment, make many copies of it, and label these copies with a radioisotope or other tag compound. If the DNA sequence copied is contained in any of the HIV genes, then the labeled copies of this DNA sequence can be used to hybridize or attach to DNA of cells that contain HIV DNA. This method of DNA probe analysis eliminates the need of searching for HIV gene products or antibodies to these products to prove that a person is HIV-infected.

At least two HIV-specific probes are on the market. One uses a radioactive sulfur label on the DNA for detection (^{35}S). This probe hybridizes to about 50% of the entire HIV genome and most specifically hybridizes to the HIV polymerase region. A second probe, also using ^{35}S, is an **RNA probe**. It is being used to detect HIV RNA in peripheral blood or tissue samples. RNA probes for in situ hybridization allow detection of one HIV-infected cell out of 400,000 uninfected cells. Specifically, the assay detects the presence of HIV in whole white blood cells as soon as the virus begins to replicate. The ^{35}S-labeled probes enter the white blood cells and combine with HIV; the procedure does not require DNA extraction and results are obtained in just over 1 day (Kramer et al., 1989).

Passive Hemagglutination Assay

There continues to be an urgent need for an inexpensive, accurate assay for anti-HIV screen-

FIGURE 13–6 HIV-antibody testing and OraSure technology. OraSure is a simple and easy-to-use, oral HIV-antibody testing technology now available to consumers through health professionals. The product does not require the use of needles or blood and is about as effective as traditional HIV blood tests. A specially treated pad attached to the handle is placed by the patient between the lower cheek and gum for 2 minutes. The pad is then placed in a vial with preservative and sent to a clinical laboratory for testing for the presence of HIV antibodies, the same way blood samples are tested.

for needle-phobic patients and in mass screening programs in which phlebotomy (drawing blood) is not readily available. A home version now being developed for marketing here should have a wide appeal (Gallo et al., 1977). Entering 1997, one urine test, **Sentinel**, was FDA approved on August 6, 1996. It is **less** sensitive and specific than blood testing. The test is available only to professional laboratories (Sax et al., 1997).

FIGURE 13–5   *(continued)*

formula 2^n, where *n* is the number of cycles. In theory, 25 PCR cycles would result in a 34 million-fold amplification. However, since the efficiency of each cycle is less than 100%, the actual amplification after 25 cycles is about 1 to 3 million-fold. The size of the amplified region is generally 100 to 400 base pairs, although stretches of up to 2,000 bases can be efficiently amplified. In HIV-infected cells, the DNA template is a specified region within the provirus (Keller et al., 1988).

Viral DNA can also be specifically amplified with some additional steps. The RNA template in infected cells is either viral mRNA or packaged virion RNA. And a different enzyme is used to amplify the RNA (Q beta replicase).

ing in the developing world. Scheffel's results (1990) indicate that the **passive hemagglutination assay (PHA)** is a good candidate. The assay is simple to perform and requires no expensive equipment or precision pipettes. The reagents appear very stable even in adverse conditions. However, the assay requires a minimum of 3 hours before a reading can be made.

The accuracy of the assay is reportedly excellent, with 100% sensitivity on some 890 anti-HIV-positive serum samples and sensitivity equal to or better than the second-generation ELISA.

The PHA uses stabilized human group O red blood cells that have been coated with HIV core protein, p24 and envelope glycoprotein, gp41. For long-term stability, the antigen-coated cells are placed in phosphate buffer and vacuumed to dryness (lyophilized). For use, the dried cells are reconstituted in phosphate buffer.

Two drops of phosphate buffer are placed in the microwell of a test plate. To this is added a small amount of a person's serum. After gentle mixing, one drop of HIV coated red blood cells (RBCs) is added, mixed, and incubated at room temperature for at least 3 hours. Hemagglutination patterns, stable for 72 hours, are read by eye and compared to a chart or scale that reads from negative to 3+ for HIV infection.

VIRAL LOAD: MEASURING HIV RNA

Recent studies have shown that a very rapid turnover of HIV RNA occurs in the plasma of infected patients, with approximately 30% of the total virus population in the plasma being replenished daily. Continual viral replication and rapid T4 cell turnover play a central role in the pathogenesis of HIV infection. High plasma HIV RNA levels have been shown to be a strong predictor of rapid progression to AIDS after HIV seroconversion, independent of T4 cell count. These findings have led to increased interest in quantitating HIV RNA in patients for prognostic purposes. HIV RNA viral load measurements will prove useful in the management of HIV-infected patients, both in predicting rate of progression and monitoring response to antiretroviral therapy (see Chapters 4, 7, and 11 for additional information on HIV RNA load). Until June of 1996, reliable measures of HIV RNA were available only in research laboratories. And, the quantitation of HIV from a clinical specimen required very expensive, labor-intensive, and difficult-to-reproduce culture techniques. Recently, however, quantitation of HIV viral load in plasma specimens has been accomplished with a variety of techniques that measure HIV RNA and are less expensive and easier to perform. Currently, three commercial assays are available: (**1**) Amplicor HIV Monitor Test, which couples reverse transcription to quantitative polymerase chain reaction (PCR) (Roche Molecular Systems); (**2**) Quantiplex HIV RNA assay, a branched DNA (bDNA) technology (Chiron Corporation); and (**3**) Nucleic Acid Sequence-Based Amplification (NASBA) (Organon) Technika). Because in June of 1996 the FDA approved Amplicor, it is briefly reviewed. In addition, the branched-DNA test will also be presented because it is near FDA approval.

Amplicor HIV Monitor Test

This multistep test includes specimen preparation, reverse transcription and PCR, and nonradioactive detection. Plasma samples ($200 \mu L$) are treated to lyse the viral particles and release RNA; isopropanol is then added to precipitate the RNA. This first step renders the sample noninfectious and safe for laboratory workers.

Because HIV is an RNA virus its RNA (the genome) must be reverse-transcribed into a double-stranded DNA molecule before it can serve as a template in a PCR reaction (Figure 13-5). Once the double-stranded DNA template is synthesized, large numbers of DNA copies are produced by PCR. After reverse transcription and PCR amplification, the person's number of HIV RNA copies in the sample can be calculated from the ratio of the HIV RNA signal to the test's internal DNA standard signal.

The Amplicor HIV Monitor Test has a three-log dynamic range; its lower limit of sensitivity is about 500 copies of HIV RNA/mL. The assay is reproducible and fivefold differences in HIV RNA copy number are easily discernible. Using stored samples for comparison, it is possible to detect the high levels of HIV RNA that occur in acute infection and the suppressed levels of circulating virus that follow seroconversion.

Branched-DNA Testing

Another new assay for measuring HIV levels directly, developed by Chiron, uses a branched-DNA (bDNA) technology to amplify a signal to indicate the presence of HIV RNA. The bDNA assay was first designed in 1989 (Horn et al., 1989) and improved upon for use in HIV detection by Urdea (1993) and Dewar (1994).

Most strategies to detect nucleic acids involve molecular amplification of the target nucleic acid (target amplification) followed by detection of the amplified product with standard, relatively insensitive methods. Although target amplification techniques such as the polymerase chain reaction, or PCR are extremely sensitive, the methods are difficult to perform reproducibly, usually require purification of the target material, and require extreme care in order to limit cross-contamination. Also, it is difficult to determine accurately the quantity of nucleic acid present in the original sample before target amplification. Using the bDNA assay nucleic acids can be detected **directly in clinical samples** by means of signal amplification. Signal amplification of HIV RNA occurs when branched oligodeoxyribonucleotides (bDNAs) hybridize to the target HIV RNA and incorporate many alkaline phosphate molecules onto the target HIV RNA. The complex of HIV RNA plus bDNA plus alkaline phosphate is then exposed to dioxetane which is then triggered by an enzyme to luminesce (give off a light that can be detected with a measuring device, a luminometer) (see Figure 13-7). The luminescence means that HIV RNA is present and the brighter the light (or signal) the more HIV RNA is present in the test sample. The current assay is sensitive to as few as 10,000 units of viral RNA/mL of sample, but another in development may detect as few as 200-500 U/mL. The bDNA assay employs 49 molecular probes, each designed to recognize and bind to specific segments within various HIV genes. After they bind to the viral RNA, a segment in each of these probes, which are made of DNA, extends beyond the HIV RNA. These overhanging probe segments link with synthetic DNA that contains branches of DNA complementary to the overhangs. As these branches are amplified during successive synthetic replication cycles, a molecular "Christmas tree" is produced. Like ornaments, copies of an enzyme can then be attached to the branches of this expanded "tree".

DETECTION OF HIV INFECTION IN NEWBORNS

Early detection of HIV infection in newborns and children is important because it may prevent unwarranted toxicity from the use of antiretroviral agents in children who are not infected, and it can allay the fears of parents with potentially afflicted but uninfected newborns. However, early diagnosis of HIV infection in children born to HIV-positive women is difficult owing to the presence of maternal IgG antibody in the newborn which may persist until the child is about 2 years old (Table 13-4). Thus serological detection of HIV infection in neonates is complicated by the presence of immune complexes, consisting of passively transferred maternal antibodies and HIV antigens. Steven Miles and colleagues (1993) have used a rapid assay designed to disrupt these immune complexes in order to permit the detection of a specific HIV antigen. Their preliminary work correctly identified p24 antigen in the blood of 29 of 29 children. These children tested HIV-positive, but when the maternal antibodies were treated to separate the p24 antigen present (the antigen would be present because the virus was present), they found p24 antigen. Children who were HIV-positive but lacked the presence of the p24 antigen were falsely positive—they contained only the mother's HIV antibodies. Although this technique is simple to perform and accurate when compared to other methods of HIV detection in newborns, additional testing of this technique is required before its adoption. If a mother is known to be HIV-infected, cells from the newborn can be subjected to HIV blood culture or polymerase chain reaction tests. These two techniques, although very accurate, are not yet ready for the screening of all newborns. They can detect the presence of HIV in the first few days of life.

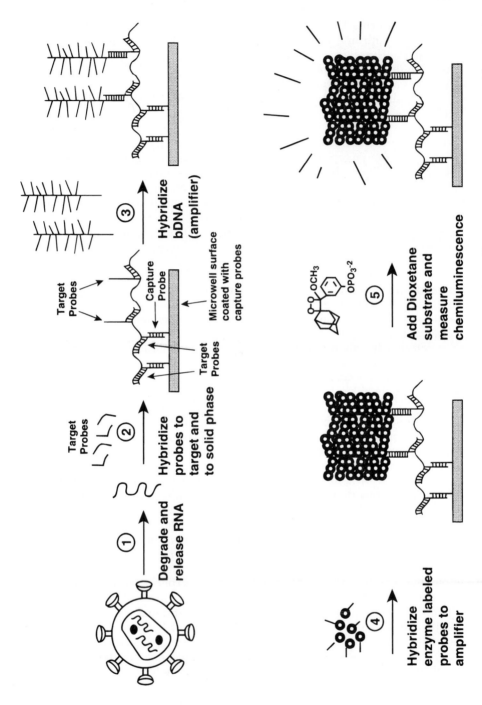

FIGURE 13-7 Branched-DNA assay for HIV RNA quantification. Schematic outline of bDNA assay. HIV is concentrated from 1-mL aliquots of patients' plasma. Pellet is then resuspended in mixture of proteinase K, lithium lauryl sulfate, and target probes. Extract is added to wells of 96-well microplate, incubated overnight at 53°C, and washed. bDNA amplifier is then added, incubated at 53°C, and washed, followed by addition of alkaline phosphatase probes, another wash, and addition of the chemiluminescent substrate. (*Adapted from Dewar et al., 1994*)

TABLE 13-4 Diagnosis of Infection in HIV-Exposed Infants

Age	Test	If Test Is Positive	If Test Is Negative
1 month	HIV culture or PCR[a]	Repeat test to confirm diagnosis of infection	Repeat test at age 3–6 months
3–6 months	HIV culture or PCR[a]	Repeat test to confirm diagnosis of infection	Test with ELISA at age 15 months
15 months	ELISA	Repeat test at age 18 months	Repeat test at age 18 months
18 months or older	ELISA	Child is infected[b]	Child is not infected[c]

[a]If HIV culture and PCR are unavailable, p24 antigen testing may be used after 1 month of age.

[b]Serological diagnosis of HIV infection requires two sets of confirmed HIV serological assays (ELISA/Western blot) performed at least 1 month apart after 15 months of age.

[c]Confirmation of seronegativity requires two sets of negative ELISAs after 15 months of age in a child with normal clinical and immunoglobulin evaluation.

(Source: El-Sahr et al., 1994).

FDA APPROVES TWO HOME HIV-ANTIBODY TEST KITS

On May 14, 1996, the FDA, which for years opposed home-based HIV testing kits because of the lack of face-to-face counseling, reversed its stance by saying the benefits of early detection of HIV infection outweigh any risks posed by the test. FDA Commissioner David Kessler said, "We are confident that this new home system can provide accurate results while assuring patient anonymity and appropriate counseling."

The FDA approved the home test **because** in a 1994 study by the Federal Centers for Disease Control and Prevention of people at increased risk of infection, like intravenous drug users and sexually active homosexual men, 42% indicated that they would use a home test. To 1994, over 60% of Americans **at risk** for HIV infection had not been tested.

Test Kit Operation

A person who buys the kit uses an enclosed lancet to prick his or her finger and places three drops of blood on a test card with an identification number. The card is mailed to a laboratory for HIV testing, and samples that test positive are retested to ensure reliability. People who use the home system do not submit names, addresses, or phone numbers with the specimen sent in on filter paper. Therefore, **the HIV test results are anonymous**. To get results, the individual calls a week later and punches into the phone his or her identification number.

If the caller's test results are positive or inconclusive, he or she will be connected to a counselor who will explain the results, urge medical treatment, and, if necessary, make a referral to a local doctor or health clinic. If the person's results are negative, he or she will be connected to a recording that will note that it's possible to be infected with HIV and still test negative, if the antibodies to HIV haven't yet developed. A counselor will be available for anyone who tests negative and wants to discuss the results.

The FDA said that the kit is as reliable as tests conducted in doctors offices and clinics.

Test Kit Availability

The first FDA-approved HIV test kit, called Confide HIV Testing Service was made available in June 1996. It was withdrawn from the marketplace in June 1997 due to poor sales. A second FDA-approved HIV home test kit went on sale nationwide in July 1996. This kit, called *Home Access Express-HIV Test* (1-800-448-8378) lets people take a blood sample at home, mail it to a laboratory, and, 3 business days later, learn by phone their results. The two tests are very similar to each other with regard to use and performance.

Pro and Con of Home-Use HIV Test (Collection) Kits

Pro— Those who favor HIV home testing point to the discouraging statistics using current HIV testing methods stating that 80% of

———— BOX 13.3 ————

HIV TESTING AT HOME

An ever-increasing number of Americans are using test kits that let them check for blood pressure, monitor cholesterol, diagnose pregnancy, predict ovulation, monitor blood-sugar levels for diabetes control, detect possible signs of colon cancer, detect possible signs of tumors, kidney stones, or prostrate problems, diagnose urinary tract infections, and now, since mid-1996, mail in a blood sample and learn by telephone whether they have been HIV-infected. Americans are growing more aggressive about making their own health care decisions. They spent more than $1 billion on home tests in 1995 and over $1.2 billion in 1996; they will most likely spend up to $1.5 billion by 1998.

CONTROLS ON USE OF AT-HOME TESTING KITS

Through mid-1997, there was no federal government policy to guide decisions on when these increasingly sophisticated tests—with their sometimes emotionally charged results—go beyond the routine and demand a doctor' interpretation.

Will patients be hurt if tests are wrong? When do they see a doctor? **Could they force a test on a family member?** More basic, are there some tests—like those that detect genetic flaws that might cause incurable diseases—that laypersons should never use.

It has become a matter of **social policy** as to what is an appropriate test for an individual to engage in themselves.

CLEARING UP THE CONFUSION OF HIV HOME TESTING VS. HOME COLLECTING KITS

Arguments will continue into the future about whether the benefits of home-based **testing** for HIV outweigh the risks. Regardless, one point should be clearly defined, that of home **testing** The two 1996 FDA-approved HIV **test** kits, *Confide* and *Home Access* (Figure 13-8) are **NOT test kits— they are home collection kits.** The term "home testing" is misleading: customers don't actually get on-the-spot results, the way they do with home test kits for glucose, cholesterol, blood pressure, or

FIGURE 13-8   Home Access Anonymous HIV Test Kit. This kit was FDA approved in July 1996 and provides access to professional counseling and medical/social service referrals 24 hours a day, 7 days a week.

pregnancy. **The HIV tests are really at-home blood collection kits to be purchased over the counter or through the mail. HOWEVER, because the literature is saturated with the term "HIV home test kit," that term will be used within this text.**

A customer pricks his or her finger with a lance provided in the kit, places a drop of blood on filter paper, and sends it to a laboratory where both enzyme-linked immunosorbent assays and confirmatory tests are performed. After a specified period, results are available over the telephone to the customer, who punches in a unique code number provided in the kit. Those who test **negative** listen to a recording informing them of the meaning of the result and offering them the option of speaking to a counselor. **Positive** results are reported by a counselor, who provides referrals to follow-up clinical services and social service agencies. Infected persons have the option of follow-up telephone counseling for a specified number of sessions.

AFTER PURCHASE OF THE KIT, the entire process is anonymous.

IS HOME HIV TESTING FEASIBLE?

Home access testing for HIV met with virtually **unanimous** opposition when it was first proposed in the late 1980s. But, in 1996, the CDC, leading clinicians, gay activists, and AIDS advocates have all **endorsed** home access testing and the FDA approved licensure of test kits from two of three companies, Johnson/Johnson and Nationwide HIV Home Test Services. The third company, Chem Trak, expects approval by early-1998.

WHAT MAKES HIV HOME TEST KITS DIFFERENT?

Home test kits differ from the traditional visit to the clinic or physician's office because: **first,** it's an easy way for people to find out if they're HIV-infected. Traditionally, getting tested for HIV has meant a trip to a doctor or clinic, getting blood drawn, then returning for results and counseling. The home testing kits save **two trips** to the doctor or clinic. It also makes testing accessible for people who live in rural areas, or inner cities where clinics are scarce, overburdened, or a long bus ride away. **Second,** home testing also affords greater **privacy.** Some people are afraid to visit a clinic or doctor's office because they fear they will be recognized by neighbors, friends, or family. In a number of studies, at-risk individuals have expressed preference for anonymous systems of HIV testing. **Home testing has the potential for complete anonymity.**

Offering another testing option is a step toward solving the national problem of inadequate HIV testing. A high proportion of those at risk (about 50%, 1997) have not been tested for HIV. Getting HIV test results early on becomes more and more important as methods of bolstering the immune system, reducing viral load using AIDS drug cocktails, and staving off opportunistic infections improve. Pregnant women are being encouraged to take voluntary HIV tests in light of studies showing that treating HIV-infected pregnant women with zidovudine (ZDV, also referred to as AZT) can reduce the rate of maternal–fetal transmission of HIV by two-thirds.

HIV TEST KIT RELIABILITY

Millions of HIV-antibody tests have been conducted using dried blood specimens. Such testing is highly accurate when laboratory protocols for confirmatory testing and quality assurance mechanisms are followed. **False-positive** results do occur in HIV testing, but at a very low rate. Some test kit blotters mailed to the lab may not have enough blood to test; telephone counselors are trained to advise customers when results are unclear or need further confirmation.

HOW PRIVATE (ANONYMOUS) ARE THE TEST RESULTS?

Each test comes with a unique identification number, which patients return to the lab with their blood samples. The lab never knows a name. When calling for results, people identify themselves by their identification.

Question: If HIV home test kit screening is so anonymous, how do people pay for the kit, especially those who order the kit by mail (using check or credit cards) or who do not have the cash to pay for it at a drugstore, etc.?

WHAT ARE PEOPLE CONCERNED ABOUT?

The proposed test kits raise a number of questions: Would they be used by people at risk for HIV infection who thus far have not been tested? Would those tested suffer because they would **not receive face-to-face counseling?** How would such testing affect public health practices? And, a positive HIV test result **does not guarantee access to needed care.** For many impoverished individuals, gaining entry into a health care and social service system by means of a ticket stamped "HIV-positive" is still a hoax.

——————— **BOX 13.3** *(continued)* ———————

After careful consideration, and taking into account the limits of the available data, the FDA concluded that the potential benefits of home access testing outweigh the potential risks.

EXPENDED ACCESS TO HIV TESTING

Central to the argument for home access testing is concern that many at risk for HIV infection **have not been tested.** The CDC has reported that about a third of the people infected with HIV were not tested until they were within 2 months of receiving a diagnosis of AIDS—about half were within a year of an AIDS diagnosis. Many women do not discover they are infected until they give birth to an infected child (Bayer et al., 1995), Given that the rate of HIV transmission can be reduced substantially by treating infected women with zidovudine during pregnancy, this is especially troubling. Although persons at higher risk have been tested and counseled to a greater degree than the remainder of the population (42%, as compared with 20% in the general population, according to the 1989 National Health Interview Survey), most people at risk have not been tested (Anderson et al., 1992).

WHO WILL USE THE HOME HIV TEST KIT: WHY?

About 50% of people in the United States who are potentially at risk for HIV infection have been tested; it is estimated that confidential testing conditions could encourage 41 million people to be tested for the first time, perhaps identifying 187,000 HIV-infected people (Phillips et al., 1995a).

Home-based HIV testing may provide reassurance to the **worried well** people for whom the risk of HIV infection may be quite remote, but are nevertheless seeking reassurance. If such individuals no longer rely on public sources of testing, resources may be freed up for more targeted interventions with those at highest risk.

Twenty-nine percent of the respondents to the National Health Interview Survey stated that they would be **very** or **somewhat** likely to use home HIV tests if they became available; 42% of those defined as at risk for infection would do so. People with fewer years of education and lower income were more likely to express an interest in home HIV testing. Blacks and Hispanics were more likely than others to say they would use home testing (Phillips et al., 1995b).

For some people, the remoteness and anonymity afforded by telephone counseling makes it easier to reveal painful feelings or embarrassing information. There is a long tradition with telephone counseling in crisis intervention and suicide prevention. People are more likely to participate in HIV testing and counseling if they believe they will not experience negative consequences in areas of employment, school admission, housing, and medical services should they test positive. Many of the estimated 700,000 to 900,000 HIV-infected people in the United States remain unaware of their infection. And finally, telephone counseling must be compared to the actual experiences of current HIV testing. For many, counseling is already inadequate or missing altogether. According to data from the National Health Interview Survey, a third of those who are tested for HIV antibodies got their results by mail (16%) or telephone (17%). Of those who seek testing at public alternative test sites, a third fail to return to find out the results (Bayer et al., 1995).

SUMMARY

The cost of the *Confide* test kit in 1997 was about $50 but it did not sell well and was taken off the market after 1 year. The cost of *Home Access Express* test kit and *Home Access* test kit were $49.95 and $39.95, respectfully (1-800-448-8378). Both had offered anonymous registration and pre- and post-test telephone counseling. *Home Access* and *Home Access Express* home testing and counseling systems allow people nationwide the opportunity to access client-centered counseling 24 hours a day, 7 days a week.

The *Home Access* test refers a predetermined percentage of persons with negative results to a counselor to deter callers from assuming such referral implies a positive result. All persons with positive or indeterminate results are referred immediately to a counselor, who reports results and offers referrals to clinics and physicians, information on partner notification services, and numbers for the National AIDS Hotline. **Individuals with indeterminate results are also offered a new kit to be used in 6 to 12 weeks, or referred to outside sites for traditional HIV testing.** Negative results are available for 30 days after the first call and positive results are available on-line for up to 1 year. Positive results are archived and available thereafter from the medical director.

WHAT A HOME TESTING KIT FOR HIV SHOULD CONTAIN

A true home test kit should contain all pre- and post-test counseling information and sample collection materials. The user purchases the test at pharmacies or by mail order, performs it at home, and has a result within several minutes.

True home testing for HIV infection should be anonymous, low cost, and accessible. However, the ramifications of receiving such information at home are unknown. It remains unclear whether persons identified as HIV-positive will enter the health care system and how public health officials will maintain surveillance. Another potential disadvantage is that individuals who test HIV-negative may not get counseling about risk modification.

people in high-risk populations are unwilling to use standard testing services. They note frequent instances of substandard HIV testing even in physician's offices, with test results delivered in brief phone calls or left on telephone answering machines. Also offered in support of home-based testing is that the existing system of testing is inefficient and wasteful because **98% of tests are HIV-negative**. Thus, there is an enormous amount of money spent on HIV-negative results that should be spent elsewhere. With respect to the need for face-to-face counseling, they cite the success of suicide hotlines and crisis counseling services in support of using home telephone HIV counseling procedures.

Con— Those against the use of home testing say that this is just one more instance of the telephone substituting for face-to-face contact in medical practice. They suggest that bad health news of this magnitude and complexity should be given in person. They also point out that these test kits will probably be used mostly by affluent people who are well but worried, while the poor at-risk people continue to remain untested. In addition, there is the risk of the tests being used coercively by employers or the police. The potential for human rights violations are great.

For a more thorough review of the issues on HIV home testing, read **"Testing for HIV at home: What are the issues?"** (Schopper et al., 1966).

Remarks— It remains to be seen just how many of the undiagnosed thousands of HIV-infected persons these home-based kits manage to capture—and at what cost—and whether the system will be more helpful than abused. WHAT DO YOU THINK WILL HAPPEN, GIVE SOME EXAMPLES OF WHAT YOU THINK WILL HAPPEN.

REPORTING HIV INFECTIONS

In April of 1992, the CDC suggested that all states consider implementing programs requiring physicians to report names of HIV-positive patients.

Reporting HIV infection is useful in directing HIV-related prevention activities such as patient counseling, partner notification, and referral for appropriate medical management. HIV infection reports are also useful for guiding pediatric medical and social support programs. Prevention activities and medical management of patients can be carried out without requiring HIV reporting, but an HIV reporting system provides a means of maintaining HIV-related prevention activities (*MMWR*, 1988b).

All 50 states and the District of Columbia require health care providers to report new cases of AIDS to their state health departments. Beginning 1997, 38 states required some form of name reporting of HIV-infected people (Table 10-4). The 38 states that require HIV reporting have over 50% of the population and accounted for over 50% of reported AIDS cases through 1996. Twenty-eight of the 38 states require the patient's name (Table 10-4). These 28 states account for over 16% of all reported AIDS cases and require information to include sex, age, and race/ethnicity; 19 states ask for the mode of transmission; six ask for clinical status and three require T4 cell count. Beginning 1997, only 11 states classified HIV/AIDS as a sexually transmitted disease and only 12 states authorized physicians to inform partners of HIV/AIDS patients (*Medical Tribune*, 1991, updated).

WHO SHOULD BE TESTED FOR HIV INFECTION?

Testing for antibodies to HIV is an important first step in establishing a diagnosis of HIV infection. Testing every person may be counterproductive. Attempts to isolate or publicly identify people with HIV/AIDS can actually fuel the spread of HIV. People outside the "tested" group may feel invulnerable, and then fail to make necessary changes in their behavior.

The effects of stimulating a false sense of security are well illustrated in Germany where, in certain towns, prostitutes are required to be checked for certain STDs every week and are given health inspection cards. Many customers think these cards guarantee against disease and so refuse to use condoms.

The problem is not confined to Germany. **A European shipbroker whose work frequently takes him to south-east Asia, where he has a regular sex partner, said: "I tell her when I'm due to arrive and she has an HIV test just before. If she has an up-to-date health card I know I'm safe."**

In fact, a negative HIV test is no guarantee the tested person is **truly** HIV-negative—he or she may be in the window period. The decision to test must be based on people's risk behaviors and/or symptoms. As to who **needs** to be HIV tested; a complete history and physical examination will give the best answer to this question. Decisions based on individual indications are often more appropriate than decisions based on one's classification (i.e., all pregnant women or all single men between 20 and 49 years of age). Initial assessment for current or past behaviors (within the past 10 years) should include:

1. Persons with **risk behaviors** such as:
   a. Anal sexual activity, male or female
   b. Injection drug use
   c. Frequent casual heterosexual activity
   d. Encounters with prostitutes
   e. Previous treatment for sexually transmitted diseases (*Condyloma acuminata* (genital warts), herpes simplex virus, gonorrhea, syphilis, *Chlamydia*)
   f. Blood transfusions, especially before 1985
   g. Sexual activity with partners having any of the above

h. Infants born to women involved in any of the above

2. Persons with symptoms such as:
   a. Fever, weight loss (unexplained)
   b. Night sweats
   c. Severe fatigue
   d. Recent infections, especially thrush and shingles (varicella-zoster)

3. Persons with **signs** (based on physical exam) such as:
   a. Weight loss
   b. Enlarged lymph nodes and/or tonsilar enlargement

––––––––––– BOX 13.4 –––––––––––

THE PHYSICIAN'S DILEMMA

While on vacation, a physician came upon a motorcycle accident. He administered cardiopulmonary resuscitation for 45 minutes to one of the riders, who was bleeding from the mouth. After the man died, the physician asked the emergency department doctor in charge, who was a personal friend, to test the deceased for HIV.

The doctor said he needed consent. The physician said, "The guy died. I have a wife and kids."

The incident prompted this physician to raise the issue of testing without informed consent. This brings up the pro and con issues on informed consent. After reading the *Pro* and *Con*, decide where you stand on the issue.

Pro: *Physician:* "Consent for every test we do is a nice luxury, but we don't do it for syphilis or hepatitis B. Only with this disease have we departed from public health policy. The majority with HIV are not aware they're infected. Not in the history of medicine have we chosen a policy to protect the infected."

Con: *Physician:* "It's extremely paternalistic. We should be trying to get patients involved in their care and give them informed choices on what is possible. I favor consent on any test. I am afraid that liberal HIV testing laws and policies are being fostered out of physician self-interest rather than patient need.

Doctors don't like HIV particularly, and they don't like people who have HIV infection. They want a way to be in control. They want to know the patient's status, and their reasons are less medical or for the patient's best interest than for the physician's."

Your Position: (class discussion)

c. Oral exam (candidiasis, oral hairy leukoplakia)

d. Skin lesions (e.g., Kaposi's sarcoma, varicella-zoster, psoriasis)

e. Hepatosplenomegaly (enlarged liver)

f. Mental status examination showing changes.

4. Pregnant women — see Point of Information
12.5.

WHY IS HIV TEST INFORMATION NECESSARY?

Thirty percent of adults who **seek HIV testing**
do so to **find out their HIV status**; 12% are
tested because of hospitalization or surgery;
16% for application for insurance; and 7% to
enter the military. Another 1% are referred
by their doctor, the health department, or
sexual partner, and 4% are tested for HIV for
immigration reasons (Hooker, 1996).

Knowledge of HIV infection status allows infected persons and their infected partners to
seek treatment with retroviral agents, prophylaxis against *Pneumocystis carinii* pneumonia,
tuberculosis skin testing and tuberculosis prophylaxis (if appropriate), and other types of
therapy and vaccines that may delay or prevent
the opportunistic infections associated with
HIV infection. Such measures have been
shown to delay the onset of AIDS in infected
persons and to prolong the lives of persons
with AIDS. Counseling and testing may help
some persons change high-risk sexual and
drug-use behaviors thereby preventing HIV
transmission to others.

Entry into Foreign Countries

An increasing number of foreign countries require that foreigners be tested for HIV prior
to entry. This is particularly true for students
or long-term visitors. Information available
through 1994, reveals that 30 of 45 foreign
countries queried require an HIV test prior to
entry, on arrival, or on application for residency. Before traveling abroad, check with the
embassy of the country to be visited to learn
entry requirements and specifically whether or
not HIV testing is a requirement. If the foreign
country indicates that U.S. test results are acceptable "under certain conditions," prospec-

tive travelers should inquire at the embassy of
that country for details (i.e., which laboratories in the United States may perform tests and
where to have results certified and authenti-
cated) before departing the United States. For
a copy of HIV Testing Requirements for Entry
into Foreign Countries, send a self-addressed,
stamped, business-size envelope to: Bureau of
Consular Affairs, Room 5807, Department of
State, Washington, DC 20520.

Testing for HIV Infection

With AIDS cases being reported from almost
all the countries of the world, and with about
650,000 to 900,000 living HIV-infected and
over 640,000 AIDS cases having occurred in
the United States beginning 1998, the question of HIV testing on either a **voluntary** or a
mandatory basis cannot be ignored. Perhaps
the decision on **who** is to be tested should be
decided by society since everyone is at risk.

The case in which a Florida dentist, David
Acer, is believed to have infected six of his patients has led members of Congress, the Senate,
and others to demand changes in HIV testing
and confidentiality procedures. Under current
policy, people are tested only with their **informed consent**. Although the **number** of people who test positive is reported to the CDC,
their names are not. No attempts are made to
track down contacts of infected individuals.

Marcia Angell, executive editor of the *New
England Journal of Medicine*, wrote in 1991 that it
was time to adopt a traditional public health approach to HIV/AIDS. She said, "Tracing and notification of the sexual partners of HIV-infected
persons, and screening of pregnant women,
newborns and hospitalized patients and health
care professionals are warranted. This should be
adopted only if steps are taken to protect HIV-
infected people from discrimination and hysteria. Jobs, housing and insurance benefits, for
example, should be protected by statute."

Regardless of protection, it has been estimated that 10% to 28% of persons in the
United States and between 18% to 30% in
Australia **choose not to be HIV-tested**. These
percentages most likely are in keeping with
personal attitudes toward HIV testing in the
other developed countries (Clezy et al., 1992).

UNITED STATES PUBLIC HEALTH SERVICE (USPHS) RECOMMENDATIONS FOR HIV COUNSELING AND VOLUNTARY TESTING FOR ALL PREGNANT WOMEN

Knowledge of HIV status is important for several reasons. **First,** women who know their serostatus can gain access to HIV-related care and therapies (such as *Pneumocystis carinii* pneumonia prophylaxis, TB screening, and antiretroviral therapy) during pregnancy and postpartum as needed. **Second**, HIV-infected women can be offered zidovudine to potentially block maternal–fetal transmission of HIV. **Third**, an obstetrician would postpone rupture of amniotic membranes and avoid scalp electrodes or other potentially invasive procedures, all of which may be cofactors for enhanced transmission of HIV. **Fourth**, zidovudine can be offered to infants of HIV-seropositive women who have recently delivered.

This report (*MMWR*, 1995) contains the recommendations of a 10-member USPHS task force on the use of zidovudine to reduce perinatal transmission of HIV. In summary, the recommendations are:

1. Health-care providers should encourage all pregnant women to be tested for HIV infection, both for their own health and to reduce the risk for perinatal HIV transmission. Four million women, in the United States, each year become pregnant.

2. HIV testing of pregnant women and their infants should be voluntary. In voluntary testing, the reason for the test, how it is administered, and the person's right to privacy and confidentiality must be explained. This allows the person the choice of taking or refusing the test and giving or not giving demographic data.

3. Health-care providers should counsel and offer HIV testing to women as early in pregnancy as possible so that informed and timely therapeutic and reproductive decisions can be made.

4. Uninfected pregnant women who continue to practice high-risk behaviors (e.g., IV-drug use and unprotected sexual contact with an HIV-infected or high-risk partner) should be encouraged to avoid further exposure to HIV and to be retested in the third trimester of pregnancy.

5. For women who are first identified as being HIV-infected during labor and delivery, health-care providers should consider offering intrapartum and neonatal zidovudine.

In Mid-1995 the CDC reported that routine HIV counseling and voluntary testing for all pregnant women has already proved effective in several communities nationwide. In one inner-city hospital in Atlanta, for example, 96% of women chose to be tested after being provided HIV counseling.

According to the Pediatric AIDS Foundation, about $350 million a year could be saved by testing pregnant women for the AIDS virus. The average hospital bill for a baby born infected with HIV is $35,000 annually for the 8 to 10 years the child lives.

Benefits of HIV Testing— Testing for the presence of HIV antibodies or antigens as early as possible when HIV is suspected can provide substantial health benefits to the individual and reduce the risk of transmitting the virus to others. The infected person can be better treated for other infections if his or her HIV status is known. For example, 2% of HIV/AIDS patients in the United States contract tuberculosis. Unless otherwise indicated, HIV-infected patients with a past or present positive TB test should receive isoniazid as early as possible because active TB may be the first sign of AIDS. If other diseases occur prior to isoniazid treatment, treatment for those diseases may interfere with the therapy for TB and vice versa.

The presence of HIV in people with syphilis may also alter the recommended therapy and follow-up. Influenza and pneumococcal polysaccharide vaccines are recommended for *all* people infected with HIV. The recommendation for pneumococcal immunization explicitly states that the vaccine be given as early in the course of HIV infection as possible to maximize antibody response (Rhame et al., 1989). In addition, the early detection of asymptomatic HIV infection provides an even more important health benefit: a chance for a lifestyle

---- BOX 13.6 ----

BOXER STRIPPED OF FEATHERWEIGHT TITLE AFTER POSITIVE HIV TEST

It took Ruben Palacio 12 years to win a world title. On the eve of his first defense, he became the first champion to test positive for HIV. The British Boxing Board of Control said, "We can't risk the life of another boxer by letting him fight. It's a kind of disease that can be spread via blood contact, and boxing is a sport where that is likely to happen."

Palacio is the first active world title holder known to have tested positive for the AIDS-causing virus. Esteban DeJesus, who held the WBC lightweight boxing title in the 1970s, contracted AIDS after his retirement and died in 1989.

HIV testing has been a routine part of the prefight medical examination in Britain for several years. In February 1990, African heavyweight champion Proud Kilimanjaro of Zimbabwe was barred from a fight with Britain's Lennox Lewis because he refused to give details of an HIV test to the British Boxing Board of Control.

His manager said, "This brings the HIV thing into perspective. Instead of going home with the largest paycheck of his life, he is going home with an HIV test result that means he will die."

Update: In March of 1996 Tommy Morrison, a former United States heavyweight contender disclosed that he is HIV-positive (see Figure 8-10). Beginning 1997 nine states require professional fighters and kickboxers, licensed in those states, to be HIV-tested.

---

change to reduce stress. This would lessen the chance of acquiring other microbial infections that may stimulate the immune system, activate HIV to reproduce and destroy T4 cells, and begin AIDS progression. However, too few of the HIV-infected are aware of their infections, and so, do not take these precautions.

Competency and Informed Consent—Competency is often used interchangeably with capacity; it refers to a person's ability to make an informed decision. For example, to consent to medical treatment, a person must be mentally capable of comprehending the risks and benefits of a proposed procedure and its alternatives. While a health care provider can assess competence, a legal finding of competency is often required based on the testimony of a mental health professional. Mental illness by itself does not indicate that a person is incompetent to make medical decisions. Various degrees of mental incapacity may occur with HIV infection, requiring an assessment of competency. AIDS dementia complex (ADC) occurs in approximately 70% of HIV-infected patients at some point in HIV disease/AIDS and may interfere with the patient's capacity to provide an informed consent.

Informed Consent

Informed consent is not just signing a form but is a process of education and the opportunity to have questions answered. The concept of informed consent includes the following components: full disclosure of information, patient competency, patient understanding, voluntariness, and decision making. The process of obtaining informed consent involves appropriate facts being provided to a competent patient who understands the information and voluntarily makes a choice to accept or refuse the recommended procedure or treatment.

When the concept of informed consent is applied clinically, complexities arise regarding both the content and the process. The concept contains ambiguous requisites such as "appropriate" facts, "full" disclosure, and "substantial" understanding. The process is affected by many variables including the communication skill and range of practice style of the physician; the maturity, intelligence, and coping strategies of the patient; and the interaction between the physician and the patient (Hartlaub et al., 1993).

Testing Without Consent

Beginning 1997, 29 states had laws that allowed HIV testing without informed consent under certain conditions. The required conditions vary and include:

1. Patient or other authorized person is unable to give or withhold consent.
2. Test result will help determine treatment.
3. Patient is unable to give consent, and physician can document that a medical emergency exists and that the test is needed for diagnosis and treatment.

4. Test is needed to protect the health of other patients, health workers, emergency or law enforcement personnel.
5. Several states require post-test counseling.
6. In 27 states, teenagers must have signed parental consent to be HIV tested. In 23 states (Alabama, Arizona, California, Colorado, Connecticut, Delaware, Florida, Georgia, Hawaii, Illinois, Iowa, Michigan, Nebraska, Nevada, New Mexico, North Carolina, North Dakota, Ohio, Rhode Island, Tennessee, Utah, Washington, Wyoming) **minors can consent** to HIV testing and treatment.

Generally, HIV antibody testing without consent is legally considered battery. Legal liability for "unlawful touching" may result from performing an HIV antibody test without consent. Such a procedure may also constitute an illegal search.

Question: **Are federal and state governments overly stressing personal privacy at the expense of prevention? (Defend your answer with examples/situations.)**

Voluntary Named HIV Testing

In voluntary **named** HIV testing, the individual freely provides his or her name. In this type of testing, an individual voluntarily seeks to learn his or her HIV status and receives a result which is known both to the individual and the test provider/testing agency. An advantage to named testing is that health care providers can contact the person tested if he or she does not return for the testing result.

Voluntary Unnamed HIV Testing

HIV testing is voluntary, but the identity of the person being tested is not placed on the blood sample or the testing form. As a result, the only person who can link the test result with an individual is the person being tested. This form of testing may encourage people concerned about the HIV infection status to obtain testing as it eliminates risk of discrimination or stigmatization. However, it places the exclusive responsibility for seeking counseling, support, and preventive measures on the individual who is infected. Unnamed testing permits reporting of test data to public health authorities without the risk of breaching confidentiality. Many public health authorities currently prefer voluntary unnamed testing to named testing.

Mandatory HIV Testing

HIV testing is **mandatory** if it is required to participate in a process or activity which is not itself required. For example, if an HIV test is required for travel to some foreign countries, or to donate blood, this is considered mandatory testing because, while the test is required, one is not required to travel or donate blood. In mandatory testing, care must be taken to ensure that people are not in fact **forced** to undergo testing. At least **in theory,** mandatory testing is a form of voluntary testing: people can decide not to participate in the process or activity for which testing is required. **In practice,** however, the degree of voluntary consent is in some cases questionable. For example, in a situation where employment is not possible unless one agrees to be tested and one needs that job, the **voluntary** nature of the test appears to have vanished (*AIDS, Health and Human Rights,* 1995).

Many people advocate mandatory HIV screening for everyone. They believe that this is the best way to stop the transmission of HIV. Perhaps this attitude is a reflection of fear. Mandatory premarital syphilis screening has often been cited as a precedent for premarital HIV screening. The logic appears to be: we screen for syphilis, but HIV infection and AIDS are a lot worse; therefore we should screen for HIV infection to prevent the spread of AIDS.

It can be answered that **syphilis is curable**; yet history reveals that syphilis screening has turned out to be ineffective and unnecessary. For example, in 1978, premarital syphilis screening found only 1% of the total number of new syphilis cases in the United States at a cost of 80 million dollars. Over the past dozen years, many of the 50 states have dropped this screening program and others have indicated that they will follow. Still, in 1988, legislation was pending in 35 states that would require premarital HIV testing. Louisiana, Illinois, and Maryland passed mandatory testing legislation; by 1989, all three states repealed that legislation.

—————— BOX 13.7 ——————

MANDATORY HIV TESTING

Historically, for each new life-threatening disease, people, motivated by a mix of emotions and ideologies, call for mandatory testing generally citing new research findings and targeting different populations. So the idea of mandatory HIV testing is nothing new. But what makes mandatory testing attractive? To many it looks like a quick fix. And if you are a politician, it makes constituents think legislators are doing something about the epidemic. Two classic examples that showed why mandatory testing is ineffective at preventing HIV transmission were the premarital screening programs in Illinois and Louisiana in the late 1980s. Both states required people seeking marriage licenses to be tested for HIV, then disclosed test results to both partners. The programs' advocates argued that knowledge of test results would prevent transmission by allowing partners to reconsider marriage, adopt safer sex practices, and make informed child-bearing decisions. These programs, however, caused many people to avoid testing, identified few cases of HIV infection, and incurred great social and financial costs.

It is uncertain whether the programs were effective in preventing people from being exposed to HIV. Many couples avoided testing altogether by marrying in another state or deciding not to marry. Since testing a population with low seroprevalence causes a greater proportion of false positives, the premarital screening programs falsely identified some people as being infected with HIV, resulting in broken engagements, aborted pregnancies, and psychologic distress. The programs had financial costs as well: Illinois spent $243,000 per positive test result.

HIV testing can be a very effective public health tool, but it 's only effective when deployed in ways that are socially, politically, and medically appropriate. If it's not, it can actually be a detriment to public health. Being identified as having HIV has caused people to lose their jobs, health and life insurance, housing, family members, and friends, and to be denied employment, medical treatment, and education. Legal safeguards such as the Americans with Disabilities Act and the Fair Housing Act have helped people with HIV fight discrimination, but discrimination remains for those diagnosed with HIV disease or AIDS.

WHEN DOES MANDATORY TESTING FOR A DISEASE MAKE SENSE?

There is a set of guidelines that were developed in the mid-to-late 1980s and incorporated into the HIV testing policies of the Centers for Disease Control and Prevention (CDC) and the World Health Organization. These guidelines require, roughly, that the level of seroprevalence in the targeted population be high enough to keep the number of uninfected people subjected to testing small; the testing be conducted in a context in which the risk of HIV transmission is high; the test results enable policymakers or health officials to take actions that could not be taken otherwise; the harm or potential harm of testing not be so disproportionate to whatever benefit that testing is unfair; and there be no means of achieving the same information in a less restrictive manner. Under these guidelines the case for mandatory testing in most situations is very weak. One exception is the screening of all blood and tissue. Actually, blood screening differs significantly from mandatory testing because screening, which allows the discarding of infected blood, is clearly effective in preventing HIV transmission. Also, blood donors are told prior to donation that their blood will be screened. So, although donors do not necessarily provide informed consent, they retain the option of not donating, thereby avoiding testing.

Another instance in which mandatory testing could be used is rape, where it could be appropriate to test the assailant. There is evidence from survivors' groups that rape victims have considerable anxiety about being infected with HIV. Therefore, it is possible that the advantages to the rape survivor override the concerns about nonconsensual testing.

In many states there is a waive of consent requirement for HIV testing under specific circumstances. In a recent 50-state survey, people tested without informed consent variously include inmates of many state and federal prison systems; health care workers; hospital patients; those arrested for or convicted of sexual assault; people charged with other sex-related crimes, such as prostitution; people charged with certain drug-related crimes; and applicants for health and life insurance. Other calls for mandatory testing have targeted children in foster care, children awaiting adoption, and professional athletes (Harvard AIDS Institute, 1995).

————— **BOX 13.7** (continued) —————

MANDATORY HIV TESTING OF NEWBORNS AND DISCLOSURE OF TEST RESULTS TO MOTHERS AND PHYSICIANS

Perhaps no call for mandatory testing has caused as much recent controversy as those requiring all pregnant women or all newborns to be tested. The results of AIDS Clinical Trials Group 076 (ACTG 076), which showed that Zidovudine (ZDV) could reduce perinatal transmission by two-thirds, have again promoted debate and prompted policymakers to take action. Most recently, on June 26, 1996, New York became the **first** state in the nation to mandate and disclose the HIV status of newborns to mothers and physicians. Governor George E. Pataki signed into law legislation known as the "Baby AIDS" bill, which authorizes the State Health Commissioner to establish a comprehensive program of HIV testing of newborns. The Governor said, "This law extends our efforts to do everything we can to reduce the number of babies born with this devastating virus. This information can be used to help mothers make important health care decisions for themselves and their children. We will no longer allow infants to be used as statistical tools in some scientific study. Today, we recognize the HIV infant as a living, breathing human being whose right to medical treatment must be respected."

The passage of this bill was immediately followed by the American Medical Association announcement endorsing mandatory testing of all pregnant women and newborns for the AIDS virus. For additional information on mandatory newborn HIV Testing and Disclosure, see Point of View 13.3.

IMPACT OF MANDATORY HIV TESTING ON PHYSICIANS AND NURSES

Physicians and nurses in 13 northern and central New Jersey hospitals responded to an anony-

mous four-page survey containing 16 questions relating to the following scenario:

"Assume a law has been passed requiring yearly HIV testing of all health care workers. Those that test positive will be prohibited from performing certain procedures and activities and, if employed by a hospital, clinic or medical school, will not be dismissed but may be reassigned. Attempts may be made to trace patients who might have contracted HIV from the health care worker."

Results: Approximately three-fourths of all surveyed health professionals stated that a mandatory testing policy would persuade individuals in their profession not to work in high-prevalence areas. Among those who currently work in high-prevalence HIV/AIDS areas, only 51% said that they would definitely or probably remain in the area should such a policy be instituted. Among those practicing surgery or performing invasive procedures, 7% currently avoid HIV-positive patients, and an additional 34% said that they would do so under the proposed testing policy. Finally, 4% of these professionals currently advise others to stop working in high-prevalence areas, and an additional 22% state that they would definitely do so if the proposed policy were instituted.

Conclusion: An HIV testing policy would create a shortage of physicians and nurses in high-prevalence HIV/AIDS areas. (Source: Passannante et al., 1993)

Update: In late 1994 new CDC guidelines called for health-care workers performing "exposure-prone" procedures to be tested for HIV and HBV, and recommended that **patients** of infected health care workers be notified of the workers' status.

Thirty-eight states have passed regulations simular to the CDC's recommendations (AIDS Alert, 1994).

Why Mandatory Testing?

Mandatory testing is for the protection of a certain group or the public at large. Although it is not anonymous, results are kept confidential on a need-to-know basis. Mandatory testing for HIV continues to be angrily debated primarily

because of the possibility of error when running large numbers of test samples, inadvertent loss of confidentiality, and lack of overall benefit to those who are found to be HIV-positive. Mandatory HIV testing is routine for blood donors, and military and Job Corps personnel.

CAN MANDATORY HIV SCREENING BE JUSTIFIED?

Paul Goldschmidt (1993) states that an argument often invoked to justify mandatory HIV screening refers to the social responsibility. The argument goes that, even if testing is of little help to those already infected, it is necessary to avoid further infection. Every effort should be made to protect others from infection; however, screening will not achieve this.

Alleviating human suffering is the common goal of medicine, and emotional support is offered in an atmosphere of confidentiality and trust. Systematic screening dramatically contradicts this principle; it may reveal information about an individual who has expressed no wish to obtain it. Furthermore, a breach of confidentiality could ultimately lead to an individual being branded as dangerous and ostracized. Instead of using knowledge to avoid suffering, it is created by confronting unwilling individuals with the possibility of developing a fatal and incurable disease.

People infected with HIV face an irreversible destruction of their immune system. **None of the attempted treatments have been shown to inhibit virus replication effectively, or to limit the destruction of the immune system.** Can mandatory screening be justified as helping those infected, when, under these circumstances, to be made aware of one's HIV infection can be detrimental. HIV-infected people face the prospect of a complete disruption of their personal and professional lives and the anguish of probable physical suffering leading to death. If the individual has given informed consent, or freely chosen to consult a physician, the medical team can be emotionally supportive. However, there is no justification for screening those who have never asked, or consented to, HIV testing.

Goldschmidt argues that mandatory screening can not be scientifically or ethically defended, so why is the pressure for mandatory screening so strong in the United States? (class discussion)

Update 1995: "The findings of the Protocol 076 (zidovudine pregnancy study) offer the hope of preventing a devastating disease in children," wrote Harold Jaffe, MD, director of AIDS research at the CDC (Jaffe, 1994). "The challenge now is to implement effective ethical, and practical public health strategies to turn the success of this clinical trial into a public health success."

The study, which involved 477 pregnant women infected with HIV, showed that just 8.3% of the infants born to the women who took zidovudine (AZT) were infected with the virus, while 25.5% of the infants born to the women who did not take zidovudine were infected with the virus.

The efficacy of zidovudine in preventing HIV transmission has changed the issue of pregnancy testing from a philosophical disagreement over patients' rights to privacy to a referendum on the responsibility of public health officials to use means at their disposal to prevent the spread of HIV. The point of contention is whether testing of pregnant women should be mandatory or voluntary.

The prevailing view among health officials is that the testing should be voluntary. But a number of vocal public health officials and medical ethicists favor mandatory, "routine" testing of pregnant women.

Arthur Caplan, MD, director of the Center for Bioethics at the University of Pennsylvania, said, "It's one thing to have voluntary testing when there are no cures, it's another matter when there's a way of preventing transmission. I don't believe that voluntary testing is going to be effective in picking up women that might be HIV-positive and don't think they're at risk. They're not going to be tested and you're not going to find them."

Opponents of mandatory testing argue that mandatory testing of pregnant women—like mandatory screening of health care workers for HIV—is inefficient and unconstitutional (AIDS Alert, 1994).

Would Paul Goldschmidt argue for or against mandatory HIV testing of pregnant women? What is your position with regard to HIV testing of all pregnant women?

Update 1996: On May 20, 1996, President Clinton signed The Ryan White Reauthorization Act. It provides federal grants to cities and states over the next 5 years to treat and assist people with HIV disease and AIDS. For 1996 it provided $758 million. Within this bill (S 641-H Rept 104-545, the section on HIV testing of newborns, there is $10 million to promote voluntary counseling, testing and treatment for pregnant women. The bill also contains an agreement that will trigger mandatory testing of newborns **unless** adequate progress is made to prevent mother-to-child HIV transmission.

The secretary of Health and Human Services will determine by September 1998 whether the testing of newborns whose mothers had declined an HIV test had become standard medical practice. If it has, then states will have to meet one of three criteria to continue to receive federal funds under the bill: (1) Show a 50% reduction by March 2000 in the rate of new AIDS cases resulting from perinatal transmission, compared with 1993; (2) show that at least 95% of mothers who had received prenatal care had been tested; or (3) have implemented mandatory testing for newborns whose mothers had not been tested.

If the secretary finds that testing has become standard practice, the criteria will not apply.

State of Florida, General Bill S474: HIV and AIDS Testing, Chapter No. 96-179—This bill became law on October 1, 1996. Section 384.31 reads as follows:

Every person, including every physician licensed under *chapter 458* or *chapter 459* or midwife licensed under *chapter 464* or *chapter 467*, attending a pregnant woman for conditions relating to pregnancy during the period of gestation and delivery shall take or cause to be taken a sample of venous blood at a time or times specified by the department. Each sample of blood shall be tested by a laboratory approved for such purposes under part I of chapter 483 for sexually transmissible diseases as required by rule of the department.

At the time the venous blood sample is taken, testing for human immunodeficiency virus (HIV) infection shall be offered to each pregnant woman. The prevailing professional standard of care in this state requires each health care provider and midwife who attends a pregnant woman to counsel the woman to be tested for human immunodeficiency virus (HIV). Counseling shall include a discussion of the availability of treatment if the pregnant woman tests HIV positive. If a pregnant woman objects to HIV testing, reasonable steps shall be taken to obtain a written statement of such objection, signed by the patient, which shall be placed in the patient's medical record. Every person, including every physician licensed under *chapter 458* or *chapter 459* or midwife licensed under *chapter 464* or *chapter 467*, who attends a pregnant woman who has been offered and objects to HIV testing shall be immune from liability arising out of or related to the contracting of HIV infection or acquired immune deficiency syndrome (AIDS) by the child from the mother.

Compulsory HIV Testing

In compulsory testing, **a person cannot refuse to be tested.** Compulsory testing may be forced onto an individual, groups, communities, or even entire populations. A court may order an individual to be tested, or a government may decree or legislate that, for example, commercial sex workers, homosexuals, prisoners, hospital patients, or persons seeking immigration must be tested.

In Colorado, Florida, Georgia, Kentucky, Illinois, Michigan, Nevada, Rhode Island, Utah, and West Virginia, HIV testing is compulsory for people convicted of prostitution. However, many prostitutes are back on the streets before their test results are in. In many cases, the prostitutes could not be found for follow-up counseling. In Duval County Florida, county judges agreed to impose a 30-day jail term for convicted prostitutes, a time period long enough to get their test results and provide counseling. Prostitutes have to sign the test results sheet. They are released as soon as they do.

Under Florida law, a prostitute who knows he or she is carrying the AIDS virus but continues to offer sexual favors can be jailed for 1 year.

At least 44 states and the District of Columbia authorize HIV testing for charged or convicted sex offenders (Hooker, 1996).

Fear of Mandatory Testing— If a massive mandatory screening test program was implemented, would it be possible to keep results confidential? What would be done with the information? For example, would the state prevent an uninfected person from marrying an infected one? Officials fear that mandatory

———— BOX 13.8 ————

FLORIDA: HEALTH CARE WORKER LEAKS CONFIDENTIAL HIV INFORMATION

As of October 1, 1996, the state of Florida mandated there be at least one anonymous and confidential HIV counseling and testing site in each of its 67 counties. As of January 1, 1997, all persons testing HIV-positive who request health services must give up their identity.

Penalties: Any person who violates the confidentiality of the new laws commits a misdemeanor of the first degree punishable by imprisonment not to exceed 1 year.

Update 1997: The state of Florida delayed the identification of HIV-positive people until they are more certain that the state can assure patient confidentiality. This concern resulted from a Pinellas County health care worker who left the office, in September 1996, with a computer disk containing the names of about 4,000 HIV-infected people. The disk included names of people with AIDS and other personal information, including telephone numbers, addresses, date of birth, information about how they got AIDS, and other health information. The disk was sent to the *Tampa Tribune* and the *St. Petersburg Times* newspapers! **Florida began mandatory HIV reporting in July 1997.**

---

testing will drive many people who might have volunteered for anonymous testing underground and away from the health care system. These people will be lost to the counseling and education that would benefit them and others. The reason for going underground would be fear of discrimination and social ostracism if found to be HIV-infected.

A case can be made that a compulsory program could maintain strict confidentiality even with large numbers of people being tested. But it would appear that the political powers and public in general are not ready for broad-scale compulsory screen testing in the United States.

Confidential, Anonymous, and Blinded Testing

Both confidential and anonymous testing involve the use of informed consent forms which are, to date, with exception of the U.S. military, Job Corps workers, and certain criminals, done on a voluntary basis. Blinded testing **does not**, because of procedure, require informed consent.

Confidential HIV Testing— A consent to HIV testing must be given freely and without coercion. The volunteer does not have to provide any information unless he or she wants to. Individuals to be tested in a state laboratory complete a HIV Antibody Form. The consent form explains in simple terms what the presence of HIV antibody does and does not signify. It explains the uncertain medical outcome and potential social and legal implications of a positive test result. The consent form assures confidentiality but **warns that the result is part of the patient's medical record, to which others may have access under certain conditions**. Some centers provide completely anonymous testing; this option is available to the patient and his or her physician.

The following example demonstrates one of the problems with confidential testing. A young homosexual male with signs of oral thrush agreed to an HIV test. Later that day, he called and asked that his blood **not** be sent to the lab. He was a teacher in a parochial school and feared the results would be revealed. His sample was set aside, but the laboratory courier mistakenly took it for testing. The result was positive, yet no one could tell the patient. A malpractice attorney said to make certain all records of the test were deleted and to send the patient a letter urging him to return for a blood test. He never appeared (Wake, 1989).

Many national public health agencies and committees favor a confidential screening and counseling program that includes all individuals whose behavior places them at high risk of HIV exposure. These agencies recommend that the following eight groups seriously consider volunteering for periodic HIV-antibody testing:

1. Homosexual and bisexual men
2. Present or past injection drug users

CIVIL LIBERTIES VERSUS SAVING LIVES

Nowhere was the trade-off between civil liberties and saving lives more vivid than in the 1994 session of the New York State Legislature. Two bills were proposed: One would have required doctors to notify parents of the results of the HIV tests now performed anonymously on all newborns. The other bill would have set up a counseling program urging mothers to find out the status of their infants. Neither was passed.

Objections to the first bill came from AIDS activists and civil libertarians who argued that, since an HIV-positive newborn always has an HIV-positive mother, telling a mother the results of her child's HIV test would violate her right to privacy. It was also opposed by a subcommittee of the state's AIDS Advisory Council, which said care cannot be mandated "through coercion."

A DIFFERENT PERSPECTIVE

Some pediatricians see the problem differently. They say that the tempo of HIV infection in ba-

bies does not offer the luxury of persuasion. At six weeks, an HIV-p[ositive infant may look normal but be desperately in need of drug treatment. Some children infected at birth are now living until age 13 or 14. If it is known that the mother is HIV-positive and the infant is also, it will not be lost in the first months. If it is not known the baby dies.

While the debate centers on testing at birth, a far better time to test mothers and inform them of the results would be during pregnancy. If HIV-positive women were identified while pregnant, found and treated, it might be possible to prevent some of their infants from becoming infected. In February of 1994, a joint French-American clinical trial showed a 67.5% reduction in transmission risk among infants whose mothers began taking zidovudine during pregnancy. The numbers are not insignificant: each year, nearly 7,000 HIV-positive mothers deliver babies in the United States, and about 25% to 30% of their infants become infected with the virus.

3. People with signs or symptoms of HIV infection
4. Male and female prostitutes
5. Sexual partners of people either known to be HIV-infected or at increased risk of HIV infection
6. Hemophiliacs who received blood clotting products prior to 1985
7. Newborn children of HIV-infected mothers
8. Emigrants from Haiti and Central Africa since 1977

The Public's Question— The situation surrounding confidentiality for patients infected with HIV is comparable to circumstances that

LEGISLATURE SURVEY OF STATE CONFIDENTIALITY LAWS (Hooker, 1996)

1. At least 39 states have laws providing for the confidentiality of HIV/AIDS-related information. At least 28 states have laws that specifically regulate medical records. The remaining states may protect confidentiality of HIV information under other statutes.

2. Almost every state allows for disclosure of HIV-related information in certain circumstances, according to a recent report on state confidentiality laws. The most frequently cited permission to disclose is given to a health care provider involved with a patient's care, to blood banks and under a subpoena or court order. Almost all states allow disclosure of data to epidemiologists and re-

searchers, with provisions for removal of information that may identify the patient. Most states have penalties for unauthorized disclosure of information.

3. Most states impose a duty on physicians and health care institutions to maintain the confidentiality of medical records. About half the states extend this duty to other health care providers. Only four states have specific legislation imposing the duty on insurance companies and few states impose a similar duty on employers or other nonhealth care institutions. Fewer than half the states have specific laws imposing a duty to maintain confidentiality of electronic or computerized medical records.

─────── BOX 13.9 ───────

LACK OF CONFIDENTIALITY AND PATIENT HARM

In 1985, I was the primary physician for a young man whose life was ruined by the inappropriate disclosure of a positive HIV test result. A physician ordered the test without consent and notified the local health department of the positive result. The health department notified the individual's employer and he was fired. The event became common knowledge in his rural Midwestern town and he was shunned. His landlord asked him to move. Ten days after testing the life he had known for the past 10 years was permanently ruined and he left town. With the loss of his job came the loss of health insurance and insurability; he has been unable to obtain health or life insurance since then.

In this case, no purpose was served by taking the HIV antibody test. The patient had been diagnosed with AIDS based on the presence of opportunistic infections 6 months earlier at a County Hospital. He was aware of his diagnosis and its implications. He had been following safe sex guidelines for the preceding 18 months and had never donated blood or semen. (A case report by Renslow Sherer, 1988.)

A similar event happened in Jacksonville, Florida in late 1990. A young man diagnosed with AIDS moved to Jacksonville and enrolled in an area HIV/AIDS clinic. Somehow his employer found out that he was visiting the clinic and receiving zidovudine. The man was fired , asked to move out of his apartment, new friends shunned him, and he had to move out of state.

In 1996, a coalition of groups that help HIV/AIDS patients in Boston went to court in an effort to stop auditors at the Department of Health and Human Services from passing on the names of patients in various AIDS programs to other government agencies.

In short, medical records contain some of the most sensitive of personal information–including sexual orientation, past drug use, and genetic predisposition to various diseases. As part of the Hippocratic oath, physicians promise to keep whatever they learn about a patient to themselves. But it's hard to keep a secret if more than a couple of people are in on it; in a typical five-day stay at a teaching hospital, as many as 150 people–from nursing staff to X-ray technicians to billing clerks–have legitimate access to a single patient's records.

Now hospitals are rushing to computerize those records, raising the fear that medical secrets could be accessed copied, and distributed with a few clicks of a mouse.

---

dictate our reporting of sexually transmitted diseases and cancer. The reason for reporting these cases to the CDC is that valuable epidemiological data may be gathered. These data can then be used to document geographical location, prevalence, routes of transmission, and those groups of people that may be at highest risk for these diseases. If these diseases are reportable for the ultimate benefit of individuals susceptible to sexually transmitted diseases and cancer, shouldn't HIV-postive people be reportable for the same reasons? It is questions such as this that are bringing about a change in public opinion concerning confidential HIV testing and use of test results.

In a mid-1989 poll taken by the Media General-Associated Press, 72% of Americans opposed strict confidentiality of HIV tests, favoring mandatory notification of spouses and health officials. In addition, 67% said the physician receiving the test results should be required to notify local or state public health officials (Figure 13-9).

The poll included 1,084 adults interviewed by telephone. Phone numbers were selected at random and the person interviewed was the adult who had the most recent birthday. About one in five of the respondents said they personally knew someone who was HIV-infected or had died of AIDS. The poll showed a growing social acceptance of individuals with AIDS compared to interviews in 1985.

About 75% said people with AIDS should be entitled to keep their jobs; and 80% said children who have AIDS shoud be admitted to school. Some 52% thought AIDS was likely to spread widely beyond current risk groups, while only 11% thought they were at great risk or some risk of getting AIDS; 23% thought they were at "not much risk" and 64% said "no risk at all." Two percent were unsure.

———— BOX 13.10 ————

CONFIDENTIALITY AND SEXUAL PARTNER BETRAYAL

This story took place in an HIV/AIDS clinic in the South. A husband and wife came into the clinic for an HIV test. They said the *only* reason for requesting the test was that they wanted to begin a family and hoped that nothing in their past would have led to either of them being HIV-positive. The test were completed.

The husband came in on a Monday; the wife came in that Friday.

Monday A.M.

Counselor: Mr. X, your test came back HIV-positive.

Reactions and counseling were similar to those presented in this chapter. Then MR. X said he wanted to be the one to tell his wife; **he insisted on it**. The counselor agreed, Mr. X left the clinic agreeing to come back for a follow-up counseling session.

Friday A.M.

Counselor: Mrs. X, your HIV test was negative.

Mrs. X: That's wonderful news. I can't wait to tell my husband. We've been waiting for my results. I want to get pregnant immediately.

Mrs. X received HIV-negative counseling and left the clinic very happy.

Quite clearly, the husband did not tell his wife the truth about his test results. A follow-up phone call to the husband went unanswered; so did a letter from the clinic. Several months later, Mrs. X called the counselor to tell her that she was pregnant!

Question: What do you think the counselor should do now?

1. Inform the woman about her husband.
2. Take no action.
3. Call the husband and discuss the situtation.
4. Threaten the husband with legal action if he does not tell his wife.
5. Your position!

Discuss the moral, ethical, and legal responsibilities of each participant.

Anonymous HIV Testing— This is also a form of voluntary testing. It differs from confidential testing only in that those who request anonymity receive a bar coded identification number. They provide no personal information and they come back at a predetermined time to find out if their test number is positive or negative. No follow-up occurs. The number of tests conducted at anonymous test sites has increased from 79,000 in 1985 to more than 2 million for each of the years 1994, 1995, 1996, and 1997.

Blinded HIV Testing— This occurs when blood or serum is available for HIV testing as a result of another medical procedure wherein the patient's blood has been drawn for analysis. In this case, the demographic data have been recorded and can be used for epidemiological studies even if the name of the individual is withheld and a bar code is used. In 1988, the CDC asked for a blinded study of all 1989 newborn blood samples taken in certain cities in 45 states for metabolic studies.

The name and other demographics of each newborn were recorded on the label of each tube. After the metabolic tests were completed, the name was changed into a bar code and leftover blood was sent to a state HIV testing center.

New York began a study of this type in 1987. Since then, New York has blind-tested about 250,000 newborns. The statewide incidence rate for HIV-infected newborns is 0.7%, or seven per 1,000. The incidence is 1.3% in New York City, between 0.1% to 0.2% for upstate New York, and close to 2% in the Bronx.

In May of 1995, and for a period of several months, the Department of Health and Human Services suspended all blinded HIV testing of newborns. The reason was that Representative Gary Ackerman, D-N.Y., introduced legislation, the Newborn Infant Notification Act (HR 1289), that would require that mothers of HIV-exposed children be told of the test results. According to Ackermen and supporters, the bill was to protect the health

The question asked was:

If a blood test shows someone is infected with HIV, should the doctor be required to notify...

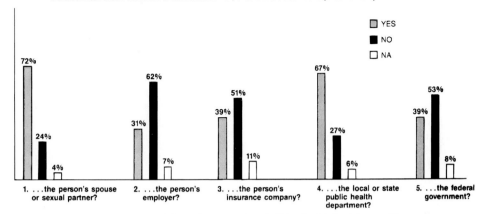

FIGURE 13-9 Confidentiality Opinion Poll in the United States. The poll was conducted by telephone for Media General-Associated Press in May 1989. The poll has a 3 point margin for error meaning that 19 times out of 20 findings should be accurate within 3 points if every adult American were asked the same questions.

and rights of the newborn/infants exposed to HIV. The pro and con arguments were many but in the end, the bill was withdrawn.

For class discussion: Present reasons for and against the Ackerman bill one of each is provided to get you started.

Pro: The state health department reports 17% of pregnant women agree to be tested, 24% know their HIV status, and the rest have unknown HIV status.

Con: Some people have argued that only mandatory testing will give mothers the information to do what's best for themselves and their babies. But, mandatory testing would not prevent HIV in children. This would be too little too late.

SUMMARY

HIV infection can be detected in two ways: first, by HIV-antibody testing prior to the signs and symptoms of AIDS; and second, by physical examination after symptoms occur.

The test most often used to screen donor blood at blood banks and individuals referred to testing centers is the ELISA test. ELISA (enzyme-linked immunosorbent assay) is a highly sensitive and specific test that determines the presence of HIV antibodies in a person's blood or serum. The ELISA test was first used in 1985 to reduce the number of HIV-infected blood units for blood transfusions.

Because the ELISA test is only a predictive test which gives the percentage chance that a person is truly positive or truly negative, serum from those who test positive is retested in duplicate. If still positive, the serum is then subjected to a Western blot (WB) test. The WB is a confirmatory test. If it is also positive, the person is said to be HIV-infected.

Other screening and confirmatory tests are available. The indirect immunofluorescent antibody assay (IFA) is relatively quick and easy to perform. Although it can be used as a screening test, it is generally used as a confirmatory test. The test is similar to the ELISA test except that the analysis is made by looking for a fluorescent color, indicating the presence of HIV antibodies, with a dark field light microscope.

The Recombigen HIV-1 Latex Agglutination test requires no special equipment and can be performed in 5 minutes. This test can be a major contribution in Third World countries that do not have the equipment or trained personnel to run ELISA and WB tests.

The polymerase chain reaction (PCR) is a process wherein a few molecules of HIV proviral DNA can be amplified into a sufficient mass of DNA to be detected by current testing methods. It can determine if newborns of HIV-infected mothers are truly HIV-positive. The branched-DNA assay offers a means of detecting the presence of HIV RNA directly within the clinical sample.

Gene probes are also being used to detect small HIV proviral DNA sequences in cells of people who are HIV-infected but not yet making antibodies.

The CDC recommends that pregnant women and people in high-risk groups volunteer for HIV testing if there is any reason to suspect they may have been exposed. Broad-scale testing in low-risk populations is not advocated because the rate of false positives rises with decreasing rates of HIV infections.

In June 1996, New York became the first state to pass legislation allowing for mandatory HIV testing of all newborns and disclosure of their HIV status to mothers and physicians. This action was quickly followed by the American Medical Association's endorsement of mandatory HIV testing of all pregnant women and newborns.

Many people have voiced opinions that HIV testing should be mandatory for all people in high-risk groups. They believe that identifying HIV carriers is the way to stop HIV transmission. However, mandatory premarital testing has failed to stop the spread of syphilis. But, nearly everyone agrees that voluntary HIV testing and counseling should be available to anyone who wants it. For those who want to be tested, there are at least two routes to consider: voluntary confidential and voluntary anonymous. In the first, people give their names and addresses and the test results become a confidential part of their medical records. In the latter, no personal identification information is asked for; a bar code (number) is used to label the blood sample.

REVIEW QUESTIONS

(Answers to the Review Questions are on page 579.)

1. What is the acronym for the most commonly used HIV-antibody test and what does each letter stand for?

2. What basic immunological assumption is this test based on?

3. Does a single positive HIV antibody result mean the person is HIV-infected? Explain.

4. Is there a specific test for AIDS? Explain.

5. What is currently the most frequently used HIV confirmatory test in the United States?

6. What is the name of one additional confirmatory test in use in the United States?

7. How is HIV antibody detected in the ELISA test?

8. True or False: All newborns who are antibody positive are HIV-infected and all go on to develop AIDS. Explain.

9. What is the greatest shortcoming of the ELISA and WB tests?

10. What are the two major problems in interpreting ELISA test results?

11. What two factors may account for false-positive and false-negative results?

12. What is the relationship between false-positive results and prevalence of HIV in the population?

13. In an HIV screening test, what is a positive predictive value? Why is it called a predictive value?

14. What is the current gold standard of confirmatory tests in the United States?

15. What is the major problem in using this test?

16. Why is the polymerase chain reaction (PCR) considered so useful in HIV testing? Name two situations when PCR can be significant in HIV testing.

17. True or False: Two home use HIV-antibody test kits are now available in the United States.

18. Using the ELISA test, when are HIV antibodies first detectable?

19. How early are HIV antigens detectable in human serum?

20. What are three benefits of early identification of HIV-infected people?

21. Name the four kinds of testing privacy available to people who want to take an HIV test.

22. What is the major difference between an anonymous and a blind HIV test?

23. Why would someone want an anonymous test?

24. True or False: The ELISA serological test is adequate to confirm HIV infection.

25. True or False: Pre- and post-HIV-antibody test counseling is recommended any time an HIV-antibody test is performed.

REFERENCES

AIDS Alert. (1994). AZT study reinvigorates debate over mandatory testing. 9:133–135.

AIDS, Health and Human Rights. (1995). Francois-Xavier Bagnoud Center for Health and Human Rights–Harvard School of Public Health, pp. 1–162.

ALLEN, BRADY. (1991). The role of the primary care physician in HIV testing and early stage disease management. *Fam. Pract. Recert.,* 13:30– 49.

ANDERSON JOHN, et al. (1992). HIV antibody testing and post-test counseling in the United States: Data from the 1989 National Health Interview Study. *Am J Public Health,* 82:1533–1535.

ANGELL, MARCIA. (1991). A dual approach to the AIDS epidemic. *N. Engl. J. Med.,* 324:1498–1500.

BAYER RONALD et al. (1995).Testing for HIV infection at home (Sounding Board). *N. Engl.J. Med.,* 332:1296–1299.

BELONGIA, EDWARD A., et al. (1989). Premarital HIV screening *JAMA,* 261:2198.

CARLSON, DESIREE A., et al. (1989). Testing for HIV risk from therapeutic blood products. In: *Pathology and Pathophysiology of AIDS and HIV Related Diseases* (Eds. Jami J. Harawi and Carl J. O'Hara), St. Louis: C.V. Mosby Co.

CLEZY, K., et al. (1992). AIDS-related secondary infections in patients with unknown HIV status. *AIDS,* 6:879–893.

CONSTANTINE, NIEL T. (1993). Serologic tests for the retroviruses:Approaching a decade of evolution. *AIDS,* 7:1–13.

CORDES, ROBERT, et al. (1995). Pitfalls in HIV testing. *Postgrad. Med.,* 98:177–189.

DEL RIO, CARLOS, et al. (1996). The use of oral fluid to determine HIV prevalence rates among men in Mexico City. *AIDS,* 10:233–234.

DEWAR,ROBIN, et al. (1994). Application of branched DNA signal amplification to monitor HIV-I type burden in human plasma. *J. Infect. Dis.,* 170:1172–1179.

EL-SADR, WAFAA, et al. (1994). Managing early HIV infection: Agency for Health Care Policy and Research. *Clinical Practice Guideline on Evaluation and Management of Early HIV Infection.* January, 7:1–37.

EL-SAHR, W., et al. (1994). *Managing Early HIV Infection: Quick Reference Guide for Clinicians.* AHCPR Publication No. 94-0573. Rockville, MD.

EMMONS, WESLEY, et al. (1995). A modified Elisa and Western Blot accurately determine anti-human HIV-I antibodies in oral fluids obtained with a special collecting device. *J. Infect. Dis.,* 171:1406–1410.

FANG, CHYANG T., et al. (1989). HIV testing and patient counseling. *Patient Care,* 23:19–44.

FRERICHS, RALPH R., et al. (1994). Saliva-based HIV-antibody testing in Thailand. *AIDS,* 8:885–894.

GALLO, DANA, et al. (1997). Testing oral secretions for HIV. *AIDS Clin.Care,* 9:26.

GOLDSCHMIDT, PAUL. (1993). Systematic screening for HIV infection. *AIDS,* 7:740–741.

HARTLAUB, PAUL, et al. (1993). Obtaining informed consent: It is not simply asking "do you understand?", *J. Fam. Pract.,* 36:383–384.

HARVARD AIDS INSTITUTE, (1995). Mandatory HIV testing: the search for a quick fix. *Harvard AIDS Letter,* May/June:4–8.

HEGARTY, J.D., et al. (1988). The medical care costs of human immunodeficiency virsu infected children in Harlem. *JAMA,* 260:1901–1905.

HOOKER, TRACEY. (1996). HIV/AIDS: Facts to consider—1996. Natural conference of State Legislatures, February, pp. 1–64.

HORN, THOMAS, et al. (1989). Forks and combs and DNA: the synthesis of branched oligodeoxyribonucleotides. *Nucleic Acids Res.* 17:6959–67.

HU, DALE, et al. (1996). The emerging genetic diversity of HIV. *JAMA,* 275:210–216.

Intergovernmental AIDS Report. (1989). Illinois court overrules mandatory HIV testing for prostitutes and sex offenders, 2:1–18.

JAFFE, HAROLD, et al. (1994). Reducing the risk of maternal-infant transmission of HIV: a door is opened. *N. Eng. J. Med.,* 331:1222.

KELLER, G.H., et al. (1988). Identification of HIV sequences using nucleic acid probes. *Am. Clin. Lab.,* 7:10–15.

KRAMER, F.R., et al. (1989). Replicatable RNA reporters. *Nature,* 339:401–402.

MACKENZIE, WILLIAM R., et al. (1992). Multiple false positive serologic tests for HIV, HTLV-1 and hepatitis C following influenza vaccination, 1991. *JAMA,* 268:1015–1017.

Medical Tribune. (1991). Beware of blanket AIDS solutions. June:14.

MERCOLA, JOSEPH M. (1989). Premarital HIV screening. *JAMA,* 261:2198.

MIIKE, LAWRENCE. (1987). *AIDS Antibody Testing.* Office of Technological Assessment Testimony To The U.S. Congress. Oct.:1–21.

MILES, STEVEN A., et al. (1993). Rapid serologic testing with immune-complex-dissociated HIV p24 antigen for early detection of HIV infection in neonates. *N. Engl. J. Med.,* 328:297–302.

Morbidity and Mortality Weekly Report. (1988a). Update: Serologic testing for antibody to human immunodeficiency virus. 36:833–840.

Morbidity and Mortality Weekly Report. (1988b). HIV infection reporting—United States. 38:496–499.

Morbidity and Mortality Weekly Report. (1992). Testing for antibodies to HIV-2 in the United States. 41:1–9.

Morbidity and Mortality Weekly Report. (1995).U.S. Public Health Service recommendations for HIV counseling and voluntary testing for pregnant women. 44:1–12.

Morbidity and Mortality Weekly Report. (1996). U.S. Public Health Service Guidelines for testing and counseling blood and plasma donors for HIV type I antigen. 45:1–9.

MULLIS, KARY B., et al. (1987). Process for amplifying, detecting, and/or cloning nucleic acid sequences. (U.S. Patent No. 4,683,195). *Official Gazette of the U.S. Patient and Trademark Office*, Volume 1080, Issue 4, July.

PASSANNANTE, MARIAN R., et al. (1993). Responses of health care professionals to proposed mandatory HIV testing. *Arch. Fam. Med.*, 2:38–44.

PHILLIPS KATHRYN, et al. (1995a).Potential use of home HIV testing. *N. Engl. J. Med.*, 332:1308–1310.

PHILLIPS KATHRYN, et al. (1995b).Who plans to be tested for HIV or would get tested if no one could find out the results? *Am. J. Prevent. Med.*, 11(3): 156.

RHAME, FRANK S., et al. (1989). The case for wider use of testing for HIV infection. *N. Engl. J. Med.*, 320:1242–1254.

ROGERS, MARTHA F., et al. (1989). Use of the polymerase chain reaction for early detection of the proviral sequences of human immunodeficiency virus in infants born to seropositive mothers. *N. Engl. J. Med.*, 320:1649–1654.

SAX, PAUL, et al. (1997). Novel approaches to HIV antibody testing. *AIDS Clin. Care*, 9:1–5.

SCHEFFEL, J.W. (1990). Retrocell HIV-1 passive haemagglutination assay for HIV-1 antibody screening. *J. Acquired Immune Deficiency Syndromes*, 3:540–545.

SCHOPPER, DORIS, et al. (1996). Testing for HIV at home: what are the issues? *AIDS*, 10:1455–1465.

URDEA, MICKEY. (1993). Synthesis and characterization of branched DNA (bDNA) for the direct and quantitative detection of CMV, HBV, HCV, and HIV. *Clin. Chem.*, 39:725–726.

WAKE, WILLIAM T. (1989). How many patients will die because we fear AIDS? *Med. Econ.*, 66:24–30.

WOFOY, C. B. (1987). HIV infection in women. *JAMA*, 257:2074–2076.

Counseling for HIV Testing, HIV Disease, and AIDS

CHAPTER CONCEPTS

♦ Some states now have mandated pre- and post-HIV test counseling for everyone who wants to take the test.

♦ Through 1998, over 21 million people ages 18 to 65 were HIV-tested in the United States.

♦ Drug abusers present special problems for HIV counselors.

♦ It is important to establish sexual preference.

♦ Counselors must prepare the counselee for both a positive and negative test result.

♦ Lack of confidentiality remains the most serious objection to HIV testing.

♦ The major problem of confidentiality is: To whom does the physician or counselor have the greater moral obligation—the HIV-positive patient or others the patient may place in danger?

♦ Does the public have a right to know who is HIV-infected?

A disease is a condition of the body **but it affects the human spirit as well**. If you live with aches, pains, stiffness, and fatigue, if you are physically limited in what you can do, if your appearance has changed, and if, in addition, you fear for your life, your thoughts and feelings about yourself and others are inevitably affected. Distressful thoughts and feelings about yourself and others can undermine your life as much as, or even more than, your illness. Emotional stress can be reduced through proper counseling.

COUNSELING FOR HIV TESTING

Perhaps more than any other disease, AIDS is about human interactions. HIV is transmitted during the most intimate moments. Diagnosis results in immediate and powerful emotional responses, often long before physical symptoms occur. At the moment, medical care and emotional and practical support are the only weapons available in the fight against HIV/AIDS.

The greatest need at the present time is effective counseling of those at both high and low risk of HIV infection. Several million Americans have already been tested for the presence of HIV antibodies. According to medical health counselors, even considering whether to be tested often constitutes a crisis in a person's life, a crisis that becomes monumental if the test results are positive. Given the complexity of the testing process and its social implications, a number of state health departments require that pre- and post-test counseling accompany all HIV-antibody testing.

State regulations on the issue of counseling HIV test clients vary widely and the definition of adequate counseling remains imprecise. HIV/AIDS counseling should cover the **purpose**, **limitations**, **risks**, and **benefits** of testing.

CDC-Supported Counseling and Testing Centers

The Centers for Disease Control and Prevention (CDC) provides support to 65 HIV-prevention programs through health departments in 50 states, eight territories, and the District of Columbia. The critical component of the CDC's prevention program is support for HIV counseling and testing services (CTS). For each calendar quarter for the 65 programs, data are collected by project areas and reported either in aggregate form or individual client records (without identifiers). Information is collected during pre- and post-test counseling sessions on: (**1**) age, sex, race/ethnicity, and risk behavior; (**2**) risk category; and (**3**) type of testing site. Sites include specialized sites for HIV CTS, sexually transmitted disease clinics, family planning clinics, drug treatment centers, and correctional facilities. Project areas determine what type and which sites provide HIV CTS. By 1994, there were over 9,000 CTS listed in the 65 project areas that provide publicly funded HIV counseling and testing.

From 1985 through 1994, the programs performed approximately 13.8 million HIV-antibody tests. About 2.4 million HIV tests were performed each year from 1995 through 1997;

1.8% were positive. In 1990, the 65 programs accounted for 1.4 millions tests; 3.7% were positive. In 1991, the federal government allocated $100 million to state and local health agencies to provide testing and counseling programs in public clinics. Additional financial support has been provided through 1998.

PURPOSE

Primary HIV Counseling Objective

Regardless of the person's HIV-antibody status, the primary objective of counseling is to provide an education that will help people avoid behaviors which may place them or others at risk of infection. Ideally, counseling should reduce anxiety, alleviate depression, lessen self-destructive impulses, and help people cope with the mental and physical stress associated with the need to be tested. A 1993 CDC report states that, although it is unlikely that a single episode of HIV counseling will result in the immediate and permanent adoption of safer behaviors, **client-centered** HIV counseling and attendant prevention services (i.e., referral and partner notification) do contribute to the initiation and maintenance of safe behaviors. A 1995 CDC report indicates that only 61% of people being tested for HIV at publicly funded sites and 28% at private sites were being counseled (*MMWR*, 1995). What will happen, with regard to the amount of testing and counseling, now that the FDA has approved **the use of home testing kits** is anybody's guess. Can telephone counseling be as effective as face-to-face counseling given at a HIV/AIDS clinic or physician's office? It may not be, but it may be enough. (See Box 13.4.)

Client-Centered Counseling

To fulfill its public health functions, HIV counseling must be client-centered; that is, tailored to the behaviors, circumstances, and special needs of the person being served. Risk-reduction messages must be personalized and realistic. Counseling should be:

1. Culturally competent (i.e., program services provided in a style and format sensitive to cultural norms, values, and traditions that are endorsed

by cultural leaders and accepted by the target population);

2. Sensitive to issues of sexual identity;

3. Developmentally appropriate (i.e., information and services provided at a level of comprehension that is consistent with the age and the learning skills of the person being served); and

4. Linguistically specific (i.e., information is presented in dialect and terminology consistent with the client's language and style of communication).

Counseling should be provided not only in **terms** and **language** that people understand, but also, it should progress at a speed that is comfortable for the individual.

HIV counseling **is not a lecture**. An important aspect of HIV counseling is the counselor's **ability to listen** to the client in order to provide assistance and to determine specific prevention needs.

Although HIV counseling should adhere to minimal standards in terms of providing basic information, it should not become so routine that it is inflexible or unresponsive to particular client needs. **Counselors should avoid providing information that is irrelevant to their clients and should avoid structuring counseling sessions on the basis of a data collection instrument or form.**

Counseling HIV-infected persons and per-

sons with AIDS can induce all kinds of feelings, including ones we do not always enjoy having—fear, repugnance, revulsion, anger, despair, resentment, hopelessness. The feelings themselves are not the problem, but a lack of awareness and understanding of these feelings means they can become obstacles to effectively and compassionately counseling those most in need.

Counseling Anecdotes on Language, Terms, and Attitudes

1. A heterosexual client at an HIV/AIDS clinic and the counselor became involved in a discussion of the client's sexual behavior. The counselor was concerned and somewhat confused when the client insisted that anal intercourse was **not** a risky sexual behavior. The counselor responded with a set of facts that led to the inescapable conclusion that anal intercourse was a **very risky** sexual behavior. The client said, "Gee, you wouldn't think that having sex **once a year** would place you at high-risk for HIV infection!" It was immediately obvious to the counselor that the client's lack of understanding resulted from confusing the words **annual** and **anal**.

2. A counselor said to a young woman during a conversation on HIV infection, "You know how one comes in contact with the virus during sex—you get it from coming into contact with **semen**. The woman responded, "Oh, I'm safe then. I don't have sex with sailors." (She obviously thought the counselor said seamen.)

3. A young woman was told by her Ob/Gyn that she was in danger of contracting HIV infection because she was **sexually active**. She responded, **"No sir, I'm not sexually active. I lie very still when I'm having sex."** (Clearly this young woman misunderstood the meaning of the term "sexually active" in the clinical setting.)

4. During the completion of a sexual behavior questionnaire, the physician asked, "Do you have **sex** with other men?" "No," said the man. The physician, not quite sure of that response, followed up with, "Has a man's penis ever entered your anus or rectum?" To which the man responded, "Oh, well, yes—many times, but that's a job for me. When I want **sex**, I have it with a woman!"

5. "At the hospital where I received treatment, the charts of HIV/AIDS clients are marked in big red letters so your confidentiality is gone. If you have

---

——————— BOX 14.1 ———————

COUNSELING MY FIRST HIV-POSITIVE PATIENT

Betty needed post-test counseling; she was HIV-positive. Sitting behind my desk, I dryly reviewed the implications of the test results and didn't let her get a word in edgewise.

She never came back for a follow-up appointment. She refused to return phone calls.

I reached Betty about a year later. She told me she had been disappointed and angry about my cold presentation of the facts and my apparent lack of interest in her feelings.

She taught me the need for better communication, and she taught me the need to be flexible in dealing with HIV-positive patients. Thank you, Betty.

---

a complaint to report, a concern about your health, often you are not taken seriously. They seem to be saying, 'Why are you complaining? What did you expect?' or 'This is nothing compared to what you'll be dealing with in the future, so why not just forget about this little problem?' Often you get no explanation about what they think is wrong or about your treatment. On one occasion, a physician and his group of residents entered my room; he looked at my chart and said, while looking at the residents rather than looking at me, **'Sex or Drugs?'** I knew he was trying to group or classify me with respect to my at-risk behavior. He repeated his dictatorial catch phrase, **'Sex or Drugs?'** to which I replied, '**Excuse me**—I don't do drugs anymore, and sex with you—I don't think so!'"

Counselors should aid people who want to be tested by reinforcing positive feelings and by encouraging them to recall successful responses to previous stressful events in their lives. These responses can then be used as signals for handling situations that may arise.

LIMITATIONS

Pre-test HIV Procedures

Pre-test HIV counseling provides an opportunity for the counselor to educate people who believe they have a need to be tested.

Front-Loaded Counseling

This means doing as much of the counseling as possible during the pre-test session. Typically some people **never** come back for **post-test** counseling. For those who do come back for test results and post-test counseling, they hear and remember only one word—**negative** or **positive**. After the result, they are likely to be overwhelmed by emotions. Pre-test procedures can be separated into three areas: **(1)** education; **(2)** taking sexual behavior and drug history information; and **(3)** counseling.

Education—Counselors should use available information on the epidemiology of HIV infection pitched at a level that can be understood. They should cover the routes of HIV transmission, methods of reducing risk, and methods of

testing. This information can be presented in a variety of ways: printed material, a group lecture format, or audio- and videotapes. The topics that ought to be presented according to the **1988 American Medical Association Physician's Guidelines** are listed in Table 14-1. This list of topics covers the spectrum of information necessary for a good education on HIV infection, the damage it creates, how it is transmitted, and how to avoid infection.

Sexual Behavior and Drug History—If more than one person is attending the general education session, after group session information is provided, participants should be told that the remaining part of the pre-test procedure

TABLE 14-1 Pre-test Educational Information

1. AIDS is caused by a virus called human immunodeficiency virus or HIV.
2. HIV infects the body and gradually damages the immune system.
3. The AIDS virus is spread by the exchange of blood, semen, and possibly vaginal secretions during sexual intercourse.
4. The concept of high-risk vs. low-risk HIV exposure situations.
5. Groups of people are considered to be at high-risk because of their sexual and drug use behaviors.
6. The AIDS virus is spread through the exchange of blood when syringes and intravenous drug needles are shared.
7. Prior to 1985, when blood screening began, the virus was spread through transfusion of infected blood.
8. Infected pregnant women can pass on the virus to their unborn children.
9. The AIDS virus is not spread by casual contact.
10. Abstinence or monogamy among partners known to be uninfected provides the surest protection against sexual transmission.
11. The more sexual partners one has, the greater the risk of exposure.
12. Unprotected sex with partners who have AIDS, who are antibody-positive, or who have engaged in high-risk behaviors is dangerous and should be avoided.
13. The proper use of a latex or polyurethane condom during intercourse provides protection because it minimizes direct contact with bodily fluids.
14. Sexual activities that could cause cuts or tears in the lining of the rectum, penis, or vagina should be avoided.
15. Having sex with male or female prostitutes should be avoided.
16. Sharing needles or syringes with anyone should be avoided.

———— BOX 14.2 ————

CULTURE-BASED COMPETENCE

ONE MALE'S EXPERIENCE: MICHAEL HELQUIST

"Nothing from my experience of 10 years of working with AIDS prepared me for the shock, confusion, and depression that came with my diagnosis of *Pneumocystis carinii* pneumonia (PCP). It wasn't for lack of familiarity that I felt so ill-equipped. I had lost a lover to AIDS in 1983—he was one of the first 100 people with AIDS in San Francisco. There have been far too many other losses since: best friends, colleagues, roommates. For many of them I had been a primary caregiver. I knew about the devastation HIV disease brings upon others. I didn't have a clue about the devastation it would bring upon me.

"AIDS, in the form of PCP, came at me like a **hard**, **cold slap** in the face that knocked me to the floor. The shock I might have expected, but I could not have anticipated the confusing and threatening mix of new emotions. Two and one half years later, I continue to be jolted by the onset of new infections and disabilities. Now, however, I am less surprised about what I do not understand. I know that I have to work very hard to grasp what is happening to someone else with AIDS, ostensibly in the same predicament but, in reality, facing a condition different from mine. I recognize that my knowledge of the emotional and psychic effects of HIV infection is limited mostly to my own experience with the disease. [Regardless of the disease, each of us deals with it separately and differently.]"

I believe that other AIDS professionals, in-cluding mental health practitioners, even those with many years of experience, may very well be in the same position. Just because we provide counseling to people with HIV disease, or lead group discussions, or write papers for publication, or generally talk AIDS does not mean we understand the experience [others are having]. In the end, I have found that familiarity with AIDS is not enough. Michael Helquist (1996) said that he feared that as providers immersed themselves in the epidemic, they may develop an overblow sense of their knowledge and fail to help others who differ. We need to help others in the context of their cultural experiences. Counselors must become culturally competent!

CULTURE COMPETENCE

Recently, counselors have begun to question whether competence in the field, that is, having the necessary and essential knowledge of the material, is sufficient to be as effective as one can be. **Competence *per se*, may not be enough.** Robert Marks (1996) suggests that counselors must take active steps toward learning about and understanding other experiences. To be most effective, counselor and client must share cultural experiences, whether it is being gay, or a woman, or African American. As an example, Stephen Ball offers a brief history of gay-affirmative counseling and relates cultural competence guidance in a situation where the counselor is HIV-positive and the counselee is HIV-negative (serodiscordant). Ball suggests in this case (or the reverse) that competence alone is not sufficient to respond to the shame and isolation faced by people who have been systematically marginalized by society.

It has been difficult for HIV-negative people living in communities hard hit by the epidemic to convince a skeptical public that they need emotional support to deal with multiple loss, post-traumatic stress syndrome, and survivor guilt. As incredible as it may seem to some, people who live through a plague face real psychological problems, and overlooking them poses a real threat to the community as a whole. Ball is suggesting that **if** the HIV-negative counselor was, in fact, a gay person of high behavioral risk or who perhaps lost a lover to HIV, the counselor would be better able to culture identify with the client. **WHAT IS YOUR OPINION ON THE CULTURE COMPETENCE APPROACH?**

AN EXAMPLE OF CULTURE-BASED NEEDS BY A COUNSELEE (CLIENT)

"As I write these words, my mind drifts towards yesterday. It was 8:00 AM. I got to work early. You know, a report always has to be completed for someone. And it must be done now! **The telephone rings.** An urgent sound that vibrated across the quietness. A startled sound.

"Can you come to the clinic right now?'
"No, there isn't anyone else here.'

———— **BOX 14.2** (*continued*) ————

"Half an hour later, a knock on the door. Hesitant. Then sharper. **THEN URGENT.**

"Later that morning, I look at my computer words sprawling across the screen. I look back. Tears are running down my face.

"I have just had my test results this afternoon. I am HIV-positive. This was not just a quiet internal statement, it is a soft cry of anguish.

"Why did I have a test?

"I recently heard this HIV-prevention presentation at a meeting. I have sex with men. It's always been, well, you know, **unsafe**. **But**, I thought since I only have sex with **Asians**, I would be safe.

"What followed for me was a period of release of pain and of fear. What do I do? I am to be married, an Asian family, arranged marriage. I am 22 years old. Who do I tell? What happens now? Thoughts of suicide enter my mind.

"The clinic offered me some sort of post-counseling, but they didn't understand my needs, my issues. Yes I can speak English, I was English educated, but my needs as an Asian are so different. My fears are different. They (the counselors) couldn't understand.

"We talk and cry together. The pain, the fear, the need. Yet my counselor fails to understand our cultural differences!"

is **confidential** and will be conducted one-on-one and face-to-face.

Sometimes a client will request permission to have another person present during the counseling session. Many people find support and added comfort in a friend's presence. In some cases, however, the client may have been coerced. The counselor may, through a series of questions, determine why the other person is present and proceed from that point.

During the **face-to-face** session, the counselor must ask specific questions about the client's sexual behavior and drug use because the counselor needs to assess the client's risk of exposure to HIV through sex and injection drug use (IDU). **NEVER IMPLY THERE IS A RIGHT ANSWER!** An opening statement such as the following could be helpful: "As you know, HIV and other sexually transmitted diseases can be "caught" or transmitted through unprotected sexual contact and IDU. In order to assess any possible exposure to HIV through sex or IDU that you may have experienced, I need to ask specific questions about your sex life and your use of drugs. **Is that all right with you?**

———— **POINT OF VIEW 14.1** ————

SEX AND HIV

Talking about sex is almost as tricky as talking about HIV and AIDS. Just imagine how difficult it is to talk about both at the same time.

Do not proceed without getting the client's permission. If the client agrees you may continue, and thank him or her. Some people have difficulty sharing intimate details, so the provider needs to appreciate the risk the client is taking and the **trust** being bestowed on the provider. It never hurts to reassure the client that all information discussed will remain confidential.

If a client does not wish to talk about personal sex life or IDU, explore why. However, **do not** push the issue. If it becomes apparent that the client adamantly does not want to talk, leave the subject(s) alone. The client might be willing to talk at a later time. It helps no one if the provider–client relationship becomes a battle over these subjects. Where the provider is concerned that the client may be engaging in risky sexual behavior or IDU, the following options can be considered.

1. Talk with the client in a more general way, e.g., "If it is all right with you, I would like to review the ways that HIV can be transmitted. As you know, AIDS is a serious disease and I am concerned about you. If you do not wish to respond, that is all right. Would you be willing to listen?"

2. If the client refuses to listen, the provider, for example, can offer written materials, offer pamphlets on safer sex and on IDU, encourage the client to look them over, and make it clear that you are available to answer any questions in the future.

SEXUAL ISSUES IN HIV/AIDS COUNSELING

POINT I

Discussing sexual issues can be uncomfortable even for the most sophisticated counselor. However, the urgent need to ensure that people stop practicing high-risk sexual behavior requires professionals to introduce sex education into their clinical practice. The issue of sexual practices should be discussed with every individual who is already sexually active, who is contemplating becoming sexually active, who is not absolutely certain that he or she has been in a sexually exclusive relationship for the past 15 years, or who is not absolutely certain that his or her partner has not used injection drugs or had a blood transfusion within the past 15 years. Thus adolescents, individuals in sexually nonexclusive relationships, newly separated or divorced adults, and anyone contemplating having sex with a gay or bisexual man, injection drug user, or transfusion recipient need to learn about safer sexual practices. It has become appropriate—in fact, essential—for therapists to ask questions such as: "How did you feel when you first heard that you might have to change your sexual behavior in order not to become HIV-infected?" or "How do you feel about the fact that HIV is sexually transmitted?" or "When you think about safer sex, what thoughts and feelings do you have?" Most important, the counselor should ask: "What are you doing to protect yourself and your sexual partners from HIV infection?" (Shernoff, 1988)

POINT II

Regardless of sexual orientation, people cannot be **absolutely** certain about the drug use or sexual history of their sex partners. Because the period of HIV latency may last for 10 or more years, people may unknowingly transmit or expose themselves to HIV, erroneously believing that they are not at risk because they are currently in a stable, sexually exclusive relationship.

Interpreting data from the studies of Kinsey and colleagues in the 1940s and those of Hunt in the 1970s, Janet Shibley Hyde (1992) found that only 2% of American men are **exclusively** homosexual during their lifetime and that 25% are bisexual at some point. These data suggest that the majority of men who are or have been homosexually active in the United States may not identify themselves as gay. Many remain in heterosexual marriages, possibly hiding their homosexuality from their wives. Thus many women may falsely assume that they are safe from the risk of contracting HIV. For example, **a woman client learned in one day that her husband of 15 years had AIDS, that her marriage had not been a sexually exclusive relationship, and that her husband's relationships outside the marriage had been with men**. The crisis was compounded by the need to decide what to tell their 14-year-old son regarding his father's illness, and worries that she herself might have been exposed to HIV.

In attempting to assess whether a client is at risk for HIV, counselors must ascertain what the client's current sexual practices are, as well as what they were in the past. Simply asking "Are you gay?" is not sufficient. Health care professionals cannot assume that a client who is not openly gay has not engaged in sex with other men. For example, a married man with numerous symptoms, who had never been transfused, who reported no history of shared needle use or other risk factors for exposure to HIV, and who stated he was not gay, baffled his physician. However, when the man was questioned by a counselor as to whether he had ever had sex with other men, he stated that he had a long history of homosexual activity (Shernoff, 1988).

3. If appropriate, the client can be referred to a confidential HIV-antibody testing program for an educational session on safer sex practices, IDU, and HIV prevention in general.

4. If all of the above fails to work, give the client the telephone number of HIV/AIDS hotlines so the client can talk to someone anonymously about sexual activities, IDU, and HIV prevention.

If, however the client is responsive, wants to become involved in the session, the questions you use must be straightforward, worded in a way that will be understood, and posed in a nonjudgmental tone of voice.

Before asking specific questions on sex and drug use, it is essential to explain why they need to be discussed, since frank, open conversation about sex and drug use does not routinely occur in a professional setting. A simple, direct statement introducing the topics and the reasons for discussing them usually clarifies the situation, reassures the patient, and permits the conversation to proceed on a professional footing.

Questions on sexual behavior and drug use will help in determining if the person is at risk for exposure or has been exposed to HIV. For some counselors, asking questions and discussing another's sexual and drug abuse behavior is uncomfortable. Yet it is crucial if there is to be any modification of that behavior. The sexual and drug abuse history are the two most important means of determining whether someone is at increased risk for HIV infection.

HIV Risk Reduction—HIV counseling is more than providing routine information. Counseling should include the development of a personalized, negotiated HIV **risk-reduction plan**. This plan should be based on the client's skills, needs, and circumstances, and it must be consistent with the client's expressed or implied intentions to change behaviors. A list of the seven major known risk behaviors for HIV infection are presented in Table 14-2. HIV counseling should not consist of the counselor **telling** the client what he/she needs to do to prevent HIV infection/transmission, but instead should outline a variety of specific **options available** to the client for reducing his/her own risk of HIV infection/transmission. The counselor should confirm with the client that the risk-reduction plan is realistic and feasible—otherwise, it is likely to fail.

When negotiating personalized risk reduction, counselors should be especially attentive to information provided by the client, especially information about past attempts at preventive behaviors that were unsuccessful (e.g., intentions to use condoms but failure to do so) and those that were successful. Identifying and discussing previous prevention failures helps to ensure that a risk-reduction plan is realistic, attentive to the client's prevention needs, and focused on actual barriers to safer behaviors. Identifying previous prevention successes (e.g., successful negotiation of condom use with a new sexual partner) offers the counselor the opportunity to reinforce and support positive prevention choices.

ESTABLISHING SEXUAL PREFERENCE. It helps to know the client's sexual preference. Counselors' assumptions about clients are often **wrong**. So, never assume that you know your client, especially when it comes to his or her sexual activities. The fact that someone is married or reports numerous sexual experiences with the opposite sex does not prove that person is exclusively heterosexual. The counselor should explore with the client whether that means that he or she has never had a homosexual experience. Many people deny a hidden part of their sexuality, even to themselves.

There are several reasons why individuals may report being heterosexual but engage in homosexual acts. The client might have been intoxicated by drugs or alcohol at the time of a homosexual act and feel that it doesn't count. Some clients report engaging in homosexual activity only for money or drugs (prostitution). Other clients report homosexual activity only while in prison. Still others, usually men, will claim that they are not homosexual, the **other** person was homosexual. Others may explain away a homosexual act as accidental or having been taken advantage of. No matter what the reason, explore the frequency of these homosexual experiences, the client's reactions and feelings, and whether he or she practiced safer sex. A client who experimented with homosexuality as a teenager is quite different from one who reports having had several homosexual encounters over the past few years as an adult.

With clients who self-identify as lesbian, gay, or bisexual, the provider may explore self-esteem issues and whether there are any problems or conflicts with personal sexuality (Dustow, 1995).

TABLE 14-2 Seven Well-Known Risk Behaviors

- Unprotected sexual intercourse (vaginal, anal, or oral) with male or female partner
- Multiple sex partners
- Sexual intercourse with partner of unknown HIV status or at high risk for HIV exposure/infection
- Intravenous drug use, especially shared needles
- Recreational drug or alcohol abuse
- History of a sexually transmitted disease
- History of blood transfusions between 1978 and 1985

In summary, with regard to sexual preference, the counselor might begin the session by saying: "In order for me to give you the very best information, I need to ask you some specific questions about your sexual lifestyle. Your answers to these questions may be embarrassing to you and even painful. They may bring back memories you wish to forget. But complete and honest answers are in your best interest. Everything said here will remain between the two of us."

The counselor may determine the client's sexual orientation by inquiring: "Do you have sex with men, women, or both?" This type of question demonstrates that (1) the counselor realizes that people have different sexual preferences; and (2) the counselor is prepared for the client's response. Questions generally asked about sexual behavior by a counselor are listed in Table 14-3.

DRUG ABUSE. On completion of the sexual activity survey, the counselor needs to address the connection between drug use and HIV transmission and finish up by stating that drug use by the client or his or her sexual partner is an important factor in evaluating the risk of HIV infection. Both IDU and non-IDU drugs are discussed because all drugs can impair the senses and may lead to a change in sexual behavior and ultimately to HIV exposure. It is difficult to practice safer sex when under the influence of drugs.

SUPPORTIVE COUNSELING FOR DRUG ABUSE.
Until recently, most drug users have been men, and their non-drug-using female partners have functioned as the glue that kept their families together, sheltering as best they could the next generation, often suffering abuse in the process.

For both sexes, drugs may be used for pleasure or to provide medication from states of depression, anxiety, restlessness, and agitation. In poor communities, men may use drugs to gain power, material possessions, or prestige. By contrast, a woman's initiation into drugs often follows rape, domestic violence, incest, or other traumatizing events including accidents, physical illnesses, or tragic losses. Drug use for women may also be connected to a relationship, as a means of capturing, pleas-

TABLE 14-3   Sexual Practice History

Questions for Men and Women:

1. Do you have a history of sexually transmitted diseases?
2. Have you had more than one sex partner in the last 14 years?
3. Do you know the sexual history of each of your sex partners?
4. Was any sex partner an injection drug user?
5. Were any of your sex partners sexually involved with an injection drug user?
6. Was any sex partner hemophilic?
7. Have you ever practiced anal intercourse? Was a condom used?
8. Have you ever practiced oral sex? Was semen swallowed?
9. Have you ever had a blood transfusion? When?
10. Have you ever had sexual intercourse with someone who was HIV-infected or who later developed AIDS?
11. Have you ever been paid for sex?

Questions for Men:

1. Have you ever had anal intercourse with another man? Were you receptive, insertive, or both?
2. Are you bisexual?
3. Have you ever had sexual intercourse with a female injection drug user (or suspected she was)?
4. Have you ever had sexual intercourse with a male or female prostitute?
5. Do you practice oral-vaginal sex?
6. Do you practice oral-anal sex?
7. Do you practice penile-vaginal sex?

Questions for Women:

1. Do you practice anal intercourse?
2. Have you ever had sexual intercourse with a bisexual male (or suspected he was)?
3. Have you ever had sexual intercourse with an injection drug user (or suspected he was)?
4. Do you practice oral-penile sex?
5. Do you practice oral-anal sex?
6. Do you practice vaginal-penile sex?

ing, or holding on to a partner, or of managing the degradation of being in a violent relationship. Relapse for women seems to be correlated with experiences.

Today, 60% of crack users are women, the majority of whom are mothers of small children and the heads of single-parent households. New York City reported a 400% increase in maternal drug use in the period 1984 to 1989, the bulk of which was the result of maternal crack and cocaine use. It is estimated that more than half of all drug-using women

———— BOX 14.3 ————

SEX UNDER THE INFLUENCE (SUI)

Have you ever been a victim of SUI? Sex under the influence can be as deadly as DUI, driving under the influence.

1. Judgment is the first capacity affected by alcohol.

2. What you do unprotected now may hurt you later.

The sentence you get if you get caught unprotected may be death (AIDS).

(This statement hangs in the counseling and testing waiting room of an HIV/AIDS clinic.)

in the major epicenters of the eastern United States are HIV-infected, and drug use among women is correlated to unprotected sex, injection drug use, and needle sharing.

Given the public health crisis of HIV diseases, it has become clear that all drug programs should target **harm reduction** rather than the **unreachable goal** of eliminating drug use (Drucker, 1995). Harm reduction seeks to maximize functioning with the understanding that drugs may continue to play a role in the person's life. By focusing on increasing the drug user's ability to carry out social responsibilities rather than focusing on drug addiction *per se*, harm reduction defines attainable goals and circumvents the cycle of failure that drives a huge percentage of people out of drug treatment. Because a woman's self-esteem depends primarily on how she perceives herself in relationships, nonblaming approaches such as harm reduction are particularly effective in reaching women (Walker, 1995).

The needs of male substance abusers—and the programs that have been designed to usher them effectively through recovery—contradict the needs of many women. The failure is twofold. First, these programs do not acknowledge the psychological differences between men and women. Second, government funding has skewed those programs that do actually consider the needs of women to focus on pregnant women and women with children. While many women with HIV disease fall

into these categories, programs that focus on this relationship risk overlooking the needs of the individuals in these relationships, primarily the women.

These issues pinpoint a critical challenge for many women with HIV disease. Also, male-centered therapeutic strategies were developed and applied to women's needs. It must be recognized, however, that just because something works for men does not mean it will work for women (Marks, 1995).

SPECIAL PROBLEMS FOR DRUG COUNSELORS AND INJECTION DRUG USERS. In a report from the First Interdisciplinary Conference on HIV Antibody Testing Counseling in 1987, it was stated that counselors face special problems in dealing with injection drug users (IDUs). IDUs may take the test but fail to return for results or counseling. Already burdened by addiction, they are unlikely to change unhealthy behaviors without substantial intervention.

Rehabilitated IDUs who test positive may refer to drugs as a means of coping with the fear of illness or death. In general, IDUs, who are impoverished and socially alienated, tend to distrust government or institution-sponsored information. Their suspicions must be offset by physicians, rehabilitation counselors, and former addicts who convey interest, consistency, and empathy.

Most important, the report pointed out the importance of realistic expectations for IDUs, setting both short-term and long-term goals, such as encouraging use of clean needles and condoms while working to control the IDU's chemical dependency. The report makes two other interesting points about IDUs. First, males and females **resist safer sex practices for different reasons**. Some men are concerned with maintaining their macho image and therefore refuse to use condoms, which they perceive as conflicting with virility. Women may be reluctant to ask their partners to use condoms for fear of jeopardizing the relationship that offers their only option for housing, food, and often human contact. Second, about 50% of pregnant IDUs who test positive complete their pregnancy despite the risk that the child will be born infected and will develop AIDS (Selwyn et al., 1989) (see Chapter 11,

———— BOX 14.4 ————

A DAY IN THE LIFE OF A DRUG USER

Janet Johnson-Wise, MSW

For most HIV providers, the lives of injection drug users are foreign at best and stigmatized at worst. This response is based both on the covert nature of drug use and on societal prejudices about drug users. A glimpse into the daily life of a "street addict" challenges these presumptions and can inform educators, counselors, and clinicians.

Street addicts, unlike more mainstream, functional drug users, often resort to theft because they have few other options for obtaining money to buy drugs and because the powerful dictatorship of addiction demands that users compromise their values in its service. Coming out of youth, poverty, and fragmented lives, street addicts often lack education and have few marketable job skills that offer alternatives to theft. Once addicted, a combination of the cost of drugs and unremitting drug craving keeps them poor and unable to compete in the job market. Even with the will to fight addiction, the social network on the street offers little support for this difficult process, and government priorities offer little hope of getting drug treatment.

The following portrait represents a "typical" day in the life of Laura, a heroin-using drug injector living in a city in the United States. Laura is a 32-year-old black single mother. After years of suffering incest, she ran away from home when she was 16. Soon she was selling her body to get money for food and shelter, and she continued to live on the streets for 2 years before becoming pregnant and then marrying. Now divorced and with three children, Laura is an unemployed high school dropout living in what appears to be an unbreakable cycle of crime, sex and drug addiction. While not all drug users fit Laura's profile, many share her fear, hopelessness, and frustration.

HUSTLING

Laura awakens with a start to face another day in the streets and immediately checks the clock. Time is critical to the addict. If it is too early the dealers won't be out yet, and the mall will not open before Laura goes into withdrawal, becoming too sick to "get a good hustle going" (steal merchandise to sell so she can buy drugs). Today Laura is relieved. It's only noon.

Laura's work team consists of three people: two shoplifters—Laura and Mary—and the driver—John—who is available to make a quick getaway. First the team visits the mall, stealing just enough to buy drugs to "take the sick off" (prevent withdrawal). Then they sell the goods, "cop" (purchase drugs), and "get off" (use the drugs). As Laura shoots her share of the drugs, she is already worrying about getting back to the stores to complete her hustling for the day.

John waits in the car ready to pick up Laura and Mary at the first sign of trouble. Today, the women return walking "all wide-legged"; they have scored big. In the car Laura and Mary raise their skirts and begin to pull merchandise from their girdles.

At this point, everybody is happy. They place the stolen clothing under the back seat of the car, drive cautiously away, and find a "fence" to buy the stolen goods.

TAKING THE SICK OFF

After using drugs for more than 10 years, Laura knows all the "dope men" (dealers) in town, who has the best dope, and who will not "burn" them (give them drugs that they later discover to be baking power or some other false substitute). Mary, a newcomer, wants to go back to the safety of her home to use the drugs. John and Laura, however, know that as soon as the drugs are in their possession, each will begin to experience pseudo-withdrawal symptoms, and the urgency to use the drugs will become overwhelming.

The team ends up in the "shooting gallery" (a place to rent drug-using equipment and inject drugs), a squalid building across the street from where Laura had purchased the dope. Each team member pays the "gallery boss" $2.00 for rental of the "hype" (the syringe) and the place.

Atop a grimy table lay about 15 or 20 syringes, several greasy jars and cups, a whole slew of bottle tops, and some bleach. John and Laura scurry about trying to clear off a small space where they can "cook" (liquefy powdered heroin or cocaine) the drugs and "fire up" (inject). They consider cleaning their needles, but there is not enough bleach, so they shoot up without using it.

———— **BOX 14.4** (*continued*) ————

NIGHTTIME

After the need to avoid withdrawal has been satisfied, the team gets back to the mall. They continue hustling until they accumulate enough to cover the rest of the day and night. This time they simply fence the goods and split the money.

Now it's everyone for themselves. Laura's kids have been home alone since they got out of school at 3:00. John has to go see his parole officer. Mary has to clean the house before her mother returns.

Laura buys more drugs. She knows to save at least $5.00 to buy hot dogs, bread, and pork 'n beans for the kids. She questions the nutritional value of these foods, but knows that her habit won't allow her to do anything else. The kids are glad to see Laura when she returns and are happy about the food she has managed to buy.

There have been many times that Laura has gotten so high that she hasn't even remembered that the kids needed food. Times when Laura has

had to have sex with guys so she could get some cocaine to mix with the heroin. On days like that, there was no money for food. Laura consoles herself with the thought that at least she has always come back to the children.

Throughout the evening Laura continues to get high, hour after hour until all the drugs are gone. At 2:00 AM, she sits on the side of the bed with tears in her eyes and wonders how long she can keep up this life. As she falls into a stupor, she thinks to herself, "Maybe it'll be over this time, maybe I won't ever have to wake up and face that jungle again. But, God, if I do wake up, please let it be by noonday."

Box 11.1). These HIV-positive pregnant women also appear more likely than male IDUs to be concerned about the health of their child and the response of their friends and family.

BENEFITS

Pre-test Counseling

Good counseling skills are essential to the outcome of the HIV-antibody testing procedure. One of the most important aspects of counseling is establishing a rapport with the counselee. Honest, nonjudgmental concern and positive regard for the counselee will create an atmosphere conducive to the open expression of his or her feelings and attitudes. The CDC recommends that individuals listed in Table 14-4 receive pre-test counseling and HIV testing. If they have received a general background presentation on HIV infection as suggested under "**Education**" and have given their sexual and drug abuse histories, the counselor may begin by asking: "Why do you feel you want to be tested?" If the counselor is faced with a person who has not received

HIV-infection education, he or she may proceed by asking: "What do you know about the AIDS virus; how it is transmitted?" For purposes of this discussion, it is assumed that the person has received the educational information.

With preinformed clients, the counselor needs to know:

1. Why they want to take the test
2. When they think they were exposed
3. How they were exposed to the virus

This information, along with a review of the person's sexual behavior and drug history, will help the counselor to assess the level of risk for HIV infection. The level of risk assessment can be useful in helping a person decide whether to take the test. Having gained some idea of the individual's at-risk behavior, use the opportunity to talk about how to **reduce** his or her risk factors, targeting the person's specific at-risk behaviors.

Prior to a final decision on whether to take the HIV test, the counselor should explain the HIV-antibody test that will be used. He or she should also explain that the average time

TABLE 14-4   Guidelines for Counseling and Testing for HIV Antibody: CDC Recommendations

1. **Persons who may have sexually transmitted diseases**—All persons seeking treatment for a sexually transmitted disease, in all health care settings including the offices of private physicians, should be routinely[a] counseled and tested for HIV antibody.

2. **Injection drug users**—All persons seeking treatment for injection drug use or having a history of injection drug use should be routinely counseled and tested for HIV antibody. Medical professionals in all health care settings, including prison clinics, should seek a history of injection drug use from patients and should be aware of its implications for HIV infection.

3. **Persons who consider themselves at risk**—All persons who consider themselves at risk for HIV infection should be counseled and offered testing for HIV antibody.

4. **Women of childbearing age**—All women of childbearing age with identifiable risks for HIV infection should be routinely counseled and tested for HIV antibody in all health care settings. Educating and testing these women **before they become pregnant** allows them to avoid pregnancy and subsequent intrauterine perinatal infection of their infants (30%–50% of the infants born to HIV-infected women will also be infected).

5. **Pregnant women at risk**—All pregnant women at risk for HIV infection should be routinely counseled and tested for HIV antibody. Identifying pregnant women with HIV infection as early in pregnancy as possible is important in ensuring appropriate medical care; planning medical care for their infants; and providing counseling on family planning, future pregnancies, and the risk of sexual transmission of HIV to others.

6. **Women seeking family planning services**—All women who seek family planning services and who are at risk for HIV infection should be routinely counseled about AIDS and HIV infection and tested for HIV antibody. Decisions about the need for counseling and testing programs should be based on the best available estimates of the prevalence of HIV infection and the demographic variable of infection.

7. **Persons planning marriage**—All persons considering marriage should be given information about AIDS, HIV infection, and the availability of counseling and testing for HIV antibody.

8. **Persons undergoing medical evaluation or treatment**—Testing for HIV antibody is a useful diagnostic tool for evaluating patients with selected clinical signs and symptoms such as generalized lymphadenopathy, unexplained weight loss, or diseases such as tuberculosis, as well as sexually transmitted diseases, generalized herpes, and chronic candidiasis.

9. **Persons who received blood transfusions or blood products from 1978 to 1985**—All persons receiving blood or using blood products between 1978 and 1985 are at risk for HIV infection, especially if the blood or blood products were collected from areas with a high incidence of AIDS. They should be counseled about potential risk of HIV infection and should be offered antibody testing.

10. **Persons admitted to hospitals**—Hospitals, in conjunction with state and local health departments, should periodically determine the prevalence of HIV infections in the age groups at highest risk for infection. Consideration should be given to counseling and routine testing in those age groups deemed to have a high prevalence of HIV infection.

11. **Persons in correctional systems**—Federal prisons test all prisoners when they enter and leave the prison system. Correctional systems should study the best means of implementing programs for counseling inmates about HIV infection and for testing them at admission and discharge from the system.

12. **Prostitutes**—Male and female prostitutes should be counseled and tested and made aware of the risks of HIV infection to themselves and others. Particularly prostitutes who are HIV-antibody-positive should be instructed to discontinue prostitution.

[a]Routine counseling and testing is a policy to provide services to clients before and after testing. Except where testing is required by law, individuals have the right to decline to be tested without being denied health care or other services. (Source: *MMWR*, 1987)

after exposure it takes for antibodies to appear in the blood is 6 to 18 weeks. In some cases that time period can be extended to over a year. A test which appears negative during this time period may be a false negative. It should be explained that the test is recommended at 3 to 6 months after presumed exposure. However, testing can be done immediately and repeated in 3 to 6 months if it will help to manage the person's fears and anxieties.

If the test is negative at 6 months, it means that the person is most likely **not** HIV-infected, but it does not mean the person is immune to HIV infection. If in fact they have been exposed and are truly HIV-negative, they have

———— BOX 14.5 ————

A COUNSELING CHALLENGE

(A letter written to Percy Ross, an internationally known philanthropist)

Dear Mr. Ross: My God—what am I going to do? I've been married for 12 years and have two children. The man I'm married to is not the man I thought I married. Imagine my horror waking up one morning to learn my spouse was a closet homosexual. That was three days ago. I didn't have a clue in the world that my husband was gay. But he's not only gay, he's also got **AIDS**! What if I have the disease too? My God, what am I going to do?

I'm confused and shocked and have never been so disillusioned with life. I kicked him out of the house and told him to seek sympathy with the man or men who gave him this decadent disease.

I have no skills, as I've been a homemaker my entire adult life. At 43, I'm faced with no hope or future for my children and myself, except the dreaded life of welfare. You've just got to help me Mr. Ross. We were living paycheck to paycheck when my husband was here and we have no savings. My household expenses are $735 a month.

I haven't been able to tell anyone about this nightmare I've been living with, I'm too ashamed. I feel like committing suicide, but my children need me. Help me. What am I going to do?

This and other scenarios continue to occur across the country. What can these people do? How can it be stopped? **CLASS OPINIONS**

won the infection gamble this time but they may not the next time.

A person should also be informed of the small chance that a test result may be a false positive. Also, that in a few cases the test is indeterminate and requires a second blood sample for repeat testing. Most important, the person must be informed that although antidiscrimination laws exist, he or she may be subjected to negative social reactions when others find out he or she has taken the test! Thus the person should be offered the choice of confidentiality or anonymity.

Test or No Test—The decision on whether to be tested can, depending on circumstances, be

very difficult to make (Figure 14-1). **Fear** is a potent emotion and one that often overrules intelligence. For some people, even considering whether to be tested constitutes a crisis—one that is exacerbated if the results are positive and by no means ended if the results are negative.

Some people may cope better with a test result, of any kind, than living with the uncertainty of not knowing their status. A positive result may enable a person to make lifestyle changes that may show the development of AIDS and improve the quality of life. In other cases, women at risk may want to use test results in deciding whether to become pregnant, complete a pregnancy, or breast-feed an infant. If the test is positive, it may also help with a medical diagnosis in people with unexplained lymphadenopathy and mononucleosis-type symptoms.

Some people have a difficult time making a decision. Counseling an indecisive person can be either directive or nondirective. Directive counseling would **assist** the person with his or her decision one way or another. Nondirective counseling would prompt the person to find a way, perhaps through additional questioning and discussion, to make his or her own decision. A moral case can be made for both kinds of counseling and is worthy of class discussion.

If a decision has been made not to take the test and the counselor feels strongly that the person is at high risk for infection, he or she can ask the person to review the information covered, and if, for any reason, he or she needs more information or reconsiders, to come back in, or if the client has moved, to visit another state or private testing facility.

If the person decides to take the test, it may be of value to have him or her explain what a positive test is and what it is not. Ask: "If the test results do come back from the laboratory positive, what do you think your reaction will be? Will you tell anyone? Will you tell your sexual partner(s), your family and your friends?" Explain that they may experience a certain amount of anxiety during the 2-week waiting period for the test results, and that if they would like, they may come back in for further discussions.

HIV Counseling and Testing Protocol

Patient asks for HIV test or
physician perceives need for test

Take history and deliver
Pre-test Counseling

Determine that testing
is necessary

Determine that testing
is unnecessary

Acquire written consent and
schedule Post-test Counseling

Initial ELISA test results ⟶ Negative

Positive or equivocal

Second ELISA and ⟶ Negative ⟶ Check for possibility of a
Western blot results   false negative (HIV infection
                             not yet causing antibody
                             production)

Positive

Post-test Counseling

Discuss the results
Begin case management
Notify partner(s)
Refer for psychological or social support

Discuss results
Stress the need to modify behavior
Schedule a follow-up and counseling
  session for 3 to 6 months later

FIGURE 14-1 Possible Scheme for HIV Pre-test and Post-test
Counseling. This is only a suggested scheme and the procedure will vary
with individual physicians and HIV/AIDS clinics.

On asking if there are any further questions, the counselor has the person sign a consent form (Figure 14-2) (individual state statutes should be consulted concerning voluntary consent forms for adults and minors), and a time is set for a post-counseling session wherein the test results will be discussed.

Post-test Counseling

Providing the results of the test is just one of the functions of post-test counseling. The counselor must also attempt to determine if the person understands the results, the prospect of continuing at-risk behavior, and

CONSENT FORM TO DO TEST FOR HUMAN IMMUNODEFICIENCY VIRUS (HIV) ANTIBODY STD, FAMILY PLANNING AND PRENATAL CLINICS — ADULTS

IMPORTANT INFORMATION REGARDING THIS TEST

This is a form that will permit the health department to test your blood for the virus that causes AIDS. The test looks for antibodies that are produced by the virus; it will not tell you if you have AIDS, or will get AIDS. The virus is called human immunodeficiency virus (HIV). For further information regarding AIDS or the HIV antibody test, please read the attached information sheet. If you still have questions about this test that the clinic staff and this form have not answered, please consult your physician or call the Florida AIDS Hotline (1-800-FLA-AIDS) between 8:00 a.m. and 5:00 p.m., before signing this form.

The antibody test is done by drawing approximately 5cc's (1 teaspoon) of blood from the arm. When the blood sample is drawn, you may have some discomfort at the site of the needlestick and a small bruise may develop. Otherwise there is no risk of physical injury.

This test is taken voluntarily. If you choose not to take the test, you will **not** lose any service to which you would otherwise be entitled. Test results will be confidential!

The test results will be available in 2 weeks, and will **only be given to you in person.** No results will be given over the telephone or by mail. A counselor may call to remind you to come to the clinic for your test result.

I understand that the test results will be part of my confidential medical record. If I am pregnant, the results of this test will also become a part of my baby's medical record. I have been informed about the AIDS (HIV) antibody test (see attached sheets). I have had a chance to ask questions which were answered to my satisfaction. I understand the benefits and risks and request this test.

Date: _____ 19____   _____
                                              (Patient's Signature)

                                          _____
                                              (Patient's Printed Name)

Date: _____ 19____   _____
                                              (Witness)

FIGURE 14-2   One Type of Consent Form, State of Florida, for HIV-Antibody Testing. Note that confidential implies a limited release of test result information.

the need for immediate medical and psychiatric care. Post-test results should, if possible, be given by the pre-test counselor and always in a face-to-face setting.

The results of the test should be given as soon as the person is settled and initial pleasantries are completed. The person has waited for 2 weeks and needs to know what the counselor knows **NOW.**

Disclosing HIV Status—When disclosing HIV status to a patient, include a face-to-face discussion of the psychosocial and medical effects of HIV infection, following a careful assessment of the person's psychosocial status. Discuss available therapies and social services and, where applicable, explain state requirements for reporting the infection. Discuss the potential advantages and disadvantages of voluntary disclosure to family, friends, and associates.

Urge patients to disclose their HIV status to significant others, particularly sex partners and needle-sharing partners. Emphasize the need to prevent further transmission of HIV infection.

Assess the need of the person infected with HIV for counseling and initial care, and make referrals for services that cannot be provided on-site (Disclosure Counseling, 1994).

The initial disclosure of HIV test results sets the foundation for the person's acceptance of his or her condition. The way in which a person accepts the information can affect the quality of life and willingness to care for themselves. Thus, the manner in which test results are communicated is very important to the formation of the infected person's future attitudes about how they will live the rest of their life. This is especially important now that the new AIDS definition has identified large numbers of **asymptomatic** people with AIDS. In the absence of overt signs and symptoms of HIV disease, it may be more difficult to believe you are HIV-infected. Thus, the asymptomatic person may be more apt to go directly into a stage of **denial** than someone who is symptomatic at the time test results are revealed. It has been shown that people in denial learn less about their illness, delay seeking help longer, and are less apt to cooperate with medical management or follow self-care or health behavior recommendations.

Denial is a coping strategy which helps the client maintain a positive quality of life. The denying client is not yet ready to deal directly or openly with the diagnosis. Denial should be challenged only when medical care or the health of others is compromised.

A Positive Test Result—A direct statement such as "**Your Test Result Came Back Positive**" is perhaps the best approach. The statement may have to be **repeated**, especially if the person implied during the pre-test session that he

or she was most likely uninfected. Allow for a time response. Many times, after hearing they are HIV-positive, **they feel like a glass ball dropped on concrete**. **Their lives have been shattered into a thousand pieces.** After allowing time for a response, the counselor may follow up by saying, "Now that you know the test is positive, can you explain what this means?" If the response is reasonably correct and he or she knows HIV antibodies are present which means HIV infection, it is reasonable to ask about feelings and thoughts. In one case, a person responded, "I lost my health—but wasn't what I really lost my freedom? How do I regain that?"

If a person does not respond after hearing the results, the counselor may say, "Now that you know that you are infected, what do you think? Can we talk about it? You're very quiet. What are your thoughts at this moment?"

If the individual appears rational, it may be possible at this point to clarify the implications of the test result and provide reassurance that the patient is not going to die immediately. Try to help the patient achieve emotional stability and accept and cope with an HIV-positive status. Explain that infection can be transmitted to others through unsafe sex, shared needles, blood donation, and contact with infected blood. Encourage condom use. If the person is an IDU, suggest cessation of IV drug use, or at least use of needle/syringe exchange programs or bleach to clean shared needles/syringes. Explain that common household contact does not transmit HIV. Stress the need to begin ongoing primary care, including care of acute infections. Explain routine care, and encourage self-education and active involvement. Encourage infected people to notify their partners. Review the risk assessment, and try to date the infection. Remind patients that HIV is a chronic disease that may not produce symptoms for 10 or more years after infection and that treatments are available and new drugs are in development.

Reactions may vary from tears to open hostility. After the patient has settled down, it must be made clear that he or she must exercise some control over what is to happen from this point on. Reactions to a positive result will continue to ebb and rise with the flow of the conversa-

---
BOX 14.6

QUESTIONS FOR THE COUNSELOR

Thousands of decisions hang on the results of a test that to most people represents a black box. Individuals who want to be tested can benefit from compassionate counseling. But counseling for this disease is not easy. **There is no cure; so how does one instill hope? It brings about a protracted and tragically ugly death; so how does a counselor encourage the patient to be happy and not bitter, up and not down?** With no other diagnosis does an individual face the stigma, the fear of rejection, the loss of friends, family, and autonomy. Even patients with incurable cancer are generally *not* subject to rejection by friends, family, or society. In addition, many patients with HIV infections are plagued by unresolved feelings about sexual preference and guilt about the possibility of having infected others.

The questions asked of the counselor vary. Some HIV-infected clients already know about the disease and ask relatively few questions. They bow their heads and their eyes fill with tears as they repeatedly clench and release their fists and rub their foreheads. Others have not received much AIDS education. To them, the virus is just one more sexually transmitted disease among several. When told that this infection has a high probability of progressing to AIDS, their eyes widen, their ill-at-ease smile fades, and their behavior changes. They usually begin by shifting in their chairs, trying to ask two questions at once; they become confused. They want to reject the counselor's bad news by saying things like "Are you kidding me?" or "Say what?" with a nervous grin. The initial rejection of the facts, the denial, usually grows into shock and reality at this point. The patient may well begin to ask the hard questions: "How long do I have to live?" "Will I suffer great pain?" "Will I be alone?" "Who is going to help me?" "Where will the money come from to pay for hospitalization and medication?" "I'm too young to die; does anybody care that I'm going to die?"

Survey of HIV/AIDS counselors finds that most persons being informed that they are HIV-positive want to ask questions. The questions usually fall into one or more of five categories: those relating to prognosis, life expectancy, and fear over loss of faculties, which are usually of greatest concern; those about work and finances; those about self-esteem and social issues; those about being lonely, having to move, or becoming sexually undesirable; and concerns about health issues. Sometimes these questions occur to the individual after the post-test counseling session.

tion. Newly informed HIV-positive people may be distraught for weeks or months. Depression often occurs and thoughts of suicide are frequent. Records of a group of HIV-positive individuals revealed that 20% considered suicide during the year following their test (Sarti, 1990).

Individual Reactions to a Positive HIV Test— In 1989, Robert, a 33-year-old San Francisco security guard, learned that his blood had tested positive for the AIDS virus. He resolved to fight, to take better care of himself. He entered a marathon.

When the homosexual lover of a Boston AIDS patient tested HIV-positive, he went home and committed suicide.

Reggie, a 38-year-old AIDS activist in San Francisco, resisted being tested until fatigue, weight loss, a tentative diagnosis of AIDS, and his partner of 7 years drove him to the doctor. He recalls, "I was holding out. In my denial and inability to accept what was happening, I took the test to prove my physician wrong. I wanted to wave the paper in his face. That didn't happen. I shut down emotionally." His partner Tim assumed that he too was HIV-infected. He quickly enrolled in a medical insurance program. California law prohibits insurers from requiring HIV-antibody testing on applicants. Tim went to an anonymous testing site, had an emotional 2-week wait, and found out he was **not infected**. The emotional reactions of the two men were quite different. Tim's first reaction was one of disbelief—there had to be a mistake. Reggie said his first reaction was to feel hurt. Reggie felt the "**Why Me?**" syndrome. He felt alone. Tim, like many others who test negative, greeted his news not with glee but with quiet relief, tinged with what might be

TABLE 14-5 Stages of a Dying Patient

Emotion	Interpretation	Stage
Denial and Isolation	No, not me	1
Anger	Why me?	2
Bargaining	Let's make a deal (God)	3
Depression	Unfinished business	4
Acceptance	Void of feelings	5

These are the five stages presented by Elizabeth Kubler-Ross in her book, *On Death and Dying*, published by Macmillan in 1969. People go in and out of the stages and may never reach stage 5. If they do, they have resigned themselves to death and only want simple companionship.

called **survivor's guilt**. Now, having been spared the infection, he affirms, "I plan to be there when Reggie needs me most." But Reggie has reason for concern. As the disease progresses, it strains the relationship. Reggie has seen other couples in similar situations break up. The decision of Reggie and Tim to take the HIV test was traumatic; like others before them, they had to face their own vulnerability.

According to interviews with people who were told they were HIV-positive, reactions were similar to those of people who were told they had terminal cancer (Table 14-5). One person, after being told that he was HIV-positive, was asked how he felt. He responded in anger. "If someone came into your home and ripped out the electrical system, loosened the plumbing and took a sledgehammer to the inner walls, you'd be furious, wouldn't you? Any if you had opened the door to that person because you trusted them, you'd feel even worse—devastated because of the destruction and **betrayal** by someone you trusted. How do you think I feel? I'm angry as hell—**I would like to hurt someone right now!**"

An AIDS patient responded in anger saying that "Loss is the critical term here. My independence is another item on a growing list of losses due to AIDS. I can't even go to a damn movie around the corner anymore! The rage and depression I feel each time an ability or choice is ripped away, or each time an example of an already lost ability rises to infuriate me, is unfathomable. **It's like a hideous auctioning off of your spirit, your freedom, at ridiculous prices. You're bankrupt and there's**

nothing you can do about it. What's doubly depressing is knowing that it will only get worse. Of course, the final loss from AIDS is the loss of life. But along the way, if one does not succumb quickly, the losses leading to the end are insidious, infuriating, and even, sometimes, humiliating" (Rowland, 1990).

PRESENTING HOPE. There is no easy way to tell a person that HIV infection is most likely forever; and based on current medical knowledge, the majority of HIV-infected people will progress to AIDS and die. But hope can be given by explaining that many people have lived without any severe illness for **as long as 15 or more years**. And that in the next 10 years, there is great hope that medical breakthroughs will save their lives. (The use of protease inhibitors in combination drug therapy is now extending some people with HIV disease indefinitely; see Chapter 4.)

In the meantime, **they must not donate blood or body organs or share personal items such as toothbrushes, razors, or anything else that might contain blood.** Sexual partner(s) should be informed of HIV status and use safer sex methods. Encourage any previous sexual contact from the time of earliest HIV exposure to go in for pre-test counseling.

In closing the post-test session, a counselor should attempt to have the person agree to take control of his or her life, not to transmit the virus to others, seek medical help through periodic medical evaluations, and confidentially inform his or her physician, dentist, and others on a need-to-know basis. Clearly the choices to be made rest with the HIV-positive person.

SUICIDE AMONG PERSONS WITH HIV DISEASE OR AIDS. Throughout history, suicide has been a uniquely human response to the misery of illness and perceptions of inescapable death. Increased rates of suicide among persons with serious illness have been well documented; these risks are especially high when the illness includes a psychiatric disorder.

Many people with HIV infection consider suicide at some point during their disease. This is not unique to HIV disease and AIDS. Jack Kevorkian has attended the deaths of peo-

————— BOX 14.7 —————

LOSS AMONG GAY MEN

Robert Marks, Editor of FOCUS

HIV researchers and educators spend a good deal of time reminding a society that prefers to partition humanity into "we" and "they" that the virus does not discriminate and that people of every stripe will respond to infection in similar physical and emotional ways. This perspective is reinforced by the societal myth that the only difference between heterosexual people and gay people—the group that has been most identified with HIV disease—is the gender of sexual partners.

In fact, being gay implies much more profound psychological differences then these approaches imply, and while they may be less relevant in treatment and prevention settings, they are central in dealing with emotional response, particularly the expression of grief. In an unusual *FOCUS* article, Herman Kaal offers insights into the psychological complexity of this response among gay men in industrialized nations. His piece provides a good example of psychological detective work, laying out in all its intricacy a range of classical psychological theories, which interpret HIV-related loss among gay men.

LOSS UPON LOSS

The most important difference between gay men and others affected by HIV disease, however, is the sociological phenomenon of multiple loss. Three factors determine the conditions that have left gay men in industrialized nations vulnerable to a never-ending grief.

First, HIV disease has killed many more gay men than people in other CDC-defined categories, and the virus has infected a higher proportion of gay men in most places than members of these other groups. Second, among these identifiable groups, gay men have weathered the epidemic for the longest period of time; and third, gay men arguably comprise the group with the strongest sense of community. As Tom Grothe and Leon McKusick point out, the most important result of a multiple loss is that it interferes with the abilities of gay men to fully grieve and heal from one loss before being faced with another and another and another. As one 23-year-old client said, "I'm sometimes glad to think that I won't be around in 10 years—because by then the only gay people left will be those whose lives were ruined by watching the rest of us die (Sullivan, 1995).

In addition, while the gay identity Kaal defines is a construct of industrialized nations, according to Grothe and McKusick multiple loss is not so limited. In fact, the most dramatic example of multiple loss is among the general population in African nations, the geographic area where the epidemic is most mature.

I suggest that grief is the most enduring aspect of the epidemic. It may be the most enduring therapeutic issue as well. Kaal, Grothe, and McKusick alert therapists—and, indeed, educators and medical professionals—to their great challenge. In the face of multiple loss, they must heal the community by healing the individual, and in this way, resurrect the sense of community fundamental to the mental health of the individual.

ple with many different chronic diseases. But the problems may be even more acute for patients with AIDS than with many other chronic, even terminal conditions. AIDS patients tend to be younger and may have already suffered the loss of many friends and lovers. Great biological and social loss and stigma exist. Furthermore, some communities, in particular the gay communities, that have been hard hit by HIV infection are now experiencing an increasing numbness, an overload of grief, and even a fatalism leading to a return to risky behavior.

The primary concern with suicide in people with AIDS, according to experts, is differentiating the person whose thoughts of suicide are associated with depression from a person who is contemplating rational suicide.

IMPACT OF HIV ON SEXUAL NEEDS

When people become infected with HIV, does it mean that sex disappears from their lives? Some people do think that those living with HIV/AIDS should never have sex again! But, they do not have to live with the virus, be asymptomatic for 10 or 15 years during the prime of their lives, and completely abstain from sex; this is an **unrealistic** expectation.

People who know they are HIV-positive, most likely, are **more worried** about transmitting HIV to others than the hundreds of thousands of people who are HIV-positive and don't know it. **QUESTION: WHO IS MORE RESPONSIBLE?** The people who don't know they are HIV-positive may be more likely to practice unsafe sexual activities. Those who have been tested most likely have received pre- and post-HIV counseling. They know they are infected. They know that the risk of transmission is greatly reduced when no penetration takes place and when condoms are used correctly.

THE IMPACT

From the moment people hear the results, an HIV-positive test, their life falls apart. It seems as though they have received a death sentence, especially if they are already ill. But most people hear the diagnosis while **they are still healthy**. Because they know they are HIV-positive, there is **confusion**; they are healthy, but just learned they will **die** early in life. It may take some time before they discover that the only thing actually different about them from **before-the-test** is that

they now **know** that they are HIV-positive. On the one hand, HIV changes their life completely while, on the other hand, they may come to the conclusion that nothing has really changed. They still are the same person and still like and dislike the same things. And suddenly they discover that they still have **sexual desires**.

People in general want to hold the HIV-positive person responsible for practicing safer sex or not to have sex at all. But isn't sex a shared responsibility? There are other STDs that can kill! Society does not now hold the same antagonism toward the **non-HIV-infected but STD-infected people—Why**? Perhaps because there are, **in proportion**, **more** HIV-infected people who have worked out a strategy of **how, where, and when** to tell their potential sexual partners about their HIV condition than there are people with other STDs who have done the same. How else can society account for the 12 million newly infected people with STDs each year in the United States and 250 million worldwide.

THE SEXUAL PRICE OF HONESTY

It is always difficult to foresee what the reaction will be. Bad experiences and cruel rejections have made HIV-positive persons very wise in this respect. They don't want compassion, they want respect. And they want to have sex for the same reasons as anyone else: because they enjoy it, they want to express love, they want to gain consolation or security. In that way, the HIV-positive person is like everyone else!

DEPRESSION AND SUICIDE. HIV/AIDS is a uniformly fatal condition. Persons living with AIDS (PLWAs) are frequently **depressed** and, in some cases, become **suicidal**. One individual who was told he was HIV-positive said, "I'm going to shoot myself" and he immediately left the counseling office. In November of 1992, a married couple did just that; both had AIDS. The husband, age 29, and the wife, age 36, died of gunshot wounds to the head. Their suicide note said they picked a spot to die together because of its natural beauty.

In 1987 through 1989, there were 165 death certificates with both AIDS and suicide listed

as causes of death. Persons with AIDS who committed suicide were 99% male, 87% white, 12% black, and 1% other races. Their median age was 35 years with a range from 20 to 69 years. There were no statistically significant differences in the age, sex, or race distribution of PLWAs who committed suicide compared with all PLWAs alive during 1987 through 1989. Suicides among PLWa were widely distributed in the United States: California (30%), Florida (11%), Texas (5%), and New York (4%) had the most cases, but suicide among PLWAs occurred in 41 other states and the District of Columbia. In 1992, male PLWAs had a suicide rate 7.4 times higher than males in the general population. Only one woman with AIDS committed suicide (Cote et al., 1992).

By the mid-1990s, it has become unclear whether an HIV-infected person is at high risk for suicide. The epidemic has changed; the reality of being HIV-infected and what that means to an individual is not the same as it was a decade ago.

Recent studies have found that most people who are HIV-positive are quite resilient. They may be sad and upset, but they do not meet criteria for depression (American Psychiatric Association, 1994). Moreover, those who are depressed often have histories of depression that pre-date their HIV infection. This suggests that HIV may be one of many possible stressors that can provoke an episode of depression, rather than being a direct cause of depression (Markowitz, 1995). The key to helping people maintain emotional balance is to ask them, at every visit, how their lives are going. How are they coping? Do they have the support they need? Are they having particular difficulties at home or at work? The impact of the disease has changed over time, and new problems have developed along with that change.

COUNSELING WOMEN WHO ARE HIV-POSITIVE: REPRODUCTIVE CONCERNS. Women who are HIV-infected should be counseled on their risk of progressing to AIDS and the risk of perinatal and sexual transmission. Infected women should be advised to refer their sex partners for counseling and testing. if a woman's sexual partner is not infected, the couple should be counseled on how they may modify their sexual practices to reduce the risk of HIV transmission to the uninfected partner. In addition, the couple should be told not to donate blood, organs, or sperm and should be discouraged from using IV drugs and advised against sharing needles and syringes. When seeking medical or dental care, they should inform those providers of their positive antibody status.

HIV-infected women should be advised to consider delaying pregnancy until more is known about perinatal transmission of the virus. Pregnant infected women may require additional medical and social support due to an enhanced risk of opportunistic infections and psychosocial difficulties during and after pregnancy. Also, HIV-infected women should be advised against breast-feeding to avoid postnatal transmission to a child who may not be infected.

A Negative Test Result—On occasion, a person hearing that his or her test was negative becomes very quiet. Some have expressed disbelief and anger because their sexual partners tested positive. An example of the kind of reaction a person goes through when told he or she is negative is in Paul Monette's book, *Borrowed Time: An AIDS Memoir*. When Paul's test came back negative, knowing that his lover Roger's test was positive, he wrote, "When my test came back negative last month, I was overwhelmed with a sadness I hadn't expected. Coming back alive is a guilt, a terrible betrayal, a necessary starting point."

Others feel a great sense of relief and are quiet because they are grateful for the reprieve. In either case, these people must be cautioned that, although a negative test means that they are not infected, it does not mean that they are immune to infection. If their risk assessment is high, they should be told that they were fortunate this time. If they wish to remain free of HIV infection, they must change their behavior and practice risk reduction. In addition, they must also be told of the test's limits—that there is a small chance the test was a false negative if they had unsafe sex or shared IV needles within the past 6 months.

Many individuals, whether their results are positive or negative, may require long-term support to reinforce and sustain changes in their behavior that must become permanent.

RECOMMENDATIONS FOR THOSE RECEIVING AN HIV-NEGATIVE TEST RESULT.
If the result is negative and risk behaviors are recent or ongoing, recommend retesting every 2 to 3 months until a negative result is obtained at least 6 months after potential exposure. Review the risk reduction strategies discussed in the pre-test session.

Disclosing HIV Infection within the Family Unit—Through 1998, there will be about 9,000 pediatric AIDS cases in the United States. The number of HIV-infected children is probably many times that, and with improving medical treatment these children are living longer. There are many more children who, although not themselves infected, have mothers and fathers who are. Unless the course of the AIDS epidemic shifts unexpectedly, the overall number of mothers, children, and adolescents infected with HIV by the year 2000 will be about 100,000. This trend intensifies the question of discussion of HIV within families.

When and how does a mother tell her child (of whatever serostatus) about her own infection? How should she tell an uninfected child about an infected sibling? These questions give rise to a range of issues within families where HIV or AIDS is present, as well as between these families and social institutions such as hospitals, schools, and churches.

Both parents and medical personnel may resist initiating discussion of HIV within the family. Often they cite the overwhelming anxiety such a revelation might bring, and children's presumed inability to understand such a devastating illness. On the other hand, children in families infected by HIV often already know the truth and give both subtle and overt signs that they want to talk.

Often it is health professionals who first urge disclosure, while family members resist. This process can begin as early as post-test counseling of infected adults. Repeated attempts may be needed to meet with people who are reluctant to hear news that the counselor **must** give. This pattern may persist, with the counselor urging greater openness, while the infected parent's initial reluctance to even know the diagnosis becomes a reluctance to tell others—especially family members.

Counselors prefer openness because of concern for the sex partners of infected patients, respect for the autonomy of infected children, and concern for the long-term well-being of uninfected children who may suddenly lose a parent or sibling to AIDS. It is often in the interests of the entire family to know about the illness of any family member. Yet, while the risk of sex partners is direct and physical, the risks of withholding such information from children are often more psychological and harder to define.

Research on pediatric cancer and bereavement in childhood has shown that relative family openness about terminal illness is beneficial. In the 1960s, cancer diagnoses within a family were frequently withheld from children, while today disclosure has become the norm. Studies of survivors of childhood cancer demonstrate that those told their diagnosis early (e.g., before age 6) grow up with better psychosocial adjustment than those told later, and that children usually know even if they are told nothing. Furthermore, other studies indicate that including children in treatment decisions improves family and individual psychological adjustment.

Although little research has been done on this issue as applied to HIV and AIDS, clinical experience has suggested that the situation is analogous. In general, it seems that even very young children (4–6 years) want to discuss family illnesses, at their cognitive level. Younger children's concerns typically focus on separation (will they be left alone?) and physical pain. Older children's questions range over such topics as the afterlife, etiology, social acceptance, and sexual issues.

Counselors who tend to apply the lessons of pediatric oncology and bereavement to HIV/AIDS should also consider HIV's unique social implications:

1. Most childhood HIV is acquired perinatally. A mother may feel guilty for having transmitted HIV to her child. Discussion would bring up not only guilt, but also grief, and render the illness and its prognosis more painfully real. Parents may also feel guilty for having an illness that threatens to remove them as parents, and shame for the high-risk activities that may have exposed them to infection.

2. For disadvantaged families, HIV may add to an already burdensome litany of issues, such as poverty, racial discrimination, divorce, crime, and drug dependence. Having often left these painful realities largely unspoken, from (partly adaptive) avoidance, such families may not address the emotional impact of HIV/AIDS with candor.

3. HIV/AIDS is associated with socially objectionable behaviors. Parents and foster parents may remain silent for fear children's questions would lead them into uncomfortable subjects. Injection drug use, sex with multiple partners, and homosexuality are topics that many families find sensitive.

4. The social stigma of HIV/AIDS is unique. Neighbors, relatives, and schools have been known to shun families in which they suspect HIV. Parents thus keep from children what they fear the children will tell others. Despite public health education, the powerful social connotations of HIV/AIDS are unlikely to vanish soon.

5. Current HIV and AIDS treatment, while not free of side effects, do not typically cause the immediate, visible changes brought on by cancer treatments such as radiotherapy, chemotherapy, and surgery. This can make secrecy more feasible and reduce pressure for disclosure for such purposes as enlisting the child's cooperation in a "fight" against the child's own disease, or explaining to the child the effects of treatment on another.

Given these constraints, it is even more important to approach disclosure issues within families carefully.

PROCESS. Disclosure is a long-term, in fact, lifelong process requiring family members to engage in repeated discussions both on their own and with a counselor. Fostering an emotional atmosphere in which this process can begin is an essential therapeutic task. Long before HIV disease or AIDS is mentioned to children, they can be engaged in discussions that focus on their own day-to-day experience. Adults' resistance to disclosure often diminishes when good rapport is established with counselors who do not try to rush the disclosure process. Parents and children alike may go through phases of secrecy, preparation for disclosure, actual moments of more open discussion, and then back to silence, in a nonlinear progression.

OLDEST FIRST. Disclosure should generally proceed from older to younger family members. Parents and grandparents need to be comfortable with more open discussion before the topic is broached with older, then progressively younger, children. Discussion should be a dialogue in which all sides communicate both facts and feelings, and information at the appropriate developmental level is provided to children. This applies when family members are in relatively good mental health; in cases of cognitive or emotional disturbance, certain aspects of disclosure may never be appropriate.

PARTICULARITY. Each family and individual has unique needs with regard to disclosure. For example, older children may acquire the added emotional burden of knowing that a parent's life is threatened. Parents may resist disclosure precisely for this reason. Counselors should address these concerns, and help parents find the right moments and words for disclosure. Using clinical sensitivity, the counselor should assess the barriers to communication in each case and decide to what degree they may be adaptive.

AWARENESS. Awareness of HIV/AIDS within the family prompts widely varying reactions. One 7-year-old boy, short since birth, responded to the invitation to discuss his disease only with questions about his height. A 10-year-old girl, whose parents finally decided on telling her, responded with outrage; she said she had known for years, "so why did everyone think it had to be kept secret?" A 10-year-old boy burst into tears after learning that his mother and younger brother were HIV-positive; he said he would be left all alone when everyone died.

It is best to approach disclosure as one aspect of a comprehensive, family-oriented medical and social service. For example, a mother may be more open to telling her children about HIV if she has support with estate and custody planning. Such social service interventions can go hand in hand with psychotherapeutic exploration of their meanings. To arrange for the children's future, a parent must contemplate his or her death, with all it signifies to the family.

Both parents and children can benefit from support groups that address the emotional and

DISCLOSING HIV INFECTION TO HIV-INFECTED CHILDREN

When do you tell a child that he or she has AIDS? When is a child old enough to understand? Who should tell the child? Is it better to "protect" a child from this knowledge? The issue of disclosure to children is not only a clinical question but an ethical one. In a legal sense, it is the parents' perogative to decide what children who are minors should be told.

According to Michael Lipson's (1995) experience at a Harlem hospital in 1991, children were **not** being told the nature of their disease. He tells of encountering a room full of children receiving intravenous treatment in the AIDS Clinical Trials Unit. These were cognitively normal children, 2 to 12 years old; none officially knew what disease he or she had. No one in the room ever mentioned HIV or AIDS, and there was no discussion between parents and children about this. Between 1985 and 1991, only 3 of 30 HIV-infected children treated at Harlem Hospital were told their diagnosis. **A number of these children died without ever being told about their illness, or even learning that they had an illness.**

There is evidence that children suffer from this state of silence. They know something is wrong, but because no one talks to them about it, they feel they cannot discuss it with anyone.

Families often participate in this kind of secret-keeping.

THE ISSUES

The issues of secrecy and disclosure within a family are universal emotional issues that cross racial and ethnic lines. Thus, **disclosure** may become the focus of a conflict between parents—who may feel guilty about their child's HIV infection and unsure of the family's future, and who want to protect the child (and themselves) from the reality of a terminal disease—and health care workers who have been specially trained and encouraged to openly discuss illness.

GUIDING PRINCIPLES FOR DISCLOSURE

The **first** guiding principle for disclosure to a child is that the patient is **never just the child**. A baby is always in a social environment, be it an orphanage, a birth home, a foster home, or a hospital. A child is always part of a familial or pseudo-familial context. Any intervention with the child must take this adult surrounding into account.

Ideally, the parents should be the ones to disclose a child's condition to him or her. They should not be forced into this but should want to do it. When health care professionals see a situation that seems wrong, they have a strong desire to right it themselves, but this is less desirable. When a child is ready to talk about feelings, nurses and doctors may not be around, but someone in the home will be, and the family needs to be open to such discussions. Too often, parents are not open to discussion because they have not come to grips with losing their child.

The **second** guiding principle for disclosure is that the child needs someone with whom it will be safe to talk about HIV and its long-term implications. Without such a long-term confidant, the child will be left at least as alone as before he or she was told the diagnosis.

The **third** guiding principle for disclosure is that disclosure should be a process with no beginning and no end. Begin speaking with children about the vocabulary and the phenomenon of their illness as soon as it is evident that they are sick.

All kinds of things are said to babies, long before they are able to understand them. There is no reason to tell a child **only what we believe he or she will understand**. Many things can be openly discussed before naming the disease. The naming of the disease is a larger problem for adults than it is for the child. If children are brought along in a constant interchange of communication about their illness, naming the disease will not be a major crisis. Once they are told about HIV disease or AIDS, that moment in time, in retrospect, becomes one event in a continuum of communication about their illness (Lipson, 1995).

social stresses of HIV infection. When parents, especially, become able to address their condition and its emotional impact in group or individual psychotherapy, they can often talk about it more readily with the family. With the guidance of a clinical psychologist or a clinical trained social worker, parents can be helped to explore their own reactions to the illness, examine the questions and topics they fear most, and learn to talk about illness with their children in ways children can understand. (This section, "Disclosing HIV Infection within the Family Unit," was adapted from Lipson, 1993; 1995.)

Reproductive Counseling

During the last decade, there has been an outpouring of literature about HIV disease, but little on HIV's special impact on women. Although most HIV-infected females are of reproductive age, a void remains in our knowledge about reproductive issues and HIV disease. Most of what has been written focuses on transmission of HIV from women to their fetuses or newborns, with some information about clinical manifestations and care of HIV-infected pregnant women.

However, counselors can use this small but growing body of information, along with the broader HIV knowledge base, to counsel patients about reproductive options. While some attention has been given to the ethics of HIV-infected women having babies, there has been little discussion of the reproductive decision-making process that HIV-infected women regularly face.

Counseling in this area is based on several assumptions:

1. Reproductive counseling is an essential part of the primary and preventive care of HIV-infected people and should begin early in the patient–counselor relationship, preferably when the female is not pregnant. Frequently, however, this counseling takes place with a pregnant woman and so must be modified and intensified.

2. Even though the CDC recommends advising HIV-infected women to delay pregnancy indefinitely, many of the nonpregnant become pregnant and many HIV-infected pregnant women choose to maintain their pregnancies. People have the right to have access to all information about HIV disease and to make their own informed reproductive decisions.

3. Because the HIV knowledge base changes rapidly and the issues surrounding reproductive decision making are intimate and complex, the counseling process should be continuous, not simply discussed once and checked off. As knowledge about HIV disease and its impact on pregnancy grows and as the woman develops her personal coping mechanisms, new issues will arise. The provider or counselor must be prepared to deal with emerging issues.

A prime example of new knowledge and emerging issues is the recent (1994) CDC announcement that the ACTG 076 study revealed that women placed on zidovudine after the 14th week of pregnancy, during labor, during delivery, and after delivery to the newborn resulted in a two-thirds reduction of HIV transmission from mother to fetus. After sharing this information, the counselor must then make it clear that, regardless of these findings, there are **no guarantees** of an HIV-negative birth.

4. Each person is unique and counseling must be individualized and shaped to each person's needs.

The framework for this counseling model is **bisocial**. With this model, the provider can support the woman as she explores the impact pregnancy, childbirth, and childrearing would have on her, her fetus and future child, and her support network. The goal is for each female to develop her own risk–benefit analysis in order to make an informed reproductive choice.

There are five essential areas of information that should be presented: (**1**) the impact of HIV infection on pregnancy, (**2**) the impact of pregnancy on HIV disease, (**3**) the effect of treatment of HIV disease on the patient and her fetus during pregnancy, (**4**) the risk of HIV transmission from the mother to her fetus or newborn, and (**5**) the course of perinatally acquired pediatric HIV infection.

To summarize information on these five points, we have incomplete knowledge about the effect of HIV infection on pregnancy and about the impact of pregnancy on HIV disease. HIV infection appears to have little effect on the course or outcome of pregnancy. In pregnancies not complicated by HIV, the T4 lymphocyte count decreases throughout pregnancy and then rises after delivery. This decrease also appears to occur in HIV-infected pregnant women, but there is some evidence that the drop in T4 count may sometimes persist after delivery. Whether this accelerates the progression of HIV disease during pregnancy is not known. Little is known about the safety and efficacy of the use during pregnancy of medications for prophylaxis and treatment of HIV-related disease. However, counselors should review these issues with HIV-infected females with reproductive capacity before instituting therapy.

After providing information, answering questions, and emphasizing that much about HIV and pregnancy remains unknown, a second stage of counseling is in order, and it may or may not be appropriate during the same visit. Use the genogram to depict visually the patient's emotional and geographic relationships with her family, and expand it to include her greater support network. Ask the patient to characterize the people in her life and her relationship with each. It is important to learn who the patient lives with, who she trusts, and who knows she is HIV-infected. Does she have a partner? Is her partner HIV-infected? Does she have any children or grandchildren? Are any of them at risk for HIV infection? One of the goals of the genogram is to help the patient identify and assess her supports and stressors. Once her network is identified, the focus can return to the patient and the biopsychosocial impact a pregnancy may have on her.

Other important questions are: What is her stage of life (e.g., adolescence, young adulthood, middle age)? In what stage is her disease? Does she have other health problems, including substance abuse? Does she have adequate housing, income, and health insurance? When was her last physical examination (try to obtain a copy before the session if one exists)?

Having done a thorough history and review of her physical examination, provide her with information about HIV and pregnancy, and draw a visual diagram of her concerns and available support groups. Then ask her to consider five possible scenarios:

1. She becomes ill during her pregnancy and must make decisions regarding treatments that may be life-saving to her and her fetus but potentially toxic to the fetus.

2. She does not know throughout her pregnancy and during the first 18 months of her child's life whether or not her child is HIV-infected, since it can take up to 18 months from birth to determine whether a baby is HIV-infected.

3. After her child is born, she remains asymptomatic, but her child becomes ill and possibly dies early in life.

4. She becomes symptomatic, needs hospitalization, and possibly dies, while her child remains healthy.

5. Both she and her child become ill, require hospitalization, and possibly die.

With each scenario, ask versions of the following question: How will you feel if ...? Who will help care for your child if...? Who will help care for you if...? How will those around you (your partner, your child or children, your family and friends) feel if...?

This is a lengthy and intense process that lends itself to role play and discussions with other HIV-infected women who have had to make similar decisions. Emotions that typically arise during the process include a sense of loss at never having been a parent or grief at losing a child, and guilt over bearing an ill child or one she can't take care of if she becomes ill or dies. Help the patient predict her emotional response to each scenario, with the goal of helping her predict how she would cope with these feelings. How has she dealt with loss and guilt before? Would she be in danger of harming herself or someone else? If she is a substance abuser, would she increase her use of drugs or alcohol? Does she have a strong, reliable support network to help her?

Each scenario and each question can raise the patient's awareness and help her explore options. As she does this, there are several self-empowering tools the counselor can help her develop and use. The counselor should emphasize safer sex practices, not only to prevent unwanted pregnancy, but also reinfection with HIV and transmission of other STDs. If the patient is a drug user and not likely to stop, safer drug use practices should be described. The counselor can support the patient in writing her living will and appointing an appropriate health care proxy; planning for child custody in the event of inability to care for her children because of illness or death; and making medical arrangements for her children and coordinating these with her own medical care and, if necessary, that of her partner. If the patient has housing or financial difficulties or other psychosocial stresses, the practitioner should see to it that she gains access to resources and, if necessary, serve as advocate for her within the larger political system.

After all this, the woman is still left with a difficult decision. Through this intensive counseling, the counselor may hope that the woman had acquired sufficient knowledge and insight to make an informed and considered decision. The counselor will also have learned a great deal, which will help in the counseling of the next patient. (This section, "Reproductive Counseling," was adapted from Bermon, 1993.)

PSYCHOSOCIAL ISSUES BROUGHT ON BY HIV/AIDS

HIV disease shares several characteristics with other life-threatening illnesses, most notably the progression toward death; the many physical, emotional, functional, and economic losses; and the process of psychological adjustment. Yet, certain issues associated with providing care for HIV/AIDS patients are unique. For example, there is the fear of contagion and social hostility toward primary HIV/AIDS risk groups—gay men and IDUs. Other issues include the stigma and blame associated with HIV/AIDS, the infectiousness (in particular, the sexual transmissibility of HIV), the epidemic nature of infection, the youth of patients, the roller coaster course of illness, and the neuropsychological impairment, especially in late stages. These issues are

irrelevant to the care of many other terminally ill persons.

Lovers and friends may distance themselves out of fear of contagion or difficulty coping with the diagnosis, or they may experience emotional exhaustion from having been exposed to too many AIDS deaths. Family members may live far away or refuse to become involved. As a result, many patients ultimately live alone. Most patients eventually deteriorate to the point of needing care on a 24-hour basis because of weakness, memory loss, confusion, diarrhea, and other impairments.

Traditional family structures are often absent, and many patients do not have the primary home caregiver required for admission to most hospice programs. For some patients, disclosing the HIV/AIDS diagnosis is tantamount to revealing to family or associates for the first time that they are gay or have used injection drugs.

Effects of Depression on HIV Disease

Accumulating evidence supports the belief held since Hippocrates that vigor, resilience, and perceived support are associated with more favorable medical outcomes. Furthermore, stress and depression have been shown to affect the immune response and, mediated by neuroendocrine mechanisms, may affect vulnerability to illnesses ranging from cancer to the common cold. So, it is reasonable to ask whether one's mental state can affect the course of HIV infection.

The clinical course of HIV disease varies widely. Some people deteriorate rapidly, while others live for years, even after AIDS diagnosis. The reasons for these different rates of decline are not known, but **psychosocial** variables are on the list of possible host factors. The notion has been that one's adaptive coping or fighting spirit might somehow delay or even prevent the progression of HIV disease and, conversely, that distress and despair might measurably accelerate progression of the disease.

Jeffrey Burack and colleagues (1993) reported that overall depression and affective depression predicted a more rapid decline in T4 lymphocyte counts. This association was not

——— BOX 14.8 ———

THE THERAPIST AND THE DYING CLIENT

Jeremy S. Gaies, Psy.D., and Michael D. Knox, Ph.D.

Psychotherapy with the dying is especially challenging when clients are young adults as are many people with HIV disease. Despite its difficulties, however, such counseling frequently offers both patients and providers opportunities for growth and for learning to live more fully.

HIV-related psychotherapy does not require special expertise. However, modifications in therapeutic approach are appropriate to meet the challenges posed by the life-threatening aspects of HIV disease. This article defines therapeutic concerns for HIV-infected people facing death, adjustments therapists must make to meet these concerns, and psychological issues for therapists treating people with HIV disease.

PSYCHOLOGICAL ISSUES OF THE PATIENT

HIV disease shares several characteristics with other life-threatening illnesses, most notably the progression toward death, the multiple physical, emotional, functional, and economic losses, and the process of psychological adjustment. Much attention to psychological responses to terminal illness has focused on stage theories, especially that proposed by Kubler-Ross.[1] While recent theorists have questioned the conception of these responses as fixed, Kubler-Ross's five stages—denial, anger, bargaining, depression, and acceptance—are of great clinical significance when viewed as positive functions of the psyche coping with the emotional demands of the illness. Denial, for example, serves a critical protective function in allowing an individual to survive the stress of catastrophic information. Allowed to progress without impediment, denial will typically and gradually fade toward realistic assimilation of complete information.

There are also striking differences between HIV disease and other terminal diseases. Among these are the intense stigma and blame associated with AIDS, the infectiousness (in particular, the sexual transmissibility of HIV), the epidemic nature of infection, the youth of patients, the roller coaster course of illness, and the neuropsychological impairment, especially in late stages.

These characteristics of HIV disease suggest psychological issues that may be grouped into three constellations. One constellation is loss, including losses of function, health, independence, financial security, standard of living, social support, sexual freedom, mental functioning, and normal life span. A second is stress, including that associated with uncertainty of information, uncertainty of prognosis, discrimination, stigma, guilt, and anger. Much of this stress is related to rational and irrational fears of rejection, abandonment, pain, disability, loss of mental control, and transmitting HIV. A third constellation focuses on issues related to terminal disease such as fear of death and dying, and existential and spiritual aspects of life and death. A client's emotional response to these concepts will affect his or her response to the later stages of disease: a person who perceives death as a peaceful escape from mortal existence will respond differently than a patient who sees death as painful, punishing, or empty nonexistence.

Within these constellations, issues may vary in importance for different individuals and in intensity over the duration of the illness. For one person, the most significant concern will be the loss of financial resources; for another it may be the experience of physical pain or the desire to plan the funeral. Issues will change over the course of disease, as will the content of specific concerns, for example, sexual relationships or mental functioning. Appreciation of the variability and range or responses and needs among clients with HIV disease is one of the most essential aspects of the psychotherapist's preparation for providing quality care. It is particularly important for the therapist to note two aspects of HIV-related care. First, patients tend to seek therapy, even at late stages, to handle immediate needs rather than chronic concerns. Second, by the time they have reached terminal stages, many patients with HIV disease have resolved philosophical issues related to mortality and are confronting practical concerns related to dying.

THERAPEUTIC OBJECTIVES

Although the focus of psychotherapy will vary over time, objectives always include fostering realistic hope, reducing stress, and helping the client to attain a measure of control. In the later stages

———— BOX 14.8 (*continued*) ————

of illness, for example, therapy may provide an opportunity for terminal care decision making, and funeral and memorial planning. Making decisions and taking charge of the final details may enhance client autonomy at a time when other aspects of life seem out of control.[2]

Because the emotional intensity of terminal HIV disease threatens the objectivity of practitioners, therapists are encouraged to use a structured assessment framework. The framework should be comprehensive, to ensure that issues regarding dying are not missed, and objective, to ensure that the framework is biased toward one view of death. Among the factors assessed in a comprehensive framework are personality profile prior to illness, coping skills and styles, hope, realistic awareness of the severity of the illness, cultural and religious background, social support, self-esteem, suicide risk and other self-destructive behaviors, compliance with care, and mental functioning. To develop a comprehensive assessment, counselors should be sure they have a thorough understanding of the key issues for people with HIV disease.

Unlike most people with terminal illnesses, a high percentage of people with HIV disease experience neuropsychological impairment.[3] Clients frequently raise concerns about loss of mental functioning. Neuropsychological assessment is often warranted to identify cognitive strengths and weaknesses and to differentiate organically based from depression-related cognitive impairment. To avoid complications related to mental incompetency, therapists should encourage clients to deal with legal, financial, and health care planning and documents, such as wills, durable powers of attorney for finances and health care, and medical directives or "living wills." With more significant impairment, the therapy process itself must change, with increasing adjustment toward supportive therapy and psychosocial case management.

ADJUSTMENTS IN PROCESS

Therapists must learn to be flexible when counseling people with HIV disease in the late stages of illness. Symptoms of terminal illness, which often make regularly scheduled weekly appointments in the therapist's office difficult, may require home visits, hospital visits, and telephone sessions. Therapy may need to be interrupted at times depending on the patient's physical condition. Lack of time precludes long-term ap-

proaches, and patients frequently require greater encouragement and direction to achieve necessary tasks of closure and planning in the limited time available.

Treatment flexibility also means being open to supplementary, alternative, and modified techniques, such as art or other creative therapies, family therapy including members of a gay client's friendship network, and the use of touch. Limited physical contact is often appropriate when clients are struggling with issues of rejection, physical disfigurement, and irrational concerns regarding infectiousness. Briefly holding a client's hand or allowing a hug at the end of a session is sometimes appropriate, while strict avoidance of physical contact can confirm a client's fears that there is a reason to reject or be afraid of him or her. Adaptable therapists may also have to assume the responsibilities of mental health case managers or advocates. This decision must be based on the specific needs of patients. In general, as patients begin to lose independence, the tasks of case management increase. These tasks may include monitoring health care, ensuring social service involvement, helping to gain access to entitlement programs, and activating and supporting family and friends to care for the patient.

Because people with HIV disease tend to become financially insolvent during the course of the illness, there is often a need at later stages to lower rates of payment and to offer free treatment when health insurance is unavailable. Since therapists, especially those in private practice, are dependent on client fees, it may be advisable to set reasonable limits on the number of people with HIV disease in treatment at any one time. If appropriate, biweekly sessions might allow continued therapy while reducing the financial burden on both the client and counselor. Whatever procedure is chosen, it is imperative that therapists raise this issue with clients at regular intervals and, at all costs, avoid any situation that may be experienced by the client as abandonment.

THERAPIST'S PSYCHOLOGICAL ISSUES

Conducting psychotherapy in general can be emotionally taxing for therapists. The additional challenges of treating clients who have a stigmatized disease and are the same age or younger than the therapist can be significant. For gay therapists, many of whom have lost loved ones to HIV disease, and for seropositive practitioners, the issue of identification is even greater. Maintaining a true sense of presence with the client while maintaining separation from the client's life is critical to the psychotherapeutic relationships. Therapists can best attain the strength to be present and the objectivity to be separate by developing and enriching their own personal lives.

This balance may be threatened as the client becomes more physically ill and nears death, and the therapist experiences some degree of anticipatory grief. Anticipatory grief is a normal reaction, even for a therapist serving in a professional capacity. It is the intensity of the grief and the adaptive response to it that should be considered. The most effective response for therapists may be to acknowledge that they have feelings about the lives and deaths of their clients. It is also essential that the therapists understand that the process of dying and the psychological response to dying (both the client's and the therapist's) are natural and should be supported rather than manipulated, avoided, or suppressed.

Therapists may benefit from practicing techniques for minimizing burnout. Burnout prevention includes setting reasonable goals for therapy and for the therapist, learning to be patient, maintaining a diversity of activities outside of therapy, and finding support in one's personal and professional life. Some form of therapist support group, including a networking or educational group with a social component, may be helpful. Employing a cotherapist for group work can be an excellent way of maintaining both support and objectivity. Other burnout prevention skills include using humor, practicing relaxation, exploring one's own feelings regarding mortality and life meaning, identifying achievable goals that add a sense of purpose to work, and focusing attention every day on personal fulfillment.

Coping with the death of a patient can be a new and threatening experience, and there is little societal support for therapists working through grief about the death of a client. The most important way to cope with this loss is for therapists to be sure that they say goodbye to clients. Saying goodbye may mean actually speaking to a client before the client's death, lighting a memorial candle, setting aside a few moments for private thoughts, or attending the client's funeral.

FINDING INSPIRATION

Providing psychotherapy to people facing the challenges of a life-threatening illness can be inspiring work, offering therapists, as well as clients, the opportunity to grow and live more fully. By sharing a client's experience of confronting the fragility of life and learning to cherish each day, for better or for worse, therapists begin to confront the vulnerability of their own lives and to acquire a deeper appreciation of living. Therapists also witness the psychological power of courage, hope, and faith. These responses awaken therapists to the great potential of human beings to adapt to life changes, an awareness that serves the therapist as an individual as well as a professional.

Jeremy S. Gaies, Psy.D., is Clinical Assistant Professor of Community Mental Health at the University of South Florida's (USF) Florida Mental Health Institute, and Staff Psychologist with American Biodyne, Inc. Michael D. Knox, Ph.D., is Professor, Chairman of the Department of Community Mental Health, and Director of the USF Center for HIV Education and Research.

REFERENCES

1. KUBLER-ROSS, E. (1969). *On Death and Dying.* New York: Macmillan.
2. KNOX, L. P., AND KNOX, M. D. (1991). *Last Wishes: A Workbook for Recording Your Funeral, Memorial, and Other Final Instructions.* Tampa, FL: Applied Science Corp.
3. MILLER, E. N., et al. (1990). Neuropsychological performance in HIV-1 infected homosexual men: the Multicenter AIDS Cohort Study (MACS). *Neurology,* 40:197–203.

———— BOX 14.9 ————

INFORMATION AND LEGAL GUIDELINES FOR PERSONS WITH HIV DISEASE/AIDS

Life expectancy after AIDS diagnosis, using the 1993 definition, is approximately 2 to 5 years. Life expectancy for those who are now on protease inhibitor combination therapy has not yet been determined. But clearly it has been extended (see Chapter 4). Like other patients with terminal illnesses, individuals with AIDS should be encouraged to express their wishes concerning the use or limitation of life-sustaining measures. Such decisions are crucial in early stages of AIDS because many patients experience moderate-to-severe neurological impairment that may deprive them of the power to understand, make decisions, or express their wishes long before they die.

Many professionals involved in AIDS care suggest that the question of using life-sustaining support be brought up with the patient as early as possible, even at the time that he or she first learns of the diagnosis. Some physicians may find it difficult to approach these questions with a patient who still appears healthy. Referral to a social service agency or group specifically concerned with AIDS may be helpful.

LEGAL GUIDELINES

Different types of legal documents expressing wishes about life-sustaining treatments are recognized by different states. Therefore, it may be wise to hire an attorney.

An attorney will be able to help in:

1. Completing an up-to-date will for distribution of assets and settling the estate. It is the best way to control the distribution of property after one dies. It is also a statement to and about people one wishes to remember.
2. Completing a living will that specifies the extent to which the patient wishes life-sustaining measures to be used in case he or she becomes mentally ill or hopelessly ill and unable to make his or her desired known.
3. Preparing a durable power of attorney to designate an individual to make medical treatment decisions, such as the withholding or withdrawal of life support, in the event of mental incapacity. (Traditional power of attorney terminates when the person issuing the document becomes disabled.) The documents may be combined in a single form.

Which document is most appropriate in any individual case may vary from state to state.

As of 1994, 41 states and the District of Columbia had legislation concerning a person's right to die. All states and the District of Columbia have legislation concerning a durable power of attorney. A living will can be executed in a state without specific legislation, because all states recognize the right of a competent person to refuse treatment, regardless of the consequences.

Durable power of attorney may be particularly important for the homosexual patient with AIDS who wishes to appoint a partner or mate as proxy for medical decisions. In the absence of specific legal provision, the authority to make decisions is usually transferred to the next of kin. Family members may not recognize the rights of a patient's partner as decision maker, and may resent the partner as representing a lifestyle of which they disapprove. It may be advisable to appoint more than one proxy, with the second to act if the first is unavailable when needed.

GENERAL GUIDELINES

1. Obtain the names, addresses, and phone numbers of the patient's physician, attorney, family, and loved ones.
2. Make funeral arrangements prior to death. Delicately determine what kind of funeral the patient wants.
3. Locate insurance policies, bankbooks, IRAs, pension funds, if any, selective service or social security numbers, safety deposit key and box, the previous year's tax return, automobile and other titles, outstanding debts, and so on.
4. Keep an account of all expenses for filing the year's tax return.
5. Specifically keep track of medical expenses—what was paid and what is still owed. The insurance company may want proof of expenses.
6. Families, friends, loved ones, or lover are not responsible for debts left by the deceased providing they have not signed on to accept debt responsibilities (**consult an attorney about specifics**).

Information about individual state laws, appropriate forms, and other matters can be obtained from your local medical society or Concern for Dying, 250 West 57th St., New York, NY 10107; (212) 246-6962. Information can also be obtained from the Society for the Right to Die, 250 West 57th St., New York, NY 10107; (212) 246-6973.

An excellent booklet called, "AIDS and Your Legal Rights," is available from National Gay rights Advocates (NGRA) which conducts litigation in the areas of AIDS, employment discrimination, freedom of speech and domestic partnerships, primarily in the western part of the country. This booklet addresses such questions as, "I already have insurance. Can my insurer refuse to pay AIDS or ARC-related claims?," "Can my employer make me take an HIV-antibody test or discriminate against me because of my results?," and "I have AIDS. What public benefits can I get?"

Because laws are constantly changing, this booklet cannot give detailed information on specific laws in every state. Your local AIDS service organization or public health department will know the current laws in your jurisdiction and may be aware of litigation on your issue. Contact NGRA at (213) 650-6200 for the booklet and for help.

---

attributable to baseline physiological differences. While the mechanisms of the association remains unknown and cannot be addressed directly by this study, the data suggest that it can be explained neither as simply a reflection of perceived somatic symptoms nor as the result of differences in recreational drug and alcohol use. Further study is necessary to determine whether treating depression can alter the course of HIV infection.

FAMILY AND FRIENDS: STRESS FACTORS WHEN THE PERSON THEY CARE ABOUT BECOMES HIV-POSITIVE

The psychosocial impact of stress on the HIV-infected is different for each individual and is-sues change during the course of the illness. Problems for asymptomatic HIV-infected individuals are not the same as those for terminal persons with AIDS. The most stress typically occurs at transition points such as confirmation of HIV positivity, the beginning of symptomatic symptoms, or when the need for institutional care develops.

For the HIV-infected, they must deal with: the stigma of HIV and associated behaviors; the real or perceived rejection by family and friends; the desire to remain anonymous because of shame or fear of rejection; not knowing how or to whom to talk about fears and concerns (Table 14-6), particularly in low-incidence areas; and few local resources in low-incidence areas or within cultures where associated behaviors are taboo.

For the family and friends, there may be a double crisis when they find out the son/daughter/friend is a drug user, homosexual, or bisexual. In this case, family/friends must cope with value conflicts as well as death and dying concerns. For parents, these revelations often force reflections on parenting practices. Parents may express guilt over permissiveness, strictness, closeness, distance, acceptance, or rejection as a way to explain or

TABLE 14-6 Common Concerns and Fears of HIV-Infected Individuals

- Leaving children behind
- Experience of real or perceived discrimination
- The possibility of having infected others in the past; continuing fears about infecting others in the future
- Loss of control over items such as who may know about one's personal choices and sexual orientation, because symptoms may reveal or raise speculation about personal matters
- A chronically uncertain future
- Fear of suffering, dying, and death
- Loneliness
- Loss of self-identity
- Loss of physical abilities
- Change in body image
- Loss of control of body functions
- Loss of independence
- Loss of mental capacity
- Bereavement—It is a mourning process for loss which typically begins at the time of an HIV-positive test result. Multiple losses are common at all stages of HIV illness.

assign blame. Parents may place blame on the lover or partner for both the HIV infection and the lifestyle. Friends often become unsure of the person they thought they knew so well and may become distant.

THE WORRIED WELL

Fear of HIV infection may bring significant psychosocial stress to uninfected individuals. Regardless of behavioral risk level, such persons are referred to as the **worried well**. In such cases, individuals have fears of infection that are disproportionate to their actual risk of infection. They can experience severe anxiety reactions leading to illness, social withdrawal or even hospitalization. In one recent event, a 35-year-old male related to the author that he had been divorced for the past 3 years and that although he is sexually aroused among women he has not had sexual foreplay or sexual intercourse since the divorce—the **reason, "I'm just too scared of becoming infected with that damned AIDS virus."** This man said he believed that most of the unmarried women who had sexual encounters carried the virus!

DEATH FROM HIV/AIDS

Never far from the surface of any interaction involving AIDS is the notion of death. In academic and public policy discussions which are often reflected in the popular media, the impact of AIDS is commonly described in terms of death rates for age and population subgroups or translated into years of potential life lost. In clinical settings, AIDS has helped to crystalize ideas and procedures long needed for other conditions, such as living wills and health care proxies. It is with individual patients and their families that these concerns come most clearly into focus (Dobkin, 1995). In brief, people with HIV disease are always living with HIV disease. It is hard to tell when an individual might start to die of it, and even harder to tell when the people around that individual should acknowledge that dying has entered the relationship. **But there is a point in HIV progression when it is no longer possi-** ble to avoid the discomfort of talking about death, the point at which someone is dying. Sometimes, even if a loved one has been in a serious and steady decline with wasting, disorientation, and a cascade of other symptoms and infections, it can be hard for the closest caregivers to see, or to admit, what is going on. It can make a tremendous difference for physicians, therapists, or friends to speak the truth, acknowledging the approach of death gently but clearly. The language and the degree of bluntness will be different for different people, but the point is, do not wait to say what needs to be said (Rose, 1996).

THE GRIEVING PROCESS

Grief is an emotional, psychological, and, often, physical response to the death of another. It is a period of time during which the normal state of one's own life (i.e., view of self and view of the world) is altered and out of balance. The grieving process for HIV disease and AIDS usually begins with a positive test result and varies in degree of intensity from one individual to another. The two major goals of the grieving process are: **(1)** restoration of the state of effective psychological functioning, and **(2)** redefining one's self in the face of loss: Who and what am I now?

The grieving process is not a linear process; grief does not occur according to a script, but there appear to be common items that contribute to the eventual resolution of grief: **(1)** the acceptance of the loss—this period is marked by a sense of unreality of the death which then gradually dissipates; and **(2)** feeling the pain of grief—grief pain may occur on a variety of levels: physical, psychological, emotional, and/or behavioral. The level and intensity of this pain varies from one individual to another. How and when this pain is expressed varies from culture to culture. In 1969, Elizabeth Kubler-Ross established her five stages of dying. Each stage is, in a way, self-explanatory:

Stage 1: Denial—no not me!
Stage 2: Anger
Stage 3: Bargaining—allow me to live to a certain point in time

Stage 4: Depression—deep sadness over the on-coming loss

Stage 5: Acceptance—it's inevitable!

The Kubler-Ross stages of death are mentioned often to patients by their counselors. (An excellent source of information on managing grief associated with HIV/AIDS is the May 1992 issue of *FOCUS*, Volume 7, or contact the National Clearinghouse for government publications on "Organizational Grief," Washington, D.C.)

HIV/AIDS SUPPORT GROUPS

Individuals who share a common problem such as a medical condition, life-threatening disease, or short-term crisis may benefit from support systems and mutual help. Over the last 25 years, there has been a proliferation of support groups for patients with a wide spectrum of medical and psychiatric conditions. These groups can be led by professionals, or they may be self-help groups directed by members. Professionally led support groups draw on psychotherapeutic principles but, like self-help groups, emphasize high group cohesion and low confrontation—no one blames anyone. Both types of groups stress the therapeutic value of universality, altruism, and hope (Levy et al., 1990).

COUNSELING FOR HIV-INFECTED TEENAGERS

To this point, counseling topics have dealt mainly with the HIV-infected adult. But there is another rapidly growing population of HIV-infected people who need caring and sensitive counseling as well—teenagers. Sex, drugs, and rock 'n roll of the 1950s and 1960s have given way to the sexually transmitted diseases, HIV and AIDS of the late 1970s, 1980s, and 1990s. Sex for the adolescent has become increasingly high-risk behavior.

As counselors, you can expect to deal with about as many adolescent males as females; the ratio of HIV-infected males to females is 2.6:1. For adults, it is about 8:1.

Teenagers are not just older children or younger adults. Adolescence is a developmental phase that occurs as one proceeds from childhood to adulthood. More changes occur between the ages of 10 and 20 than during any other period, and these may include dramatic shifts in biological and cognitive functioning. Psychosocial development shows even greater diversity as teenagers develop their own identities, experimenting with an array of sexual, moral, vocational, and political paths. This diversity frames the experience of teenagers with HIV disease, which complicates this already challenging period.

For seropositive teenagers, HIV infection can be a terrifying and mysterious intrusion into life, and teenagers react to HIV infection in a variety of ways. As with HIV-infected adults, seropositive and at-risk teenagers form a diverse group, one for which a single, formulaic approach to treatment and care is sure to result in failure. Similarly, reactions to HIV disease depend upon each youth's stage of illness, life history, social and familial support system, and levels of cognitive development, moral development, emotional maturity, and self-acceptance.

In response to these factors, counselors should pay special attention to two issues: the level of understanding and rapport. First, while many teenagers, particularly older ones, are psychologically sophisticated, counselors should assume, until proven otherwise, that they have not reached mature levels of thought. Second, as with adults, counselor rapport with teenagers is crucial to success. Achieving rapport is especially challenging, since teens may see counselors as authority figures and feel that they have been forced into talking with them about something that they find terrifying or shameful.

Four specific issues that require special emphasis when counseling teenagers are: **(1)** disclosing HIV infection status, **(2)** how they respond to the news of HIV infection, **(3)** coping with disease progression, and **(4)** approaching their death.

Disclosing Infection

The issue of when and to whom to disclose the fact that they are HIV-infected is one of the first major decisions teenagers must face. Many teenagers face greater pressure to disclose because they are more likely than adults to live with family, who assume an entitlement to this knowledge, and because they are less likely than adults to have learned the resourcefulness necessary to access help. In addition, disclosure to family may be potentially more difficult among teenagers because families are legally and socially able to exert greater control over minors. Like adults, many teens fear the loss of support from family, friends, and present and future sexual partners.

For some teens, disclosure is twofold. Those teens who became infected through male-to-male or female-to-female sexual activity effectively "come out" about homosexual experimentation or orientation at the same time they disclose HIV infection status. Some support systems can tolerate the reality of HIV disease, but cannot tolerate homosexuality.

Telling a parent may be more difficult than telling a friend. The decision should be based on a thorough exploration of potential consequences. Are the parents likely to support or reject the teenager? Will they provide emotional and financial support? Are they capable of providing such support? Does the teen want to tell his or her parents, or does he or she feel compelled to do so? If a youth decides to tell a parent, it may be useful to role-play the conversation to help him or her prepare for parental reactions. It may also help the teen for the counselor to be with him or her during the disclosure, and to have follow-up meetings to help the family adjust to the news. Referral for family therapy is another good option.

It is worth mentioning that while the involvement of a supportive adult is ideal, informing parents may not always be in the best interests of teenagers and may even be dangerous. This is particularly relevant in cases of runaway or throwaway youth.

Responding to Seroconversion

The only generality that can be made about teenagers is that each will, either overtly or covertly, have a strong reaction to the news that he or she is HIV-infected. Reactions may include anger, guilt, anxiety, depression, suicidal or homicidal ideation, numbness, or terror, and, in all likelihood, all of these will be present to one degree or another.

Teenagers may have difficulty confronting HIV disease for reasons similar to adults. Unlike adults, however, many teens—particularly younger ones—have difficulty, in the absence of overt signs of infection, understanding and believing they are HIV-infected. This can be frustrating to counselors in that it adds to the difficulty of motivating changes in risk-related behaviors and ensuing compliance of medical regimens and prudent care.

Teenagers who do not fully acknowledge the implications of being HIV-infected may simply be confused or in denial. Many teens have not yet achieved the cognitive maturity level whereby full acceptance and understanding is even possible. The ability to think in abstract terms occurs slowly during the adolescent years. Until the capacity for mature thought is achieved, they frequently perceive themselves to be immortal, are predominantly egocentric, and view the world in very concrete terms.

What may be common knowledge or basic information to most adults may be new to HIV-infected youth, especially if they are disenfranchised from the mainstream due to homelessness, ethnicity, or sexual orientation.

Teenagers also tend to be less deliberate in what they do or say and are less likely to follow through on actions; their impulse control and frustration tolerance may not yet be developed to the point where they can behave in a manner that ultimately serves their best interests. It is vital that counselors be ready to provide adolescents with a more mature perspective and necessary structure when the capacity to provide it for themselves is not operating. They can do this by helping teens to verbalize feelings and explore the consequences of planned actions. This approach will discourage acting out in potentially self-destructive ways, such as suicidal gestures, revenge towards others, or refusal to keep appointments or to take medications—behaviors that may function to camouflage feelings of fear, anger, and despair.

Finally, it is critical during this period to assist teens in disentangling reality from fantasy and to correct distortions stemming from internalized fears and judgments. For example, it can be difficult for teenagers to make the fine distinctions required to understand that the desire to engage in oral, anal, or vaginal intercourse did not lead to infection; the act of sexual intercourse without barrier protection did.

Coping with Disease Progression

Teenagers tend to think in a concrete manner, to believe that a fixed T-helper cell number implies a specific serious illness or impending death. The idea that T-helper cell counts are a barometer of immune system function is a difficult concept for teenagers to grasp. Therefore, T-helper cell counts should not be discussed in an isolated manner; such a discussion should always be in the context of current medical status and level of functioning. To help teens negotiate these issues, counselors should focus on the concept of the spectrum of HIV-related illnesses, and not on fixed cutoffs for disease diagnosis and progression.

It is equally essential to provide a safe, nonjudgmental forum for teenagers to voice fears and concerns if and when T-helper cell counts fall, particularly since they may be doing everything they can to stave off such a deterioration of health. In general, teens are less able to permanently integrate this information without intense fear, anxiety, and defensiveness distorting their perceptions of reality, and they often require repetition of basic facts regarding their illness. In response, counselors should repeatedly explain concepts in different ways.

As teenagers develop symptoms, they may be jolted from the denial about the severity of their symptoms. Counselors should fully explore the subjective meanings and implications of each symptom and should seek to validate these impressions while simultaneously correcting misconceptions. In particular, teens may need help in putting symptoms into perspective, to understand that not all infections are equally serious and not all are AIDS-defining.

Approaching Their Death

Perhaps the most agonizing area of adjustment for teens and counselors involves confronting the possibility of death. Teenagers, many of whom lack the capacity for this abstract thought, have fixed ideas about death, and this lack of flexibility may raise anxiety. As with adults, teenagers may respond to this anxiety with subtle verbal and nonverbal cues. Counselors should be particularly aware of cues such as crying, anger, silence, or anxious fidgeting, which may indicate discomfort.

Discussions of death should be preceded by a thorough exploration of any preconceived notions about dying. From that base, counselors can gently and compassionately help teenagers prepare for death.

Ironically, a conversation about death is frequently a relief for teens. It may be a topic they have thought about, but have been afraid to verbalize for fear of upsetting family, loved ones, and friends. In keeping silent, teenagers, sensing the discomfort of others, may have actually been taking care of parents and counselors. (This section, "Counseling for HIV-Infected Teenagers," was adapted from Elliot, 1993.)

LIVING WILLS

The fact that HIV disease is not considered a terminal illness in over half of states in the United States makes it difficult for HIV-infected people to implement living wills. According to a review of the U.S. law surrounding this issue, the right to refuse treatment is often related to whether refusal is in response to a terminal illness. People with HIV disease face the challenge of proving that HIV disease is terminal. If they cannot, states may stop the implementation of their living wills.

Statutory definitions of what constitutes a terminal condition and a life-sustaining treatment tend to be circular. In most statutes, withdrawal or withholding of life-sustaining treatment can proceed only after several physicians certify that the person is in a terminal condition. A condition is defined as terminal only if "life-sustaining procedures" are employed to postpone the moment of death but do not improve life. Many common HIV-related treatments do not meet this definition.

Many HIV-related treatments do not meet other aspects of these definitions. In 11 states, a life-sustaining procedure is defined as that which "sustains, restores, or supplants a vital function." Medication is specifically excluded from these definitions in 19 states and the District of Columbia. HIV disease is not considered terminal in 11 states because death must be "imminent," and recovery from opportunistic infections occurs too often to meet this requirement (Kortlandt, 1991).

The federal courts have frequently defined the right to die in broader terms than state statutes would imply. Case law, based on judicial decisions, has tended to be more flexible than statutory law. The federal courts have viewed the right to die in terms of the individual's right to privacy versus the state's need to prevent suicide, protect third parties, maintain the integrity of the medical profession, and preserve life. They have used the state's right to prevent suicide as a means of investigating the motives of those rejecting treatments and have ruled against withdrawal of treatment if such a decision appears to be irrational.

The federal and state courts appear to be moving toward expanding privacy rights by letting mentally incompetent as well as competent patients die. Family members and patient-designated medical decision makers are being allowed to decide to withdraw treatment. The 1990 Supreme Court decision in *Cruzan v. Harmon* established a patient's right to die if there is clear and convincing evidence that the patient would forgo treatment if men-

—————— BOX 14.10 ——————

MAKING TERMINAL CARE DECISIONS

Jeannee Parker Martin, R.N., M.P.H.

People with HIV disease should consider their options for terminal care early in the disease process to avoid the pressures of medical complications, such as AIDS dementia complex, and psychosocial concerns, such as diminishing financial resources. It is generally accepted that a patient is "terminally ill" when disease prognosis is 6 months or less, so the notion of terminal care should not be limited in conception to the last few weeks of life. If considered early enough, people with HIV disease may have several options about where they die and under what conditions, including in hospitals, at home, and in group residential facilities.

FACTORS TO CONSIDER

Where does the individual want to die? The place where someone dies may be determined by factors out of a patient's control. A good first step is to identify, through direct questioning, whether a patient has a preference about where he or she dies. Caregivers may find that patients will be relieved, instead of dismayed, by a direct approach to terminal care issues.

Does the patient want aggressive curative therapy or palliative hospice care during the final months of life? Patients in the terminal phases of illness may choose to seek curative therapy that will extend life, even when practitioners predict that these therapies will have little effect, or patients may choose only palliative care, aimed at reducing discomfort but not at fighting disease progression. Patients seeking a curative therapy may have fewer options about where to die because treatment may require special equipment and care. On the other hand, palliative therapy, which forms the basis of the hospice philosophy of care, can be provided in the patient's home, as well as in hotels, group residential settings, hospitals, skilled nursing facilities, and other sites.

What type of insurance or financial resources does the patient have now and expect to have during the final 6 months of life? The type of insurance coverage a patient has, and whether or not it changes over the course of illness, will allow access to different care options. Private insurance policies cover medically necessary care in hospitals, and increasingly, in home care settings. Most private insurers want to provide appropriate, cost-effective care and will consider options—such as home, hospice, and residential care—even if they are not specified in their policies.

Low-income or indigent patients may become eligible for Medicaid (Medi-Cal in California), which pays for acute hospital services, skilled nursing facility care, and intermittent home health care. In some states, Medicaid may pay for group residential care, extended hour attendant or nursing care, and hospice care. Older and disabled patients may be eligible for Medicare, which covers acute hospital services, short-term skilled nursing facility care, intermittent home health care, and hospice care, but does not pay for group residential care, or extended attendant or nursing care.

Loss of job-related income, costly medications, and routine expenses such as food and shelter may diminish financial resources. Assets such as cars and homes may be sold to help pay for insurance premiums or other health-related expenses, but patients should consider how much sacrifices will affect quality of life.

What human resources are available to assist as the patient's physical or mental status deteriorates? Patients who prefer home care may be able to facilitate this care, even without insurance coverage, by organizing friends and relatives to provide round-the-clock support. This type of care requires a cohesive and reliable network of volunteers, as well as one or two individuals who are available to help organize and run this network. In addition, patients and their caregivers should consider how support services from community programs can provide additional assistance.

What cultural and religious distinctions should be considered? Patients should give credence to their own cultural and religious beliefs about death and where to die. Lack of adherence to these cultural mores may make the dying process difficult and have lasting emotional consequences for survivors.

HOSPITAL INPATIENT CARE

Before they die, people with HIV disease may experience multiple episodes of acute illness requiring repeated hospitalizations. Although the focus of hospital care is generally rehabilitation to prior level of functioning, some individuals require hospital care as disease progresses and conditions deteriorate. To deal with the needs of dying HIV-infected patients, hospitals may offer designated specialty units, skilled nursing facilities for patients with long-term inpatient need, and inpatient hospice units.

Because hospitals offer care around the clock, some may feel that this is the safest environment for people whose conditions are deteriorating. They may also find a medical setting, where expert care is readily available, to be comforting and may fear that, if a patient remains at home, family members will not provide the "right" care to deal with medical emergencies, pain, or death itself.

HOME CARE

When offered adequate physical care and emotional support by either family, friends, or professional caregivers, most individuals choose the familiar surroundings of their homes for terminal care. Whether receiving short-term, intermittent care, extended nursing care, or hospice care, home care is most often provided by a coordinated professional health care team.

This team generally consists of the patient's attending physician, nurses, social workers, home health aides, attendants, and counselors, and addresses both physical and psychosocial needs. Specialty services, such as intravenous therapy, total parenteral nutrition, and respiratory care can be provided by most home care agencies and may be needed even during terminal phases. While family or friends may provide all or part of necessary terminal care, they usually require professional instruction and supervision.

GROUP RESIDENTIAL CARE

Some communities have developed group residential hospice facilities. These homelike facilities are cost-effective because they consolidate services, such as round-the-clock attendant and nursing care, and deliver them to patients who would otherwise have to use more expensive hospital settings. Despite this, group settings often are not covered by public or private insurance programs. Skilled nursing facilities and nursing homes, while appropriate for terminal care, provide limited access to people with HIV disease.

CONCLUSION

Under the best circumstances, individuals will make terminal care decisions while they are mentally competent and with the help of health care professionals. They should also assign to trusted friends or relatives decision-making rights under durable powers of attorney for health care and include these people in terminal care planning. This preparation is important, because the practical aspects of terminal care are as influential in determining a patient's comfort with dying as is his or her spiritual approach to death.

tally competent. This "substituted judgment test" and the "best interests approach"—by which the court makes decisions based on the best interests of the patient—mark an expansive trend in the law that may make it easier for people with HIV disease to have their living wills implemented (Kortlandt, 1991).

SUMMARY

In a few states, HIV testing is preceded by counseling on HIV infection, its transmission, and the type of tests available to detect HIV antibodies. Regardless of whether results are positive or negative, the person is counseled to practice safer sex and to strive to change any behavior that led to his or her visit to the testing center. Based on interviews of counselors at testing centers, the hardest client is the past or present injection drug user. Past IDUs, if positive, may revert to drug abuse with reckless abandon—a kind of suicidal behavior. The present IDU, if positive, believes he or she has **no sane reason to give up drugs**. They feel they are going to die either way.

With regard to those who take an HIV test, strict confidentiality is of the utmost importance. The literature is replete with examples of people being persecuted for taking the test—after all, if they had reason to take the test, they must be doing something wrong. In many cases, males are immediately labeled homosexuals because of the high incidence of HIV infection and AIDS in the homosexual population. Individuals who have been identified as HIV carriers and patients diagnosed with AIDS have lost their jobs, friends, families, lovers, and homes and have been denied insurance policies, bank loans, and home mortgages. Confidentiality appears to be a must in the success of any HIV testing program. It has been shown repeatedly that lack of confidentiality is driving high-risk people who might be HIV-infected away from testing centers.

REVIEW QUESTIONS

(Answers to the Review Questions are on page 580.)

1. What are the three components of HIV pre-test procedure?

2. Name the two forms of counseling that can be offered when a person is indecisive about taking an HIV test.

3. What is post-HIV test counseling for?

4. People finding out that they are HIV-positive enter a stage of _____. What other stages may they go through?

5. Patients who test HIV-negative may still need counseling, because they _____.

    A. need reassurance

    B. feel guilty

    C. may become suicidal

    D. all of the above

6. Most patients will undergo testing if _____.

    A. a sexual partner is HIV-seropositive

    B. their physician recommends such and ensures confidentiality

    C. they have shared needles/syringes

    D. their physician explains their behavior has put them at risk

7. Who is primarily responsible for informing an HIV-positive patient's contacts or partners?

    A. the patient

    B. the physician

    C. a public health service agency

    D. the state health department

8. True or False: The pain associated when grief is expressed will vary from culture to culture.

9. True or False: The homosexual individual often replaces his or her family of origin with a family of choice, which may consist of lovers and close friends.

10. True or False: Support groups for HIV-infected homosexual or bisexual men should be as heterogeneous as possible with regard to disease stage.

REFERENCES

AMERICAN PSYCHIATRIC ASSOCIATION. (1994). *American Psychiatric Association Diagnostic and Statistical Manual of Mental Disorders*, ed. 4[DSM-IV]. Washington D. C.

BERMAN, NANCY. (1993). Family and reproductive issues. *AIDS Clin. Care*, 5:45–47.

BURACK, JEFFREY, et al. (1993). Depressive symptoms and CD4 lymphocyte decline among HIV-infected men. *JAMA*, 270:2568–2573.

COTE, TIMOTHY, et al. (1992). Risk of suicide among persons with AIDS. *JAMA*, 268:2066–2068.

Disclosure Counseling. (1994). *JAMA*, 271:492.

DOBKIN, JAY. (1995). Death and AIDS. *Infect. Med.* 12:300.

DRUCKER, ERNEST. (1995). Harm reduction: a public health strategy. *Curr. Issues Public Health*, 1:64–70.

DUSTOW, CHRISTOPHER. (1995). Sex, sexuality, safer sex and HIV. *AIDS Clin. Care*, 7:53–55, 59.

ELLIOT, ALAN. (1993). Counseling for HIV-infected adolescents. *FOCUS*, 8:1–4.

HELQUIST, MICHAEL. (1996). Living with therapy. *FOCUS*, 11:1–4.

HUNT, MORTON. (1974). *Sexual Behavior in the 1970s*. Chicago: Playboy Press.

HYDE, JANET SHIBLEY. (1992). *Understanding Human Sexuality*. New York: McGraw Hill.

KINSEY, ALFRED C., et al. (1948). *Sexual Behavior in the Human Male*. Philadelphia: W.B. Saunders.

KORTLANDT, C.E.M. (1991). AIDS and living wills. *AIDS Public Policy J.*, 5(4):157–166.

KUBLER-ROSS, ELIZABETH. (1969). *On Death and Dying*. New York: Macmillan.

LEVY, RUTH SHIPTON, et al. (1990). A group intervention model for individuals testing positive for HIV antibody. *Am. J. Orthopsychiatry*, 60:452–459.

LIPSON, MICHAEL. (1993). Disclosure within families. *AIDS Clin. Care*, 5:43–44, 47.

LIPSON, MICHAEL. (1995). Disclosing HIV status to HIV-infected children. *AIDS Reader*, 5:200, 205–208.

MORKOWITZ, JOHN. (1995). Treating HIV-associated depression with psychotherapy. *AIDS Reader*, 5:95–98.

MARKS, ROBERT. (1995). Editorial: women, men and drugs. *FOCUS*, 10:4.

MARKS, ROBERT. (1996). Editorial: cultural competence. *FOCUS*, 11:2.

MONETTE, PAUL. (1988). *Borrowed Time: An AIDS Memoir*. New York: Harcourt Brace Jovanovich.

Morbidity and Mortality Weekly Report. (1987). Public health service guidelines for counseling and antibody testing to prevent HIV infection and AIDS. 36:509–515.

Morbidity and Mortality Weekly Report. (1993). Technical guidance on HIV counseling. 42:11–17.

Morbidity and Mortality Weekly Report. (1995). HIV counseling and testing–United States. 44:169–174.

PERRY, SAMUEL. (1993). Depression and HIV: how does one affect the other? *JAMA*, 270:2609–2610.

ROSE, AVI. (1996). HIV and dying: the challenges of caring. *FOCUS*, 11:1–4.

ROWLAND, CRAIG. (1990). Losing it. *PAACNOTES*, 2:99–100.

SARTI, GERALYN M. (1990). Asymptomatic patients with HIV infection. *Postgrad. Med.*, 87:143–154.

SELWYN, PETER A., (1989). Knowledge of HIV antibody status and decisions to continue or terminate pregnancy among intravenous drug users. *JAMA*, 261:3567–3571.

SHERER, RENSLOW. (1988). Physician use of the HIV antibody test. The need for consent, counseling, confidentiality, and caution. *JAMA*, 259:264–265.

SHERNOFF, MICHAEL. (1988). Integrating safer sex counseling into social work practice. *J. Contemp. Social Work*, 69:334–339.

SULLIVAN, PATRICIA. (1995). The second decade of AIDS—a book review. *FOCUS*, 11:1–2.

Summary Report. (1993–1994). HIV counseling and testing in publicly funded sites. U.S. Department of Health and Allied Services. Atlanta: Centers for Disease Control and Prevention, March 1996.

WALKER, GILLIAN. (1995). Supportive counseling for HIV-infected drug using women. *FOCUS*, 10:1–4.

Images of the AIDS Pandemic: Knowledge, Attitudes, and Behavior

CHAPTER CONCEPTS

♦ The HIV/AIDS "devastation" is here.

♦ Inaccurate journalism leads to public hysteria.

♦ Vignettes on AIDS.

♦ Over 15 years later, what do we know about HIV/AIDS?

♦ Use of explicit sexual language on TV and in journalism.

♦ Goal of sex education: To interrupt HIV transmission.

♦ Education, just say know.

♦ The Red Ribbon.

♦ Education is not stopping HIV transmission.

♦ Students still have misconceptions about HIV transmission.

♦ The general public and homophobia.

♦ Employees are not well informed and fear working with HIV/AIDS-infected co-workers.

♦ Teenagers are not changing sexual behaviors that place them at risk for HIV infection.

♦ First World AIDS Day observed in 1988.

♦ Orphaned children due to AIDS-related deaths.

♦ Physician–patient relationships in the AIDS era.

♦ Educating employees about AIDS.

♦ Placing the risk of HIV and infection in perspective.

Acquired Immune Deficiency Syndrome (AIDS) is an illness now characterized, according to CDC criteria, as the presence of antibody to HIV and a T4 cell count of less than $200/\mu l$ of blood, and by the presence of certain opportunistic infections and diseases that affect both the body and brain.

BLAME SOMEONE, DÉJÀ VU

The greater **hostility** and greatest **stigma** tends to be assigned to diseases in which individuals are seen as responsible for having the disease; in which the disease's course is fatal; in which fear of transmission is a major issue; and in which the disease leads to highly visible and frightening physical expressions. All the above conditions are associated with HIV disease and AIDS. With AIDS more than any other disease in history, people have found verbal mechanisms for distancing themselves from thoughts of personal infection. Worldwide, from the onset of this pandemic, people have learned in a relatively short time to **categorize**, **rationalize**, **stigmatize**, and **persecute** those with HIV disease and AIDS. AIDS statistics are published in categories to identify how many gay or bisexual men, injection drug users, persons with hemophilia, and so on, have developed AIDS. Also listed are the countries, states, and cities with the highest incidence of the disease, along with which racial and ethnic groups are highest among reported AIDS cases. **By focusing on categories of people, have we made it possible for society to rationalize that AIDS belongs to somebody else? Have we made the thought of HIV/AIDS somewhat impersonal? HAVE WE FOUND A WAY TO BLAME SOMEONE ELSE?**

Placing blame does not always require reason and tends to focus on people who are not considered normal by the majority. Thus minorities and foreigners are often singled out to blame for something, sometimes anything. Epidemics of plague, smallpox, leprosy, syphilis, cholera, tuberculosis, and influenza have historically focused social blame onto specific groups of people for spreading the diseases by their "deviant" behavior. Blaming others leads to their stigmatization and persecution.

While the Black Death, an epidemic of bubonic plague, swept across Europe in the 14th century, blame was variously attached to Jews and witches, followed by the massacre and burning of the alleged culprits. In Massachusetts between 1692 and 1693, some 20 people were hanged or burned at the stake after being accused of having the powers of the devil. Eighty percent of those accused were women. And when Hitler blamed Jews, communists, homosexuals, and other "undesirables" for the economic stagnation of Germany in the 1930s, the result was death camps and ultimately the second World War. Now there is a new plague—HIV/AIDS. What blame comes packaged with this new disease?

Jonathan Mann, former head of the World Health Organization's Global Program on AIDS, points out that there are really three HIV/AIDS epidemics, which are in fact phases in the invasion of a community by the AIDS virus.

First is the epidemic of silent infection by HIV, often completely unnoticed. **Second**, after a period of incubation/clinical latency that may last for years, is the epidemic of the disease itself, with an estimated 8 million AIDS cases worldwide beginning 1997.

Third, and perhaps equally important as the disease itself, is the epidemic of social, cultural, economic, and political reaction to HIV/AIDS. The willingness of each generation to place blame on others when believable explanations are not readily available simply recycles history. We have been there before; we have placed blame on others and it will continue. With respect to the HIV/AIDS pandemic, blame has been disseminated among nations. And, there is no shortage of political, economic, social, or ethical issues associated with this **new** disease.

PANIC AND HYSTERIA OVER THE SPREAD OF HIV/AIDS IN THE UNITED STATES

With the 1981 announcement by the U.S. Public Health Service and the CDC that there was a new disease, AIDS quickly became a symbol for our darkest fears. Responsible public officials gave out conflicting messages: **reassurance** on one hand and **alarm** on the other. Public panic and hysteria began.

People with HIV disease and AIDS are still abused, ridiculed, and maligned. Some people believe that AIDS is divine retribution for immoral lifestyles. People who have not indulged in high-risk lifestyles (e.g., newborns and recipients of blood products) continue to be labeled as innocent victims, implying that other HIV-infected individuals are guilty of the behavior that led to their infection and therefore deserve their illness.

Families and communities continue to be divided on their beliefs and acceptance of HIV/AIDS patients. Federal and state agencies

DO PEOPLE REALLY TRUST SCIENCE?

The essence of science is to find **TRUTHS**. To attack **IGNORANCE**! Sounds good—but most science as presented in scholarly works is difficult for the lay person to understand. And scientists themselves do little to make their work more easily understood. Then there is the news media's constant clamor to expose scientific fraud and to overplay scientific reports to sell copy. Note the 1997 explosion of media events following the announcement of **cloning sheep**. But what the news media didn't say was **more important**, that the technique for cloning sheep had been used some 45 years ago to clone frogs. But suddenly, our society was at risk? Earlier there were the announcements of **electromagnetic fields** causing cancer and a "**tremendous breakthrough**" at Fusion Research Laboratories that would virgually solve the **world's energy problems**. The media hype, then too, was out of proportion to the available known facts and this turned out to be a fraud. And remember, President Nixon promised a cure for cancer in the 1970s! These and many, many other accounts of media-hyped scientific promises may be the cause of public **distrust** (?) or at the very least the public's hesitancy to believe in science. How do we know lay persons are hesitant about science? **here we are in 1998**, and we live in a country in which half of the people believe that our earth is no more than 10,000 years old, and where many people still believe the earth is **flat**, that humans never landed on the moon, or that Sojourner rolling across the martian surface is really a series of photographs of a battery-operated toy moving over rocky earth terrain! Yet, the majority of people believe in paranormal phenomena! The fact that most newspapers carry a daily column on astrology but not on astronomy gives us a strong indication of where the public's faith lies. To add to this confusion, with respect to HIV/AIDS, are the headlines and TV programs that continue to provide a wide array of opinions, by some reputable scientists, physicians, and politicians that declare H IV does not cause AIDS. (See Chapter 2 for a discussion of this material.) Is it any wonder that millions of people, worldwide, do not believe what scientists are saying about the HIV/AIDS pandemic?

stand accused of a lack of commitment and compassion in the war against AIDS. The bottom line is that **value judgments** are associated with HIV/AIDS because the disease involves the most private areas of people's lives—sex, pregnancy, drug use, and finances.

The Fear Factor

Worldwide the media political, medical, and legal communities set out to scare people about a new disease called AIDS. The result has been to scare people into fearing other people rather than the disease. For example, a 1990 survey of 1,000 black American church members in five cities found that more than one third of them believed the AIDS virus was produced in a germ warfare laboratory as a form of genocide against blacks.

Another third said they were "unsure" whether the virus was created to kill blacks. That left only one third who disputed the theory.

The findings held firm even among educated individuals, said one of the authors of the 1990 survey. Rumors that AIDS was created to kill blacks have circulated in the black community for years, and the belief is endorsed by some black leaders. **The message to everyone now is to encourage public compassion**.

A poster in the Swiss STOP AIDS Campaign focuses on how we think about people with AIDS:

> For the doctors, I am HIV-positive; for some neighbors, I am AIDS-contaminated; for my friends, I am Claude-Eric.

Soon after young homosexual men began dying in large numbers, a barrage of frightening rhetoric began filling the airwaves, television, the popular press, and even the most reputable scientific journals. The AIDS disaster was here. One health care administrator stated "We have not seen anything of this magnitude that we can't control except nuclear bombs."

In 1986, Myron Essex of the Department of Cancer Biology at the Harvard School of Public Health noted,

> The Centers for Disease Control and Prevention (CDC) has been trying to inform the public without overly alarming them, but we outside the government are freer to speak. The fact is that the dire predictions of those who have cried doom ever since AIDS appeared haven't been far off the mark . . . The effects of the virus are far wider than most people realize. It has shown up not just in blood and semen but in brain tissue, vaginal secretions, and even saliva and tears, although there's no evidence that it's transmitted by the last two.

In 1987, columnist Jack Anderson reported that the Central Intelligence Agency (CIA) concluded that in just a few years heterosexual AIDS cases would *outnumber* homosexual cases in the United States. Also in 1987, Otis Bowen, former Secretary of Health and Human Services, said AIDS would make the Black Death that wiped out one-third of Europe's population in the Middle Ages pale by comparison. In 1988, sex researchers William Masters, Virginia Johnson, and Robert Kolodny stated in their book, *New Directions In the AIDS Crisis: The Heterosexual Community*, that there was a possibility of HIV infection via casual transmission— from toilet seats, handling of contact lenses from an AIDS patient, eating a salad in a restaurant prepared by a person with AIDS, or from instruments in a physician's office used to examine AIDS patients.

In contrast to these reports is the 1988 article by Robert Gould in *Cosmopolitan* reassuring women that there is practically no risk of becoming HIV-infected through ordinary vaginal or oral sex even with an HIV-infected male. The vaginal secretions produced during sexual arousal keep the virus from penetrating the vaginal walls. His explanation was: "Nature has arranged this so that sex will feel good and be good for you."

ACTIONS OF COURAGE

There are far too many heroes of this pandemic to list here. And the heroes come from every walk of life and profession. So many have

---

BOX 15.1

AN EXAMPLE OF UNCONTROLLED FEAR AND HOSTILITY

In 1986, a very ill AIDS patient on an airline flight spilled some urine from a drainage bag on the seats and carpet. After the patient deplaned, several rows of seats around the area were taped off; the contaminated area would be removed. Crew members and airline union leaders expressed outrage at the exposure of passengers and crew to this threat. The clean-up crew refused to remove the carpet, even using rubber gloves.

BUT WE HAVE LEARNED SINCE THEN, RIGHT? **WRONG!**

In April 1993, an American Airlines flight crew requested that all pillows and blankets be changed on a plane that carried a group described by an internal communication as "gay rights activists." A representative for American Airlines apologized saying that such action was completely and totally inappropriate and that American Airlines has a strict policy against discrimination of any individual or group. **But it happened.**

Well, that is behind us, not to worry, **it will not happen again—certainly not in 1995** when we have all been exposed to so much AIDS education- RIGHT? **WRONG AGAIN!** In June of 1995 a delegation of 50 gay and lesbian elected officials was met at the White House by uniformed Secret Service officers wearing rubber gloves. The officers were apparently concerned about the risk of infection from HIV.

CAN IT HAPPEN AGAIN? September 1997— His sister told ambulance personnel that her sick brother had AIDS and had to go to a specific county hospital. They said they could **not** go outside their county line. She called a multi-county ambulance service. After arrival, neither ambulance service personnel would go near her brother. Her young daughter held an oxygen mask on him while she drove him to the hospital. He died later that evening. The sister filed an AIDS discrimination suit against the ambulance services. (Case pending)

---

answered the call for help, for compassion and human kindness. But there are a few examples that might be considered either sufficiently different or unusual enough to mention. And although unusual, even these actions have been demonstrated by many.

First, in 1979, when gay pride was rising, a teenage male took a boy to the prom in Sioux Falls, South Dakota. The national media were there to record the moment; the camera lights glared as he and his date danced; gay activists were elated. It was the first time a same-sex couple had been allowed to attend an American prom. This male couple faded into obscurity—until January 1993. His death from AIDS was reported to the CDC.

The next examples of courage are about two courageous teenagers. He was a husky eighth-grader from Missouri who wore a peace symbol around his neck and was diagnosed with HIV in the summer of 1991. He recalled the day his mother called him into the house to give him the news. "I was getting ready to play baseball. I said, 'Does this mean I'm going to die?' She said, 'Not today.' I said, 'Can I go play baseball now?'".

He had only one problem with prejudice. A few parents in neighboring towns didn't want their children to play against his baseball team. **"I quit the team because I didn't think it was fair for them to not get to play because of me."**

A 13-year-old girl in Detroit who goes by the nickname of Slim has very grown-up responsibilities at home.

"It's hard, but I won't show you or let you see my pain," she said. "I was always taught to be strong."

She's had to be. Her mother, a single parent, is infected with HIV. At the same time, she learned that her sisters were also infected.

One sister died in April of 1993 at age 9. Then in November, her 6-month-old sister died. Now, another sister is battling HIV.

Through it all, she has been responsible for giving medications and intravenous feedings to everybody, around the clock.

"I want people to know what's going on. But I don't want anyone's pity."

WHOM IS THE GENERAL PUBLIC TO BELIEVE?

Because of the complexity of HIV disease, a great deal of press coverage of AIDS issues reflects what scientists say to journalists. A journalist's responsibility is to check that the facts are accurate, but not necessarily to judge their overall merit. Why should a good story be spiked just because other scientists disagree with the data interpretation? When scientists say contradictory things to the public, how can the public assess whom to believe? Science has a duty to inform and educate the public, but it must neither frighten people unnecessarily nor give them unjustified expectations. Claims of "AIDS cures" in the popular press need to be based on much more than just test tube data. **Whatever the need to attract research funding, is 5 minutes of fame ever worth a day of fear or weeks of false hopes for many?** The popular press has provided HIV-infected persons with a roller coaster ride between hopelessness and fantasies of imminent cure.

As a result of journalistic promises, there was and still is a range of emotions that run from real hope of a cure to public panic and hysteria. In at least five states, children with AIDS were barred from attending local public schools. The case of 12-year-old Ryan White of Kokomo, Indiana was made into a TV movie, *The Ryan White Story*, in 1989. Many parents fail to place HIV infection in perspective. In reality, automobile accidents, voluntary and involuntary exposure to tobacco smoke, drugs, and alcohol present greater risks to their children than does casual contact with an HIV-infected person.

In some localities, police officers and health care workers put rubber gloves on before apprehending a drug user or wear full cover protective suits when called to the scene of an accident (Figure 15-1). In other communities, church members, out of fear of HIV infection, have declined communion wine from the common cup.

Since the epic announcement in 1981, HIV/AIDS has refashioned America. It is not the first epidemic to alter history; measles, smallpox, bubonic plague, leprosy, polio, cholera, and other diseases have ravaged their eras. But HIV/AIDS is a disease molded to the times, one that has wedged apart the thinly concealed fault lines of American society by striking hardest at the outcasts—gay men, injection drug users, prostitutes, and impoverished whites, blacks, and Hispanics. HIV/AIDS

FIGURE 15-1 Ambulance Workers Protecting Themselves from the AIDS Virus at the Scene of an Accident.

Early on, the federal government and its public health apparatus showed little interest in the HIV/AIDS epidemic. **Former president Ronald Reagan never once met with former Surgeon General C. Everett Koop to talk about AIDS despite Koop's pleas.** Koop said, "If AIDS had struck legionnaires or Boy Scouts, there's no question the response would have been very different."

By the time, former president of the United States, Ronald Reagan, delivered his **first** speech on the AIDS crisis in **1987** over 36,000 men, women and children had been diagnosed with AIDS and over 25,000 Americans had died of AIDS. It took 9 years and over 200,000 AIDS cases before the U. S. Congress and former president George Bush enacted the nation's first comprehensive AIDS-care funding package—the Ryan White CARE Act (1990).

Misconceptions About AIDS Linger

Despite widespread reports that casual contact does not spread the virus, families have walked out of restaurants that employed gay waiters and hospital workers have quit rather than treat HIV/AIDS patients.

has brought forth uncomfortable questions about sex, sex education, homosexuality, the poor, and minorities. The disease has inevitably polarized the people, accentuating both the best and worst worldwide. Many churches, schools, and communities have responded to the new disease with compassion and tolerance; others have displayed hate and reprisals of the worst kind.

As Camus wrote in *The Plague,* **"The first thing (the epidemic) brought . . . was exile."** Anyone who carried the disease could inspire terror. They became pariahs in society.

Hate-mongers torched the house of the Ray family and their three HIV-positive hemophilic children in Arcadia, Florida. And someone shot a bullet through the window of Ryan White's home to let the teenager know he should not attend the local high school. After he died, his 6 foot 8 inch gravestone was overturned four times and a car ran over his grave!

――――――― **POINT OF VIEW 15.2** ―――――――

A SOUTHERN UNIVERSITY STUDENT'S EXPERIENCE

A southern university student taking a senior semester course on HIV/AIDS in 1996, experienced first-hand the fear-related ignorance that still exists.

This student had accompanied her friend to the office of a physician in a nearby small town. While the student was in the waiting room, she was using the time to read the given class assignment in her textbook, **AIDS Update 1996**. People coming into the office would **look over** at the empty chairs on each side of her—then look at her and decide to sit elsewhere. Even as the office filled and fewer and fewer seats were available, no one chose to sit near her. She said, "People took one look at the book and chose another seat some distance from me." She said, "So much for education on nontransmission of HIV by casual contact!!"

In 1989, a man was barred in Anderson, Indiana from coaching his daughter's intramural basketball team because he had been diagnosed with AIDS. The 37-year-old father received the virus in a blood transfusion during open heart surgery in 1984.

Each example points out that regardless of education, the public still assumes the virus can be casually transmitted. **It is fear that is being transmitted by casual contact—not the virus**. How would you react if a good friend, classmate, or co-worker told you he or she was HIV-positive? What if you found out that your child's schoolmate, a hemophiliac, had AIDS? What if you were told this child had emotional problems or a biting habit? What if your work put you in direct physical contact with people who might be HIV-positive?

An AIDS diagnosis for one person resulted in his physician's refusal to treat him, his roommate left him, his friends no longer visited him, his attorney, advised him to find another attorney and his clergyman failed to be there for him. They were all afraid of "catching" AIDS. In another case, a mother whose young son has AIDS sent cupcakes to his classmates on his birthday. School officials would not permit the children to eat the cupcakes. The elementary school principal said the school had a policy against homemade food because it could spread diseases such as AIDS.

In Jacksonville, Florida, Leanza Cornett (Miss America 1993) using her reign as a national platform to teach about AIDS, was told by public school officials not to use the word **condom** while addressing student groups. In Bradford County, Florida she was told she could not mention the name of the disease (AIDS) in three elementary schools she planned to visit.

In Hinton, West Virginia, one woman was killed by three bullets and her body dumped along a remote road. Another was beaten to death, run over by a car, and left in the gutter. Each woman had AIDS and told people so. And each, authorities say, was killed because she had AIDS. Lawyers and advocates for AIDS patients say the similar slayings, two counties and 6 months apart, illustrate AIDS' arrival in the American countryside and the fear and ignorance it can unearth.

What Do We Know?— Beginning 1998, and nearly 17 years of the AIDS epidemic it is clear that the scare headlines and tactics lack substance. From what has been learned about the biology of HIV, it appears that the virus is not casually nor easily spread and will not reach the magnitude of the great plague.

The social and medical history of the AIDS epidemic parallels the syphilis epidemic. It was feared that syphilis was casually transmitted via pens, pencils, toilet seats, toothbrushes, towels, bedding, medical procedures, and kissing. Immediate concern about casual transmission indicates the depth of human fears about disease and sexuality. Concerns about hygiene, contamination, contagion, pain, and death are expressions of anxieties that reveal much about contemporary society.

Fallout from AIDS— The biggest difference between HIV/AIDS and other diseases is the large amount of social discrimination. Society does not reject those with cancer, diabetes, heart disease, or any other health problems.

The AIDS pandemic has taught people about risk behavioral groups, homosexuals in particular. In some, this has promoted tolerance and understanding; in others, it has reinforced feelings of hatred. Information on HIV disease and AIDS, how it is spread and how to prevent becoming infected has, over the past 16 years, become a part of TV talk shows, movies, TV advertisements, and newspaper and magazine articles.

Phil Donohue, host of a popular TV show, said "On ***Donohue***, we're discussing body cavities and membranes and anal sex and vaginal lesions. We've discussed the consequences of a woman's swallowing her partner's semen. No way would we have brought that up five years ago. It's the kind of thing that makes a lot of people gag."

The language, photography, and art work used by the media are explicit and have upset certain religious groups. They believe that open use of language about condoms, homosexuality, anal sex, oral sex, vaginal sex and so on promotes promiscuity. **Question:** How can people learn to prevent HIV infection and AIDS without talking about sexual behavior

————— BOX 15.2 —————

HOW SOME PEOPLE RESPONDED AFTER LEARNING THAT SOMEONE HAD AIDS

VIGNETTES ON COMMUNITY BEHAVIOR AND AIDS

In **Colorado Springs, Colorado**, Scott Allen's wife Lydia had contracted HIV from a blood transfusion hours before son Matthew was born. A second son Bryan was also born before Lydia learned of her HIV infection. Scott wasn't infected, but was **dismissed** as minister of education at First Christian Church in Colorado Springs, when he sought his pastor's consolation. Matt was **kicked out** of the church's day-care center and the family was told to find another church.

When the family moved to Dallas and moved in with Scott's father Allen and his wife, church after church refused to enroll Matt in Sunday school. Allen, a former president of the Southern Baptist Convention wrote in his book, *Burden of a Secret: A Story of Truth and Mercy in the Face of AIDS*, "Good churches. Great churches. Wonderful People. Churches pastored by fine men of God, many of whom I had mentored. Nobody had room for a boy with AIDS."

Bryan, an infant, died in 1986, Lydia died in 1992, and Matt died in 1995.

In **Ohio**, a man was erroneously diagnosed as being HIV-infected. Within 12 days of learning the test results, he lost his job, his home, and he almost lost his wife. The error almost cost him his life: He had planned to commit suicide on the very day he received notice that he had received the wrong test results!

In **Maryland**, a court of appeals upheld a lower court's ruling permitting courtroom personnel to wear gloves to prevent picking up the AIDS virus. The court did suggest that the gloves were unnecessary.

In **New York**, a minister said that he was in a religious "Catch-22": He wanted to show concern and compassion for AIDS patients, but there are definite biblical injunctions against homosexuality. "How," he asked, "can I support these people without supporting homosexuality?"

In **Florida**, Mrs. Ray, the mother of three hemophilic HIV-infected sons (Ricky, 14; Robert, 13; and Randy, 12) turned to her pastor for confidential counseling. He responded by expelling the family from the congregation and announcing that the boys were infected. As a result, the boys were not allowed to go to church, school, stores, or restaurants. Barbers refused to cut their hair. Some townspeople interviewed said they were terrified at having the boys in the community. They had to move to another town! Ricky Ray died of AIDS on December 13, 1992 at age 15. Robert, age 14, was diagnosed with AIDS in 1990; Randy, age 13, was diagnosed with AIDS in May of 1993.

In **Florida, Broward County** parents packed school meetings and teachers filed a class action grievance saying a student's presence endangered their health. District officials determined that the 17-year-old mentally handicapped boy with AIDS would be educated by a teacher in an isolated classroom in the school. The student received 3 1/2 years of isolated education. For the 1 1/2 years, maintenance people would not walk into the portable classroom. Instead, they would leave packages or supplies in the doorway. The teacher and an assistant got used to doing their own cleaning. The one student cost over $50,000 per year to educate.

In **Duval County, Florida** (1990), the foster parents of a 3-year-old AIDS child who was infected by his mother, were forced to leave their church because other parents insisted that the child not be allowed to attend the church nursery. The pastor went along with the majority. When presented with CDC findings that HIV is not casually transmitted, one parent scoffed. "I called the CDC for information and they asked me what I was going to use it for." He then asked the congregation, "How can you believe anyone like that?"

In **California**, a young man arrived home one evening to find that the locks had been changed. A few days later he discovered that everything he had ever touched had been thrown out—clothes, books, bed sheets, toothbrush, curtains, and carpeting. Even the wallpaper had been stripped from the walls and trashed. The day before, he had told his friends he had AIDS. "Overnight, I had no friends. I slept on park benches. I stole food. I passed bad checks. No one would come near me. I was told that I had 14 weeks to live."

In a second California incident, volunteer fire fighters refused to help a 1-year-old baby with AIDS at a monastery that cares for unwanted infants. The baby was reported to be choking. Although the fire department has agreed to respond to such calls in the future, one fire fighter quit, saying he was frightened because he had not been trained to deal with victims of acquired immune deficiency syndrome.

———— **BOX 15.2** (continued) ————

In **New Jersey**, a bartender could not tell his parents or friends he had AIDS. It meant confessing that he was gay. He feared it might also mean the loss of family, friends, lovers and insurance. He was expressing signs and symptoms and paying out of pocket for medical bills rather than file an insurance claim.

In **Charlotte, North Carolina**, 1993, a bride wore an ankle-length chiffon dress, white above and flowered black below. She'll wear the dress again, at her husband's funeral. The groom was diagnosed with progressive multifocal leukoencephalopathy (PML), a relentless viral infection that attacks the nervous system and causes brain lesions. About 4% of people with AIDS contract the disease. No treatment exists.

A legal marriage would make the groom ineligible for Medicare and Medicaid, which he can't afford to lose. So their wedding had to be symbolic and legally nonbinding.

Both wanted a wedding as a sign of commitment. He also wanted it for psychological support: It tells him that his wife will be there as things get worse.

PML has already begun to separate the newlyweds. He has developed speech problems. Sometimes he doesn't remember what he's doing.

From the wreckage, they have clutched love. "Love is — period," she said "We don't qualify it. We don't distinguish between heterosexual and homosexual. When love is there, the physical form it takes is just a detail."

In **Charleston, West Virginia** in July of 1995, a 10-year postal mail carrier who refused to deliver mail to a couple with AIDS was indefinitely suspended with pay after an educational class failed to change his mind. The mailman said he was afraid of cutting himself on the home's metal mail slot and becoming infected from envelopes or stamps the couple had licked. Postal sources said the mailman would eventually be fired.

In **Texas**, a father with AIDS cried while praying that his three children would not be treated as cruelly. The man, in his mid-20s, was mugged because he looked too weak to fight, hit with rocks by people who found out he had AIDS, and in one incident a man broke a bottle over his head screaming that he was out to kill AIDS. During one beating, an attacker said, "After we kill you, we will kill your wife and children in case they have AIDS."

Almost daily, similar senseless acts of violence and cruelty occur across the United States as a response to AIDS. Such episodes of panic, hysteria, and prejudice are perpetuated by the very people society uses as role models: clergy, physicians, teachers, lawyers, dentists, and so on. Philosopher Jonathan Moreno said, "Plagues and epidemics like AIDS bring out the best and worst of society. Face to face with disaster and death, people are stripped down to their basic human character, to good and evil. AIDS can be a litmus test of humanity."

THE LIFE OF RYAN WHITE

In Kokomo, Indiana, Ryan White was socially unacceptable. He was not gay, a drug user, black, or Hispanic. He was a hemophiliac; he had AIDS. His fight to become socially acceptable, to attend school, and to have the freedom to leave his home for a walk without ridicule made Ryan a national hero (Figure 15-2).

FIGURE 15-2 Ryan White was diagnosed with AIDS in 1984 and died on April 8, 1990. This young male became another teenage AIDS tragedy. He gained the respect of millions across the United States before he died of an AIDS-related lung infection. (*Courtesy AP/Wide World Photos*)

Ryan's short life was a profile in courage and understanding. Like many other people with AIDS, Ryan tried to change the public's misconception of how HIV is transmitted. Ryan suffered most from the indignities, lies, and meanness of his classmates and his classmates' parents in Kokomo, Indiana. They accused him of being a "fag," of spitting on them to infect them with the virus, and other fabrications. Ryan said he understood that this discrimination was a response of fear and ignorance. Ryan got the virus from blood and blood products essential to his survival. Ryan's wish was to be treated like any other boy, to attend school, to study, to play, to laugh, to cry, and to live each day as fully as possible. But AIDS was an integral part of his life. AIDS may not have compromised the quality of his life,

as much as the residents of his community. One day, at age 16, as Ryan talked about AIDS to students in Nebraska, another boy asked Ryan how it felt knowing he was going to die. Showing the maturity that endeared him to all, Ryan replied "It's how you live your life that counts." Ryan White died, a hero of the AIDS pandemic, at 7:11 A.M. on April 8, 1990. He was 18 years old.

Gregory Herek and colleagues (1993) determined via telephone interviews that HIV/AIDS stigma is still pervasive in the United States. They interviewed 538 white adults and 607 African-Americans. Nearly all respondents indicated some stigma. Regardless of race, men were more likely than women to support preventive policies such as quarantine and said they would *avoid* persons with AIDS.

—————— POINT OF VIEW 15.3 ——————

HATRED EXPRESSED

In April 1996, a youth traffic safety program coordinator with the Florida Department of Transportation received a pledge form requesting a donation for the Florida AIDS Ride, an Orlando to Miami Beach bike race to raise money for AIDS programs. The person responded to the pledge form by writing to the race organizers that AIDS "was created as a punishment to the gay and lesbian communities across the world. As far as the gay and lesbians of this world . . . let them suffer the consequences!"

—————— POINT OF VIEW 15.4 ——————

NEWSPAPER HEADLINE
SHOCKS READERS

On June 7, 1996, a large bold print headline of the Jacksonville, *Florida Times Union* newspaper, a **very** conservative Southern newspaper, read:

STUDY: ORAL SEX POSES HIV
INFECTION RISK

This headline, in this newspaper, would **NEVER** have happened in this author's lifetime without the 15-plus years of HIV/AIDS history. During this time, declarations involving all types of sexual behavior and drug use appeared during prime time TV programming and voluminous publication of such topics in all types of regional, state, and federal pamphlets, magazines, journals, and public reading materials. Yet, this newspaper received 124 phone calls from people angry about this headline in their newspaper. Their main objection concerned the use of the words "ORAL SEX." Many others objected but did not call— some dropped their subscription! **How do you feel about this headline appearing in your hometown newspaper? (Class Discussion)**

and injection drug use? Does it seem at times as if opponents of sex education would rather have people suffer with AIDS than have them learn about sex?

Regardless of who is correct, few could have predicted in 1980 the casualness with which these topics are presented in the media. If the AIDS pandemic has done nothing else, it surely has affected the nature of public discourse. In 1987, prior to the TV broadcast of the *National AIDS Awareness Test*, viewers were warned of objectionable material. By 1990, few if any such viewer warnings were given. It is as if to say that no one can afford to be ignorant of this information because it may save your life.

How Can Information Help?— There is great hope that information will lead the nation past its social prejudice and forward to compassion for those who are HIV-infected or have AIDS. More than any disease before, AIDS has proved

——— BOX 15.3 ———

WHEN ONE WITH AIDS COMES FORTH

Father Paul made the decision to preach on AIDS because of a phone call he had received informing him that a former parishioner was coming to Jacksonville. "George has AIDS. He will be in Church on Sunday. With your permission, he will be receiving Communion."

Father Paul granted permission and welcomed George's attendance. He sensed, however, that some might not agree to have George in church or receive Communion. In his parish a number of people refuse to believe that HIV is not transmitted by saliva from the lavitha (Communion cup).

By Sunday morning's sermon, over 60% of the congregation had learned of George.

Father Paul began his sermon, "Today's Gospel lesson, Luke 10:25-37, tells us the Parable of the Good Samaritan . . . The Parable challenges us to take stock of who our neighbors are who have needs that we can meet. . . . is it not also true that our neighbors are being harmed by AIDS? . . . Many Orthodox Christians are good about reaching out to the needy and indigent. But we are not so willing to reach out to those with AIDS."

Father Paul said that he would be dishonest if he did not admit having concerns about people receiving Communion after George. "I did not fear for myself, I feared for them, and especially for my two daughters who receive Communion regularly."

Father Paul reminded everyone about the faith of The Church. He addressed the question, "Can AIDS be contracted through casual contact and specifically from the Eucharistic Chalice?" He said, "Communion is the Body and Blood of our Lord. In the Gospel of John, chapter 6, Jesus speaks to us of His Body and Blood as being agents of life, NOT of sickness and death. Similarly, St. Ignatius of Antioch alludes to Communion as the `medicine of immortality' which allows one to eternally abide with God. To believe, therefore, that one can contract sickness and AIDS from Holy Communion is blasphemy against the Holy Spirit. It is also to render everything that the Bible and the Church teaches about Communion meaningless."

As he spoke, he saw George near the back of the Church. Though only 47 years old, George looks 60. George was weak, abnormally thin, spoke with a rasp, and walked with a cane.

Before Sunday's Liturgy, Father Paul had discussed with George his pastoral concerns about the people's anxieties. Without asking, he proposed a solution, he would receive Communion last.

Father Paul introduced George to the congregation and announced that he would be receiving last.

At Communion time, several of the congregants assisted George to the front of the church. Then, the same individuals and several others lined up behind him.

About 10 people received Communion after George. Father Paul asked one why he did it. "Father, did you not tell us in your sermon that we had to be Good Samaritans. It would have been a very unloving and discriminatory act to allow George to go last."

George died several weeks later in New York City. The news was received with sadness.

George, thank you for coming to Jacksonville. God brought you to us to help us grow. May God remember you in his Kingdom.

(Adapted with permission from Father Paul Costopoulos, Jacksonville, Florida)

FREEDOM FOR COMPASSION: CHILDREN AND AIDS

Charlie the doll was pressed against the antique glass case. Jeff, a blue-eyed, blond-haired boy of 10, looked at him closely. "Someday Charlie will leave this cage," he pondered, "and someday he will be free."

A few visits later, Jeff devised a plan to buy Charlie. He began his task by seeking employment as a leaf raker, a car washer, and the best of panhandlers among friends. After a while his hope faded and his energy waned, but he did not despair. He had met adversity before, in fact, for most of his life. When Jeff was 4 years old, he had contracted AIDS.

The family of John Calvin Presbyterian Church met Jeff because other congregations had turned him away, telling his family that Jeff's illness was a punishment from God. Jeff planned his own memorial service, but five different congregations ignored him by making excuses that the songs he had chosen from the play, "Peter Pan," and the balloons he had requested would not be appropriate.

One Sunday morning as I was beginning my sermon, Jeff's mother wheeled him down the main aisle to a front pew. I wondered what would happen if this church rejected him, too? How would the other children treat him? Could this congregational family risk enough to love Jeff and his family in the same way in which God loved them? But my fears were relieved after church at the coffee fellowship. Parents introduced themselves to Jeff's mother and the children included Jeff within their circle of games. People earnestly gathered to accompany Jeff and his family on their special journey: members ran errands, provided transporta- tion, and brought in food. This outpouring of help came at a crucial time: Jeff's mother had given up her own business to take care of Jeff, emotional pressures contributed to Jeff's parents' divorce, the family lost their home to bankruptcy court, and Jeff's brother and sister suffered from the prejudice of schoolmates and others.

A few weeks prior to Jeff's death, I bought Charlie the doll. As Jeff's fragile hands began to untie the shiny silver ribbon that secured the purple box, large tears began to trickle down his sunken cheeks. When he discovered what was inside, Jeff smiled and said, "Now he's free . . . and someday I will be, too."

Jeff's freedom arrived on March 2, 1988. Those of us who knew him have gained freedom as well. Jeff, and others, have introduced us to a new appreciation of life. Through them we have been reminded of how fragile we are and of our precious responsibility to live each moment fully. Together we have discovered the gift that no person, no circumstance, no condition—even the AIDS virus—can take from us. We have discovered God's gift to us in Jesus Christ.

John Calvin Presbyterian Church is now a better-educated congregation. Jeff helped to teach us the importance of risking and reaching out. Our church has adopted a resolution stating that we are committed to minister intentionally with people with AIDS and their families. We provide office space to the Tampa AIDS Network, an advocacy, support, and fund-raising group serving the Tampa Bay area. A number of members and I are part of a growing coalition of volunteers serving on task forces, care-giving programs, and support groups.

In the midst of our congregation's activity we are still keenly aware of the continuing apathy, ignorance, and prejudice permeating much of the religious community. Many underestimate the possibility of this disease intruding into their lives and communities. Much work remains to be done with few to accomplish it.

Jeff's memorial service was just as he had planned it. The sanctuary of the church was filled with the nurses and doctors who had worked with him, the many hospice volunteers who had given him solace, his buddies from the Tampa AIDS Network who had held his hand, the many other friends he had made on his journey. Hundreds of brightly colored helium balloons were released into the sky at the end of the service. We celebrated Jeff's life—and ours as well. Our celebration continues as we minister with others who are traveling this very difficult path. Our strength and hope are renewed with each encounter, for we have been given the freedom for compassion.

(Adapted from Rev. Jim Hedges, pastor of John Calvin Presbyterian Church, Tampa, Florida, in *Church and Society*, Vol. 79, No. 3(January/ February 1989). Reprinted with permission.)

that ignorance leads to fear and information can lead to compassion. The need for compassion is great.

Admiral James Watkins, Chairman of the 1988 Presidential Commission on the HIV Epidemic, reported that "33% to 50% of physicians in some of our major hospitals would not touch an AIDS patient with a ten-foot pole."

A friend of a dying AIDS patient who was in the hospital with pneumocystic pneumonia went to visit him. As he was leaving, his dying friend said, "Thank you for coming—thank you for touching me." He said, "I can't even imagine being at a point in my life that I would be so grateful for someone touching me, that I would have to say thank you."

It would appear that although biotechnology has provided methods of HIV detection, new drugs, and hope for a vaccine, human emotional responses have not changed much from those demonstrated during previous epidemics like the plague, cholera, influenza, and syphilis.

AIDS EDUCATION AND BEHAVIOR

I said education was our "basic weapon." Actually it's our *only* weapon. We've got to educate everyone about the disease so that each person can

CHANGING ATTITUDES

A January 1996 opinion poll on public attitudes concerning HIV/AIDS revealed that to some degree people, through education, are changing their beliefs about HIV/AIDS.

In 1985, 31% of adults believed children with HIV disease or AIDS should be barred from school. In 1996, only 6% held that belief.

In 1985, 6% of adults knew someone with AIDS. In 1996, 40% of adults know someone with AIDS.

In 1985, 70% of adults believed that AIDS was the nation's greatest health problem. In 1996, 37% held that belief.

In 1985, 33% believed it was unsafe to associate with someone who had AIDS. In 1996, 15% still held that belief!

In 1990, 30% of randomly picked adults feared they would become HIV-infected. In 1996, 15% had the same fear.

In 1996, 73% of adults polled favored spending tax dollars to treat people with AIDS.

THE WAY WE ARE

The young man worked alongside a 35-year-old woman helping to teach the disabled to function. She was very attractive with a wonderful sense of humor He watched her every movement - he was in love from a distance; she inspired him to new heights in his work and thoughts about his future. She understood his emotions so she was not surprised when, after work one evening, he offered dinner and a moonlight walk around the lake. During the walk, she could tell from the conversation that his young hormones were flowing - as were her own. In the awkwardness of saying goodnight she said, "I know you want me - I would like that very much." As his broad face glowed she said, "I must share something with you. I have been diagnosed with AIDS but there are no outward signs yet." The love that moments before surged through his body crashed down around him; he felt ill yet sympathetic - his urge for sex vanished. He could not bring himself to look at her as he said, "Please forgive me, I just can't." She nodded her understanding and explained it was either a blood transfusion in 1984 following an auto accident or death. **"I made the choice for life and whatever comes with it."** The young man cried as he walked home. He left the job the next morning.

take responsibility for seeing that it is spread no further.

C. Everett Koop
Former U.S. Surgeon General

For some, the occurrence of over 40,000 new HIV infections in the United States each year is evidence that HIV education and prevention efforts have failed. If HIV prevention programs are held to a standard of perfection and are expected to protect 100% of people from disease 100% of the time, the efforts are by definition doomed to failure. No intervention aimed at changing behaviors to promote health has been or can be 100% successful, whether for smoking, diet, exercise, or drinking and driving. For example, even though warnings regarding the health effects of smoking were issued in 1964, warning labels on cigarettes were not mandated until 1984, and smoking-related illness still remains a major cause of death.

Because some of the behaviors and activities that need to change in order to avert HIV infection are pleasurable, it should be no surprise if short-term interventions do not lead to immediate and permanent behavior

changes. An important difference between HIV infection and other life-threatening diseases is that HIV can be contracted by a single episode of risk-taking behavior. Once HIV-infected there is no second chance—no giving up the behavior, like drinking alcohol or smoking, that will make any difference; HIV disease progresses to AIDS. The adverse effect of smoking, alcohol or diet on health usually manifests after years of smoking thousands of cigarettes or after years of drinking or poor dietary choices.

But education appears to be working. More than a dozen years of experience with HIV has demonstrated that lasting changes in behavior needed to avoid infection can occur as a result of carefully tailored, targeted, credible, and persistent HIV risk-education efforts. Given experience in other health behavior change endeavors, no interventions are likely to reduce the incidence of HIV infection to zero; indeed, insisting on too high a standard for HIV risk-reduction programs may actually undermine their effectiveness. A number of social, cultural, and attitudinal barriers continue to prevent the implementation of promising HIV risk-reduction programs. The remote prospects for a successful prophylactic vaccine for HIV and the difficulty in finding effective drug treatments have underscored the importance of sustained attention to HIV prevention and education (Stryker et al, 1995).

The goals of educating people about HIV infection and AIDS are to promote compassion, social understanding and to prevent HIV transmission. To achieve these goals, accurate information must be provided that makes people aware of their risk status. People at minimum risk can continue their safer sexual lifestyles. People at high risk should determine their HIV status, alter behaviors, and practice safer sex.

This sounds so easy: Educate people and they will do the right thing. **Wrong.** Knowledge does not guarantee sufficient motivation to change sexual behavior or stop the biological urge to have sex. Education has not stopped teenage pregnancy, nor has the threat of lung cancer stopped people from smoking.

Perhaps the reason education is not as effective as it could be is because the public receives its education by daily doses from the mass media. With so much going on in the world, people have become more or less dependent on the media for information essential to their well being. Gordon Nary (1990) said, "The public wants to know what's right or wrong in five three-second images or 25 words or less. It wants simple problems with simple solutions. It wants *Star Wars* with good and evil absolutely defined. The media often responds to these demands."

Mathew Lefkowitz (1990) says that the word AIDS has been infused with an irrational fear that has nothing to do with the illness. He states that the word AIDS has been politicized in such a way that it can and has been used as a weapon. Lefkowitz relates the parallel between today's use of the word AIDS with Eugene Ionosco's classic absurdist play *The Lesson*. In the play, a professor stabs a girl to death with the word *knife*—not with a knife but with the **word knife**. It appears that today the word *AIDS* is being used to stab those whom we fear; namely the HIV-infected. How long will it take the educational process to work? **THE VIRUS IS NOT AS MUCH OUR ENEMY AS OURSELVES.** For example, in Washington, D. C., 1995, because a national public radio commentator was furious at U. S. Senator Jesse Helms of South Carolina for having the audacity to suggest that the government spends too much money on AIDS research, said, "I think he ought to be worried about what's going on in the good Lord's mind because if there is retributive justice, he'll get AIDS from a transfusion—or **one of his grandchildren will get it**."

Perhaps zealots need to realize that the purpose of civil exchange is to arrive at wisdom through reasoned debate, not to verbally intimidate those who differ into silence. **WHAT IS YOUR OPINION?**

Public AIDS Education Programs

The 1988 Presidential Commission on the Human Immunodeficiency Virus Epidemic stated:

> No citizen of our nation is exempt from the need to be educated about the HIV epidemic. The real challenge lies in matching the right educational approach with the right people. During the last year, there has been a great deal of debate over the content of HIV/AIDS education. The Commission is concerned that, in the promotion of the personal, moral and political values of those from both ends of the political spectrum, the consistent distribution of clear, factual information about HIV transmission has suffered. HIV/AIDS education programs, for example, should not encourage promiscuous sexual activity; however, they need to be explicit in nature so that there is no confusion about how to avoid acquiring or transmitting the virus. The Commission firmly believes that it is possible to develop educational materials and programs that clearly convey an explicit message without promoting high-risk behaviors.

West Coast health officials told this same Presidential Commission that the censorship of sexually explicit materials is hampering the fight against AIDS. Many of those who testified before the Commission expressed frustration about the barriers posed by government bureaucracy. Several representatives of AIDS organizations told commissioners of the difficulties they have experienced in trying to produce effective educational materials and programs. They said that state officials prohibit the use of certain language when they fund educational programs. It is sometimes necessary, however, to use slang or sexually explicit language in order for readers to understand the material. As an example, they cited women who had given birth but claimed they had never had "vaginal intercourse." They did not know what **vaginal** meant, but they did know what *cunt* meant. Educational material must use recognizable language to be effective.

Over the years many millions of dollars have been spent by federal and state health departments to inform the public about cardiovascular risks, health risks associated with sexually transmitted diseases (STDs), smoking and lung cancer, chewing tobacco and oral cancer, drug addiction, alcohol consumption, and seat belt use to name just a few. In some cases these campaigns were eventually supported by specific state and federal legislation. Tobacco advertisements were outlawed on TV and drivers in some states who are not buckled up must pay a fine. But even with laws to support these educational programs, the majority of adults have failed to change established behavior patterns. In the larger cities, educators must combat the fear that AIDS is a government conspiracy to eliminate society's "undesirables"—minorities, drug addicts, and homosexuals. They must overcome cultural and religious barriers that prevent people from using condoms to protect themselves.

Another problem is that educational programs are not preventing individuals from acquiring one or more STDs, using drugs, drinking to excess, driving drunk, failing to use seat belts or motorcycle helmets, and smoking. It might also be added that there have always been educational programs against crime, but in 1989 through 1996 more new jails were built in the United States than ever before. And this expanding jail-building program continues! In short, educational programs on TV, radio, in newspapers, and in the popular press have achieved only limited success in changing peoples' behavior.

It is not that education is unimportant; it is essential for those who will use it! But that is the catch. Although education must be available for those who will use it, too few, relatively speaking, are using the available education for their maximum benefit. In general, people, especially young adults, **do not do what they know. They sometimes do what they see, but most often do what they feel.** In short, knowledge in itself may be necessary but it is insufficient for behavioral change. A variety of studies have failed to show a consistent link between knowledge and preventive behaviors (Fisher, 1992; Phillips, 1993)

Costs Related to Prevention— The assertion that spending more money on educational programs will ensure disease prevention for the masses, as the examples given above suggest, may not be the case. In particular, peoples' behaviors regarding the prevention of HIV infection do not appear to be changing significantly despite the hundreds of millions of dollars being used to produce, distribute, and promote HIV/AIDS education. The major educational thrust is directed at how not to become HIV-infected. Most of this information is being given out to people from age 13 and up.

The problem with AIDS education is that communicating the information is relatively easy but changing behavior, particularly addictive and/or pleasurable behavior, is quite difficult. Most cigarette abusers know that smoking causes lung cancer and would like to quit or have tried to quit. Likewise, many alcoholics have tried to quit. But both cigarettes and alcohol are pleasurable to those who use them. The mass media have provided near saturation coverage of key AIDS issues and it is very unlikely that significant numbers of future HIV infections in the United States will occur in individuals who did not know the virus was transmitted through sexual contact and IV drug use. Yet new infections and AIDS cases continue to increase.

Evidence accumulated between 1983 and 1987 indicates that homosexual and bisexual males modified their sexual behavior and this resulted in a drop in AIDS cases among them. There is also evidence that some IDUs have begun wearing condoms. But recent evidence suggests that some of these people are being drawn back to their former practice of unprotected sex and needle sharing. The disease is

THE RED RIBBON

We were sitting in a small Italian restaurant. I had just come back to town from a presentation on AIDS. The jacket I wore still had the red ribbon on the lapel. As we enjoyed our meal I noticed a woman at the next table who appeared to be glaring at me and making statements to her companion. At one point her voice became loud enough for us to hear her say, "I am sick and tired of those people trying to push the lifestyle of homosexuals down our throats" as she was looking right at me. She then said, "That red ribbon is a sign of a sick person trying to make all of us sick too. That ribbon and all that it stands for ruins my day." With that she and her companion left the restaurant.

That outburst left my family and me embarrassed and confused. My children deserved an explanation. I don't think I have ever explained the idea of the red ribbon to anyone before. Like so many things we observe in life, after a while they become understood by each in his or her own way. This woman expressed her way rather forcefully. To my children I said that the ribbon is a symbol to call attention to a social problem that needs a solution. I went on to say, "Do you recall the song 'Tie A Yellow Ribbon Round the Old Oak Tree' in 1973 and what that meant? And, do you recall the ribbons tied around trees, on car antennas, mailboxes and so on while our 56 service men were held captives in Iran in 1980 and again for out captives in the 1991 Persian Gulf War? Remember the first lady Nancy Reagan's campaign using red ribbons for 'Just say no to drugs' and more recently the pink ribbons for women against breast cancer and most recently the purple ribbons for stoppng violence in our schools? These are all symbolic gestures to show support for those enduring suffering and pain. All of the ribbons then and now serve to connect people emotionally, to help unite people in a common cause, to help people feel less isolated in a crisis."

I explained to my children that the problem with the red ribbon now is similar to what occurred over the long time period our soldiers were in captivity—people begin to wear the ribbon as an accessory.

The Author

showing signs of a resurgence in the gay community as health workers struggle to get their message to a new generation and to older gays who seem to have lost the motivation to protect themselves.

In 1982, there were 18 new HIV infections for every 100 uninfected gay men in San Francisco. That rate dropped to 1 per 100 in 1987 but rose to 2 per 100 in 1993. For gay men younger than 25, it is 4 per 100.

Although humans are capable of dramatic behavioral changes, it is not known what really initiates the change or how to speed up the process.

Public School AIDS Education: JUST SAY KNOW

Some information relevant to AIDS education can be learned from educational programs that have been designed to reduce pregnancy and the spread of STDs among teenagers. However, data from a variety of high school sex education classes offered across the country indicate that teenagers are learning the essential facts but they are not practicing what they learn. **They do not do what they know.**

Risky sexual behavior is widespread among teenagers and has resulted in high rates of STDs. Over 25% of the 12 million STD cases per year occur among teenagers. One teenager is infected with an STD every 10 seconds in the United States. One in six teens has been infected with an STD. Over 50% of sexually active teenagers (11 million) report having had two or more sexual partners; and fewer than half say they used a condom the first time they

——— BOX 15.5 ———

ANECDOTE: FATHER AND SON EXCHANGE SEX INFORMATION

"Son, I think it's time we had a talk about sex."
"O.K., Dad, what do you want to know?"

had intercourse (Kirby, 1988). A National Research Council panel (1989) stated that 75% of all female teenagers had sexual experience and that 15% had four or more partners.

Teenage Perceptions About AIDS and HIV Infection in the United States— A recent survey run by People magazine indicated that 96% of high school students and 99% of college students knew that HIV is spreading through the heterosexual population; but the majority of these students stated that they continued to practice unsafe sex. Combined data from surveys performed in 1988-1989 indicate that among sexually active teenagers, only 25% used a condom. Peter Jennings stated in a February, 1991, AIDS Update TV program that 26% of American teenagers practice anal intercourse. Data such as these have prompted a number of medical and research people to express concern for the next generation. If HIV becomes widespread among today's teenagers, there is a real danger of losing tomorrow's adults. Available data suggest that teenagers have not appreciably changed their sexual behaviors in response to HIV/AIDS information presented in their schools or from other sources (Kegeles et al., 1988).

Teenagers at high risk include some 200,000 who become prostitutes each year and others who become IDUs. About 1% of high school seniors have used heroin and many from junior high on up have tried cocaine (Kirby, 1988). A large number of children from age 10 up consume alcohol. Is it possible that too much hope is being placed on education to prevent the spread of HIV? Beginning 1998, teenagers made up about 0.5% of 646,000 AIDS cases, or about 3,232 cases. Teenagers must be convinced that they are vulnerable to HIV infection and death. Until then, it only happens to someone else. The World Health Organization estimates that worldwide, through 1997, there were between 3 and 4 million HIV-infected teenagers.

Teenagers, like adults, must be convinced of their risk of infection but not with scare tactics. Behavior modification as a result of a scare is short lived. However the information is given, it must be internalized if it is to be of long-term benefit.

College Students— Everyone must know and act on the fact that a wrong decision about having sexual intercourse can take away the future. For example, a young college student had a 3-year nonsexual friendship with a local bartender. She was bright, well educated, and acutely aware of AIDS. After drinks one evening, as their friendship progressed towards sexual intercourse, she asked him if he was "straight" (a true heterosexual) and he said yes. But he was a bisexual! It was a single sexual encounter. She graduated and left town. She found out that the bartender died of AIDS 3 years later. She did not think much of it until she was diagnosed with AIDS 5 years after their affair. **This young, talented, bright, and personable girl lost her future.** This brings home the point that it is difficult to change something as complex as personal sexual behavior regardless of knowledge. It also brings up at least one other important point in personal relationships: **telling the truth**.

During the 1988 Psychological Association Convention, the following facts were presented with respect to telling the truth or lying in order to have sex. The data come from a survey of 482 sexually experienced southern California college students:

1. 35% of the men and 10% of the women said they had lied in order to have sex.

2. 47% of the men and 60% of the women reported they had been told a lie in order to have sex.

3. 20% of the men and 4% of the women said they would say they had a negative HIV test in order to have sex.

4. 42% of the men and 33% of the women said they would never admit a one-time sexual affair to their long-term partner.

Adult Perceptions About HIV Infection and AIDS in the United States— R.J. Blendon and colleague (1988) summarized the results of telephone surveys and personal interviews with a large number of adults. They provide an insight into adult knowledge and emotions regarding transmission of the AIDS virus. The data may also serve as a potential indicator for

——————— BOX 15.6 ———————

HIV-RELATED BELIEFS, KNOWLEDGE, AND BEHAVIOR
AMONG HIGH SCHOOL STUDENTS

"Education concerning AIDS must start at the lowest grade possible as part of any health and hygiene program. The appearance of AIDS should bring together diverse groups of parents and educators with opposing views on the inclusion of sex education in the curricula. There is now no doubt that we need sex education in schools and that it must include information on heterosexual and homosexual relationships. The threat of AIDS should be sufficient to permit a sex education curriculum with heavy emphasis on prevention of AIDS and other sexualy transmitted diseases."

Up to 500,000, of those infected with HIV in the United States are **under** the age of 25, making HIV/AIDS a major concern for young adults. And, about half of all new HIV infections now occur among people under age 25. About 20%, or one in five people, who have AIDS are in their twenties. A large proportion of these individuals become infected during adolescence. It is clearly time to place a special emphasis on teenagers and AIDS.

Reported data suggest that HIV-related beliefs, knowledge, and behaviors among the students surveyed in 32 states and 10 cities in 1990 were generally similar in 1997. Many students incorrectly thought that HIV infection could be acquired from giving blood, using public toilets, having a blood test, and from mosquito or other insect bites. Most students knew intercourse and injection drug use could result in HIV infection.

STATE MANDATED POLICY ON HIV/AIDS EDUCATION

Elementary and secondary school students in Nevada need written permission from their parents to participate in the state-mandated HIV and AIDS education program. In Minnesota, state law requires schools to target high-risk adolescents for education programs. But in California, where the incidence of AIDS is second highest in the country, an AIDS education law has not been passed.

These three policies represent the broad spectrum of approaches states have been taking toward HIV and AIDS education through 1993. By the end of 1997, at least 40 states had mandated some form of HIV/AIDS education in their school systems. Twenty-eight of these states determined that such education must be given during regularly scheduled classes in health, family life, or sex education. Only Washington state mandates that HIV/AIDS is to be presented specifically as part of a required course on sexually transmitted disease. Seven states do not, by law, specify the context in which HIV and AIDS education is to be presented (Voelker, 1989). Without a statewide policy, school districts may devise their own HIV/AIDS curricula. Because of a lack of national policy, students are receiving different HIV/AIDS educations. For example, even though all 40 states require discusssion of HIV/AIDS prevention and 18 states stipulate that sexual abstinence be stressed, only three require discussion of condom use and only two require a discussion of homosexuality. Seven states require giving information on the risks of IV drug use and sharing needles.

Fourteen of the 40 states have requirements for training or for the credentialing of instructors who will teach HIV/AIDS programs. While some require unspecified training for the "appropriate" staff, others require teachers to have completed specialized in-service training. Nine states require some in-service training for school employees' the requirements vary from specialized health education training to attending annual AIDS awareness programs. In 1990, the CDC gave an average of $250,000 to each state to develop HIV and AIDS education programs, but only seven education departments received funds from their state budgets.

discrimination against HIV-infected people. Of the adults surveyed:

General Public—

1. Over 50% felt that the AIDS pandemic has lead to increased homophobia (fear of homosexuals) and discrimination.

2. 10% actively avoided social contact with homosexuals.

3. 20% said AIDS was punishment against immoral homosexual behavior and that the punishment was deserved.

4. 29% said HIV-infected people should wear a tattoo or other means of identification to warn the public.

5. 30% supported the idea of quarantine for HIV-infected and AIDS patients.

6. 40% believed that HIV-infected school employees should be fired.

7. 33% said they would keep their child out of school if a student there were HIV-infected or had AIDS.

The Workplace— With AIDS now the second leading cause of death in all Americans between the ages of 25 and 44, if a person is **not** working near or beside someone who is HIV-positive, they will be relatively soon! But they may not know it because a person's right to privacy prevails over an employee's right to know.

Recently, 2,000 adult employees were phone interviewed during a national survey concerning their attitudes about AIDS." The survey (Hooker, 1996) revealed that:

♦ AIDS is the **chief health concern** among 20% of U. S. employees (cancer, was the primary concern of 32%; heart disease, of 7%).

♦ 67% of employees predicted that their co-workers would be uncomfortable working with someone with HIV or AIDS.

♦ 32% thought an HIV-positive employee would be fired or put on disability at the first sign of illness.

♦ 24% said that an HIV-positive employee should be fired or put on disability at the first sign of illness.

♦ 75% of employees said they wanted their employers to offer a formal AIDS education program.

AIDS can have a variety of impacts in the workplace. The obvious one, of course, is on the individual employee who is diagnosed with HIV. The probability of sickness and death obviously affects the individual and his or her ability to continue to contribute to the organization's activities and goals.

Employees fear AIDS can create a widespread loss of teamwork and productivity, and create an environment that is inhumane and insensitive toward the infected employee.

As the incidence of HIV and AIDS increases, the impact on organizations will obviously increase as well. While there are important log-ical and moral reasons for ensuring that infected people are not discriminated against, there are also practical reasons for addressing the employee HIV/AIDS problem.

An educated work force, aware of the facts regarding diagnosis, testing, treatment, and transmission of HIV, can have a positive impact on the overall health of all employees. People are more inclined to openly acknowledge their HIV status and to seek treatment when assured of a supportive workplace environment. This increases productivity.

The results of a survey of people in the workplace by Blendon and Donelan (1988) revealed that:

1. 25% believed HIV was transmitted by coughing, spitting and sneezing.

2. 20% believed HIV infection could occur from a drinking fountain or toilet seat.

3. 10% believed touching an HIV-infected or AIDS patient was dangerous.

4. 25% refused to work with an HIV-infected or AIDS person.

5. 25% believed employers should be able to fire people who were HIV-infected or had AIDS.

Whether additional public education will change these attitudes over time is unknown. The Surgeon General's brochure, "Understanding AIDS" (Figure 15-3), was sent to 107,000,000 homes in 1988 at a cost of 22 million dollars. Fifty-one percent of those who received the pamphlet did not read it because they did not remember getting it or they chose to ignore it (Eickhoff, 1989).

A recent Georgia Tech survey found that workers who received educational brochures or pamphlets about the disease were more likely to have negative feelings toward HIV-infected co-workers than employees who received no information. The results suggest companies should be more concerned about the kind of messages workers receive. By focusing only on practices that can transmit the disease, many educational materials neglect to deal with the social, emotional, and humanitarian aspects of the problem. Education may be the key, but we need to look closely at what kind of education that should be.

What You Should Know About AIDS

Facts about the disease
How to protect yourself and your family
What to tell others

AMERICA
RESPONDS
TO AIDS

An Important Message from the U.S. Public Health Service
Centers for Disease Control

FIGURE 15-3 Understanding AIDS. This public health pamphlet contains eight pages of HIV/AIDS information. It was sent to 107 million homes in the United States in 1988. Fifty-one percent of those who received the pamphlet did not read it!

THE CHARACTER OF SOCIETY

Rumors of Destruction

Today, friends are asked on street corners, at social gatherings, or over telephones: "Did you hear that he/she has AIDS?" Or: "Do you believe that he/she might be infected? You never know with the life they lead!" Some of the fa-mous people *rumored* to have HIV/AIDS are Madonna, Elizabeth Taylor, Burt Reynolds, Richard Pryor, and Joe Penny from the TV show *Jake and the Fatman*.

Rumors ruin lives. People suddenly subtly lose services; the lawn boy quits, no reason given. Quietly job applications are turned down or car and homeowner insurance poli-cies are canceled, and so on. In one case, after rumors of HIV infection spread in a small town, a man, if he was served in local bars at all, received his drinks in plastic cups. A health club refunded his membership dues. His apartment manager asked him to leave and when his toilet backed up the maintenance man came in wearing a hat over a World War II gas mask, deep water fishing boots, raincoat, and rubber gloves. In frustration, he had an HIV test. The results were negative and he gave copies of the test to every "joint" in town, his physician, dentist, theater manager, grocery store manager... He felt this approach was better than running. **Do you agree?**

In another case in Brantly County, Georgia, population 11,077, the 22-year-old mother of a 2-year-old son was the subject of a rumor that she was HIV-infected. The rumor also stated that she had had intercourse with 200 men in the past year. To convince the townspeople, she took the HIV test and was not HIV-infected. This young woman had to circulate the results of her blood test around town, but it was still not enough to stop the rumor. A newspaper in nearby Waycross quoted an unnamed source saying that this woman was HIV-positive. The rumor goes on!

There was the case of a compassionate person who opened a home for helping AIDS patients. Rumor quickly spread that the entire neighborhood was in danger, especially after the mail carrier refused to deliver mail and was ordered to wear rubber gloves and return to the post office for disinfection! To help the neighborhood understand AIDS and stop unfounded fears, a seminar was held at the AIDS home, but no one would enter the house.

A young person with AIDS reluctantly returned home—it meant revealing that he was gay to his family—and to the community. He said to his parents, "I have good news and bad. The bad is that I'm gay. The good is I have AIDS. I won't be around long enough to interfere with anyone." Once the word got out a catering service refused to do the annual family Christmas party. They could not hire a practical nurse. Family and friends who used to drop in stayed away. People whispered that the son had gay cancer . . . that it was lethal . . . that it could be caught from dishes, linens, a handshake and breathing in the same air he breathed out.

THE RIGHT TO PRIVACY

Arthur Ashe died of AIDS in February of 1993; he was *forced* to go public about having AIDS. Did that affect his life? Yes. He had to alter a lifestyle he was trying to live with his family. He could no longer live a normal day with his family.

The immediate defense from the press, which forced Arthur Ashe to go public, is that it serves the public interest to identify prominent people with AIDS. The news media says that it increases awareness—and therefore, theoretically, action—to fight back against AIDS. **DO YOU AGREE?**

Organizations can write and broadcast about HIV/AIDS any time, about anybody they want to. **IS THIS MORALLY RIGHT?**

Some defenders of the news media say that a public figure cannot have it both ways—cannot deliberately keep himself in the limelight with sports-equipment endorsements, and so forth, and then turn around and say, "I want to be a private person." But what is public and what is private?

As Ellen Hume asks, "Is there no moment of a public figure's life that is not open to prurient exposure? Does being a political officeholder or, as in Ashe's case, a sports champion, mean that the public owns all of your life, including your life in the bedroom, the doctor's office, the church confessional or the psychiatrist's couch?" **WHAT IS YOUR REPLY TO HER?**

Ms. Hume asks, "Should journalists end their scrutiny of public figures?" She thinks not. But she says, "Not every revelation serves the public interest. No American president and few athletes, astronauts, journalists or other heroes could have survived this Spanish Inquisition. Isn't it time for the press to develop a more sophisticated sense of priorities and ethics to go along with its extraordinary new power?" **WHAT IS YOUR REPLY?**

In Athens, Alabama, the headline of the town's newspaper read, "Athens doctor: 'I don't have AIDS.'" This doctor, a prominent pediatrician in this town for 18 years, had to produce a public defense to dispel the gossip that he had AIDS. Because in a small town everybody knows everybody, the rumor spread with lightning speed to the town hospital, grocery store, hair salon, school, newspaper, and so on. The doctor offered a $2000 reward for any information about who began the rumor. To date no one has collected the money, but the townspeople have gathered to support him.

Mathilde Krim of the American Foundation of AIDS Research said, "From the beginning, the people with AIDS have been a disposable group—gays, blacks and drug users. People don't care about them. They'd rather they wouldn't be here anyway." When the National Gay Rights Advocates asked the nation's 1,000 biggest companies whether employee medical plans covered AIDS-related expenses, one anonymous answer read, "Just enough to defray the cost of the bullet." However, HIV has spread to infect most other groups of society and attitudes are slowly changing.

Good News, Bad News, and Late News

Good News— Good news is thinking and believing you're HIV-infected and you're not. There must be a reason to think you're infected, so not being infected is, as some would say, a new lease on life. All too often that feeling is soon forgotten and many people continue lifestyles that place them at risk for infection.

Bad News— Bad news is thinking you're HIV-infected and you are. It is difficult to predict what a person sees, hears, or does after being told he or she is HIV-positive. For example, some have contemplated suicide, some have committed suicide, others have become completely fatalistic and proceeded to live a reckless and careless lifestyle that endangered others. Some have said it's like death before you're dead.

You are never prepared to hear the bad news regardless of how sure you are that you're infected. For example, one man who had suffered from night sweats, fevers, weight loss, and other classic symptoms just knew he was infected. Yet when told of the positive test results he said "I got so angry, I ripped a shower out of the wall." Being told you are infected is totally devastating, said another infected person. "You feel that everyone is looking at you, everyone can tell you're dirty." Another person said, "The fact that I'm HIV-positive completely

dominates my life. There is not a waking hour that I do not think about it. I feel like a leper. I live between hope and despair." Still another said, "I did not leave the house for two days after being told I was HIV-positive. The initial shock was that I was contaminated—unhealthy, soiled, unclean. I carried this burden in isolation for over two years. After all, I had met people who had AIDS but never a person who said—I'm HIV-infected."

The bad news is not confined to those hearing they are HIV-infected; it touches everyone they know—lovers, family, friends, and employers. Nothing remains the same. The more symptomatic one becomes, the greater the social and human loss. One symptomatic mother said, "Whenever I tell my four-year-old I am going to the doctor, he screams because he knows I could be gone for weeks." I try to put him in another room playing with his sister when they come for me." This woman has died. Relatives care for her children.

Late News— Late news is remaining **asymptomatic** after infection. Asymptomatic can be defined as when no clinically recognizable symptoms appear that would indicate HIV infection. During this time period, the virus can be transmitted to sexual partners. By the time either antibodies and/or clinical symptoms appear, the news is too late for those who might have been spared infection had their sexual partner tested positive or demonstrated clinical symptoms early on.

When People Pretend to Be HIV-Positive or to Have AIDS

As Hector Gavin wrote in 1843 in his 400-page history *Of Feigned and Factitious Diseases*, "The monarch, the mendicant, the unhappy slave, the proud warrior, the lofty statesman, even the minister of religion . . . have sought to disguise their purposes, or to obtain their desires, by feigning mental or bodily infirmities."

Donald Craven (1994) reported that a growing number of people may pretend to have AIDS either because of emotional disorders or because they want to gain access to free housing, medical care, and disability income. In one case, seven patients with self-reported HIV infection were treated for an average of 9.2 months in a clinical AIDS program before their sero-negative status was discovered at the hospital (in general, hospitals in the United States do not require a written copy of the HIV test results proving that someone is HIV-positive). Craven noted that "because patients with AIDS often have preferred access to drug treatment, prescription drugs, social security disability insurance, housing and comprehensive medical care, the rate of malingering may increase and reach extremes."

Another doctor who treats many AIDS patients said that he and his colleagues have seen many patients who repeatedly come to their offices fearing that they have AIDS, even though multiple tests have shown that they do not (Zuger, 1995).

An Oklahoma physician has written about the AIDS **Munchausen's syndrome**—an emotional disorder in which people pretend to have the disease simply to get attention from doctors. Confidentiality requirements make AIDS a "perfect" illness for people suffering from Munchausen syndrome, because the laws shield them from being discovered.

Physicians' Public Duty: A Historical Perspective of Professional Obligation

Physicians enjoy a virtual monopoly on medical care, social status, and generous financial remuneration. Thus the medical profession is uniquely entrusted with the knowledge to care for those with HIV disease/AIDS or any other contagious disease and has a clear responsibility to do so, absent compelling considerations to the contrary. A fair and reasonable share of medical risk just naturally goes with the professional territory.

Robert Fulton and Greg Owen (1988) stated that throughout history, plagues and pestilences have challenged humankind. In his book, *Plagues and People,* William McNeill (1976) cited the many death-dealing epidemics in Europe. He wrote that one advantage the West had over the East in the face of deadly epidemics was that caring for the sick was a recognized duty among Christians. The effect of a prolonged epidemic more often than not strengthened the Church when other

social institutions were discredited for not providing needed services. McNeill further observed that the teachings of Christianity made life meaningful, even in the immediate face of death: Not only would survivors find spiritual consolation in the vision of heavenly reunion with their dead relatives or friends, but God's hand was also seen in the work of the life-risking caregivers.

The United States has also had its share of plagues and epidemics; one of the most notable was the outbreak of yellow fever in Philadelphia in 1793. Thousands of citizens of the capital city perished. William Powell (1965), in his book *Bring Out Your Dead,* describes Philadelphia at the time of the yellow fever plague: the dying were abandoned, the dead left unburied, orphaned children and the elderly wandered the streets in search of food and shelter. Nearly all who could fled the city, including the President, leaving the victims of the fever to their fate. Among those who remained, however, were Benjamin Rush, M.D., the mayor, a handful of medical colleagues and their assistants, and a number of clergy. With the help of a small group of laborers and craftsmen, they undertook the enormous tasks of maintaining law and order, providing medical care, food and shelter to the sick and helpless, as well as gathering up and burying the dead.

Dr. Rush and the others remained at their posts because of their overriding sense of professional obligation along with a conviction inspired by the precept of the New Testament "Blessed are the merciful, for they shall obtain mercy" (Matthew 5:9).

But this vision, shared by Christians for centuries, along with a sense of professional commitment, may not be sufficient to persuade contemporary health care workers to stay at their posts.

The baby boom generation, well-educated and self-oriented, has learned to blame AIDS on groups whom society defines as deviant: homosexuals, prostitutes, and drug abusers. There is a significant probability, therefore, that today's young health care practitioner may turn away from HIV/AIDS patients despite the fact that a 1981 Gallup Poll of the religious beliefs and practices of 14 countries showed that the United States leads the world not only in church membership but also in charitable services.

According to an article in the November 13, 1987, issue of *The Wall Street Journal,* Arthur Caplan, a director for the Center of Biomedical Ethics at the University of Minnesota in Minneapolis, believes that doctors and nurses who refuse to treat AIDS patients do so out of disapproval. "They know how to deal with violent patients and infectious diseases like hepatitis." So why not treat someone with AIDS? "It's more than fear. They're making a value . . . judgment about AIDS victims. They're saying they won't treat people (they find) disgusting." Others refuse to place their lives at risk for someone who became HIV-infected through immoral behavior. C. Everett Koop said the refusal by some medical personnel to treat AIDS patients "threatens the very fabric of health care in this country." **DO YOU AGREE?**

Medical Moral Issues

HIV/AIDS represents a new era in medicine, one in which physicians are faced with complex moral issues. When the American Medical Association (AMA) issued a statement to the effect that it is unethical to refuse to treat HIV/AIDS patients, that statement reflected a deep concern in the medical community about the possibility of their becoming infected by treating patients with HIV/AIDS.

The AMA statement for an ethical call to arms is unprecedented in this century. It is the result of a spreading fear that HIV/AIDS is too contagious to tolerate in spite of the knowledge that the virus is not transmitted via casual contact. **Emotions**, not education, are in control of those whose fears exceed reality. But these emotions are real and they are having an impact on the medical community.

There is an ongoing dilemma concerning the rights of the physician and other health care workers to practice medicine in a safe environment as opposed to the rights of HIV-infected and AIDS patients to receive care and medical support. Although the risk of HIV transmission through medical occupational exposure appears to be quite low, the fact that it is possible at all, coupled with the uniformly fatal prognosis associated with AIDS, suggests that physicians,

nurses, and other health care workers have legitimate concerns about risk to their health.

In a recent report by C.E. Lewis and colleagues (1992), almost half of the primary care physicians in the Los Angeles area had refused to treat HIV-infected patients or had planned not to accept them as regular patients.

In a more recent survey of American doctors in residency training, 39% said that a surgeon or other specialist had refused to treat a patient with AIDS in the resident's care. In Canada, only 13% reported a specialist had refused to treat a patient with AIDS; in France, only 8% said a specialist had rejected care.

Further, 23% of American doctors would not care for AIDS patients if they had a choice as compared with 14% of Canadian physicians and 4% of French doctors.

The survey results may be a disturbing indicator of how American physicians view their work and a reflection of cultural and political attitudes here that view with veiled hostility those with AIDS.

To combat that fear, medical schools are now providing their students with disability insurance that covers AIDS. Hospitals have adopted policies that require physicians to treat AIDS patients or face dismissal.

AIDS Influencing Medical Students' Choices

Nathan Link and colleagues (1988) surveyed 250 first, second, and third year interns in two medical and two pediatric residency programs. Twenty-five percent said they would not continue to care for AIDS patients if given a choice. These data represent a significant degree of fear of contracting AIDS from patients.

A 1989 survey of 120 students in their second and third year of medical school (66% male; 91% had no experience with AIDS patients) revealed the following:

1. 75% worried that they might contract AIDS if they had to work with AIDS patients.
2. 25% felt that AIDS patients should be quarantined.
3. 25% said they would be afraid to care for AIDS patients.

4. 15% said they were morally offended by AIDS patients.
5. 33% said they would avoid caring for AIDS patients.
6. 50% said hospital personnel should not be required to care for AIDS patients.
7. 27% said they had considered changing their careers because they might be required to care for AIDS patients.

In another study, a survey on the attitudes of 1,045 internal medicine staff physicians revealed: (1) 63% said that they did not intend to treat people with HIV; (2) 17% had no objection to caring for HIV/AIDS patients; (3) about 66% stated that they would withhold life-saving measures from a patient if they felt there was a 1-in-100 chance that they themselves might become infected. Such attitudes can be found in virtually all medical specialties (Driscoll, 1990; Kindig et al., 1994).

Collectively, these data suggest that medical students and practicing physicians are deciding, on some level, whether they want to continue on in medicine. This decision has important ramifications for everyone. It would be interesting to know how many students decide against entering medical school because of the HIV/AIDS pandemic.

HIV-Infected Physicians

The fact that medical students and residents fear contracting HIV infection and AIDS can be tied to the reality that by mid-1991, 720 physicians were reported to the CDC as having AIDS. This number is probably underreported by 20% to 50%. At least 5,000 physicians were HIV-infected by 1990 (see Chapter 10 for additional information on HIV-infected health care workers) (Breo, 1990). The question residents and medical students are asking is: How did so many become infected?

Along with the recognition of infected physicians come many disturbing questions on whether they should be permitted to continue their medical practice. In 1987, a Gallup Poll (as reported in January 1989 in *The Wall Street Journal*) asked that very question, and 57% of the general public said **not under any circumstances.**

─────── **BOX 15.7** ───────

PHYSICIAN SHORTAGE—WHO SUFFERS?

A 1991 survey of physicians throughout the United States revealed that there is only one primary care physician for every 2,857 residents in rural areas compared to 1 for every 614 residents nationally. And there are 111 rural counties in 22 states with no physician at all. Texas has 18 counties without a physician. Rural America needs at least 35,000 more general practitioners.

Senator Max Bacus (Dem., Montana) said that in his state, eight counties have *no* physicians and 18 counties have no one qualified to deliver babies. He said, "There currently are 50 vacancies for family practice doctors in Montana. Thirty of our 56 counties are designated 'health-professional shortage areas.' In Montana, where we have no medical school, we have an additional disadvantage in that young doctors do not spend their learning years or their residencies anywhere in our state." Montana is only one of many states that face physician shortages in smaller cities, towns, and outlying areas. If HIV-infected physicians, whose numbers continue to climb, are denied the right to practice, the physician shortage will become worse. If physicians who are HBV-infected (carry the hepatitis B virus) or are infected with other serious sexually transmitted diseases are included among the HIV-infected, a very serious physician shortage would occur not only in the rural areas, but also in the larger cities.

Discussion Questions: At what point or for what reason should physicians and other health care workers be denied the right to practice?

Can these physicians still save lives even though their own may be forfeited?

Medical experts say the public should not be worried about patients contracting the virus during a routine physical examination or through casual contact with an infected doctor or hospital worker.

But the public does worry about what might happen during surgery and procedures involving contact with mucous membranes (Table 15-1). For example, some medical experts fear that if an infected surgeon is accidently cut in the operating room, the surgeon's blood could cause an infection. Because of the controversial

TABLE 15-1 Poll on Revelation of HIV Status

A. Should the following health care workers who are HIV-infected be forbidden to practice?

	Yes	No
Surgeons	63%	28%
All physicians	51%	42%
Dentists	60%	33%
All health care workers	49%	43%

B. Should patients be required to inform their physicians, dentists and other health care workers whether they are HIV-infected?

Yes	No
97%	2%

(Source: *Newsweek*, July 1, 1991)

─────── POINT OF INFORMATION 15.2 ───────

HIV TRANSMITTED BY AUSTRALIAN SURGEON

A breakdown in infection control procedures is being blamed for the transmission of HIV to five patients of an Australian surgeon. It's believed the virus was transmitted from one patient to four others during minor skin surgery on a single day in November, 1989. Health officials say one patient, a gay man, is believed to have been the infection source. The CDC calls the case the first known patient-to-patient transmissions of HIV in a health care setting (*American Medical News..* 1994 37:2.) Similar to the more recent dentist-Bergalis case, the source of HIV, will most likely, never be documented to everyone's satisfaction.

dentist-to-patient HIV transmission that occurred in Florida, the CDC has convened its advisors to help revise CDC guidelines for infection control. A major question under review is whether any HIV/AIDS professional who performs invasive procedures should be allowed to continue. Restriction of HIV-infected surgeons and dentists would greatly curtail or even destroy their practices. It was suggested by one consultant to the CDC that any restriction would lead to mandatory screening of all health care workers. At the moment, the CDC says that the question of whether an infected physician or dentist should be allowed to perform invasive procedures (those in which bleeding may occur) can only be answered on a case-by-case basis.

Risk Protection of the Patient: Political Dimensions— The American Medical Association's position is that HIV/AIDS doctors "should consult colleagues as to which activities the physician can pursue without creating a risk to patients."

There must be a rational relationship between the degree of risk, the morbidity and mortality of the disease, and the consequences of policies and procedures implemented to reduce the risk. Invasive surgery involves many risks. There is an overriding ethical obligation to reduce these risks in ways that do not create more harm than good. The justification of policies to prevent life-threatening illnesses with a risk fac-

tor of 1 in 10,000 is significantly greater than those with a risk factor of one in 100,000. More lives can be saved by innovative approaches to preventing the kind of injuries that have accounted for 75% of all cases of occupationally related HIV infection than by preventing HIV-infected health care workers from performing invasive surgery.

The risk of HIV infection by an HIV-infected surgeon is only one-tenth the chance of being killed by lightning, one-fourth the chance of being killed by a bee, and half the chance of being hit by a falling aircraft. The 1 in 100,000 risk of transmission from an infected surgeon equals the probability of death we face bicycling 2 miles each way to school for 1 month, or commuting 15 miles round-trip by car for a year.

Similarly, our chance of dying from anesthesia during an operation is roughly 10 times our chance of being infected by a surgeon known to be infected with HIV. A mother who approves a penicillin injection for her toddler with pharyngitis accepts a 1 in 100,000 risk of death from anaphylactic shock. In one study, the most successful coronary artery bypass graft surgeon surveyed had a 1.9% mortality rate, while the least successful had a 9.2% mortality rate. Patients selecting the least successful surgeon thus face 7,300 times the extra risk of death posed by an HIV-infected surgeon. The risk to a person undergoing invasive surgery by a surgeon of **unknown** HIV status is about 1 in

20 million of becoming HIV-infected (Daniels, 1992). The CDC estimates the risk to a patient by an HIV-infected surgeon to be between 1 in 42,000 and 1 in 420,000 (Lo et al., 1992).

Patients' Right to Know if Their Physician Has HIV/AIDS— In a 1987 Gallup Poll, 86% of those polled felt that they had the right to know if a health care worker treating them was HIV-infected. Many lawyers also take this position. The courts appear to be moving toward an interpretation of the doctrine of informed patient consent as **"what a reasonable patient would want to know,"** rather than **"what a reasonable physician would disclose."** Because it is so difficult for surgeons to avoid occasionally cutting themselves during surgery, it has been suggested that the best solution is not to have HIV-infected surgeons perform surgery at all.

Public anxiety on HIV/AIDS and medical care is becoming increasingly tinged with hysteria. A national Gallup Poll undertaken for *Newsweek* (June 20, 1991) asked a representative sample of 618 adults, "Which of the following kinds of health care workers should be required to tell patients if they are infected with the AIDS virus?"

The answers were: surgeons 95%; all physicians 94%; dentists 94%; all health care workers 90%.

Clearly, people do not differentiate between doctors who perform invasive procedures and those who do not. However, the patient could ask what the probability is of a single dentist (Acer) infecting six of his patients (Bergalis, Web, and four others). Extremely low, **yet it did happen!** The lowest of probabilities and best of guidelines and precautions do not stop the fire of fear. It must also be mentioned that the same *Newsweek* poll found that 97% of those interviewed felt that HIV-infected patients should tell their health care workers that they are infected (Table 15-1B).

There is one important aspect related to this poll that needs to be addressed. That is, many of the people interviewed stated that if they knew their surgeon was HIV-infected, they would "get another surgeon." This *switching dilemma* may, at some point, have the majority of the population needing surgery standing in

line for the uninfected surgeons. Services provided by the reduced number of surgeons, it could be claimed, at some point, result in increased costs and diminished quality.

Physician–Patient Relationships

In most states, physicians may **not test** a patient for HIV antibodies without written permission from the patient. Physicians can run tests for any other infectious diseases without written permission.

Do you think this is fair and equal medical practice?

Because the majority of HIV-infected patients are asymptomatic, there is no way of telling **who is** or **is not** infected. Therefore, for the protection of health care workers, everyone must be treated as though they were HIV-infected.

HIV is the silent medical threat of the 1980s and 1990s. Whenever blood is drawn, a wound is examined, a dressing is changed, or anything that involves blood, needles, or surgery is done, there is an unspoken fear that HIV might be present. The patient sees this preventive attitude of physicians and other health care workers by the new look of the 1980s and 1990s: wraparound smocks, gloved hands, and masks. The patient wonders whether his or her physician is an HIV carrier and the physician assumes that the patient may be a carrier. A recent Associated Press article presented some

─────── **BOX 15.8** ───────

MY FIRST AIDS EXPERIENCE

"A man was waiting for his mother in my office while she consulted me about a back problem," reports a family practitioner in a Gulf state city. "He had a grand mal seizure, bit his tongue and bled quite a bit. I put a tape-wrapped tongue depressor into his mouth to keep him from further injuring his tongue and then just supported him until the seizure was over. Later the physician who had been caring for him at a hospital clinic called to ask that I confirm the seizure, adding, "By the way, this man has AIDS." I never gave a thought to AIDS in this situation," continues the family practitioner. "It was my first experience in dealing with an AIDS patient" (Polder et al., 1989).

examples of how the AIDS pandemic has changed doctor–patient relationships:

1. In many operating rooms, doctors and nurses wear wraparound glasses in case of blood splashes.
2. In many emergency rooms, health care workers cover themselves with caps, goggles, masks, gowns, gloves, shoe covers, and blood-proof aprons.
3. Infection control specialists must spend time convincing hospital workers it is safe to enter an HIV/AIDS patient's room to perform normal duties ranging from picking up dinner trays to fixing the plumbing.
4. At some hospitals, all emergency room trash, no matter how innocuous, is treated as hazardous waste.
5. Many doctors and nurses routinely pull on gloves whenever they give an injection or draw blood.
6. Mouth-to-mouth resuscitation is simply not done at many hospitals. Instead a mask and valve device is used to avoid direct contact with the patient's mouth.
7. A surgeon at San Francisco General Hospital takes the AIDS drug zidovudine whenever he operates on people he thinks are infected.
8. Physicians are increasing life insurance policies to provide for their families in case they become HIV-infected.

The health care professionals' fear of getting AIDS will persist as long as there is a risk that HIV can be transmitted in the workplace. The goal is not to eradicate that fear, but to prevent it from compromising the quality of patient care and from threatening the health professional's own well-being (Gerbert et al., 1988).

In early 1990, Lorraine Day quit her post as chairperson of the Orthopedics Department at San Francisco General Hospital and abandoned her surgical practice because of her fear of exposure to HIV. "I have two children to think about and operating was too dangerous. If I was a skydiver, people would say I was an irresponsible mother, but to me, surgery now, it was just as risky."

Dr. Day said during a TV interview, "Our risk is one in 200 per single (needle) stick with AIDS blood and it can be the first one—it doesn't take 200. And I ask you, if you came to work every day and flipped the light switch on in your office and only one out of 200 times you were electrocuted would you consider that low-risk?"

While Dr. Day has been called a scaremonger, many surgeons in private conversations call her a "hero" for raising the risk issue.

Physicians with AIDS

According to Mandelbaum-Schmid (1990), one overriding issue facing physicians who become HIV-infected is that there is no support system to compensate them once they become too sick to work (Figure 15-4). For example, a 32-year-old gastroenterologist, claimed she was infected with HIV in 1983 when she accidently pricked herself with a needle that an intern had used to draw blood from an AIDS patient. She was working at the time at Brooklyn's Kings County Hospital.

She tested HIV-positive in 1985. On subsequent consultations with physicians at the

FIGURE 15-4. Together for Now: Judy (37), Andy (39), Robbie (10), and Amy (6) Lipschitz. In 1986, during his residency, Andy was asked to work with an AIDS patient. He inserted an arterial line into the patient's arm. After withdrawing the needle from the catheter, he accidentally punctured his thumb. Several weeks later Andy had severe flu-like symptoms. He demonstrated *Pneumocystis carinii* pneumonia in mid-1992—he had AIDS. His ever-changing regimen of ZDV, ddI, ddC, and d4T all cause side effects. He is hoping a successful drug will soon be available. ©Shonna Valeska 1995.

————— BOX 15.9 —————

THE PHYSICIAN'S RIGHT TO KNOW IF THE PATIENT IS HIV/AIDS-INFECTED

PRO:

Recently there have been calls for attention to the rights of health care providers to know when they are being exposed to HIV-infected patients (Hagen et al., 1988; Fournier et al., 1989; Rhame et al., 1989).

(*A letter from a practicing nurse to the editor of a large southeastern newspaper*)

"Perhaps the physician's letter was a bit too harsh in the opening sentence when he stated that he was 'sick and tired of AIDS patients and their rights.'

However, I don't think this doctor is hysterical or ignorant. I can only speculate on his feelings, but I assume that he is like other health care professionals who want to help, but think they also have rights to protect themselves.

We all use or are instructed to use universal precautions. These precautions can easily be violated when a patient with alcohol or drug withdrawal bites someone or a needle goes through a gloved hand.

I have been spat on, bitten, clawed and urinated on, among other things, in my years of nursing. It is not glamorous, but, at least, I knew if the patient had hepatitis or tuberculosis. Why shouldn't I know if he has AIDS?

We can't work as a team if we don't know what we're dealing with. When someone develops a sudden increase in temperature, we don't have to go through mounds of red tape to do cultures to determine the cause of illness. When the patient goes to the doctor with a symptom, he expects the doctor to make a diagnosis. What's the physician supposed to do if he suspects AIDS but can't confirm it because the patient has rights?

This disease should be treated like any other, beginning with a diagnosis, followed by treatment, concern and confidentiality among the patients and health care professionals.

Eventually, these people will realize that when they stop fighting us we will have the same genuine compassion for them that we have for all patients".

Behind physicians' anxiety about HIV/AIDS is anger about being obligated to take risks in an atmosphere of uncertainty. They feel that AIDS is an infectious disease that is not being treated like one. And according to law, HIV/AIDS is *not* an infectious disease, it is considered a disability. (See Chapter 16 for legal definition.) Most physicians feel it is absurd that they do not have the right to find out whether or not a patient is HIV-infected. The recommendation that doctors treat every patient as if he or she had HIV/AIDS is unrealistic in the hospital setting, especially in hospital emergency rooms. Currently, there is great pressure from the health care community to obtain legislation for health care workers' *right to know* patient HIV status.

CON:

There is another side to this conflict of rights, the side that says universal patient testing will not be useful. J.D. Gostin, executive director of the American Society of Law and Medicine says that there are no data to indicate that physicians would reduce their risk of exposure if they knew the HIV status of their patients (Mandelbaum-Schmid, 1990). Gostin believes that patients have a moral obligation, although not a legal one, to be retested after a health care professional is exposed to their blood. "It's true that a few patients may not consent," he concedes, "but the overwhelming majority will. One can't develop a policy of testing everyone in the country because of a hypothetical case where a doctor might be stuck, the patient won't disclose, and zidovudine might be effective. That is too speculative a basis for taking away people's rights."

THE COMPROMISE:

Sanford F. Kuvin, M.D. (Vice Chairman, Board of Trustees, National Foundation for Infectious Diseases, Washington) is of the opinion "all health care professionals involved in invasive procedures should have themselves tested for HIV and make their status known to their patients. Similarly, patients who will be undergoing invasive procedures should be tested and make their status known to those treating them."

THE QUESTION:

Are federal and state governments overstressing the need for privacy at the expense of prevention?

THE SECRET

In 1992, a 40-year-old gay family practice doctor had to decide on whether to tell his patients he had HIV disease. If the doctor tells his patients he has the virus, he will lose his business. At least that has been the case for the doctors, dentists, nurses, pharmacists, and surgical technicians who have come forward so far. If he lost his profession he could face the last years of his life not only grappling with a devastating and expensive illness, but also be deprived of income, health insurance, and the solace of employment. If he concealed his infection and continued to work, his infection could be revealed and his practice destroyed anyway, through lawsuits. That was the experience of one doctor who publicly announced he had AIDS in 1990, *after* another doctor reported him to the state board of medical examiners. This doctor was subsequently sued by 24 former patients for malpractice and personal injury. In another case, a Johns Hopkins University surgeon died of AIDS disease in 1990, since then, two patients have filed suit against his estate, claiming damages because they were so horrified to find they had been operated on by a doctor with the virus and because they now face the prospect of repeated HIV tests. About 50 more of this doctor's patients are contemplating similar actions. However, the charges against him were dismissed because the claimants couldn't show any actual damages. In addition, some hospitals and institutions have dismissed all medical or health care workers who were HIV-positive.

In a survey by the Medical Expertise Retention Program, a San Francisco-based program that helps infected health workers sort out their options, 67% of HIV-positive doctors said they have avoided, or plan to avoid, seeking treatment or submitting insurance claims because they fear their **secret** will be told.

Before this doctor died, he decided that "there were no good solutions." Left to his own conscience and reasoning, the doctor came to the conclusion that his doubts were based on emotion, not science—just like the fears of his patients. Technically, he decided, there was no way he could give the virus to a patient. "If there was the slightest possibility I could give it to them it would be their right to know I'm HIV-positive," he says. "But there is no conceivable way. So it is absolutely not their business. My patients like

me, love me, depend on me. But if they find out I have HIV, they're going to leave me. How many are going to stay? Three out of ten? Why should they take the chance? Why should they be crusaders? They won't." (Adapted from Japenga, 1992)

QUESTION: Should the patient have the choice as to whether they wish to become a crusader? Compare your immediate response to the responses of physicians who read "The Secret".

RESPONSE from physicians who read this story, "The Secret":

1. "Thank you for your story 'The Secret.'" I, too, am a physician who learned of my HIV infection one year ago. I have experienced many of the same feelings as the doctor you profiled in the article.

    For the past year, I have lived much of my life "in secret." I am afraid to tell even my closest friends for fear of divulging my status to the hospital and medical school for which I now work. I have had to worry about who I might meet at a support group, about whether I might run into my patients at community meetings about HIV/AIDS, and about losing my job and health insurance if my employer finds out.

    Just as other infected people, I have fought guilt, shame, fear, anger, and hopelessness. However, as a physician at an inner-city hospital, I am also responsible for a large number of patients with HIV/AIDS. Although I enjoy my work and feel fulfilled, it has been very difficult for me to care for people who are at a later stage of the same disease that I have, and watch as they decline mentally and physically.

    Perhaps someday we may not have to keep this important part of our lives such a secret.
    NAME WITHHELD

2. "My situation as a physician with HIV infection is complicated by the fact that I am a surgeon". I went through virtually the exact decision process as the doctor profiled in `The Secret' but I arrived at a different conclusion, and have been devastated by the results.

    I told my chief of service, in confidence, of my diagnosis. Within two days, my privileges

———— **BOX 15.10** (*continued*) ————

were suspended, and the hospital sued to get permission to disclose my condition to all patients I had treated while at the hospital, to the press, and to any other hospital I applied to. The court granted the request. My practice evaporated, and the hospital has made certain that my efforts to build an alternative non-operative practice would fail.

The doctor in `The Secret' made the right decision: Since he's not a danger to his patients, he should say nothing, and get on with his life.

The irony is that all this can be prevented: This 'crisis' is driven not by medical fact or necessity, but by the hospital industry's fear of being sued."

NAME WITHHELD

3. Bravo for publishing 'The Secret.' I am an HIV-positive operating room nurse, and I know this story all too well. I did what I thought was the moral and ethical thing to do: I disclosed my status to my supervisor. From

that point on, all confidentiality went out the window. I discovered that confidentiality is only rhetoric.

After review by the hospital's 'expert review panel'—which did not include a peer or anyone else from the department of surgery—my practice was restricted. I could no longer work as a scrub nurse. No one ever noticed that I was the **only** one in my operating room who followed impeccable infection control and universal precautions.

Yes, doctor keep your mouth shut, and practice impeccable infection control. The review panel I dealt with provided no counseling, no follow-up, and even less support. To quote from one survey of high-risk and HIV-positive hospital workers like myself, 'Let us not forget that HIV-positive health care providers have saved and continue to save thousands of lives every year.'"

NAME WITHHELD

National Institutes of Health (NIH), she was told that she was a healthy carrier of the virus who could become ill. She continued training at Kings County, completing a residency in internal medicine and a fellowship in gastroenterology.

She became symptomatic in 1987. A year later, she filed a 175 million dollar lawsuit charging that the hospital's negligence had caused her illness. At the time of the trial, her life expectancy was estimated at less than a year. Following a stormy 2-month trial that challenged the integrity of all the physicians and expert witnesses who testified, she reportedly settled for just under 2 million dollars.

Another pressing issue pointed out by Mandelbaum-Schmid is that HIV-infected doctors are not protected against discrimination. The experience of an otolaryngologist who died of AIDS in June, 1989, at the age of 46, set an unwelcome precedent. Before his illness, he had a thriving practice in Princeton, New Jersey. He believed he was infected in 1984 after being splashed in the face with blood while performing an emergency tracheotomy. He became ill with an undifferentiated pneumonia in 1987. Physicians per- formed a bronchoscopy and gave him an HIV test without telling him.

Word of his positive HIV test soon spread through the hospital and soon after into his community. By the time he was released from the hospital, his telephone lines were jammed with calls from hysterical patients. He eventually lost about half his practice. When he tried to schedule operating room time, the hospital's president convened an emergency meeting of trustees. They made the unprecedented decision that he may operate but only with the informed consent of his patients.

He filed a lawsuit based on breach of ethics and doctor–patient confidentiality—his diagnosis had been leaked by the hospital laboratory—and violation of antidiscrimination laws. In April, 1991, New Jersey Superior Court Judge Philip S. Carchman ruled that the Medical Center of Princeton, after learning the doctor had AIDS, made a "reasoned and informed response" in barring him from performing surgery without informed consent of his patients.

The last example of the plight of a physician with AIDS involves a physician at Johns Hopkins Medical Center. He contracted an HIV infection from a patient in 1983 while working as a resident in the bone marrow transplantation unit, he had an accident with the blood of a young leukemia patient who had been transfused many times. The accident was followed 3 weeks later by an acute febrile illness with cough, sore throat, rash, and lymphadenopathy. After this, he was in good health for the next 3 years. He completed his residency and became a chief resident and a fellow in cardiology. He married, and had a daughter. In November of 1986, unexplained weight loss led him to be HIV tested. He tested positive for HIV.

The hospital's reaction was unexpected. He had to sue the institution and some members of the faculty in an effort to defend his reputation and obtain appropriate benefits. After endless months of legal battle, Johns Hopkins proposed a settlement 3 weeks before the trial date.

He said, "By actions like this, medical institutions send an awful message to the health care worker: we ask you to be in the front lines,

but if something happens to you, we will not stand behind you, you will be abandoned, and you will be deprived of the privilege of practicing medicine" (Aoun, 1990). He died of AIDS in February of 1992, 9 years after becoming infected with HIV.

SUMMARY

In 1981, AIDS was announced as a new disease affecting the homosexual population. Many religious people believed this was a sign that homosexuality should be punished. The few facts available at that time gave rise to a great deal of fantasy and fear. Affected people were either innocent victims or they deserved the disease. Contracting AIDS labeled a person as less than desirable, a homosexual or one who practiced deviant forms of sexual behavior. But even the so-called innocent victims, the children, the hemophiliacs, and the recipients of blood transfusions were not spared social ostracism. If you had AIDS, you were twice the victim—first of the virus and second of the social behavior.

Children were barred from attending school, adults from their jobs, and both from adequate medical care. For example, there are still relatively few dentists who will treat AIDS patients and a significant number of surgeons refuse to operate on AIDS patients. Fourteen years have passed, but many misconceptions about HIV/AIDS linger on.

Fear is being casually transmitted rather than the virus. A significant number of people, after 14 years of broad scale education, still believe that the AIDS virus can be casually transmitted from toilet seats, drinking glasses, and even by donating blood.

The fallout from the fear of the AIDS pandemic has been a major change in sexual language in TV advertisements, magazines, and radio. Condoms once spoken about only in hushed tones in conversations and kept under the counter in most drug stores, are now spoken of everywhere as a means of safer sex. AIDS, perhaps more than any other disease, has demonstrated that ignorance leads to fear and knowledge can lead to compassion.

To achieve understanding and compassion, people must be educated as to their HIV risk sta-

---

────── POINT OF INFORMATION 15.3 ──────

CURRENT VIEW OF HEALTH CARE WORKERS WHO ARE HIV-INFECTED

The legal system traditionally has been reluctant to challenge the professional autonomy of physicians by removing or altering their choice of medical decisions. In this light, neither the courts, legislatures, nor public health agencies have produced clear, binding rules for the treatment of HIV-positive health care workers (HCWs). The legal developments of the last several years return the question of HIV-infected HCWs to the HCWs themselves, to the institutions that employ them, and therefore to the colleagues and professional organizations with whom HIV-infected HCWs are associated.

What Is the Medical Profession Doing with This Authority Relative to HIV Infection/AIDS?

Individual HCWs have evidently concluded that they should keep their infections secret for as long as possible, while **many institutions seem to have adopted a "don't ask, don't tell" policy**. When a HCW's HIV infection is discovered, most institutions evaluate the worker under applicable guidelines and negotiate a mutually acceptable course of action, all in strict confidence. Few institutions go public; in some cases the HCW has no option but to sue (Burris, 1996).

---

tus and how they can keep it low. Many hundreds of millions of dollars have been spent to inform the public of the kinds of behavior that either place them at risk or reduce their risk for HIV infection. The problem is that although people are getting the information, too many refuse to act on it. Former Surgeon General C. Everett Koop's office mailed 107 million copies of the brochure "Understanding AIDS" to households in the United States. Fifty-one percent of those who received it said they never read it. But even among those who read the brochure, are those who refuse to change their sexual behavior. Old habits are difficult to break.

To date, the hard evidence shows that only the homosexual population has significantly modified their sexual behavior as evidenced by the drop in the number of new cases of AIDS among them from 1988 through 1997.

A major problem looming on the horizon is the prospect of HIV being spread in the teenage population. Large numbers of teens use drugs and alcohol, have multiple sex partners, and believe they are invulnerable to infection.

The AMA stated in 1988 that physicians may not refuse to care for patients with AIDS because of actual risk or fear of contracting the disease. Some physicians get around this through referral to other physicians who will treat AIDS patients. There is one area of medicine that takes issue at having to treat AIDS patients. That area is surgery. Because it is difficult not to accidently get cut during surgery, surgeons have been the leading advocates for HIV testing of all surgical patients so they will know their risks before performing surgery.

On the other hand, patients feel they have a right to know if their physician, especially a surgeon, is HIV-infected. Surveys indicate that most people would not want to be treated by an HIV-infected physician.

REVIEW QUESTIONS

(Answers to the Review Questions are on page 580.)

1. Name three major sources of information that contributed to the early panic and hysteria about the spread of AIDS.

2. Give three examples of unfounded public fears to AIDS infection.

3. Fear of the casual transmission of AIDS parallels what other earlier STD epidemic?

4. What evidence is there that it is difficult to get people to change their behavior even though they know it is harmful to their well being?

5. What is the major thrust of AIDS education in the United States?

6. If education is the key to preventing HIV infection and new cases of AIDS; and most people interviewed say they have been 'educated,' why is it not working?

7. Why are today's teenagers in danger of contracting and spreading HIV?

8. Yes or No: Do physicians have a right to refuse to treat AIDS patients? Support your answer.

9. Do patients have a right to know if their physician is HIV-infected or has AIDS?

10. What is the primary means of offsetting the bias toward people with AIDS in the workplace?

REFERENCES

American Medical Association News. (1991). Ruling fuels debate over HIV-infected doctors. May:1,41–43.

AOUN, HACIB. (1990). A handful helped us. *Medical Doctor,* 34:31–32.

BLENDON, R.J., et al. (1988). Discrimination against people with AIDS: The public's perspective. *N. Engl. J. Med.,* 319:1022–1026.

BREO, DENNIS L. (1990). The slippery slope—handling HIV-infected health care workers. *JAMA,* 264:1464–1466.

BURRIS, SCOTT. (1996). Human immunodeficiency virus-infected health care workers. *Arch. Fam. Med.,* 5:102–106.

CRAVEN, DONALD, et al. (1994). Factitious HIV Infection. *Ann. Intern. Med.,* 121:763–766.

DANIELS, NORMAN. (1992). HIV-infected professionals, patient rights and the 'switching dilemma'. *JAMA,* 267:1368–1371.

DRISCOLL, CHARLES E. (1990). AIDS: Issues for every woman and her physician. *Female Patient,* 15:11–12.

EICKHOFF, THEODORE C. (1989). Public perceptions about AIDS and HIV infection. *Infect. Dis. News,* 2:6.

FISHER, J.D., et al. (1992). Changing AIDS risk behavior. *Psychol. Bull.,* 111:455–474.

FOURNIER, A.M., et al. (1989). Preoperative screening for HIV infection. *Arch. Surg.,* 124: 1038–1040.

FULTON, ROBERT, et al. (1988). AIDS: Seventh rank absolute. In *AIDS: Principles, Practices and Politics.,* Inge B. Corliss, et al., eds. Bristol, PA: Hemisphere.

GERBERT, BARBARA, et al. (1988). Why fear persists: Health care professionals and AIDS. *JAMA,* 260:3481–3483.

HAGEN, M.D., et al. (1988). Routine preoperative screening for HIV: Does the risk to the surgeon outweigh the risk to the patient? *JAMA,* 259:1357–1359.

HEGARTY, JAMES D., et al. (1988). The medical care costs of HIV-infected children in Harlem. *JAMA,* 260:1901–1909.

HEREK, GREGORY M., et al. (1993). Public reaction to AIDS in the United States: A second decade of stigma. *Am. J. Public Health,* 83:574–577.

JAPENGA, ANN. (1992). The secret. *Health,* 6:43–52.

KEGELES, S.M., et al. (1988). Sexually active adolescents and condoms: Changes over one year in knowledge, attitudes and use. *Am. J. Public Health,* 78:460–461.

KINDIG, DAVID, et al. (1994). How will graduate medical education reform affect specialties and geographic areas? *JAMA,* 272:37–42.

KIRBY, D. (1988). The effectiveness of educational programs to help prevent school-age youth from contracting AIDS: A review of relevant research. United States Congress.

LEFKOWITZ, MATHEW. (1990). A health care system in crisis: The possible restriction against HIV-infected health care workers. *PAACNOTES,* 2:175–176.

LEWIS, C.E., et al. (1992). Primary care physicians' refusal to care for patients infected with HIV. *West. J. Med.,* 156:36–38.

LINK, R. NATHAN et al. (1988). Concerns of medical and pediatric house officers about acquiring AIDS from their patients. *Am. J. Public Health,* 78:455–459.

LO, BERNARD et al. (1992). Health care workers infected with HIV. *JAMA,* 267:1100–1105.

MANDELBAUM-SCHMID, JUDITH. (1990). AIDS and MDs. *Medical Doctor,* 34:33–40.

MCNEILL, WILLIAM H. (1976). *Plagues and People,* Garden City: Anchor Press.

MICHAELS, DAVID, et al. (1992). Estimates of the number of youth orphaned by AIDS in the United States. *JAMA,* 268:3456–3461.

Morbidity and Mortality Weekly Report. (1990). HIV-related knowledge and behavior among high shool students—Selected U.S. cities, 1989. 39: 385–396.

NARY, GORDON. (1990). An editorial. *PAACNOTES,* 2:170.

PHILLIPS, KATHRYN A. (1993). Subjective knowledge of AIDS and Use of HIV testing. *Am. J. Public Health,* 83:1460–1462.

POLDER, JACQUELYN A., et al. (1989). AIDS precautions for your office. *Patient Care,* 23:161–171.

POWELL, JOHN H. (1965). *Bring Out Your Dead.* New York: Time-Life Inc.

RHAME, FRANK S., et al. (1989). The case for wider use of testing for HIV infection. *N. Engl. J. Med.,* 320:1242–1254.

ROWE, MONA, et al. (1987). *A Public Health Challenge: State Issues, Policies and Programs, Volume 2.* Intergrovernmental Health Policy Project, George Washington University.

STRYKER, JEFF, et al. (1995). Prevention of HIV infection *JAMA,* 273:1143–1148.

VOELKER, REBECCA. (1989). No uniform policy among states on HIV/AIDS education. *Am. Med. News,* Sept.:3,28–29.

ZUGER, ABIGAIL. (1995). The high cost of living. *Sci. Am.* 273:108.

The AIDS Industry: Economics of HIV/AIDS

CHAPTER CONCEPTS

♦ There is an AIDS industry.

♦ The medical cost of treating AIDS patients is in the billions of dollars.

♦ The direct or true costs for HIV disease and AIDS.

♦ The indirect costs for HIV disease and AIDS.

♦ The costs for AIDS research, education, and prevention.

♦ Public backlash to the high cost of the AIDS industry.

♦ Hospital space available for AIDS patients.

♦ Thirty-seven million people in the United States do not have health care insurance.

♦ Commercial health care insurers are leery of writing policies for HIV-infected people.

♦ Commercial life insurance carriers want to test for HIV infection before writing a policy.

♦ Funeral directors charge higher rates for burying the AIDS-related dead.

WORLDWIDE ECONOMIC FORECAST-YEAR 2000

HIV disease and AIDS are producing a global economic challenge. According to Jennifer Oldham, by the year 2000, the total cost to the global economy of the HIV/AIDS pandemic could reach $514 billion and, in the worst-case scenario, rob the world of 1.9% of its gross domestic product—the equivalent of wiping out the economy of Australia. In addition to the tremendous cost of health care, HIV disease and AIDS is directly affecting business around the world. The majority of cases strike adults in their most productive years, the early twenties to late forties. Gross domestic product (GDP, previously called gross national product or GNP) losses due to AIDS cases by the year 2000 worldwide can be seen in Table 16-1. Worldwide, the GDP may experience a 2%

TABLE 16-1 Global Loss of Gross Domestic Product Because of AIDS by Year 2000

Maximum	Loss in GDP (%)[a]	
	Countries	Minimum
United States	0.9	1.1
Canada	0.8	1.0
Africa, Middle East	2.4	4.6
Southeast Asia	1.7	2.3
Japan	0.7	0.8
Latin America	0.8	1.4
Europe	0.8	1.0
Rest of the world	1.8	3.1

Percent of GDP loss is based on projected low and high numbers of AIDS cases.

[a] In 1994, the term gross national product or GNP was changed to gross domestic product or GDP.

(Source: Jennifer Oldham, 1995)

TABLE 16-2 Forecasting Medical Care Costs for People with HIV Disease and AIDS, United States, 1991–2000

Year	Costs in Billions
1991	5.8
1992	7.0
1993	8.5
1994	10.3
1995	12.5
1996	15.1
1997	18.1
1998	21.8
1999	26.3
2000	31.7
Total	157.1

Costs calculated from data provided by Fred Hellinger (1991–1993). Average cost/year of treating an adult person with HIV disease, $5,150. Average cost/year of treating a person with AIDS, $32,000. Lifetime cost for medical care for an AIDS patient, $85,333. Adult costs from HIV infection until death, $119,000.

The costs of care of an adult AIDS patient during the last 6 months of life increase dramatically to $9,098 a month, five times the cost of care for less severely ill people with AIDS. Even though more patients are choosing to die at home, the medical costs do not change.

The annual costs of care for an HIV-infected child without an AIDS diagnosis is $9,382. The annual cost of medical care for a child with AIDS is $37,928.

(Source: Agency for Health Care Policy and Research, July/August, 1995)

drop, while Africa and the Middle East may lose 4% to 5% of their GDP! The medical care costs for people with HIV disease and AIDS in the United States from 1991 through the year 2000 can be seen in Table 16-2.

Cost of AIDS in the United States vs. Developing Countries

The cost of AIDS to developing countries such as in Africa is not measurable on the same scale used in the United States. The cost of treating 100 patients with AIDS in the United States is greater than the entire health budget of the majority of sub-Saharan African countries (Tables 16-3 and 16-4). The cost of treating an AIDS patient until death in Africa has been estimated to be $150–$400 compared with an average per capita expenditure on health of $15. In some of these countries, AIDS treatment may be the equivalent of up to 4% of the gross domestic product, which is already in a state of decline in many countries as a result of the ravages of drought and war. Aggravating the economic plight even further is the greater likelihood for the virus to infect preferentially the educated and economically more productive young men in the community, those with greater disposable incomes who are able to pursue more active sexual lifestyles. Involvement of women has similar devastating economic implications as they form the bulk of the agricultural workforce on which

many African economies are so dependent. The growing problem of AIDS orphans in Africa, currently estimated to be over 2 million but projected to exceed 10 million by the year 2000, will be responsible for an even greater load on the existing health care and further reduce available human resources for agriculture and other economic developments.

DREADFUL DUALITY

The United States and other developed nations have vast sums of money with which to pursue costly and sophisticated drug therapies (see Chapter 4). Clearly, poor countries, such as Africa, where over 90% of new HIV infections now occur, **cannot** afford these new or even the older drugs. As Peter Piot, head of the United Nations Program on AIDS (UNAIDS) noted, current drugs that now cost

TABLE 16-3 Annual Direct Costs of HIV/AIDS Related to T4 Cell Counts

T4 Cell Count/μL Blood[a]	United States Dollars[b] (/month)
Over 500	1,934 (161)
499–200	6,015 (501)
199–50	9,031 (753)
Less than 50	25,239 (2,103)

[a] Much of the cost of treating HIV infection is concentrated in the period immediately preceding death due to the intensity of services used throughout the terminal period.

[b] Resource use costs were derived from the published literature, insurance database, Medicare fee schedules, surveys, and the Physician Panel.

(Source: Gable et al., 1996)

TABLE 16-4 Annual Direct Costs of the More Common Opportunistic Diseases

Disease	United States Dollars
Esophageal candidiasis (yeast)	2,194
Tuberculosis (TB)	2,924
Cryptococcal meningitis (CM)	17,264
Toxoplasmosis	17,631
Mycobacterium avium complex (MAC)	20,153
Non-Hodgkin's lymphoma (cancer)	22,329
Wasting syndrome (weight loss)	26,676
Central nervous system lymphoma (cancer)	27,333
Pneumocystis carinii pneumonia (PCP)	
Mild	3,545
Moderate	4,889
Severe	32,609
Kaposi's sarcoma (KS)	
Mild/moderate	5,902
Severe	10,744
Cytomegalovirus (CMV) retinitis (blindness)	100,337

Based on 1995 dollars. Resource use costs were derived from the published literature, insurance database, Medicare fee schedules, surveys, and the Physician Panel.

(Source: Gable et al., 1996)

$20,000 a year per HIV-infected or AIDS person, in the developing nations, even if brought down to $5,000/year/person would still be out of reach for about 90% of the world's HIV-infected population. Also noteworthy is that even at $5,000/person/year for current drug therapy, for 1998, it would cost about $132 billion/year to treat the 26,400,000 people living with HIV worldwide! It appears that the economic impact of HIV disease and AIDS will become as serious as the pandemic itself.

NATIONAL HEALTH CARE SPENDING: UNITED STATES, 1993–1998

Health care spending in the United States will top $1 trillion, 400 billion in 1998. This figure represents about $5,000 for every man, woman, and child. This exceeds any other country's spending on health care, either per capita or as a percentage of gross domestic product. It costs about $75 billion a year just to treat the infectious diseases. And this item is increasing by $3 billion to $6 billion a year (Perkin, 1993).

Former Health and Human Services secretary Louis Sullivan said in 1991 that health care costs were growing at an unsustainable rate and that something had to be done (Packer, 1991).

In 1998, Americans will spend about $4 billion a day on medical care. That is twice what they spent 6 years ago. For the federal government, **medical care** has become the fastest growing item in the budget, increasing at about 6% annually. Health care spending is expected to rise by at least 6% annually through the year 2000. For corporate America, health care has become a crippling expense. General Motors paid out $3.2 billion in 1990—more than it spent on steel—to provide medical coverage for 1.9 million employees, dependents, and retirees. Unchecked, the cost of medical care will reach $2 trillion in the next 10 years, crowding out spending for other needs.

Medicaid

Medicaid is a form of combined federal and state financing of health care for the **disadvantaged.** Within certain broad federally determined guidelines, states decide who is eligible; the amount, duration, and scope of services covered; rates of payment for providers; and methods of administering the program. Medicaid provides health care services for certain low-income persons. Medicaid does not provide health services to all poor people in every state. It categorically covers participants in the

FINANCIAL HELP FOR THOSE WITH SYMPTOMATIC HIV DISEASE OR AIDS

Financial problems can be one of the most stressful aspects of living with symptomatic HIV disease or AIDS.

Several government entitlement programs are available to people with symptomatic HIV disease or AIDS. The rules and regulations for applying may seem overwhelming, but once you have a basic understanding of the programs you can make the system work for you. It is important to seek advice and information so that you will receive the maximum benefits available.

The best time to plan for disability and other entitlement programs is before you leave work. Although you cannot apply for benefits until you have stopped working, **start to educate yourself now.**

Available benefit programs are:

State Disability
Social Security Disability (SSD)
Supplemental Security Income (SSI)
Income Support (IS)
Medicaid
Food Stamps
Division of AIDS Services (DAS)

State Disability

State Disability is generally a short-term benefit for people who have left, or must leave, their jobs due to illness or disability. If you are currently working but need to leave your job because of your health, or if you have recently left your job, or if you are receiving Unemployment Insurance Benefits, you may qualify for benefits from your state. Contact your state agency for information or application deadlines and potential benefits.

Social Security Disability (SSD)

SSD pays monthly checks to people who have worked and paid into the Social Security program and are now disabled. If you have worked on the books or paid FICA taxes most of your working life, you can apply for SSD. You can apply at the same time you apply for state disability benefits.

Deadline for Applying—There is no filing deadline for SSD. Try to file within 6 months after you become disabled. The easiest way to file for SSD is to apply by phone using the SSA Teleclaim number, (800) 772-1213.

It is very important that you indicate on your application the very first date you were unable to work because of your HIV-related illness. Even if your employer paid you after this date, your eligibility begins the first day you physically could not work or your normal work pattern became disrupted. Social Security will then base the 5-month waiting period on that date rather than on the date you stopped working or receiving a salary.

Required Documents—These include: a certified birth certificate; Green Card or Naturalization Papers; W-2 forms or tax statements from last 2 years you filed taxes; Social Security Card; and last (most recent) paycheck stub.

Benefits—Your SSD benefits are determined by a formula based on the amount of money you paid in FICA taxes during certain periods of on-the-books work. If you receive SSD payments for more than 2 years, you automatically become eligible for Medicare benefits. If your application is denied, or your benefit amount is lower than you think it should be, you can appeal. Once you receive your award letter stating when your checks will begin and how much you will receive, you may be eligible for Food Stamps, the Medicaid Surplus Spend-Down Program, or benefits from the Division of AIDS Services.

Supplemental Security Income (SSI)

SSI is a federal program run by Social Security. It pays monthly checks to people who are disabled and have few assets and low income. If you do not have more money and/or assets than allowed, you can apply for SSI benefits at the same time you apply for SSD benefits. Even if you do not qualify for SSD benefits, you may qualify for SSI. If you are married or live with your family, the allowances are different.

Deadline for Applying—There is no deadline, but the sooner you file a claim the better. SSI claims are based on the date you file—your "protective filing date." This date affects the amount of money you will get. Be well informed before filing in order to get the maximum benefits to which you are entitled.

The easiest way to file for SSI is to apply by phone using the SSA Teleclaim number, (800) 772-1213. Later, you will receive a computer printout confirming your application and the assets you reported. You will sign this paper verifying it is correct.

Required Documents—These include: all of those documents described under Social Security Disability and original copies of your three most recent checking/banking statements; all passbooks of any savings accounts you own or share; original copy of your apartment lease or a letter from your roommate; diagnosis letter from your doctor; rent receipt or canceled check; and electric and other utility bills.

Benefits—You will receive money, medical benefits, and possibly Food Stamps. The amount of money you get is based on your living arrangements and other sources of monthly income. The maximum benefit paid in 1993 was $520 per month for a single person in New York State. You will automatically get Medicaid benefits without applying for them separately. You will be eligible for Food Stamps, but you must send in a separate application for them. You may also be eligible for money from the Division of AIDS Services.

SSI benefits will continue for as long as you are disabled and your assets remain below the allowance listed. SSI benefits will stop when SSD or other benefits begin (if these benefits are higher than your SSI award). Your SSI benefits may also be adjusted to account for any other benefits you receive. Benefits are paid monthly.

Income Support (IS)

Also called "Public Assistance" or "Welfare," Income Support is issued as an intermediary program for individuals who have no other source of income and who have applied for SSI and/or SSD. You may also be eligible if you owe back rent and are facing possible eviction. Most often, your IS benefit will continue only until SSI/SSD starts.

Required Documents—These include: all those documents described under SSD and SSI, plus any SSI, SSD, or other benefit award letter you may have.

Benefits—Income support creates a monthly budget—usually $354 for a single person—plus a Medicaid card and $60–$80 in Food Stamps. Of this amount, $215 is considered as a rent allotment; the remaining $139 is for utilities and other expenses.

As a person with symptomatic HIV or AIDS, you may be eligible for an "enhanced shelter allowance." Instead of the standard $215 for rent, you may be able to get up to $480 for rent from IS.

Medicaid

Medicaid is a program that pays medical bills for eligible individuals and families who cannot afford medical care. Medicaid pays for hospital inpatient and outpatient services, laboratory tests and X-rays, some physician's services, home nursing services, and private health insurance premiums.

You can obtain Medicaid in any of three ways: (**1**) A hospital may arrange for it; (**2**) you get it automatically with SSI or Income Support; or (**3**) you can apply directly for Medicaid.

Medicaid is a complex program. As with other benefit programs, educating yourself in advance will save much time and energy.

Required Documents—These include: a birth certificate or other proof of age; 8 weeks of wage stubs (if you were/are working); Social Security card; documentation of your income from SSI, VA, retirement funds, etc.; insurance policies (especially health insurance; three recent bank statements/savings account passbook; lease, letter from landlord, rent receipt, or canceled check; heat/utility receipt.

Eligibility—You are probably eligible if your maximum assets (money and property) do not exceed: (**1**) your home (primary residence only, not a second or vacation home); (**2**) your automobile (if valued at under $4,500); (**3**) your clothing, personal effects, furniture, and appliances; (**4**) home, term, group, or other insurance with no face (cash) value; (**5**) a burial fund not exceeding $1,500.

(*continued*)

—————— **POINT OF INFORMATION 16.2** ——————

BEHAVIORS ARE EXPENSIVE

Drug and alcohol abuse, smoking, failure to use seat belts, unsafe sex, and sharing contaminated needles are all behaviors that account for more than one-fourth of the billions of dollars that Americans spend on health care each year. It is estimated that over $250 billion of the dollars spent on health care in this country is attributable to unhealthy lifestyles (Health Insurance Association of America, 1994, updated).

AID to Families with Dependent Children program and in the Supplemental Security Income program. In most states it also covers certain other people deemed to be medically needy. The program was authorized in 1965 by Title XIX of the Social Security Act (Figure 16-1).

As increasing numbers of people infected with HIV exhaust their private insurance, lose their insurance, or become reliant on Medicaid, the problem of financing their health care becomes a pressing public policy issue. The 1997 federal Medicaid budget was $104 billion, and for 1996 it accounted for 60% of all AIDS care.

Obstacles to Medicaid Funding— An obstacle to medical care for persons with HIV disease and AIDS who qualify for Medicaid is the low reimbursement rate. Stunning examples of Medicaid physician compensation rates far below those by private insurance or Medicare were presented during a recent commission hearing. For example, a new patient intermediate office visit in New York City is compensated by Blue Cross at $78, by Medicare at $80, and by Medicaid at $7. One witness indicated that physicians in New York with large AIDS practices were reluctant to refer Medicaid patients for specialty consultations because of low levels of reimbursement—levels so low that several physicians said that the few dollars at stake per office visit were not worth the time and paperwork to bill the Medicaid program. Overall, however, Medicaid pays for the health care of at least 40% of all adult/adolescents with AIDS and 90% of all pediatric AIDS cases (Kent, 1995). But AIDS patients represent less than 1% of Medicaid beneficiaries. The estimated combined federal and state Medicaid expenditures for people with HIV and AIDS will be $4.5 billion in FY 1998; it was $4 billion for 1997, $3.5 billion in 1996, and $3 billion in 1995 (Medicaid and AIDS and HIV, HCFA, October 1995; Medicaid's Role for Persons with HIV/AIDS, The Kaiser Commission on the Future of Medicaid, 1995, updated).

Twenty-nine percent of AIDS patients are **uninsured** and those with private health insurance often have limited benefits or high out-of-pocket costs (Levi, 1994). While it is clear that some type of health reform will occur in 1998/1999, how well this reform plan will address the medical problems of people with HIV disease and AIDS is presently unknown.

Percentage of Americans Who Receive Medicaid or Do Not Have Health Insurance

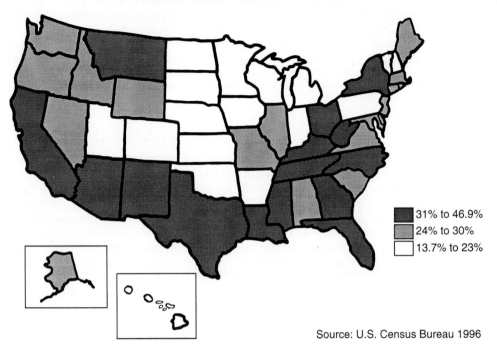

31% to 46.9%
24% to 30%
13.7% to 23%

Source: U.S. Census Bureau 1996

FIGURE 16-1   Health Care Costs. For 1996, in spite of Americans spending 13.7% of the Gross National Product, or over $1 trillion on health care, millions of Americans depend on Medicaid because they can not afford health insurance!

Medicare

This is a nationwide health insurance program providing health insurance protection to people 65 years of age and over, people entitled to social security disability payments for 2 years or more, and people with end-stage renal disease, regardless of income. The program was enacted July 30, 1965, as Title XVIII, Health Insurance for the Aged of the Social Security Act, and became effective on July 1, 1966. It consists of two separate but coordinated programs, hospital insurance (Part A) and supplementary medical insurance (Part B). Beginning 1997, there were 38 million people in the United States on Medicare. For 1996, Medicare accounted for about 13% of all AIDS care. In 1997, this $189 billion program which started out in 1965 with a budget of $5 billion was designed to provide medical care for those 65 and older and some people in exceptional medical categories. **But the program gives the same benefits to those who are well-off as to the poor.** Although the elderly do pay some of the costs, nearly 90% of Medicare funds come from income taxes. As a result, the burden falls partly on working people who often have no health insurance of their own.

The burden on younger Americans continues to increase as the population ages, bringing with it the responsibility of caring for millions of elderly with expensive medical needs. **There are now about seven Americans under the age of 65 for every person over, compared with 11 to one in 1960.** And one of those seven is unemployed and two are children. That leaves about four workers to support each elderly American. And one of them does not have his or her own health insurance (Castro, 1991).

Medicare AIDS Expenditures—It is estimated that Medicare will spend approximately $880 million in federal funds during FY 1998 for direct medical care for people diagnosed with AIDS. In 1996, $690 million was spent on people diagnosed with AIDS (Medicaid and AIDS and HIV, HCFA, October 1995, updated).

HEALTH CARE INDUSTRY

As a disease increases in incidence, it demands greater expenditures for research, testing, education, and setting up a network of health care services to meet the needs of patients. In other words, a disease over time gives rise to its own medical industry. There are health care industries that focus on the brain (psychiatric disorders), cardiovascular disease (heart), and bone and eye diseases. The largest health care industries are those that deal with cancer and infectious diseases. **NOW THERE IS THE AIDS INDUSTRY**.

Financing the AIDS Industry

Federal—In 1990, the United States Congress did something quite rare: **it allocated money specifically for the treatment of one disease—HIV/AIDS.**

In some ways the increased commitment of federal and state government to cancer research and treatment in the early 1970s is similar to what has happened in the war on AIDS in the 1980s. In both decades, there was a major funding surge to stimulate research, therapy, and prevention. A major difference, however, is that dollars for cancer came more slowly over a longer time period that began well before the 1970s. With AIDS, federal funding began in 1981 (Figure 16-2) and has increased at an unprecedented rate.

During the 16 years from 1982 to 1998, federal spending on AIDS-related projects increased from $8 million in 1982 to $6.2 billion in 1994, and $8 billion for 1997, and is estimated to be $9 billion for 1998. Ending 1996, the Presidential Advisory Council on HIV/AIDS provided the President with six AIDS goals that will be funded with the $8.04 billion 1997 federal budget for AIDS. The goals are to:

(1) develop a cure; (2) reduce/eliminate new infections; (3) guarantee care/service for the HIV-infected; (4) fight against HIV/AIDS discrimination; (5) quickly translate scientific advances into improved care/prevention; and (6) provide support for international AIDS efforts. Figure 16-3 demonstrates the 1998 allocation of federal dollars for AIDS and non-AIDS programs within just three of the federal agencies allocating AIDS dollars: the Centers for Disease Control and Prevention (CDC), the National Institute of Allergy and Infectious Disease (NIAID), and the National Institute on Drug Abuse (NIDA).

In 1989, the federal government spent $1.3 billion, or about 33% of total dollars spent, on AIDS-related projects. The other 67%, or $3.9 billion, came from the private sectors. In 1990, $2 billion was allocated by the federal government for AIDS projects. In 1992, the federal government spent $4.5 billion, in 1993, $4.9 billion, in 1994 $6.2 billion, and for Fiscal Year 1997 $8 billion (Figure 16-2). In addition, the private sector also spends about $4 billion a year. By the end of 1997, the federal government spent over $50 billion for HIV/AIDS-related work, and the private sector spent, from 1990 through 1997, $30 billion. In reality, adding in unspecified federal dollars that went to AIDS-related projects and the dollars spent in the private sector prior to 1990 would most likely bring the total AIDS-related expenditures to **$100 billion. If not, it will certainly exceed this number by the end of 1998!** Through 1997, only two states, Wyoming and West Virginia, provided **no** state funding for HIV/AIDS programs. Both states rely 100% on federal government funding for all HIV/AIDS programs.

AIDS Costs as a Percentage of the National Health Care Budget Placed in Perspective

The $9 billion estimated for 1998 represents about 1% of the $1.4 trillion federal health care budget. For any given year the total expenditures for HIV/AIDS is less than 2% of the U. S. health care budget. To place health care and AIDS expenditures in perspective, in 1989 the federal government allocated $159

——— BOX 16.1 ———

AIDS INDUSTRY SPIN-OFFS

1. Sale of "AIDS-Free" Certificates

In Jacksonville, Florida, an entrepreneur promoted a service that would have allowed patients to know the names of doctors and dentists who have tested AIDS-free. Many medical community leaders thought the service would promote hysteria.

The president of Jacksonville-based National Free of AIDS Identification Service said he was going to recruit doctors, dentists, and other health care professionals for HIV testing (1991). His plan was that those who paid the $189 fee and who tested HIV-negative would be issued "Free of AIDS" certificates.

Prospective patients will be able to call the service's 24-hour information line and, for a $2 fee, get a list of doctors and dentists who have received the certificate.

List the major problems involved with this enterprise: biological (e.g., how might this list promote/prevent HIV transmission?) and the moral-social aspects. Is the idea based on good biology?

2. Clothier's Exploitation of the HIV/AIDS Pandemic

An apparel maker shrugged off complaints of exploitation and said it was having no problem finding U.S. magazines for a new advertisement that shows a person dying of AIDS and his grieving family. The trendy fashion concern is pinning its United Colors logo on previously published news photographs. The advertisement appeared in issues of *Vogue, Vanity Fair, Interview, Details, Elle, Mademoiselle, Us,* and *Spin* magazines.

3. Investors Promised Profits from AIDS Patient Insurance Policies

Investors around the country are invited to buy the life insurance policies of AIDS patients—and the sooner the patient dies, the better for the investor, who then collects the insurance.

Newspaper, wire, and staff reports that one company is giving would-be investors a patient list to help them pick people who will die soon. The list predicts how many months each patient is supposed to live, based on the health of their immune system, and the amount of insurance they have.

In a nutshell, the companies line up investors to buy the insurance policies of the dying, typically at a 33% discount from face value, and pay the premiums until the insured dies. Then the investor collects the money. The promotion is as follows: A non-HIV/AIDS persons takes out, for example, a $100,000 policy. He or she is later diagnosed with AIDS. An investor may be able to buy that person's policy for, say, $65,000, most of which is used to pay for the person's medical expenses. After death, the investor, who became the beneficiary of the policy, collects the $100,000 for a net profit of $35,000. AIDS persons and potential investors are urged to contact their state insurance commissioner's office to be certain that this activity is legal.

4. Sale of AIDS-related Products

A few companies have begun to sell AIDS-related products of questionable taste. For example, one AIDS promotional kit reads: "RED RIBBONS ARE NOT ENOUGH!" And then it proceeds with an attempt to sell name tags or dog tags—"polished silverstone, military-style dog tags, inscribed with 'ALWAYS REMEMBER,' " and the name of a lost loved one. Cost $25. It continues, "Red ribbons offer **no monetary donations to the fight against AIDS.** With a *Remembrance Tag,* you can remember the one you love while contributing to the defeat of the virus."

A second promotional package, for $25, describes a Director's Handbook that teaches one how to make a memorial videotape of oneself. It provides questions that "you don't want to forget to answer." It provides a format for telling your personal history. It also says, "Be remembered as *you* want to be remembered.

A third company offers a video package for mothers. "Leave a message for your children." (Cost not given)

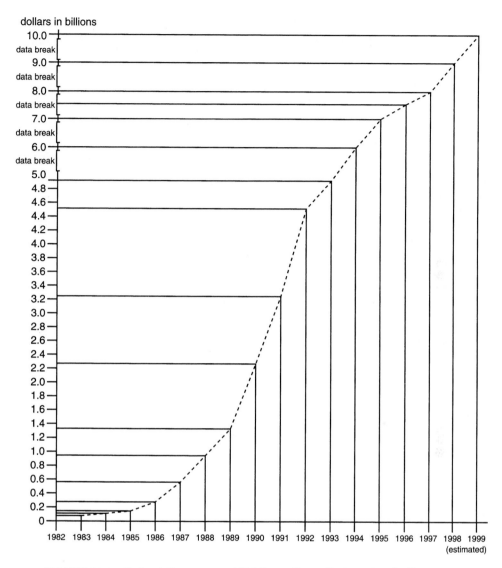

FIGURE 16-2 Federal Government AIDS Expenditures Projected to the Year 1998. Note that the sharp rise in monies spent on AIDS-related projects by the Public Health Services, 1998 and 1999, are estimated. Federal expenditures were $1.3 billion in 1989, $4.5 billion in 1992, $5.3 billion in 1993, $6.3 billion in 1994, $7.1 billion for 1995, $7.5 billion in 1996, and $8 billion in 1997, and are estimated to reach $9 billion in 1998 and $10 billion in 1999.

billion to "bail out" the savings and loan industry over the next 10 years; however, along the way through 1994, another $7 billion was added. It is estimated that $500 billion will be needed over the next 40 years. In 1989, the Department of Energy estimated it would take $128 billion to clean up nuclear weapons plants. But in 1994, it was estimated that it will take 30 years and over $300 billion. In 1995 it was estimated that the cost to clean up nuclear waste dumps across the United States would be $1 trillion (*Nature*, 1995). The government

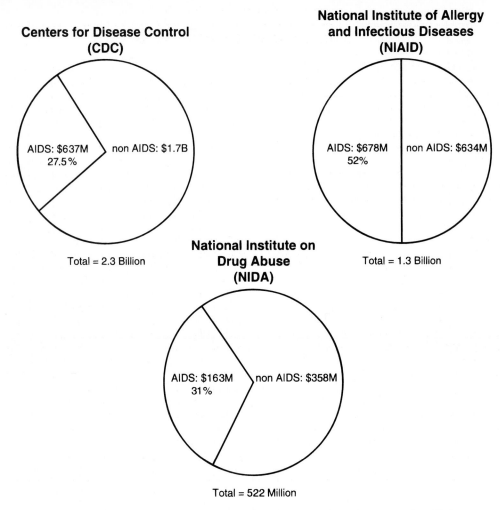

Centers for Disease Control (CDC)

AIDS: $637M
27.5%

non AIDS: $1.7B

Total = 2.3 Billion

National Institute of Allergy and Infectious Diseases (NIAID)

AIDS: $678M
52%

non AIDS: $634M

Total = 1.3 Billion

National Institute on Drug Abuse (NIDA)

AIDS: $163M
31%

non AIDS: $358M

Total = 522 Million

FIGURE 16-3 Three Major Federal Health Agency Budgets for 1998. The CDC receives its own separate budget while the NIAID and NIDA receive their funding from the Department of Health and Human Services.

spends about $300 billion annually on its military machine.

Costs Related to Care—Right now, there is one HIV-related death about every 12 minutes in the United States (estimated: over 450,000 deaths through December 31, 1998). These data raise questions as to whether more money invested in AIDS research will slow the death rate and whether the money already spent was spent effectively. Timothy Murphy (1991) wrote that all the money spent so far on the HIV epidemic has not ensured adequate medical care for all people with HIV-related conditions. This is especially true for the poor and homeless. Neither have the dollars spent on HIV research produced a cure. Treatments with nucleoside analogs (ZDV, ddI, ddC, d4T, and 3TC) have proved ineffective for long-term care and there are still many unresolved questions about their short-term use. (See Chapter 4 for a discussion on the effectiveness of nucleoside analogs and other drug treatments.)

———————— BOX 16.2 ————————

THE COST FOR TREATING HEMOPHILIA—UNITED STATES

Before the blood supply in the United States became contaminated with HIV, the **cost per unit** of **blood factor VIII** was about 12 cents. The new technologies that are needed to establish and maintain a safe supply of factor VIII drove the price so high that it is jeopardizing the lives of patients. While some hemophiliacs are covered by private health insurance, many are not. Those who must depend on Medicaid and other state-supported programs are often forced to limit family income to maintain their eligibility, and it is not unheard of for husbands and wives to divorce in order to meet the requirements for this kind of aid.

In 1992, the television program "60 Minutes" interviewed people who had children with hemophilia. The cost of treatment was staggering—it may run as high as $200,000/year/child.

In order to stop a bleeding episode, hemophiliacs need an injection of a blood clotting factor (factor VIII). Clotting factor is isolated out of the blood of donors, concentrated, and sold. A batch of clotting factor may be separated out from the donated blood of 20,000 or more people. It is estimated that up to 50% of the 20,000 individuals affected by inherited bleeding disorders who used blood component therapy prior to 1985 are infected with HIV. In 1989, AIDS replaced hemorrhage, central nervous system (CNS) bleeding, and liver disease as the leading cause of death among hemophiliacs.

The reporter interviewed one family who had a 13-year-old son who was hemophilic. His condition was discovered at age 3, at a time prior to recognizing that much of the blood supply in the United States was contaminated with HIV. Somewhere along the way, he was injected with HIV-contaminated clotting factor. He now has AIDS.

The parents of this young man said that their expenses for HIV/AIDS therapy were between $45,000 and $50,000 a year. But that was small compared to the cost of the clotting factor. In April 1992, just 1 month, his bill for clotting factor came to $24,000. One vial of clotting factor, enough for one infusion, cost $1,000. Their son, in one episode, used two vials per day for 10 days. This family has been trying to pay bills like this for the past 5 years. Friends help with food and mortgage payments, but they owe too much to pay the 20 to 30 medical bills coming in each month. Because of their financial burden, the parents have considered divorce. This would allow their son to receive free medical benefits under Medicaid, and Social Security benefits.

The reporter interviewed a second family with a similar story: cost of clotting factor, $200,000/year and about $50,000 for AIDS treatment. In this case the husband and wife divorced so the son could receive the medical benefits.

Update 1997—Biotechnology has produced a recombinant factor VIII and it is currently being evaluated in patients. If acceptable, the price of factor VIII should drop significantly!

AIDS Expenditures Compared to Other Major Diseases

Federal spending for AIDS research, educational programs, counselor training, testing, and prevention programs has been compared with federal spending for other diseases (Table 16-5). There is a discrepancy between the total federal dollars spent on certain diseases and the number of deaths they cause. In 1997, with about 40,000 deaths, HIV/AIDS received $8 billion. That's equivalent to **$200,000** per AIDS-related death! In 1997, cancer caused about 560,000 deaths (about 1,500 people/day) and received $2.3 billion or about $4,100/death. During the same time, there were 1,170,000 new cases of cancer in the United States; 183,000 were new cases of breast cancer and there were over 46,000 breast cancer-associated deaths. One in seven to nine women will get breast cancer. Heart disease, which caused some 950,000 deaths in 1997 (43% of all deaths for the year), received less than $1 billion or about $1,000/death. Some 2 million Americans require insulin injections for type I diabetes and perhaps as many as 10 to 12 million have type II diabetes (diet controlled). Diabetes, a severe progressive disorder, received $315 million, or about 4% of the AIDS budget in 1997 or about $1,200/death. It is estimated that 260,000 people will die because of diabetes complications. Stroke, which affects millions of Americans and

TABLE 16-5 Federal Monies Spent on Five Major Diseases

Diseases	Millions of Dollars	Deaths[a] in 1997
Cancer	2,300	560,000
AIDS	8,000	40,000
Heart disease	900	950,000
Diabetes	315	260,000
Stroke	186	160,000

1997 Federal expenditure figures are for research, education, and prevention programs and may underestimate actual amounts.

[a] Deaths in the United States (Source: Monthly Statistics Report, U.S. Dept. Health and Human Services, CDC. April, 1997; A. Cancer J. Clinic, 1997, 47:7–26)

Note: The total **global expenditures** on **malaria research** in 1993 were US$84 million, equivalent to $42 for every death; for tuberculosis $13. For HIV/AIDS research, $3,274 was invested in **research** for each death (O'Brien, 1996).

is involved in about 160,000 deaths per year, received $186 million or $860/death. Overall, between 1981 and the end of 1997, while 623,000 people died of AIDS, 11.5 million died of heart disease and 6.7 million died of cancer.

Justification for AIDS Expenditures—William Winkenwerder and colleagues (1989) pointed out that if federal dollars for HIV/AIDS projects continue to increase at current rates, it will become difficult to justify the expenditures. They point out that over 63 million Americans have cardiovascular diseases and about 30% of the population will eventually have some type of cancer. Smoking, a preventable health risk, is associated with an estimated 400,000 deaths annually. Alcohol abuse is linked to premature death, accidents, crime, and lost productivity, with an associated cost estimated at over $150 billion a year.

Winkenwerder and colleagues also point out that **spending more money on AIDS does not necessarily mean progress or a cure, and may, in fact, be wasted.**

Through 1997, it will be 26 years and $38 billion since President Richard M. Nixon signed into law the National Cancer Act. With it, a "**war on cancer**" was declared. Funding for cancer research was made a national priority, and the budget of the National Cancer Institute, the cancer research arm of the National Institutes of Health, the premier government-funded biomedical institute in the world, was increased to an all-time high. This allocation of federal dollars was based on the assumption that a cure could be found if enough money were available to support basic research. But many years and billions of dollars later, a cure for cancer still eludes our best scientific efforts. In fact, it is now believed that in the year 2000 cancer may be the leading cause of death in the United States, surpassing heart disease, the nation's number one cause of death. **However, the cause of AIDS and means of its prevention are known.** With many diseases such as diabetes, heart disease, stroke, and cancer, cause and prevention are complex and not as easily defined. The questions now being asked by legislators are: How much money is enough for HIV/AIDS projects? What about all the other diseases that have to be funded?

DEFINING AND MEASURING THE COSTS OF THE HIV/AIDS PANDEMIC: UNITED STATES

Social costs include **direct costs**, the resources used in providing health care, and **indirect costs**, the resources lost to society as a result of the epidemic. Costs to business include illness-based employment costs, caregiver costs, and nonmonetary costs. Not all social costs are borne by business, and businesses may incur costs that are not traditionally measured from the social perspective. Most published estimates of the costs of the HIV/AIDS pandemic have been developed from the social viewpoint, and they include direct and indirect costs.

AIDS: Direct Costs of HIV Disease and AIDS

Direct costs are the medical and nonmedical expenditures associated with screening for HIV infection, counseling those who are infected or at high risk for infection, and diagnosing and treating infected persons until their death. In 1991 the Department of Health and Human Services' Agency for Health Care Policy and Research determined that between 1991 and 1994, the costs of treating all people with HIV

——— BOX 16.3 ———

QUALITY VS. QUANTITY AND ECONOMIC COSTS OF AIDS THERAPIES

The care of patients with HIV and AIDS presents the medical profession and the public with a tangled web of competing obligations to prolong survival, to improve quality of life, to contain costs, and to promote equity. Often, there is an irreconcilable conflict between the clinician's duty to do what is best for the patient and the public policymaker's obligation to promote the collective safety and well-being.

IMPROVED SURVIVAL: INCREASED COSTS

Improved survival fuels the hope that HIV illness may one day be treated as a persistent, chronic condition. Yet, the gains that have been made to date in reducing AIDS-related morbidity and mortality come at a price. Most experts agree that the **lifetime direct medical costs** of HIV illness and AIDS have grown more than 50% in real terms since 1985. Moreover, existing therapies are generally associated with serious medical side-effects and toxicities. **Gains in survival, therefore, involve an explicit trade of cost and quality of well-being in exchange for quantity of life.** Progress in reducing AIDS-related morbidity and mortality imposes another, less obvious burden: increased exposure to competing risks. As patients live longer with more advanced immune dysfunction, previously rare opportunistic infections are becoming more common. For example, the success of prophylaxis and therapy in controlling *Pneumocystis carinii* pneumonia incidence and death means that many more patients are progressing to *Mycobacterium avium* complex, cytomegalovirus, toxoplasmosis, and fungal infections than ever before. These end-stage complications generally carry with them seriously increased levels of discomfort and disability, as well as economic cost.

The policy dilemma is clear. **Preventing the early symptoms buys marginal improvements in life expectancy while exposing patients and society to a host of potentially painful and expensive downstream consequences.** At a time of serious budgetary compressions and continuing spread of infections nationwide, it is important to ask whether the benefits of AIDS therapies justify the many alternative, life-prolonging opportunities forgone.

IRRECONCILABLE DIFFERENCES

The question of priority setting and resource allocation among competing AIDS interventions boils down to a tragic choice that pits the interests of the individual against those of the general population. At the heart of the dilemma is an irreconcilable tension between two deeply rooted human convictions: the Rule of Rescue vs. Utilitarianism.

The Rule of Rescue

Pulling us in one direction is the ethical sense of duty to the identified life in peril, a conviction that has been labeled the "Rule of Rescue." It is a natural human predisposition to focus on highly visible individuals in danger, even when actions to rescue them risk the potential loss of a greater number of unseen, "statistical" lives. This inclination is what drives us to spend tens of thousands of dollars to treat those who have not taken an available vaccine or those with tobacco-related illness.

Utilitarianism

Pulling us in the other direction is a utilitarian conviction that society ought to set its priorities and allocate its scarce resources in a manner that confers the greatest possible benefit to the greatest number, subject to resource constraints. Rising health costs, growth in the size of the uninsured population, and the proliferation of new medical technologies have all served to heighten social concern with issues of fairness and efficiency in the health sector. A more informed, more sophisticated, and more distrustful public detects some perversity and unfairness in the Rule of Rescue when applied at the population level. Simply stated, we cannot afford to provide every possible form of care, to every patient in need, without regard to severity, equity, or the forgone alternatives.

As a basis for global resource allocation, the Rule of Rescue is both inequitable and financially disastrous. At the patient care level, however, it will almost invariably trump the more "rational" utilitarian view.

(Adapted from David Paltiel, 1995)

HAVE HIV/AIDS FUNDS BEEN WASTED? PROBABLY!

There are numerous anecdotes in the literature about whether too much or too little money has been allocated for the fight against HIV/AIDS. Data provided within this chapter indicate that more money has been allocated for this **singular disease AIDS** in the United States than for any other disease and, over a much shorter time period (over $80 billion through 1998, 17 years). Some AIDS medical, economic, and research personnel have stated to the effect, that the vast sums of money available for all imaginable ways to obtain AIDS dollars **is equivalent to throwing gasoline on a fire—it creates a lot of flash and a lot of waste!**

Here are just two of the hundreds of ways in which AIDS dollars have been wasted in the large variety of HIV/AIDS programs funded in part or in whole with **federal dollars**.

Mark Harrington, policy director of the New York-based **Treatment Action Group** said, with respect to **misspent AIDS dollars,** that within the National Cancer Institute, with an AIDS budget approaching $300 million, "anything related to the drug Taxol was called AIDS, although that is a drug being studied for many cancers. Across all

of the NIH, we found examples where money was being miscoded [misspent]. Perhaps it was spent on meritorious research, **but it was not AIDS research**" (Voelker, 1996).

Laurie Garrett, author of "The Coming Plague" wrote an article about misspent AIDS research dollars in *Newsday* (1996). She stated that according to a study committee involving AIDS research money, that of $9.5 million to the National Institute of Alcohol Abuse & Alcoholism for AIDS research, **only $391,000** went to research to prevent the spread of the virus that causes AIDS. The rest went to study alcoholism in general. And, $35 million to the National Heart, Lung & Blood Institute to develop artificial blood, which the panel says is no longer needed because of competent U.S. blood screening. The author, as a member of two separate HIV/AIDS committees that received federal money for prevention and for care/treatment, witnessed sufficient waste within each committee's allocation/use of these dollars to speculate that the waste of federal dollars collectively from all federally funded programs must be, within the last 16 years, **over a few billion dollars**.

---

disease/AIDS would increase 21% each year. In 1998, about $22 billion will be spent on people with HIV disease/AIDS (Table 16-2).

Lifetime Costs for Treating People with HIV Disease/AIDS

Fred Hellinger's (1993) study on the lifetime costs of treating a person with HIV disease/AIDS assumes that an individual is identified and treated for HIV immediately following infection (Table 16-6). The study presents data from a large multistate survey that collected data directly from persons with HIV from March 1991 through August 1992. Data in Table 16-6 indicate that the mean survival time of a person diagnosed with AIDS in 1993 is 25 months. Multiplying this figure by the average monthly cost of $2,764 indicates the lifetime **cost after**

AIDS diagnosis until death in 1993 will be $69,100. Lifetime cost from HIV infection until death is estimated to be $119,274.

Table 16-7 presents hospitalizations, costs of those hospitalizations, and the total cost of care during **all** stages of HIV disease. Gable et al. (1996) estimated the average medical costs for an HIV-infected person with a T4 cell count of less than 200/µL to be about $753/month. The medical costs for an HIV-positive person with a T4 cell count greater than 200/µL but less than 500/µL was estimated to be $501/month. And for an HIV-positive person with a T4 cell count of 500/µL or higher, $161/month (Table 16-3). The lifetime costs of treating a person with HIV may be calculated by multiplying the average monthly cost of care in each of the four stages by the corresponding mean occupancy time (i.e., the average number of

QUALITY OF LIFE: FOR WHOM? WHAT COST IS ACCEPTABLE?

Concerned with the quality of life, the United States and other affluent democracies are prepared to commit public resources to fight devastating diseases that afflict small numbers of people. At the same time, critics charge, there is no serious public dedication to programs that would alleviate the plight of many, many more whose prospects are blighted by social and environmental causes. What accounts for the difference? If our fundamental goal is to promote the quality of human lives, does it matter that the potential is lost because of a human malfunction, because of negligent and abusive parents, or through the other hostile forces of a slum?

These questions have been an important part of public debate. Enthusiastic rhetoric about the marvels of tomorrow's medicine, which makes it appear that tackling HIV disease is **the** important problem, invites critics to present seemingly uncharitable comments. For example, Adrianne Appel (1995) reported that, "Heart, lung, and blood diseases account for half of the deaths in this country, yet they receive only 7.2% of NIH's budget. We spend $295 per patient on cancer research, $158 per patient on multiple sclerosis, $93 on heart disease, $54 on Alzheimer's, $26 on Parkinson's—and $39,000 per AIDS patient on research." The point is that more money is being spent on AIDS research than on any other of the higher incident and deadly diseases. However, if one looks at total federal funding, FY 1997, including money for treatment under Medicare and Medicaid, then AIDS ($8 billion) trails behind heart disease ($40 billion) and cancer ($19.5 billion).

In 1995, North Carolina Republican Senator Helms said he wanted to reduce funding for AIDS sufferers because they had contracted the disease through "deliberate, disgusting, revolting conduct." He also complained that AIDS is overfunded compared with heart disease and cancer, which strike far more Americans. He hopes to reduce spending on AIDS and "get some equity for people who have had heart trouble."

EACH DISEASE DESERVES AN INDEPENDENT LEVEL OF FUNDING

The tragedy of cancer and other diseases cannot be denied. But should the distribution of funds be based on the number of people dying from a disease? It would appear that this type of judgment may be short-sighted because the cause of each disease must be taken into account. AIDS is caused by a transmissible virus: **It can be spread geometrically!** There is a real chance to prevent HIV infection. Can we say that about most other diseases whose cause is vague and not associated with a microorganism? The point is that each disease needs funding sufficient to service the needs of that particular disease spectrum. Money for one disease should not be taken from a pool of money needed to combat another disease. Funding for disease prevention should be taken out of the political arena; there should be no "pet" diseases sponsored by a single physician or group of politicians. People must resist the divisive effort to pit one disease group against another and to compare one disease against the other, simply because such comparisons are so often dealing with "apples and oranges." Instead, people fighting against all those life-threatening illnesses must band together and seek more money for use against all diseases. The monetary obligation to each disease should be determined by those who research and treat it.

TABLE 16-6 HIV Disease, Stage, and Lifetime Treatment Cost (in 1992 Dollars)

Disease Stage	Mean Occupancy Time (mo.)	Cost per Month ($)	Total Cost of Care During Time in Disease Stage ($)
HIV-positive without AIDS (T cell count ≥0.50 × 10⁹/L)	67.3	282 (216–348)	18,978 (14,537–23,420)[a]
HIV-positive without AIDS (T cell count ≥0.20 and <0.50 × 10⁹/L)	44.0	430 (353–507)	18,920 (15,527–22,308)
HIV-positive without AIDS (T cell count <0.20 × 10⁹/L)	12.4	990 (842–1,138)	12,276 (10,441–14,111)
With AIDS	25	2,764 (2,610–2,918)	69,100 (65,250–72,950)
Total Lifetime Cost of Care	148.7	802	119,274 (105,760–132,789)

[a]Numbers in parentheses are 95% confidence intervals.

(Source: Hellinger, 1993)

months an infected person spends in a given stage before proceeding to the next stage) and summing the four products (Table 16-6).

AIDS: Indirect Costs or the Human Capital Approach

The human capital approach to the cost of AIDS takes into account the usual life cycle patterns of the labor market and potential earnings. Indirect cost is lost productivity due to premature death. Most people dying from AIDS are in the 20- to 45-year-old age bracket. The expected lifetime earnings of a 29-year-old male are $727,000. If he dies at age 29, society loses $727,000 worth of productivity.

Indirect costs are about five times higher per person than direct costs. For example, in 1986 direct costs for AIDS patients were $600 mil-lion, while the indirect cost of lost economic productivity was about $3 billion. Projections of all direct costs for 1991, with about 100,000 living AIDS patients, were about $11 billion and indirect costs were projected at $55 billion. For 1998, direct cost estimates just for medical services are $21.8 billion (Table 16-2) with at least 5 times (depending on the country, indirect costs may be 5, 10, or even 20 times direct costs) that amount in **indirect** costs or $109 billion. While the direct costs of AIDS are about equal to those of cancer and heart disease, the indirect costs are much higher because AIDS is primarily a disease of the young and middle-aged. Heart attacks, and strokes in particular, are associated with older people with less economic potential. The future earnings of a 67-year-old male are estimated at $30,000 (Caldwell et al., 1988).

TABLE 16-7 Estimated Monthly Cost ($) of Treating a Person with HIV by Disease Stage

Service Component ($)	Persons with AIDS	HIV-Positive without AIDS (T Cell Count <0.20 × 10⁹/L)	HIV-Positive without AIDS T Cell Count ≥0.20 × 10⁹/L and <0.50 × 10⁹/L	HIV-Positive without AIDS (T Cell Count ≥0.50 × 10⁹/L)
Inpatient	1,890 (68)	456 (46)	119 (28)	54 (19)
Outpatient visits	380 (14)	344 (35)	191 (44)	151 (54)
Home health	174 (6)	80 (8)	21 (5)	10 (4)
Drug costs	265 (10)	110 (11)	99 (23)	67 (24)
Long-term care	55 (2)	0	0	0
Total	2,764	990	430	282

Charges in 1992 dollars. Percentage of total charges shown in parentheses. HIV, human immunodeficiency virus; AIDS, acquired immunodeficiency syndrome. Percentages may not total 100 due to rounding.

(Source: Hellinger, 1993)

Federal Funding for HIV/AIDS in Jeopardy?

During 1997, the United States will begin the attempt to balance the national budget. Legislators will look for ways to trim **$1.3 trillion** over the next 7 years. There is a growing concern that the HIV/AIDS appropriations will be among the first to be cut. A primary reason for the cut in the HIV/AIDS appropriation comes from the lowered estimates of those now believed to be HIV-infected in the United States. The **estimate** is now from 600,000 to 900,000, down from 800,000 to 1.2 million, a 25% decline in the estimated number of HIV-infected.

Shifting Risk Groups

The downward trend **does not mean the number of new infections has significantly decreased,** only that statisticians are making more accurate projections and updating their estimates accordingly. Studies continue to show a disturbing rise in infection rates in certain population groups, including adolescents, gay men, minority women, and residents of rural areas, where there had not been significant representation before.

Shifting Funding Targets Can Help Offset Financial Needs

Sifting data resulting from nationwide HIV/AIDS prevention programs, it has become quite clear that continued saturation of the airwaves, newspapers, journals, public service announcements, sides of public busses, and so on, with HIV/AIDS-prevention messages has not, since the early 1980s, lowered the annual number of new HIV infections in the United States. This is why private foundations are laying plans to redirect potentially millions of dollars in AIDS-prevention money to groups highest at risk for the disease. For example, Funders Concerned about AIDS—which works with about 1,800 U.S. foundations that contribute money to combat AIDS—says that advocating **targeted prevention programs** has become a top priority for 1997 and beyond.

A number of organizations decided to target their funds after reading an article in the *Wall Street Journal* that showed that a dispro-portionate amount of public **AIDS-prevention** money in the United States has been spent on the **low-risk** general population. The *Journal* was essentially saying that while it is true that anyone can become HIV-infected, funds must go to the populations where the disease is most prevalent!

Targeting Geographic Areas

In addition to focusing on specific high-risk behaviors, funding dollars are also increasingly being directed at **geographic areas with high HIV concentrations**. The Prudential Foundation in 1997 will deploy **all** of the approximately $400,000 a year it spends on AIDS in the greater Newark, New Jersey area, where about half of New Jersey's AIDS cases are clustered. The idea is to focus the money where it will have the greatest impact.

INSURANCE INDUSTRY AND AIDS

Insurance is, by definition, a spreading of the risk, and HIV disease and AIDS most affects the age group that had previously been the healthiest and therefore the least likely to use health benefits. Because the cost of treating an AIDS patient is high (and group health and life insurance premiums are based in part on a group's loss-claims experience with its insurance carrier and also on actuarial tables, which forecast the probable cost of medical treatment for an age group), insurance costs have risen (and continue to rise) even for those companies in which no employee has contracted AIDS or an HIV-related illness. However, the cost for treating an individual with AIDS is actually less in many cases than treating an employee for cancer.

Fifty-nine percent of health care in America is financed primarily through private insurance and uninsured people who pay their own expenses. Forty-one percent is financed through public sector programs at the federal, state, and local levels. The problem of providing care for people with HIV infection and AIDS has financially strained the health care system.

Barriers to health care for HIV/AIDS patients include: (**1**) refusal by private insurers to underwrite individual policies for people who

——————— BOX 16.4 ———————

PUBLIC BACKLASH TO AIDS

Because of TV, plays, magazine articles, newspapers, radio talk shows, phamplets in physicians' offices, and courses in schools and universities, the public is feeling AIDS anxiety. Perhaps because they have been told repeatedly that the majority of people affected are homosexuals, bisexuals, IDUs, and prostitutes. Many people might think, "I'm not one of them. I just want to be left alone. The problems they have could be prevented if they wanted to."

PLACING THE BLAME

The AIDS pandemic has provided individuals with a platform from which he or she can blame someone else for a disease. During the 14th century, Jews were burned at the stake for causing the plague. In the 19th century, cholera was called God's wrath on the poor and immoral. In the 20th century, polio in America was believed to be caused by Italian immigrants. Now it is AIDS, and some evangelists and politicians say it is God's condemnation of the homosexuals, injection drug users, and prostitutes. California Senator Jim Neilson said in 1989 that AIDS may be God's way of visiting a plague upon mankind (Silverman, 1990).

Former U.S. Surgeon General C. Everett Koop said he feared the American public may turn against AIDS patients as their numbers increase and the taxpayer has to pick up the tab for their health care.

> Such a public response would be tragic, but it is not unexpected among health professionals. Retribution may come about in the 1990s as Americans grow to resent the cost of caring for AIDS patients, estimated now at over $10 billion a year, and as health workers burn out from the pressures of watching young people die. There is a public mood of retribution as evidenced by the spread of no-smoking areas aimed at smokers, as well as the crackdown against drunk drivers, against teenage pregnancies, wife beaters, and drug addicts.

For whatever reasons, fund raisers say that almost none of the largest foundations in the United States have given a cent to fight AIDS. William Freeman, director of Institutional Affairs for the National AIDS Network said that because 44% of AIDS patients are minorities, he fears that within the next 3 years AIDS will be considered just another disease of the poor.

An example of how individuals perceive the HIV/AIDS epidemic can be found in a letter to a newspaper columnist.

> In a recent column you said 47,000 people died of AIDS since the early '80s. You didn't say how many people died of cancer during the same period.
>
> When I saw that quilt commemorating AIDS victims on Ted Koppel's *Nightline* I was infuriated. My brother had just died of cancer. He was 44, didn't smoke, didn't drink and lived for his wife and three kids. According to the American Cancer Society, a half-million people like him will die this year. But federal funding for cancer research is being cut back because there isn't enough money to go around.
>
> I realize that AIDS is a terrible disease. But homosexuals who are monogamous do not get AIDS. I am also aware that some babies are born with AIDS and that a bad blood transfusion can result in AIDS. I am not talking about these people, I am talking about homosexuals who are promiscuous.
>
> I realize that people who have AIDS, from whatever source, are gravely ill and need our compassion and our sympathy, but skip the quilt. Just remember that AIDS is avoidable. Most cancer is not.

RESENTMENT GROWS

As the economic and medical impact continues to increase, resentment may grow in proportion. The burden of dealing with the AIDS pandemic

(continued)

is moving from the federal government onto city, state, and voluntary agencies, placing the issues of how much to spend and on what directly in the hands of the voters.

Aran Ron and David Rogers reported that:

> The majority of new AIDS diagnoses are in injection drug users, their sexual partners, and infants born to these couples. More than 80% of these patients are black or Hispanic and almost all are poor. These groups, along with homosexual AIDS patients and substance abusers who don't have AIDS, are already placing great demand on limited hospital resources. It is becoming more difficult to arrange admission for patients with acute illnesses requiring hospitalization. There are anecdotal reports of patients who wait days in emergency departments before a hospital bed becomes available, and elective admissions are also becoming more difficult to arrange. If care for persons with AIDS is perceived as interfering with the health care of others, bitter conflicts between those with and without AIDS and acts of discrimination that may fall along racial lines seem likely. (Ron et al., 1988)

test positive for HIV; (**2**) loss of employment-related group health insurance; (**3**) variable coverage and eligibility policies of state Medicaid programs; (**4**) reimbursement by private insurance and public programs at levels that do not encourage use of services and facilities commensurate with need; and (**5**) lack of coordination between health care and social service systems. There is the additional problem of over 37 million uninsured individuals who do not qualify for public health care (Friedman, 1991). It should be mentioned that although the number, 39 million, of uninsured in the United States has been used repeatedly in all types of forums, Katherine Swartz (1994) argues that the number is very misleading. Her statistics describe the dynamics of people moving in and out of particular insurance situations. Swartz writes that a large proportion of the uninsured pick up insurance within relatively short periods, but a significant number of people are uninsured for very long periods of time. For many people (at least 21 million in 1993), being without health insurance is not a temporary or transitory phase in their lives.

Over the course of a year, many more than 37 million Americans will be uninsured for 1 to 11 months, but not during the single month that the Census Bureau counts the uninsured. That 1-month survey is the basis for the point-in-time figure of 37 million. In fact, the number of Americans who are uninsured during a given year is closer to 58 million; about one-quarter of the nonelderly population is uninsured.

─────── **POINT OF INFORMATION 16.4** ───────

HEALTH INSURANCE COVERAGE BY STAGE OF ILLNESS

Claudia Schur and colleagues (1994) reported on a 1991 health insurance survey of 5,811 people aged 13 and older in 10 major cities who were patients of hospitals, clinics, and private physician practices. Their survey showed that for people with HIV, there was a variation in insurance coverage by stage of illness. People with no symptoms were less likely to have public coverage and more likely to have no other form of coverage than the study population as a whole. For those with HIV infection but no symptoms (asymptomatic), 31.4% had private insurance coverage, 37.3% had public coverage, and 31.4% had no health insurance coverage. For HIV-positive people with symptoms but not diagnosed with AIDS (symptomatic non-AIDS), 29% had private insurance, 49.5% had public insurance, and 21.4% had no coverage. For people with an AIDS diagnosis, 25.9% had private insurance, 62.3% had public insurance, and 11.9% had no coverage.

About 36% of this total are uninsured for the entire year, some 21 million Americans. Thus, when the point-in-time estimate of 37 million is used, it represents 16 million people who will be uninsured for less than a year and 21 million long-term uninsured.

In 1988, of 31 million adolescents between ages 10 and 18, one in seven had no health insurance. In 1994, one in three had no health insurance (*Hastings Center Report*, 1991, updated). Between the ages of 18 and 44, 25% lacked health insurance (Diaz et al., 1994).

For the medically disenfranchised, there is no access to a system of care. For those who have no doctor, no clinic, and no means of payment, access to health care services is most often through the emergency room door of one of the few hospitals the community that treats people with HIV infection and AIDS. Five percent of the nation's hospitals treat 50% of the people with AIDS.

As new therapies are developed, the gaps in the system may present even greater problems. In addition to the direct cost of therapy, prolonging life may result in additional costs. If new therapies are effective for asymptomatic HIV-infected people, who may outnumber other clinic patients by 20 or 50 to one, the financial implications will be profound. Moreover, as HIV/AIDS patients live longer, many may become eligible for Medicare, having outlived the 24-month waiting period following determination of disability. As patients live longer, many more will also outlive insurance coverage (*Public Health Reports*, 1988).

Is Insurance Obtainable and/or Affordable?

Industry trade groups estimate that health insurance claims and death benefits paid in AIDS-related cases will total over $20 billion through 1998.

Life insurance companies typically require individuals to take a blood test before writing a policy for a large amount of money. Insurance officials say they deny coverage to people who test positive for HIV because the odds are that those people will get AIDS and die, absorbing large claims or benefits after paying only a small amount in premiums. The insurance companies feel that if they continued paying those high claims, they would not be able to continue coverage for other customers and remain financially sound.

The American Council of Life Insurance and the Health Insurance Association of America conducted a survey of 325 insurance companies. All of these companies said they would refuse coverage to someone who had tested HIV-positive.

As a response to this, 14 states have set up a pool of money to help care for the uninsurable. Other states are considering such pools. California, the District of Columbia, and Maine have passed controversial bills concerning AIDS and insurance companies. These bills **prohibit** companies from requiring anyone to take the HIV-antibody test or inquiring if they have had such a test. They also restrict the companies from basing rates or other aspects of coverage on whether a person has had such a test.

The latest trend among companies is an attempt to control, rather than avoid, the cost of AIDS care. In the earlier stages of illness, AIDS patients do not usually require acute care. Less expensive home or hospice care is an alternative to hospitalization. Insurance companies that do not normally cover this sort of care are beginning to investigate such alternatives.

As reported, over 39.7 million people in the United States are without health insurance (*American Family Physician*, 1996). These people are not all poor and unemployed. Some make respectable wages but have simply been priced out of the private insurance market, and their employers refuse to cover them in a group plan because the cost of group insurance is sky-rocketing. Some individuals are not insurable because they have certain illnesses such as cancer or diabetes.

Between 1980 and 1983, health insurance premiums increased 50% while the average income went up only 17%. The rates are leveling off somewhat, but are still beyond the reach of many millions of Americans.

Profile of the Uninsured

The General Accounting Office recently drew a profile of the uninsured population. Nearly three-quarters are employed, but most work at

FIRST NATIONWIDE LIFE INSURANCE AVAILABLE TO HIV-POSITIVE PEOPLE

Acknowledging the recent advances in anti-HIV drug therapy, Guarantee Trust Life Insurance, in April 1997, began, on a trial basis, selling insurance to HIV-infected people. The company president said "from a life insurance risk perspective, we believe many otherwise healthy HIV-positive individuals are more appropriately viewed as having a treatable chronic illness rather than a terminal disease." Guarantee Trust Life is the **first** in the nation to actively insure HIV-positive people. The cost of this insurance is about 6 times higher for the HIV-infected than for the noninfected.

part-time jobs where insurance is not part of the package. The growth of employment in retail and construction has contributed to the number of uninsured workers because those industries traditionally are less likely to offer coverage.

Risk Classification for the Insured

From the insurance industry's point of view, the issue is one of risk classification. Life insurers have always used medical information to try to predict how long customers are likely to live. In a process known as underwriting, a company groups people with similar risk—based on factors such as age, current health status, family medical history, occupation, and lifestyle—and charges each member of a group the same rate, which is proportional to the amount of risk the company assumes in insuring them. In this way the industry attempts to keep healthier individuals from subsidizing people with greater risks.

Depending on a physical examination and answers to specific questions asked by a physician, an individual may be able to obtain a policy by paying a higher than normal premium or by accepting a policy that contains a waiver (insured but not for a certain condition). There are, however, a number of health problems for which individuals are denied an insurance policy (Table 16-8). Diagnosed HIV infection and AIDS are both reasons for health care and death benefit insurance policy denial. In fact, the insurance industry is still reacting to a study in late 1987 indicating that a 35-year-old man who is infected with HIV is 51 times more likely to die prematurely than a healthy male of the same age. Insurance applicants who are more than five or six times as likely to die prematurely are usually too expensive to underwrite. For example, a 35-year-old male with coronary heart disease would be five times as likely as a healthy applicant to die a premature death.

ONE IN SEVEN AMERICANS DO NOT HAVE HEALTH INSURANCE

According to a report in the January 5, 1996 issue of *Hospitals & Health Networks*, 39.7 million persons (one in seven) in the United States do not have health insurance. The statistics were released by the U.S. Census Bureau. Of those Americans with health insurance, 70% were covered by private insurance plans, about 13% were covered by Medicare, 12% by Medicaid, and 4% by military policies. Young adults aged 18 to 24 were the most likely group to not be covered. Most elderly persons have health insurance under Medicare. Employers provide over one-half of the nation's 139 million workers with health insurance.

Susan Dentzer (1996) reported that at any given moment, about 41 million Americans, 10 million of whom are children, are without medical coverage. The number of uninsured may reach 60 million in the year 2000.

———————— BOX 16.5 ————————

THE RIGHT TO HEALTH INSURANCE?

A physician shared his concern over patients' rights this way: "You have the right to remain silent or to request that I not record any part of your medical history."

If abusive practices by insurance companies do not cease, this medical equivalent of a Miranda criminal rights statement could become necessary so physicians could warn their patients that what they say could be used against them—often unfairly.

To obtain private health insurance, the health consumer has no choice but to sign his or her name, allowing insurance companies to obtain medical records from any physician or health provider.

In the past, this would consist of a brief summary form completed by the physician. Now increasingly, insurance companies photocopy every page of the patients' medical records, opening their most intimate, nonmedically pertinent secrets to scrutiny.

It is not uncommon for insurance companies to turn down single men who happen to be waiters, decorators, or hairdressers for fear that some might be gay and more prone to AIDS. Even married men have been scrubbed because an unreliable test for AIDS falsely tagged them as HIV-positive. In 1991, the 5th U.S. Circuit Court of Appeals in New Orleans ruled that employers who provide **self-insured health plans** for their workers have the right to substantially reduce medical benefits to those with AIDS-related illnesses. The ruling stems from a case where a Houston company cut its plan for $1 million in lifetime health coverage to $5,000—but only for workers with AIDS. This is the first federal appeals court ruling of its kind to become law in Louisiana, Texas, and Mississippi, unless overturned by the U.S. Supreme Court. In November 1992, the United States Supreme Court refused to hear an appeal of the 5th Circuit Court ruling. This decision may be used to reduce insurance coverage for many other illnesses. However, similar reduction in coverage for other such cases has now been ruled discriminatory under the Americans with Disabilities Act. (See ADA rulings in Chapter 17.)

Commercial Health Insurers

In 1988, Jill Eden and colleagues reported the results of a survey on AIDS and health insurance for the Office of Technological Assessment (OTA). The survey was sent to 88 commercial insurers, to 15 of 77 available Blue Cross/Blue Shield (BC/BS) plans, and to the 50 largest local and national Health Maintenance Organizations (HMOs). Sixty-one commercial insurers, all 15 BC/BS, and 39 of the HMOs responded to the survey. Several questions from that survey are presented along with the respondents' answers:

Question: Do health insurers attempt to identify applicants exposed to HIV?
Answer: Forty-one commercial insurers currently test applicants for HIV infection—10 are planning to test. If the applicant tests positive for HIV, he or she will be denied insurance.

Question: How do insurers screen applicants for HIV exposure?
Answer: Not all health insurers concerned with the applicant's HIV status demand HIV testing. Those that do not test rely on a review of the applicant's medical history questionnaire and the attending physician's statement (APS) to assess the risk of HIV exposure. Thirty-four of the 41 commercial health insurers have AIDS-related questions on the medical history form. The AIDS-associated questions vary with the insurance company. Some companies ask about AIDS-related signs and symptoms; some ask whether the applicant has ever been HIV tested and what test he or she has had (Table 16-9).

Beginning 1997, at least 24 states (Arizona, California, Colorado, Connecticut, Delaware, Florida, Illinois, Iowa, Kentucky, Maine, Minnesota, Missouri, Montana, New Hampshire, New York, Ohio, Oregon, Pennsylvania, Rhode

TABLE 16-8 Some Commercial Health Insurers: Classification of Risks

Higher Premium	Exclusion Waiver	Denial
Allergies	Cataract	AIDS
Asthma	Gallstones	Ulcerative colitis
Back strain	Fibroid tumor (uterus)	Cirrhosis of liver
Hypertension (controlled)	Hernia (hiatal/inguinal)	Diabetes mellitus
Arthritis	Migraine headaches	Leukemia
Gout	Pelvic inflammatory disease	Schizophrenia
Glaucoma	Chronic otitis disorders	Hypertension (uncontrolled)
Obesity	Spine/back disorders	Emphysema
Psychoneurosis (mild)	Hemorrhoids	Stroke
Kidney stones	Knee impairment	Obesity (severe)
Emphysema (mild/moderate)	Asthma	Angina (severe)
Alcoholism/drug abuse	Allergies	Coronary artery disease
Heart murmur	Varicose veins	Epilepsy
Peptic ulcer	Sinusitis, chronic or severe	Lupus
Colitis	Fractures	Alcoholism/drug abuse

Island, Texas, Vermont, Virginia, Washington, Wisconsin) have insurance laws regarding HIV testing. At least 16 states require written and/or informed consent, and at least 20 contain confidentiality provisions. The states of California, Connecticut, Florida, Hawaii, Maine, and Washington, D.C. prohibited HIV testing as a condition for life and health insurability. Similar HIV testing bans for insurance applicants in New York, Wisconsin, and Massachusetts have been invalidated. Although California does not allow HIV testing, it does allow a T cell count to determine if the individual has a properly functioning immune system. Insurers and gay rights activist groups nationwide are escalating their fight over AIDS issues, with testing foremost in the struggle.

The insurers say that if they are not allowed to test, then other policyholders will have to subsidize the costs. Gay activists say that those who most need access to health insurance are least able to get it.

Another effort by gay activist groups is to ban the limiting of AIDS-related coverage. By 1988, 19 states had already prohibited the practice.

Insurers say that if HIV testing is prohibited, they may experience **adverse selection.** As insurance companies raise their premiums, low-risk individuals will stop buying insurance. But individuals at high risk of developing AIDS will continue to want full coverage, and the percentage of AIDS patients among those insured will rise. As a re-

TABLE 16-9 Commercial Insurers, BC/BS Plans, and HMOs Screening for Exposure to HIV

Method(s) Used to Identify AIDS Exposure	Commercial Insurers[a] (n = 50)		BC/BS Plans[a] (n = 11)		HMOs[a] (n = 9)	
	Number	Percent	Number	Percent	Number	Percent
Question on application	44	88	11	100	9	100
Attending physician statement	42	84	9	82	6	67
T cell subset study	17	34	0	–	0	–

BC/BS, Blue Cross/Blue Shield; HMOs, health maintenance organizations (25% of medically insured Americans have BC/BS plans; BC/BS offers 69 different medical plans across the United States).

[a]Data included only those insurers or plans that screen or intend to screen for AIDS exposure.

(Adapted from Office of Technology Assessment, Eden et al., 1988; updated 1994) sult, insurance companies will again raise their premiums and more low-risk individuals will drop their coverage. Finally, only those individuals with the highest risk of developing AIDS will want to buy insurance at rates they may not be able to afford.

Testing is already affecting low-risk insurance applicants. A long-married Florida resident with two children had a chance to save $300 a year by switching life insurance carriers if he took the AIDS test the insurer now requires for policies of $250,000 or more. Rather than risk a false-positive result that would go on his record, he remained with the old insurer.

Question: Which applicants are to be tested?
Answer: Of the 61 insurers responding to the survey, 31 routinely tested applicants. Seven of the 31 companies tested every applicant, 14 of 31 tested those who admitted to a lifestyle that placed them **at high risk** ("high risk" was defined differently by each company). Ten companies tested applicants depending on criteria such as residence, medical history, homosexuality, job, and amount of the policy. Three insurers stated that all applicants living in high HIV prevalence areas such as large cities in New York, California, and Florida were tested. Some insurance companies stated that they did not insure IDUs or hemophiliacs.

Question: What are the future plans of the 61 responding insurance companies to offset the financial impact of AIDS?
Answer: Only one insurer, an HMO, plans to withdraw from the marketplace. Thirty-four percent of the commercial insurers and 40% of BC/BS insurers plan to reduce individual and small group health markets (use more restrictive underwriting guidelines). Thirty-three percent of commercial insurers plan to expand HIV or other types of testing for applicants. Nine companies will add questions on AIDS to their medical history forms. Seven BC/BS companies plan to exclude HIV/AIDS and other STDs from individual health coverage. One commercial insurer plans to establish a 2-year waiting period for AIDS before the policy takes effect. And two commercial insurers plan to limit the dollar value for AIDS claims.

In summary, private insurance covers a large part of the medical cost of AIDS patients. AIDS patients without private insurance coverage must pay for treatment themselves. After they

---

BOX 16.6

NEW YORK'S NEW INSURANCE LAW—1992

In July 1992, the New York State Legislature passed the Community Rating Bill. This law is a major victory for all people with HIV disease, AIDS, and chronic illnesses. It widely expanded the opportunity of buying insurance, and helps people hang on to coverage they already have.

"Rating" is insurance-speak for the way the insurance company sets the cost of the premium.

"Community Rating" means that the insurance company spreads the cost of claims across the community. All claims from all policyholders are added up and the average of the cost of providing coverage at the end of the year becomes the new premium. No one is penalized for being in poorer health or punished for using their health insurance by getting a huge increase at the end of the year.

When this law took effect on April 1, 1993, people were allowed to change jobs without fear of losing their coverage or having an additional "preexisting condition waiting period" imposed. In short, if you have the money for the policy, commercial insurers, through an **open enrollment,** must sell it to you. This means you can go **shopping!** Maybe you'd like a policy with better prescription coverage, or more home health care, a higher lifetime maximum, or a lower deductible. This is not to say that a perfect "dream" policy is out there, or that it is within your price range, but it means that people of New York State won't have to worry about being rejected because of their age, sex or health status, sexual orientation, etc.

have spent nearly all their assets and are indigent, they become eligible for Medicaid coverage in most but not all states. Also, income and asset limits for Medicaid vary across states. The federal government pays 50% to 77% of Medicaid costs, depending on per capita state income, with the state governments, and in some instances, local governments paying the remainder.

Commercial Life Insurers

Life insurance companies say they need to be allowed to test for HIV because people who know they are HIV-infected can pool resources and take out large policies. In 1986, $20 billion worth of individual policies and $15 billion worth of group policies were written for HIV-infected people. If left unchecked, increased premium payouts for AIDS deaths could bankrupt many insurers. The gay community argues that to test for insurance purposes would breach individual confidentiality. The insurers argue that they have a right to protect their financial stability. They say that they are allowed to withhold insurance for certain health problems, to increase premiums for people who practice destructive lifestyles such as smoking or alcoholism, and to stipulate exclusion waivers. Why should it be different for HIV-infected or people with AIDS?

Finally, insurance companies are suspected of denying coverage to people who live in certain neighborhoods, in same-gender households, or who work in certain professions. Sometimes insurers cancel policies or refuse to pay on grounds of preexisting conditions, fraud, or the experimental nature of treatment.

There may be laws in your state which prohibit insurance companies from asking certain questions, requiring an HIV/AIDS test, denying coverage, or engaging in other discrimination. Federal law also prohibits certain practices.

If you have an insurance-related problem, you probably will need legal help if your state insurance department cannot provide it.

Insurance Breakthrough: Collection of Benefits Before Death

Insurance experts estimate that one in five deaths will be due to AIDS by the year 2000.

The cost of these AIDS-related deaths to life insurance companies may reach $50 billion to $100 billion. In mid-1989, in a move praised by gay rights activists and members of the medical and health care communities, the Canadian branch of Prudential Life Insurance started a program in which victims of acquired immune deficiency syndrome can get benefits from their life insurance policies before they die. The **viatical program** allows patients access to 40% to 70% of their death benefits to pay for health care. Other insurers are now following this practice (see Box 16.7).

How It Works: 1997—

1. **The Policyholder**—A person with a terminal illness decides to sell a $100,000 insurance policy to get money to live on before he or she dies. He or she receives $65,000.
2. **The Broker**—A broker finds an investor willing to buy the policy and arranges its legal transfer to the investor. The broker receives $15,000.
3. **The Investor**—An investor pays the dying policyholder a percentage of the face value of the policy, as well as paying the broker's and legal fees. In return, when the original policyholder dies, the **investor gets the full death benefit**, or **$20,000 profit.**
4. **The Dilemma**—Because the amount the investor receives when the original policyholder dies is fixed, the investor's rate of return depends on how long the dying person lives.

If the dying person lives . . .	the annual return is . . .
1 year	25.0%
2 years	12.5%
3 years	8.3%
4 years	6.3%

A Right to Treatment

Some hospitals, nursing homes, and doctors may deny treatment to **persons** living with AIDS (PLWA) or provide less or inferior care than they provide to other patients. Health care discrimination against PLWAs may be

———————— BOX 16.7 ————————

VIATICALS: INCOME FROM THE SALE OF LIFE INSURANCE POLICIES

In 1989, insurance companies began to purchase life insurance policies from the terminally ill to allow them to collect benefits before they die. **This new industry offers cash—a "viatical settlement" help to a person in danger of death, in return for being named the irrevocable beneficiary of a life insurance policy.** Viatical settlements offer people with HIV disease disposable income that would otherwise accrue to their beneficiaries.

Viatical companies or private investors typically purchase life insurance policies at 60% to 80% of face value; this payment increases if life expectancy is shorter. Companies generally acquire policies valued at $50,000 to $500,000 and are reluctant to buy a policy if minor children or other dependents are reliant on the policyholder for financial support.

To meet the requirement of a viatical settlement, terminally ill people must release their medical records for review to the viatical company, which will use these records to estimate life expectancy. Group life insurance coverage can be viaticated only after it has been converted to an individual policy, but some group policies preclude viatication. The entire viatication process can take 3 to 4 months.

Viatical settlements are considered taxable income. Receiving a viatical settlement also disqualifies recipients from any means-based entitlements such as Medicaid or Supplemental Security Income (Peterson, 1992).

UPDATE 1997: NEW TREATMENTS A CAUSE FOR RECALCULATING VIATICALS

A longer life means a lower return to the industry that buys life insurance policies from terminally ill patients at discount prices and profits by collecting the death benefits. So recent breakthroughs in AIDS therapies (protease inhibitors and drug cocktail mixes—see Chapter 4) are intensifying the industry's search for new areas of growth, hoping to attract people with cancer and other diseases.

Since information of the dramatic effects of protease inhibitors on viral load appeared in 1996, the prices being paid to AIDS patients for their policies have fallen by 5% to 10% and may decline even further.

One company, Dignity Partners, Inc. of San Francisco, which does 95% of its business with people who have symptomatic HIV disease or AIDS has temporarily stopped processing new applications.

Executives of other companies said they had already been doing slowly what Dignity did precipitously: weaning their business from an almost exclusive dependence on people with AIDS and broadening their appeal to those with other terminal illnesses.

ONE EXAMPLE OF A VIATICAL SURVIVOR ENJOYING HIS JACKPOT

To those who bet $100,000 on his quick death, one AIDS person became a viatical nightmare.

For the last 2 years, he has defied the laws of AIDS, surviving on a T4 cell count of less than 200.

And thanks to his viatication, in which investors paid him a portion of his life insurance money for the rights to the policy's proceeds, he has a lot of money.

For premium payments totaling $857 a year, he wound up with $100,000 in cash from a viatical investor. He said, "You go through this guilt thing at first. You know they are making money off your death."

In 1990, Baez began negotiating with three viaticals, receiving offers of $75,000, $85,000, and $100,000 before selling his $150,000 policy to the top bidder.

Immediately, he went on a spending binge: two new cars, home redecoration, and college tuition for his siblings.

"Since I sold my policy, I haven't thought about AIDS. What more can you ask for than that you forget about your disease?"

The settlement led to other fortuitous events. Baez had never gone near the stock market before. But his settlement put him in a gambling mood. He plunked down $30,000 on assorted stocks, betting on their 1-day rise. A year later, he had $300,000.

"Most people that I know are living longer and are happier," he said. "That is the bottom line: Happiness creates longevity."

Baez is ready to viaticate his second policy. It has a face value of $500,000. He says he will probably get $350,000.

fought under a number of federal and state laws. The following are some examples. They are not intended to give legal advice. It is important that you contact your state department of health or county welfare program to determine if you are eligible for benefits or protection under these laws. If you encounter difficulties in obtaining the protection described or you think you have legal problems, you should consult your local AIDS organization, ACLU legal services, or bar association. Assistance may also be obtained from:

NATIONAL HEALTH LAW PROGRAM
2025 M Street, N.W.
Suite 400
Washington, D.C. 20036
(202) 887-5310

Section 504 of the Rehabilitation Act—This prohibits discrimination against the handicapped, in certain situations, by hospitals, nursing facilities, and state agencies which receive federal funds. AIDS has been determined to be a handicap for these purposes. Other recipients of federal funds may be covered under this act.

Hill-Burton Act—Hospitals and nursing homes which receive federal funds to build and operate their facilities may be challenged for discrimination in certain circumstances.

Anti-Dumping Laws—New federal law and some state laws require hospitals to examine, treat, and stabilize people in need of emergency care before discharge or transfer to other facilities.

State Anti-Discrimination, Privacy, or Civil Rights Laws—Many states have new or existing laws which prohibit discrimination against the handicapped, invasion of privacy, and violation of civil rights.

Funeral Expenses

Funeral directors in some cities will not knowingly handle AIDS deceased. Others are charging $300 to $1,000 extra for handling the bodies. The directors explain that they often must hire outside embalmers and other additional personnel to prepare the bodies. They also point out that after working on the bodies, they must disinfect their labs and throw away gloves and other items that may be contaminated.

SUMMARY

AIDS is an expensive illness. The average cost of treatment per patient from diagnosis to death is about $69,000. Because many health care services are required to treat this pandemic, there has evolved an AIDS industry. For 1997, it is estimated that over $18 billion will be spent on the care of people with HIV disease/AIDS; and the cost is expected to continue to rise throughout the 1990s. In terms of number of deaths from a given disease and the federal dollars spent on it, AIDS is receiving a disproportionately large sum. For example, in 1997, $8 billion in federal funds was allocated to AIDS projects.

The fact that so many federal dollars are being used in AIDS programs, seemingly at the expense of other projects, and that the majority of affected people are homosexuals, bisexuals, and injection drug users has spawned a public backlash. There are an increasing number of low-risk Americans who resent the expenditure of vast sums of money on these people when so many others need those same federal dollars. The situation may worsen as more hospital beds are occupied by AIDS patients and non-AIDS patients experience shortages. This is particularly true for public hospitals that already have a high caseload of indigent patients. As the number of AIDS patients increases in the 1990s, fewer and fewer hospital resources will be available for non-AIDS patients. In addition, there may be a physician and nurse burnout—they may simply get tired of treating AIDS patients.

The high cost of AIDS therapy and hospitalization is now being met by individual insurance, group insurance, Medicaid, and Medicare. But insurance companies are looking for ways to deny policies to people who might be HIV-infected. Applicants are asked to fill out forms that ask specific questions about their lifestyles and whether they have ever been HIV-tested. Insurers believe they have a right to stay solvent. They feel they owe it to those who are insurable. Some insurers have, since the AIDS pandemic started, raised their life insurance premiums because they will have to pay claims on many people who were HIV-infected prior to obtaining a policy. Life insurance companies estimate that the cost of AIDS- related deaths may reach $50 billion by the year 2000. In that year, they project that one in every five deaths will be due to AIDS. Even funeral directors have added extra charges for embalming.

REVIEW QUESTIONS

(Answers to the Review Questions are on page 581.)

1. What is the average cost of medical care for an AIDS patient in the United States? Is that significantly higher than for patients who die of cancer, chronic heart disease, or diabetes?

2. What are indirect costs with regard to AIDS; and do they amount to more than direct costs?

3. With respect to AIDS, what is the irony of the health insurance industry?

4. What is the major concern of life insurance companies?

5. Who is responsible for your not becoming HIV-positive?

REFERENCES

American Family Physician. (1996). One in seven Americans do not have health care insurance. 53:1026.

APPEL, ADRIANNE. (1995). Future of AIDS office threatened. *Nature,* 376:206.

BAUM, RUDY M. (1992). Progress fitful on understanding AIDS, developing therapies. *Chem. Eng. News,* 70:26–31.

CALDWELL, JACQUES R., et al. (1988). Economic stresses of AIDS: Lessons for the United States and Florida. *Florida M.A.,* 75:449–452.

CASTRO, JANICE. (1991). Condition critical. *Time,* 138:34–42.

DENTZER, SUSAN. (1996). For mercy's sake, let's cover kids. *U.S. News and World Report,* Oct. 21:69.

DIAZ, THERESA, et al. (1994). Health insurance coverage among persons with AIDS: Results from a multistate surveillance project. *Am. J. Public Health,* 84:1015–1018.

EDEN, JILL, et al. (1988). AIDS and health insurance: an OTA survey. *OTA, United States Congress,* 20510–8025.

FRIEDMAN, EMILY. (1991). The uninsured: From dilemma to crisis. *JAMA,* 265:2491–2496.

GABLE, CAROL, et al. (1996). Costs of HIV/AIDS at CD4+ counts disease stages based on treatment protocols. *J. Acquired Immune Deficiency Syndromes and Human Retrovirology,* 12:413–420.

GARRETT, LAURIE. (1996). Misspent money/study: AIDS funds often go elsewhere. *Newsday,* March 13, p A05.

Hastings Center Report. (1991). A generation at risk. 21:3.

HEALTH INSURANCE ASSOCIATION OF AMERICA. (1994). Source book of health insurance data 1993. Washington, D.C.

HELLINGER, FRED J. (1991). Forecasting the medical care costs of the HIV epidemic: 1991–1994. *Inquiry,* 28:213–225.

HELLINGER, FRED J. (1993). The lifetime cost of treating a person with HIV. *JAMA,* 270:474–478.

Intergovernmental AIDS Report. (1989). Non-medical funds for HIV patient care. George Washington Univ. 2:1–18.

KENT, CHRISTINA. (1995). Medicaid threatened by reform. *Am. Med. News,* 38:1,57.

LEVI, JEFFREY. (1994). The AIDS agenda and reform. *FOCUS,* 9:4–6.

MURPHY, TIMOTHY F. (1991). No time for AIDS backlash. *Hastings Center Report,* 21:7–11.

Nature. (1995). Task force turns on sponsor (DoE). 373:457–458.

O'BRIEN, CLAIRE. (1996). Malaria research suffering relative neglect, study claims. *Nature,* 383:286.

OLDHAM, JENNIFER. (1995). The economic cost of AIDS. *Los Angeles Times,* Oct. 13. v114, p D1, col 2.

PACKER, JUDY. (1991). 1990 Health Tab—666.2 billion. *Modern Health Care,* 21:3.

PALTIEL, DAVID. (1995). Risk in perspective: the human and economic costs of AIDS therapies. *Harvard Center For Risk Analysis,* 3(3), May.

PERKIN, JUDY. (1993). Facing the health policy challenge of HIV infection. *Natl. Forum,* LXXIII:45–47.

PETERSON, D. (1992). Viatical settlements: Living benefits for the insured, terminally ill patient. *The Bulletin (New York City Association of Life Underwriters),* April 1–4.

Public Health Reports. (1988). Report of the work group on patient care/health care needs. 103:80–87.

RON, ARAN, et al. (1988). New York City's health care crisis: AIDS, the poor, and limited resources. *JAMA,* 260:1453.

SCHUR, CLAUDIA, et al. (1994). Health insurance coverage of persons with HIV-related illness: Data from the ACSUS screener. *AIDS Cost and Services*

Utilization Survey (ACSUS) Report, No. 2, AHCPR Pub. No. 94-0009, Rockville, MD: Agency for Health Care Policy and Research.

SILVERMAN, MARVYN F. (1990). The social and political impact of the AIDS epidemic. *AIDS Patient Care*, 3:3–6.

SWARTZ, KATHERINE. (1994). Dynamics of people without health insurance. *JAMA*, 271:64–66.

VOELKER, REBECCA. (1996). Politicians, AIDS experts wage budget debate. *JAMA*, 275:1390–1391.

WEISSENSTEIN, ERIC. (1993). Health spending hits $838 billion in 1992. *Modern Healthcare*, 23:2–3.

WENNEKER, MARK B., et al. (1990). The association of payer with utilization of cardiac procedures in Massachusetts. *JAMA*, 264:1255–1260.

WINKENWERDER, WILLIAM, et al. (1989). Federal spending for illness caused by the human immunodeficiency virus. *N. Engl. J. Med.*, 320:1588–1603.

Legal Aspects of HIV/AIDS: A Review of Legislation and Court Decisions in the United States

The information in this chapter is general in nature and not intended as legal advice. Always seek legal counsel with regard to specific questions and situations in your state.

Many articles have been published in the United States on the legal aspects of the HIV/AIDS epidemic. A few of these articles are presented with permission.

INTRODUCTION

The history of the HIV/AIDS pandemic is one of remarkable scientific achievement. A search of the literature does not reveal a single life-threatening disease where so much has been learned in so short a time. AIDS was clinically described in June 1981, its epidemiology was known by 1983, the course of the disease was reported by early 1984, a blood test for anti-bodies to the virus was commercially available by June of 1985, and in late 1986, zidovudine was being used to treat people with AIDS. Since then, a series of new drugs, those used in the treatment of opportunistic infections and those used to inhibit HIV replication, have been FDA-approved and have slowed the advance of HIV disease progression to AIDS. However, 17 years into this modern-day plague, there is still **no cure** for those who are HIV-infected or have AIDS. Nor is there a clinical means of preventing the spread of infection. A vaccine is probably years away. In the meantime, it is estimated that 40,000 Americans became HIV-infected

in each year of the 1990s in the United States; **worldwide there are 9,000 new HIV infections each day!** And the number of new HIV infections is expected to increase as the pool of HIV-infected people becomes larger. The majority of these people do not know they are HIV-infected. There are between 650,000 and 900,000 HIV-infected people living in the United States. Beginning 1998, there were about 240,000 people living with AIDS in the United States.

A QUESTION OF RESPONSIBILITY

HIV/AIDS investigators say that the vast majority of HIV/AIDS cases could have been prevented. HIV infection is caused by a virus that in most cases is sexually transmitted, transmitted via blood or blood products, or by HIV-contaminated needles during injection drug use. Therein lies many of the legal and ethical problems that must be confronted. Bernard Dickens (1988) and others raise questions such as: Because people behave in a manner that causes their infection, should they be compelled to be tested and test results be made known to protect others? Should everyone be HIV-tested? What about surgical patients? If they refuse, does a surgeon have the right to refuse to perform surgery? What are the obligations to prevent health care workers from being HIV-infected or from infecting their patients? What about confidentiality—who is responsible for it? Should confidentiality be preserved at any cost? Who may inform a spouse that his or her sexual partner is HIV-infected? Is it the responsibility of society to pay the medical costs of those who have been educated about HIV/AIDS and become infected anyway? Who is responsible for HIV-infected children? Who pays the medical bills? What if the child gets the virus from a blood transfusion? Who is liable—the blood bank, the hospital, the doctor who ordered the transfusion? And who pays—the insurance company or the taxpayer?

Questions such as these have spawned more HIV/AIDS-related lawsuits than have been associated with any other disease. But many of the court decisions appear to be based on fear and stereotype rather than fact. For example,

---

POINT OF VIEW 17.1

RIGHT TO PRIVACY IN THE AIDS ERA

The AIDS epidemic has joined the threat of a lethal viral infection to the most intimate behaviors, those behaviors typically engaged in in private settings beyond the scrutiny of even the most pervasive surveillance. As such, every advanced democratic society has been required by the epidemic to confront the problem of how to protect the public health while respecting the right to privacy.

THE RIGHT TO DIE?

For the last 100 years, at least, some people feel that under the right to privacy, they should have a right to die—it's no one's business how they choose to die. But a problem occurs when a person choosing to die requires assistance. In a most recent challenge to the idea of assisted suicide, a Central Florida judge ruled in February 1997 that a totally disabled AIDS patient could receive the assistance from his physician. The physician would be held harmless. The judge said this person **"HAS A CONSTITUTIONAL RIGHT TO DECIDE TO TERMINATE HIS SUFFERING AND DETERMINE THE TIME AND MANNER OF HIS DEATH."** The Attorney General appealed the ruling. In July 1997 the Florida State Supreme Court reversed the lower court's decision. "It is clear that the public policy of this state as expressed by legislature is opposed to assisted suicide."

jurors have been influenced to find for the prosecution in cases against HIV-infected people who bit or spit on someone. These jury decisions occurred even though there has only been one documented case that showed a bite was a means of transmitting HIV. Brian McCormick (1992) cites a case in which the jurors were shown evidence labeled **"DO NOT TOUCH—AIDS EVIDENCE."** An appeals court refused to overturn a guilty verdict, ruling that the display was not discriminatory and did not prejudice the jury.

David Schulman (1988) in his article "Remembering Who We Are: AIDS and Law in a Time of Madness" wrote that

Fear and ignorance divide people. They pit infected against uninfected, threatening once again the web of relationships which enable us to understand each other as people. Law is rarely thought of as a healing social force, yet in the AIDS epidemic it can remind us of our highest ideals concerning ourselves, how we wish to treat others and would wish to be treated.

This chapter presents an overview of some major areas of legal concern in which the HIV/AIDS epidemic in the United States is having an impact. Where appropriate, legal concerns in foreign countries are presented.

———— **POINT OF VIEW 17.2** ————

HUMAN RIGHTS AND HIV/AIDS

Understanding the significance of human rights in relation to HIV/AIDS requires both a practical approach and an understanding of the principles at stake. Yet the response of many people to HIV disease and AIDS prevention is to call for strict measures: compulsory testing, obligatory screening of so-called risk groups, criminal punishment for spreading infection, and quarantine if at all possible. These are, after all, common responses to past plagues and epidemics.

Those who are better informed should explain why such measures are **ineffective, counter-productive**, and **harmful** in the global struggle against HIV/AIDS. It is unlikely that a time ever existed when strict quarantine for HIV infection could have worked; if it ever did, that time has long since passed. Global travel spreads HIV to the most remote communities. Testing and screening are expensive and also ineffective in the window period before antibodies show up. Further, these measures may alienate and stigmatize people whose confidence must be won if they are to be open to receiving information and counseling on behavior change. And behavior modification is essential for HIV/AIDS prevention.

HUMAN RIGHTS

Human rights occurred as a global movement after World War II. Concern for human rights has

since been expressed in the U.N. Universal Declaration on Human Rights (1948) and the International Covenants on Human Rights (1966). **These basic tenants to uphold human rights include the following**:

- the right to privacy, now held to extend rights to sexual privacy and one's own sexual orientation
- rights to health care, including preventive health education and self-protection
- rights to shelter and housing
- the right to protection from oppressive laws and policies of the State
- the right to due process of the law
- rights to employment without discrimination
- rights for children to have the basic information necessary for their protection, health, and life
- the right of women to dignity of their person
- rights of all persons without distinction to protection against vicious conduct and hate attacks

THE AIDS PARADOX

All of these and other rights are relevant to HIV/AIDS, although people do not always see this. The explanation involves a **paradox. Unless people combat the second epidemic of discrimination and retaliation against people who have (or are believed to have) HIV, the virus will continue to spread unchecked across the globe**. No other current strategy promises a chance of convincing people to avoid unprotected sex, to use condoms, to avoid injection drug use, or to use only sterile equipment. Only a full appreciation of the HIV/AIDS paradox will secure from governments, the health industry, the media, and the community in general the effective measures which offer a chance of providing protection to all.

THE RIGHT TO HEALTH: A BASIC RIGHT

When HIV/AIDS first arrived, the period of mandatory screening, quarantine, and criminal laws led to confrontation between health officials and human rights advocates. Now, however, many of-

ficials, led by the World Health Organization, recognize the AIDS paradox and the need to supplement public and health prevention measures with attention to human rights. We now realize that the right to health is, itself, a basic human right.

Understanding the global principles of human rights helps put strategies to combat HIV/AIDS and other STDs in a context of basic universal principles designed to defend and uphold the human dignity of each individual. Recognizing this, the International Commission of Jurists in Geneva has adopted the human rights of persons living with HIV/AIDS, human rights concerning sexual orientation, and human rights of drug-dependent persons and drug users as items for its program.

(Adapted from Justice Michael Kirby, 1996)

——— BOX 17.1 ———

LEGAL HIV/AIDS VIGNETTES—UNITED STATES

New Jersey—In July 1997, the New Jersey Supreme Court ruled in favor of allowing people to sue for emotional distress caused by fear of having contracted HIV, **even if no actual exposure took place**. The unanimous decision came in a case brought by a cleaning woman who had pricked her finger on an improperly discarded surgical instrument in a medical office 6 years ago. In 1993, she sued the three doctors who run the office for emotional distress, even though she continues to show no evidence of infection.

New Orleans, LA—In August 1996, a federal appeals court ruled against a widow who contended that an insurance company should have told her husband that his blood test was positive for the virus that causes AIDS.

The United States Court of Appeals for the Fifth Circuit affirmed a federal judge's decision that the insurer was not required to release the test results.

This woman, of Vienna, VA, sued the Jackson National Life Insurance Company of Mississippi after her husband died in 1991 from AIDS-related complications.

Her husband, a lawyer, took a blood test in 1988 as part of a routine examination required to increase his insurance coverage. The company advised him he was medically unsuitable, but did not tell him why until 9 days before his death.

In the meantime, his wife said she was exposed to repeated unprotected sex. Tests have shown that she was not infected.

In court papers, Jackson National Life Insurance Company argued that Mississippi law permitted it to withhold the results of the test. The couple lived in Mississippi when the husband became ill.

The lower court ruling affirmed by the appeals court said Mississippi law **did not** require an insurance company to disclose blood test results if the information was used only to determine coverage eligibility.

At least 21 states have laws similar to Mississippi's. A federal disclosure bill is pending before Congress.

Portland, OR—An AIDS-infected man under court order to abstain from sex for 5 years has been charged with attempted murder for previously having unprotected sex with a 17-year-old teenager. The man was sentenced, in December 1992, to 9.4 years in prison.

Pensacola, FL—An HIV-positive parolee who allegedly raped his former girlfriend and injected her with his blood because he wanted her to know what it was like to be HIV-infected, killed himself. He had a history of crime and drug abuse. (1992)

Jacksonville, FL—A 30-year-old gay male faces charges of first-degree attempted murder

——— **BOX 17.1** (*continued*) ———

and sexual battery after he was accused by a former lover of infecting him with the virus that causes AIDS. He is being held in lieu of $1 million bail. In a second case, same city, a 22-year-old man was arrested and charged with attempted second-degree murder and knowingly engaging in heterosexual intercourse while infected with HIV. He has been sentenced to 4.5 years in jail and to serve 13 years of probation during which time he must do 1,950 hours of community service. In a third case (January 1994), same city, a 42-year-old male was charged with attempted murder for engaging in unprotected heterosexual intercourse while knowing he was HIV-infected. To date, six women who had sex with him after he became HIV-positive have been contacted. The man now has AIDS. (Case is pending)

Jacksonville, FL—In April 1995, a 13-year-old girl was given a sentence of 5 years probation and extensive residential therapy for making prank phone calls to seven people who visited a medical center's emergency department over a weekend, and telling them they tested HIV-positive. The teenager got the names from her mother's computer screen when her mother was not looking (she had gone to work with her mother who worked at the medical center and was fired for breach of confidentiality after the incident). In one call, the teenager told a young woman that she tested pregnant and HIV-positive. This woman became hysterical and searched for a gun to kill herself. Her husband and father calmed her before she located the father's gun.

Gainesville, FL—During the arrest, ensuing scuffle, and deliberate bite, the man looked at the officer, smiled and said, "I have AIDS." The officer told the court about the anguish of not knowing for months whether he had been HIV-infected. He has since tested negative. (January 1995)

Miami, FL—A former exotic dancer was ordered to pay her ex-husband $18 million for knowingly infecting him with the AIDS virus. The award was described by an attorney as the largest U.S. civil verdict of its kind. (1993)

Miami, FL—An HIV-positive 32-year-old male was sentenced to five consecutive life terms in prison for kidnapping, sodomizing, and trying to kill three boys in 1991. It is the first case in the country of a rapist with HIV being convicted of attempted murder. Ending 1994, the boys remain HIV-negative.

Miami, FL—For 2 years, a Miami woman thought she was dying of AIDS. She would not let her children hug her. Friends would not visit. Family members refused to speak with her.

She gave legal custody of her three teenage children to her mother—who would wash her daughter's dirty dishes with bleach. Finally, she returned to her hometown in Georgia, where her attorney said she planned to kill herself when the disease made her seriously ill. But she never became seriously ill, because she was not HIV-infected!

A Circuit Court jury in September of 1994 ordered the state Department of Health and Rehabilitative Services to pay the Miami woman $390,000 for her pain and suffering after the agency misread her HIV test. The physician who prescribed anti-HIV medication was required to pay $250,000.

Philadelphia, PA—In October 1992, he was working for a top Philadelphia law firm, billing clients $150 an hour to handle complex commercial litigation and antitrust suits, just 3 years out of law school. By early 1993, the attorney identified in court papers as Scott Doe, Esq. had learned he was HIV-positive. He stated that his employer told him to find a new job within a year.

A bad situation grew worse when his employer learned Doe planned to sue for disability discrimination. An office administrator promised Doe "could kiss his legal career goodbye," Doe asserts, and he had to stand by as his belongings were packed. Doe said the firm's senior partner demanded his keys to the building and watched until he left. Doe sued for discrimination under the Americans with Disabilities Act and a similar Pennsylvania law. The federal law prohibits employers from discriminating against people with disabilities, including HIV disease and AIDS.

The case has haunting similarities to the fictional movie, "Philadelphia," in which a new law partner is drummed out of his prestigious firm after a colleague notices a tell-tale sign of AIDS. The case was settled out of court, in Scott Doe's favor, on October 31, 1994, for $1 million plus costs.

Oakland, CA—A man convicted of having unprotected sex with a 22-year-old woman in order to give her AIDS was sentenced to 3 years in prison. (1991)

Riverside, CA—In March 1995, a judge ordered 4 years in prison for a woman who hung up the telephone as her son tried to report that his little sister, who is now infected with the AIDS virus, was raped by their new stepfather. The Superior Court judge rejected the prosecution's recommendation for a year in jail and criticized the mother, who is also HIV-positive, for actions he said will kill the child.

"The court's primary concern and compassion is for a 7-year-old girl . . . who will not be with us long. All the good [the mother] did prior to that day . . . cannot balance the evil that was done to her child on that date."

Boston, MA—Wendy Doe (a pseudonym used in court papers) is a nurse struggling with AIDS. But she is also involved in a fight of another sort against the Lahey Clinic of Burlington, MA, where she worked for 6 years in the 1980s.

The clinic is contesting her claim for workers' compensation benefits based on her belief that she contracted AIDS while working for the clinic, and denies she was routinely exposed to blood.

Ms. Doe's lawyer says the clinic is lying about her exposure, and has filed a lawsuit in Middlesex Superior Court accusing the health care institution of behavior that "shocks the conscience and violates the law."

Rarely sick throughout her life, Ms. Doe's first symptoms appeared in 1986. But they were not diagnosed as AIDS until 1990, 4 years and nine doctors later, she says. The test results came 3 weeks before her wedding. (Case pending, 1993)

Muskegon, MI—A woman quarantined by Michigan officials after having unprotected sex without telling her partners she is infected with the virus that causes AIDS, agreed to stay home for a month. No charges were filed against the woman, 31, who has an IQ of 72 and lives in an adult foster home. The case will be reviewed monthly.

Boston, MA—The U.S. government refused to appeal a $3.8 million judgment awarded to an HIV-infected marine whose wife and son died of AIDS after she received HIV-tainted blood at a Navy hospital.

The ruling ended a 5-year court battle for the Marine, who is hospitalized and sought the money for his 8-year-old daughter.

The Marine charged in his lawsuit that doctors at the Long Beach, CA, Naval Hospital botched his wife's pregnancy in 1981 by failing to give her a cesarean section. She was 2 weeks late delivering the baby and required a blood transfusion. The blood was infected with HIV.

The infant was stillborn. The couple had another son, who died of AIDS at age 13 months. His wife died of AIDS in 1987.

The U.S. District Court judge ruled in 1991 that if a cesarean section had been performed in time, a transfusion would not have been necessary.

Denver, CO—Jurors, who did not know a woman had died the day before, ordered a blood bank to pay her $6.6 million for providing a transfusion tainted with the virus that causes AIDS. Her husband was awarded $1.5 million for loss of companionship.

The woman had contracted AIDS from a 1983 transfusion that came from United Blood Services of Albuquerque, NM. She died in a hospital as her attorney presented closing arguments in her case. (Case is on appeal, 1992)

Portland, OR—The American Red Cross settled out of court on a $10 million lawsuit. A man claimed he received HIV in blood supplied by the Red Cross. (1993)

San Diego, CA—A woman who became HIV-positive after being injecting with a syringe that had been used on an AIDS patient in a hospital mix-up 2 years ago has settled her lawsuit against the hospital for $1 million—receiving $600,000 at the time of the settlement and $2,300 a month for life. (1991)

San Francisco, CA—The California Supreme Court let stand a ruling that says convicted prostitutes and their customers must submit to HIV tests. The court declined to review a state appeals court ruling upholding the constitutionality of a 1988 law. A San Francisco public defender challenged the law on behalf of 11 prostitutes, who claimed it unfairly singled them out and subjected them to privacy violations. A state appeals court upheld the law, saying that the prostitutes' constitutional rights were outweighed by the danger to society of spreading HIV through multiple sex partners. (1990)

Charleston, WV—The state Supreme Court upheld a $1.9 million award to a security guard who sued a hospital after being bitten by a person infected with the virus that causes AIDS. (1991)

Jacksonville, FL—In 1991, a Jacksonville man who is HIV-infected was awarded $59,000 by a jury that found he was turned away from a homeless shelter because of his disease. His lawsuit was the first major test of a 1988 Florida law that forbids discrimination against people who have AIDS or the virus that causes AIDS.

Orlando, FL—In December 1992, a 21-year-old woman with AIDS was arrested for the attempted murder of her 2-year-old daughter via multiple bites. The woman said she bit the child to infect her to prevent her grandmother from caring for her. The girl is now in the custody of state health officials.

Texas—In July 1992, a mid-level appeals court **affirmed** the conviction and 99-year or life, whichever is longer, sentence of a man who has

AIDS and spit on a prison guard. The man was charged with attempted murder. Ruth Harlow, staff attorney for ACLU AIDS Project said, "his sentence is to die in prison for the crime of spitting." During the trial, Texas prosecutors relied on the testimony of two "expert" witnesses to win a conviction. One witness has made a career of testifying against litigants who are gay or who are associated with AIDS. During the trial, he (erroneously) testified that not only could AIDS be transmitted by spitting, but he also said that it could be transmitted by mosquitoes and through the air. The Texas Court of Appeals has been petitioned to reverse the lower court decision. (Outcome pending)

Martin, TN—In 1991, when her fiancee collapsed from a heart attack, a woman rushed desperately to a stranger and pleaded for help. She didn't say the dying man had AIDS. Because the woman knew the man had AIDS, she faced felony charges for not warning rescuers. The officer who administered mouth-to-mouth resuscitation fears he was infected. The woman, an unemployed nursing assistant, was jailed for 5 days. She was freed on $2,500 bond. A county grand jury later found her innocent of intentional wrongdoing.

Wilmington, DE—In 1988, the state's Attorney General ordered one of the state's largest pediatric institutions to recind a controversial policy of not treating AIDS patients.

The order targeted a 90-bed pediatric hospital. The Attorney General stated that the hospital's policy violated the state's public accommodation policy.

New York City, NY—In February 1994, a data supervisor at the New York City Health Department was charged with changing the computerized result of an AIDS test from positive to negative. The supervisor knew the person whose test result he had changed.

The data supervisor's lawyer said: "He was trying to do a good deed. It was a matter of trying to protect the confidentiality of a patient or a testee." (Trial is pending.)

Albany, NY—In July 1992, Court of Claims judge ordered the state to pay $5.4 million to a nurse and her husband. She became HIV-infected after being stuck with a needle used on an HIV-infected prisoner who became uncontrollable. She had sued the state for $10 million, claiming that the guards should have helped control the inmate. The state claimed the guards were under no legal obligation to help. The state attorney said the state was liable and willing to pay $3 million

but would appeal the remaining $2.4 million as excessive. (Outcome pending)

Bridgeport, CT—A mistrial was declared in the case of a man who beat his girlfriend to death with a hammer. The judge learned during the trial that the man demonstrated AIDS dementia. A competency examination was ordered. (Case pending, 1993)

Salt Lake City, UT—Two women with AIDS have filed suit in July 1993 to overturn a Utah law that bars those with the disease from marrying. Utah is unique in having such a law. The women are requesting immediate action on their suit. They feared that their families could lose financial benefits if they died before the law was revoked because their marriages could be ruled invalid. (Case pending)

Chicago, IL—Ruling for the first time that a dentist's office is a public accommodation and is therefore subject to the Illinois Human Rights Act, the chief judge of the State of Illinois Human Rights Commission decided that a Chicago dentist broke the law in 1987 by refusing to continue treatment of a long-time patient solely because the patient disclosed that he was HIV-positive. In the October 1994 ruling, the chief administrative law judge concluded that the plaintiff is handicapped due to his HIV status (a precedent in Illinois law) under the Americans with Disabilities Act. Under the Act, a dental office is a place of public accommodation and the dentist acted in a discriminatory fashion. The judge awarded the patient $8,048, primarily for the emotional damages suffered due to discriminatory treatment.

In 1992, 1993, and 1994, a number of insurance companies in the United States attempted to reduce coverage after a person became HIV-infected or was diagnosed with AIDS. One case is cited herein—it aptly represents at least 50 such cases that have already been litigated.

St. Paul, MN—The health plan of Local 110 of the International Brotherhood of Electrical Workers in St. Paul and the electrical contractors' association agreed to lift a $50,000 ceiling on payments for AIDS-related diseases. The health plan provided insurance up to $500,000 for other catastrophic conditions.

Settling charges that it had discriminated against members with AIDS, the union welfare fund also agreed to pay $100,000 to the estate of a 36-year-old construction worker who died in November 1992. **This was the first large award in a case involving an AIDS-related denial of**

health insurance under the Americans with Disabilities Act. (1993)

These vignettes cover selected episodes that were written up in the newspapers in 13 states. Note that although the events vary, they are all concerned with who is or was responsible for HIV transmission. There are countless incidents and legal cases of HIV/AIDS-related events in the United States. Most likely there are countless similar legal cases occurring in other countries.

By the end of 1995, there were over 450 arrests made against persons who deliberately attempted to use their HIV infection as a weapon against (to harm) others. Charges range from first- to third-degree felony depending on the state. For example, North Dakota statutes provide remedies for dealing with HIV-infected individuals who may be putting the health of others at risk. Individuals violating 12.1-20-17 are guilty of a first-degree felony which carries a sentence of 20 years and/or a $10,000 fine. Individuals violating 23-07.4-01 may be ordered by the state health officer to stop the activity which could be putting others at risk.

In contrast, in the state of Florida the same individual would be guilty of a third-degree felony statute 796.08, 5 which calls for up to 1 year in jail. Numerous charges have also been filed against workers' unions and insurance companies for discrimination against persons with HIV diseases.

POINT OF INFORMATION 17.1

DNA AND AMINO ACID SEQUENCING OF HIV REVERSE TRANSCRIPTASE CONVICTS RAPIST: STOCKHOLM DISTRICT COURT

The male, a Swedish injection drug user, was HIV-positive. The woman he raped tested HIV-positive several weeks after the rape. Much of the trial evidence that led to his conviction was based on direct DNA sequence analysis of their HIVs. His and her viruses were "highly DNA homologous." Further, amino acid analysis of both individuals' HIV-produced reverse transcriptase were identical at six positions. Control samples taken from injection drug users and gay males in the same geographical region showed no more than two of the six amino acids to be similar.

This is believed to be the first case ever where DNA and amino acid sequencing of HIV was used to help in a conviction (Albert et al., 1993).

Over 25 states now have laws on the books making it a misdemeanor or felony for an HIV-positive person to spread HIV through methods ranging from sexual contact to the exposure of blood. Such laws in Louisiana carry a maximum punishment of a $5,000 file and 10 years in prison.

FIRST HIV/AIDS LEGISLATION: SWEDEN

Sweden was the first country to introduce legislation on AIDS. Passed on March 8, 1983, regulations made mandatory the reporting of confirmed and suspected AIDS cases to the National Bacteriological Laboratory. Sweden also adopted the first legislation dealing with protection against HIV transmission in the health care environment. In March 1985, Sweden's National Board of Occupational Safety and Health issued general recommendations concerning protection against AIDS in the course of the care and administration of patients along with highly detailed measures to be taken in work entailing a risk of infection with HIV.

As of September 1988, approximately 70 countries had introduced some form of legislation concerning AIDS and HIV infection, a significant number of which addressed specific issues concerning health care workers (HCWs). The following countries, among others, have addressed hospitals or HCWs in their legislation: Australia (New South Wales), Austria, Belgium, Brazil, Canada (Alberta), Chile, Chi-na, Dominican Republic, Greece, Guatemala, Indonesia, Luxembourg, Malta, Norway, Pana-ma, Peru, Rwanda, South Africa, Spain, Sweden, Switzerland, and Turkey (Fluss et al., 1989).

LEGAL FRAMEWORK

The Congress of the United States has demonstrated its concern about the HIV/AIDS epidemic by approving the expenditure of billions of dollars for educational programs, research, and medical care. But most of the legislative activity surrounding the issue of HIV/AIDS has been at the state level. Since 1987, state legislators have enacted over 200 bills addressing HIV/AIDS-related issues such as testing, blood bank screening, confidentiality, housing, insurance, prisons, informed consent, counseling, and medication programs (Rothstein, 1989).

Lawrence O. Gostin, J.D. (Juris Doctorate) has written a series of papers discussing legislative and regulatory policies regarding HIV/AIDS in the United States (Figure 17-1).

In his report "Public Health Strategies for Confronting AIDS," Gostin presents evidence that, although state legislatures have responded well to health care and research, they have also been susceptible to attitudes that the primary modes of HIV transmission are immoral, even criminal. He says that both federal and state statutes, by placing special emphasis on warning against extramarital intercourse and drug use, choose to ignore that these behaviors have historically persisted. He writes that there is political pressure on legislators to use the coercive powers of the state to deal with the HIV/AIDS epidemic. And legislation for compulsory HIV screening, quarantine, and criminalization for behavior that spreads HIV has proceeded in some states without evidence that it would be effective.

In a follow-up 1989 article, "The Politics of AIDS: Compulsory State Powers, Public Health and Civil Liberties," Gostin reviews the various risks involved in the transmission of HIV and concludes that the risk of transmission from biting, spitting, or splattering blood is negligible. The risk of sexual transmission is much greater. Mr. Gostin is opposed to coercive or compulsory public health measures because they are likely to be ineffective and violate human rights. He reviews various suggestions, such as isolation of the infected in AIDS care facilities, modified isolation based on behavior, and criminalization of HIV transmission, all of which he thinks are inappropriate. He urges focused education, testing, counseling, and treatment for drug dependency.

In 1990, Gostin examined public policy on AIDS. **His exceptional two-part article reviews AIDS-related litigation and Human Rights Commission decisions in the United States since 1981 (Gostin, 1990a).**

Part I

Gostin reports in his "AIDS Litigation Project, Part I," that sharp differences in perception of public health, ethics, and civil liberties have created the largest body of legal cases attributable to a single disease in the history of American jurisprudence. He reviews the areas of law that encompass 469 cases (cited in the bibliography), and of over 1,000 cases decided or pending, and notes that they show conflicts of values that will likely require legislative and policy resolution. But he also shows that there has been significant progress in addressing HIV/AIDS in school and the workplace. The

FIGURE 17-1 Photograph of Lawrence O. Gostin, J.D.

courts have affirmed that a child with HIV/ AIDS has a right to public education, and in most cases this has meant attendance in his or her usual classroom. Similarly, the right of employees with HIV/ AIDS to remain on the job has been repeatedly upheld. In both areas, reasonable accommodations are made for the affected individual.

Most of the cases Gostin cites have escaped the attention of the public health community. They contain important information for everyone—health workers, blood bankers, policymakers, attorneys, legislators, and perhaps most of all, people with HIV/AIDS and people at risk.

In presenting legal and policy controversies in light of public health imperatives, Gostin's articles are significant for their potential to prevent enactment of unfounded HIV/AIDS legislation and to promote freedom from discrimination.

In Part I of the review, Gostin also examines court and Human Rights Commission decisions since the start of the AIDS epidemic in 14 subject areas. These include AIDS education, testing, criminal law, state regulation of bathhouses, private tort actions, confidentiality, and AIDS in prison populations.

Perhaps the most valuable lessons in Part I may be found in examples of sound and unsound public health policies and their consequences. Reasonable policy based on scientific fact promotes the public health, as is demonstrated by laws that require the testing of blood products, semen, and donated organs. In most cases, these laws followed, rather than preceded, the standard of practice. Similarly, laws that require AIDS education clearly serve the best interests of the public.

Unscientific or irrational policy, on the other hand, may harm the public health. For example, restrictions on HIV/AIDS educational content inhibit the ability of organizations to produce accurate and effective programs; as a result, more people may become infected. Laws and policies that compromise confidentiality may jeopardize efforts to prevent infection and provide early intervention to those infected by discouraging them from seeking care (Sherer, 1990).

Gostin addresses the futility of measures to prevent immigration and free travel of people with HIV/AIDS. Such measures are discriminatory and have no convincing public health rationale (Duckett et al., 1989; Gilmore et al., 1989). The Immigration and Naturalization Service can authorize HIV-antibody testing on visitors to the United States or, through the Justice Department, bar their entry. This regulation was issued by the Justice Department in 1988. It was temporarily lifted in 1990 to permit HIV/AIDS-infected people to attend the Sixth International Conference on AIDS. Because the law is still in effect, sponsors for the Eighth International Conference on AIDS (May 24–29, 1992) moved it from the United States to Amsterdam.

Health workers may take particular interest in the section on private tort actions that involve health professionals. One clear lesson from this section is the imperative for all health workers, physicians in particular, to learn as much as possible about HIV/AIDS. Physicians who order HIV-antibody tests without patient consent or who misdiagnose or improperly treat HIV-related disease may put themselves at risk for liability.

Part II

In Gostin's "The AIDS Litigation Project, Part II: Discrimination" (1990b), he reports on the most controversial area of human rights. He points out that public health and medical organizations that have issued HIV/AIDS papers have unanimously condemned discrimination as unjust and detrimental to public health. Case identification (testing, reporting, and partner notification) is of growing importance as the benefits of early intervention become clearer. Gostin looks at the 149 cases of discrimination reported by municipal and federal agencies and reviews the major areas of discrimination litigation: education, employment, housing, insurance, and health care. The bibliography includes citations to the discrimination cases. Gostin's report should be read with care as it explains why HIV/AIDS patients are considered handicapped even though HIV infection leads to an infectious, contagious disease. That is, the mental picture that one holds of a handicapped person (person living with disabilities, PLWD) is usually different from the legal definition. Take a moment. Think of the words **handicap** and **disability**. Form a mental image of a disabled or handicapped person. In a compelling review of these cases, Gostin concludes that there has been a critical mass of discriminatory behavior that warrants government action in the form of comprehensive federal antidiscrimination legislation. These cases underscore the imperatives of confidentiality and full, written, informed consent prior to HIV-antibody testing.

In order to better understand Gostin's review of HIV/AIDS discrimination cases, it should be understood that people with HIV/AIDS have been disabled by the disease. Because of the disability imposed on those who have HIV disease and AIDS, they are said to be handicapped. As such, they receive the civil protection of the federal statutes regarding discrimination against the handicapped.

You are encouraged to read the excellent review of **"Discrimination on the Basis of Handicap" (Box 17.2)** for a better understanding of the key statutory language of the federal legislation on handicap, clarification of who is to be considered a handicapped or disabled person, and who qualifies for federal protection from discrimination under the New Americans with Disabilities Act of 1990.

The Americans with Disabilities Act of 1990

The Americans with Disabilities Act (ADA) addresses the concern that society has been inclined to segregate individuals with disabilities. The ADA is a mandate to eliminate discrimination against those with physical and mental disabilities in **all** aspects of their lives. An employer, program, or health care provider must evaluate each person's ability to perform a given task and make **reasonable** accommodations that would allow the disabled person to perform.

Nondiscrimination obligation can be found in Section 504 of the Vocational Rehabilitation Act passed in 1973. The ADA is modeled after Section 504 and, for the most part, the difference between Section 504 and the ADA is a change in terminology from "otherwise qualified handicapped individual" to "otherwise qualified individual with a disability."

Every court case deciding on the HIV/AIDS discrimination issue has found that HIV-positive individuals are protected as handicapped under Section 504. Section 504 and the ADA protect not only the people with actual impairments, but also those with a past history of an impairment and those **perceived by others** as being impaired, despite the fact that the individual has no past or present impairment at all (Palma, 1992). To demonstrate the extent of coverage in Section 504, Palma cites a recent AIDS discrimination case against Beth Israel Hospital. A resident teaching M.D. of a hospital refused to perform surgery on an HIV-infected patient. The court held that because the hospital received Medicare and Medicaid funds for services rendered, the hospital was liable under Section 504. However, the court dismissed the claim against the physician because he could not receive federal funds as a resident teaching M.D. The ADA eliminates such exclusions.

Discrimination Laws Have Social Limits— Discrimination laws provide a legal foundation for the rights of people with HIV infection and AIDS, but this foundation is not really adequate to ensure that they receive the humane treatment to which everyone is entitled as a basic human right. The statutes provide limited remedies, and their administration frequently takes more time than people with HIV infection or AIDS can afford. This means that the ethical issues must take precedence if true justice is to be done.

First Federal ADA Case—The first federal case of HIV/AIDS discrimination since the implementation of the ADA was filed against Westchester County Medical Center, Valhalla, New York in April 1992. According to an opinion issued by Department of Health and Human Services administrative law judge, Westchester did discriminate against a pharmacy job applicant, an HIV-infected pharmacist, under the Rehabilitation Act of 1973, and sanctioned the hospital from receiving Medicare and Medicaid payments until it "complies" with the act. The pharmacist was awarded $30,000 and the job without restrictions.

In defense, the hospital states that the pharmacist stated on his application that he had no infectious conditions. But the hospital learned— because the applicant was being treated at the facility—that he was HIV-positive. Following a policy the hospital has had in place for years barring employees with infectious diseases from preparing intravenous solutions, the hospital offered him a position with the provision that he could not prepare IVs. The applicant took action against the hospital through state and federal agencies, charging that he was discriminated against based on his HIV status.

The *Westchester* case illustrates the challenges that confront hospitals in dealing with HIV-positive health care workers, and the difficulties they face in trying to **balance the protection of patients with the rights of workers**. A spokesman contends that the hospital acted reasonably and fairly. "It's ridiculous to take what has always been a fundamental right of hospitals in this country and carelessly cast it aside based on someone's handicapped status." The spokesman also said that the hospital is one of 12 AIDS management centers in New York and acts as a clearinghouse for all AIDS activity in the surrounding counties. He adds that the center has a full-service dental clinic for HIV-positive patients, one of the few in the nation. "We know how difficult it is to cope with this disease. We know some of the social stigmas attached to it; we know how it is transmitted. Further, the applicant was offered a job with the same rate of pay and opportunities for advancement that anyone else in the pharmacy would have (Lumsdon, 1992).

On January 11, 1993, Westchester County Medical Center agreed to hire the HIV-infected pharmacist without restriction. Failure to comply would have cost the hospital $107 million in Medicaid and Medicare reimbursement.

What is your initial reaction to this situation? If you were the presiding hospital officer, how might you decide—was the applicant discriminated against? Would you have employed him because of federal/state pressures? Why?

ADA as Civil Rights Legislation—The ADA is the most sweeping piece of civil rights legislation since 1964. The goal is to remove barriers to employment, shopping, travel, and entertainment for the nation's 43 million disabled people.

The guidelines cover more than 5 million public facilities. Companies have begun making changes to their premises. They must do so as long as the changes can be done without excessive expense. The act is estimated to cost business as much as $2 billion.

ADA Highlights, First Phase, which began on January 26, 1992 include the following:

• Public accommodations may not discriminate on the basis of disability.
• Physical barriers in existing facilities must be removed if possible. If not, other methods of providing services must be offered. Alterations to existing facilities must be accessible.
• Public transit systems must provide comparable paratransit, such as vans, to people who cannot use a fixed-route bus service. New busses and rail vehicles must be accessible.

ADA Access Time Line—
• **January 26, 1992**: Organizations must take steps to assure that people with disabilities have access to existing public areas so long as such accommodations would not pose an unreasonable hardship. New buildings and renovations undertaken after this date must meet more stringent guidelines. Physicians may be sued for refusal to treat patients solely because of disability.
• **July 26, 1992**: Employers with 25 or more people on the payroll must make sure that persons with disabilities are not discriminated against in any employment practice. Takes effect July 26, 1994, for companies with 15 or more employees; those with fewer than 15 are exempt.
• **July 26, 1993**: Requires that states provide unrestricted telephone service for individuals who use telecommunications devices for the deaf.
• **July 26, 1995**: Providers of commuter rail transportation must have at least one passenger car per train readily accessible to individuals with disabilities.

The ADA will eventually apply to **all** employers with 15 or more employees. It will impact nearly every local government. For large cities, the impact began in January 1992; for smaller towns, 1994. ADA will underscore the rights of the HIV-infected worker by utilizing the same criteria for coverage that is currently used in Section 504 of the 1973 Vocational Rehabilitation Act. But ADA goes beyond existing legislation and strengthens the rights of HIV-infected employees in several ways. First, it is the specific intent of Congress to include HIV/AIDS as a handicap covered by ADA. Second, the legislation provides concrete examples of reasonable accommodation. Third, with the exception of drug testing, ADA will also prohibit employers from using pre-employment medical examinations as a screening device. Employers will still be able to impose job-related physical examinations, but only after they have extended job offers to applicants. Moreover, HIV-infected people will benefit from the heightened stature of ADA in that its implementation and monitoring will now fall under the auspices of the Equal Employment Opportunity Commission (Slack, 1991). Key statutory language of ADA 1990 can be found in Box 17.2.

Legal Rights and Obligations

In an attempt to place legal rights and obligations during this HIV/AIDS epidemic in perspective, Bernard M. Dickens provides us with some legal insight in his report "Legal Rights and Duties in the AIDS Epidemic" (1988). In this report, Dickens reviews the rights of infected individuals with regard to testing, treatment, and confidentiality, and looks at discrimination in access to health care, employment, housing, education, and insurance. He outlines the obligation an infected person has to prevent transmission of the virus, including liability for contaminated blood. The author also considers the rights of the uninfected to protection, the rights and duties of health professionals and health authorities, and international legal developments outside the United States. This is a must-read article if you are interested in legal rights and obligations.

Confidentiality Laws

The word **confidential**, according to Webster's dictionary, means **private or secret, to entrust (information) with confidence**. In medicine this means that a patient's records, including name, address, phone number, medical history, and so on must be kept confidential. This means the results of an HIV test may not be released without the patient's written consent or a court order. All states have laws on the books to protect medical and public health records from unauthorized disclosure. But some believe that these laws are inadequate and vulnerable to court orders for the release of

---

——— **BOX 17.2** ———

"DISCRIMINATION ON THE BASIS OF HANDICAP"

I. FEDERAL STATUTES REGARDING HANDICAPPED DISCRIMINATION

Congress has enacted two federal laws designed to eliminate discrimination on the basis of handicap. These two laws are known as the Rehabilitation Act of 1973 and the Americans with Disabilities Act of 1990. As its name indicates, the Rehabilitation Act of 1973 has been in effect for 28 years. The Americans with Disabilities Act of 1990 did not become effective until July 26, 1992. Those provisions of each Act which are of particular interest to colleges and universities are set out below.

A. The Rehabilitation Act of 1973

Section 504 of The Rehabilitation Act of 1973, 29 U.S.C. Sec. 794, was designed to eliminate dis-

crimination on the basis of handicap in any program or activity receiving financial assistance from the federal government. Because most colleges and universities receive some form of financial assistance from the federal government—whether in the form of grants, loans, or contracts—most colleges and universities have been subject to the provisions of the Rehabilitation Act of 1973.

1. The Key Statutory Language

The key language of Section 504 reads as follows:

> No otherwise qualified individual with
> handicaps . . shall, solely by reason of
> her or his handicap, be excluded from

the participation in, be denied the benefits of, or be subjected to discrimination under any program or activity receiving federal financial assistance . . .

Section 504, thus, protects otherwise qualified handicapped persons from discrimination based on their handicapped status.

2. Who Is an "Individual with Handicaps"?

An individual with handicaps is any person who has a physical or mental impairment which substantially limits one or more of the person's major life activities. Any person who has a record of having such a physical or mental impairment or who merely is regarded as having such an impairment is also protected by the statute as a handicapped person. 29 U.S.C. Sec. 706(8).

a. What Is a "Physical or Mental Impairment"?

A physical impairment is any physical condition or disorder which affects a major system of the body. The term "physical impairment" includes orthopedic, visual, speech, and hearing impairments, cerebral palsy, epilepsy, muscular dystrophy, multiple sclerosis, cancer, heart disease, and diabetes. A mental impairment includes disorders such as mental retardation, emotional or mental illness, and specific learning disabilities. 45 C.F.R. Sec. 104.3.

b. What Is Meant by "Substantially Limits"?

A determination as to whether a person is "substantially limited" by his or her handicapping condition depends upon the nature and severity of the condition. Courts, for example, have held that fear of heights and left-handedness do not qualify persons as "handicapped" because such conditions do not substantially limit major life activities.

c. What Is a "Major Life Activity"?

A major life activity means a function such as caring for one's self, performing manual tasks, walking, seeing, hearing, speaking, breathing, learning, and working. 45 C.F.R. Sec. 104.3.

d. Who Has a "Record" of Having an Impairment?

A person will be protected by Section 504 as a handicapped individual if the person has a history of, or has been formally classified as having, a physical or mental impairment which substantially limits one or more major life activities.

e. Who Is Merely "Regarded" as Having an Impairment?

A person will be protected by Section 504 as a handicapped individual **even if the person has no handicap** if the person is perceived and treated by others as a person with a physical or mental impairment which substantially limits one or more major life activities.

3. Who Is an "Otherwise Qualified" Individual with Handicaps?

A person is not entitled to protection under Section 504 just because the person has a handicap; the person also must be "otherwise qualified" to perform the essential requirements of the job or program in question in spite of the handicap. In the employment context, an otherwise qualified handicapped person is a person who, **with reasonable accommodation**, is able to perform the essential functions of the job in question. In the student context, an otherwise qualified handicapped person is a person who, in spite of his or her handicap, is able to meet the academic and technical standards for admission to and participation in his or her institution's educational programs. 45 C.F.R. Sec. 104.3.

a. What Is "Reasonable Accommodation"?

Reasonable accommodation is a concept that is central to handicap law. It essentially requires that institutions adopt a reasonable and flexible attitude toward handicapped applicants, employees, and students. Reasonable accommodation does **not** require that institutions undertake accommodations which fundamentally alter the nature of their academic programs, which lower or substantially modify their academic standards, which result in safety risks to the handicapped individual or others, or which impose undue administrative or financial burdens on the institution.

In the employment context, reasonable accommodation might entail making facilities

——————— **BOX 17.2** (*continued*) ———————

readily accessible to and usable by handicapped employees, restructuring jobs to eliminate duties that are peripheral to the position in question but which eliminate handicapped persons, permitting part-time or modified work schedules, or purchasing specially modified equipment. In the student context, reasonable accommodation might entail modifying building access routes to permit entrance by wheelchair, permitting light course loads or additional time to complete exams, or providing readers, interpreters, or special tutors.

b. Court Decisions Interpreting the "Otherwise Qualified" Standard

(1) Tuberculosis-Infected Teacher

A federal court held that a schoolteacher with tuberculosis was "otherwise qualified" to remain on the job, since the court concluded that she posed no threat of transmitting tuberculosis to her students. *School Board of Nassau County v. Arline*, 692 F. Supp. 1286 (1988).

(2) HIV-Infected Teacher

A federal court held that an elementary schoolteacher with AIDS was "otherwise qualified" to remain on the job, since the court concluded that the teacher posed no threat of transmitting HIV to his students. *Chalk v. U.S. District Court*, 840 F.2d 701 (9th Cir. 1988).

(3) Hearing-Impaired Nursing Student

The U.S. Supreme Court held that a hearing-impaired nursing student was **not** "otherwise qualified" to perform the essential aspects of a nursing program because of concerns about patient safety. With a hearing aid, the student could hear gross sounds occurring in the listening environment. However, to understand speech, she relied on lip-reading. The student proposed that she be given individual faculty supervision when attending patients directly and that certain required courses be dispensed with altogether since it was unnecessary that she be trained to undertake all of the tasks a registered nurse is licensed to perform. The Supreme Court held that Section 504 does not require colleges and universities to make fundamental alterations in their academic programs or to lower or substantially modify their academic standards in order to accommodate a handicapped individual. *Southeastern Community College v. Davis*, 442 U.S. 397 (1979).

(4) Hand-Function-Impaired PT Student

A Texas court held that a physical therapy student with deformed fingers was **not** "otherwise qualified" because he could not perform the manipulations required for graduation from the physical therapy program. *Samelson v. Texas Woman's University*, (not reported) (S.D. Tex. 1989).

4. Can an Institution Find Out if an Individual Has Handicaps?

a. Employment Context

As a general rule, the regulations do not permit an institution to make a pre-employment inquiry as to whether an applicant for employment is handicapped or to conduct a pre-employment medical examination. An employer may, however, describe the functions of an open position and ask if the applicant is able to perform those functions. For example, an employer may not ask if an applicant is visually impaired, but may ask if the applicant holds a current driver's license—if a license is a necessary qualification for the position in question. In addition, an employer may condition an offer of employment on the results of a medical examination to be conducted after the offer is extended but before the first day of work, **if but only if,** (**1**) such an examination is administered to all entering employees, (**2**) the results are used in accordance with the laws on handicapped discrimination (which means that the results cannot be used to deny employment unless the revealed conditions indicate that the person is not "otherwise qualified") and (**3**) the results are treated on a confidential basis. 45 C.F.R. Sec. 104.14.

b. Student Context

As a general rule, the regulations also do not permit an institution to make a preadmission inquiry as to whether a prospective student is an individual with handicaps. **After** admission, however, an institution may inquire on a confidential basis as to whether a newly admitted student has handicaps that may require accom-modation. 45 C.F.R. Sec. 104.42.

B. The Americans with Disabilities Act of 1990

The Americans with Disabilities Act of 1990, 42 U.S.C. Sec. 12101 et seq., extends the reach of federal protection for people who are disabled. Whereas the Rehabilitation Act of 1973 only applies to federal contractors and programs and activities receiving federal financial assistance, the Americans with Disabilities Act (popularly known as the ADA) will eventually apply to all private employers with 15 or more employees. Colleges and universities already in compliance with Section 504 of the Rehabilitation Act of 1973 will need be make sure that they will also be in compliance with the ADA.

1. The Key Statutory Language

The key language of the ADA is contained in Section 12112 which reads as follows:

> No covered entity shall discriminate against a qualified individual with a disability because of the disability of such individual in regard to job application procedures, the hiring, advancement, or discharge of employees, employee compensation, job training, and other terms, conditions, and privileges of employment.

Section 12132 similarly prohibits public entities from discriminating against qualified individuals with a disability. Section 12182 prohibits discrimination on the basis of disability in the full and equal enjoyment of places of public accommodation such as schools, hospitals, banks, and gas stations.

2. Who Is an Individual with a "Disability"?

The ADA's definition of an individual with a "disability" is almost identical to the Rehabili-tation Act's definition of an "individual with handicaps." The term "disability" is used, however, instead of the term "handicap." An individual with a disability is an individual who has a physical or mental impairment that substantially limits one or more of the major life activities of the individual. An individual with a record of such an impairment and an individual merely regarded as having such as impairment are also considered to be individuals with a disability.

3. Who Is a "Qualified Individual with a Disability"?

Under the ADA, a "qualified individual with a disability" is an individual with a disability who, with or without reasonable accommodation, can perform the essential functions of the employment position that such individual holds or desires. "Reasonable accommodation" under the

ADA is defined in substantially the same way that it is defined under the Rehabilitation Act.

4. Can an Institution Find Out if an Individual Has a Disability?

Under the ADA, an employer will not be permitted to use qualification standards, employment tests, or other selection criteria that screen out or tend to screen out an individual with a disability or a class of individuals with disabilities unless the standard, test, or other selection criteria is shown to be job-related for the position in question and consistent with business necessity. As a general rule, an employer will neither be permitted to make pre-employment inquiries as to whether an applicant for employment has a disability or to conduct pre-employment medical examinations. An employer may, however, describe the functions of an open position and ask if the applicant is able to perform those functions. In addition, an employer may condition an offer of employment on the results of a medical examination to be conducted after the offer is extended but before the first day of work, **if but only if**, (**a**) such an examination is administered to all entering employees in the same job category, (**b**) the results are treated on a confidential basis, and (**c**) the results are used only in a manner consistent with the provisions of the ADA. This means that an employer may withdraw an offer of employment on the basis of medical examination results only if the revealed conditions are job-related, consistent with business necessity, and no reasonable accommodation is possible. 42 U.S.C. Sec. 12112(c).

II. CONTAGIOUS DISEASES AND FEDERAL LAW

A. Specific Statutory Provisions

1. Individuals with a "Currently Contagious Disease"—The Rehabilitation Act of 1973

In 1986, the Rehabilitation Act was amended. The amended statute specifically provides that, in the employment context, the definition of an "individual with handicaps" does **not** include an individual who has a currently contagious disease and who, by reason of such disease or infection, would constitute **a direct threat to the health or safety of other individuals** or who, by reason of the currently contagious disease or infection, is unable to perform the duties of the job. 29 U.S.C. Sec. 706(8) (C). Thus, in cir-

————— **BOX 17.2** (*continued*) —————

cumstances where a person with a currently contagious disease poses a direct threat to others, the infected person will not be deemed to be "handicapped" within the meaning of the statute and will not be entitled to Section 504's protection.

2. Individuals Who Pose a "Direct Threat"— The Americans with Disabilities Act

Under the ADA, an employer will be permitted to require that an individual not pose a direct threat to the health or safety of other individuals in the workplace. 42 U.S.C. Sec. 12113. The ADA defines "direct threat" to mean "a significant risk to the health or safety of others that cannot be eliminated by reasonable accommodation." 42 U.S.C. Sec. 12111. According to proposed regulations, in order to reject an applicant or employee on this basis, an employer must consider (a) the duration of the risk, (b) the nature and severity of the potential harm, and (c) the likelihood that the potential harm will occur. The employer's decisions in this regard must also be based on either valid medical analysis or on other objective evidence individualized for the particular individual and job. 56 Fed. Reg. 8578 (Feb. 28, 1991).

B. Application of the Law

1. Is AIDS or HIV Infection a Handicap/Disability?

a. AIDS

AIDS has been found to be a "handicap" under the Rehabilitation Act of 1973. In *Chalk v. U.S. District Court*, 840 F.2d 701 (9th Cir. 1988), a federal court of appeals ruled that AIDS was a handicap covered by the Rehabilitation Act and held that the dismissal of a elementary school teacher because he had AIDS violated the Act. There have also been a number of federal suits involving elementary school children with AIDS. In virtually all of these cases, the courts have deemed the children to be protected by the Rehabilitation Act and the federal Education for All Handicapped Children Act and have ultimately ordered school systems to permit such children to attend school in normal classroom settings. See *Thomas v. Atascadero Unified School District*, 662 F.Supp. 376 (C.D. Cal. 1987).

b. Asymptomatic HIV Infection

The analysis is more difficult as to whether HIV infection alone is a "handicap" or "disability." Many people who are infected by HIV appear to be healthy; they have no physical or mental symptoms which incapacitate them. Nonetheless, the Rehabilitation Act and the ADA protect not only individuals who are handicapped, but also individuals who are perceived to be handicapped. It is safe to assume that, in most cases, asymptomatic HIV infection—like AIDS—will be deemed a "handicap" or "disability" protected under federal law.

2. Is an Individual with HIV Infection or AIDS "Otherwise Qualified"?

In order to fall within the protection of federal law, it is not enough to be an "individual with handicaps"; one must also be "otherwise qualified." The U.S. Supreme Court has stated that **"[a] person who poses a significant risk of communicating an infectious disease to others in the work place will not be otherwise qualified for his or her job if reasonable accommodation will not eliminate that risk."** *School Board of Nassau County v. Arline*, 480 U.S. 273, 287 (1987). Thus, in evaluating whether an employee or student with HIV infection is "otherwise qualified," a two-step analysis is required.

a. Significant Risk

First, an institution must decide if the employee or student poses a significant risk of communicating HIV to others. The U.S. Supreme Court has enumerated four factors that must be considered in determining whether a person poses a "significant risk" of transmitting a communicable disease to others. Those four factors are as follows:

(1) The nature of the risk (how the disease is transmitted);
(2) The duration of the risk (how long the carrier is infectious);
(3) The severity of the risk (the potential harm to the third parties); and
(4) The probability that the disease will be transmitted and will cause the varying degrees of harm.

In evaluating these factors, sound medical advise should be sought. It was important to the Court that decisions in this area be based on reasonable medical judgments.

b. Reasonable Accommodation

Second, if there is a "significant risk" to others, an institution must determine if reasonable accommodation would eliminate that risk. Accor-ding to the Supreme Court in *Arline*, an accom- modation will not be deemed reasonable, if it either (**1**) poses undue financial and administrative burdens on an institution, or (**2**) requires a fundamental alteration in the nature of the institution's programs.

3. Can an Institution Find Out if an Employee or Student Is Infected with HIV or Has AIDS?

a. Employment or Academic Setting

Under the federal laws prohibiting discrimination on the basis of handicap or disability, an institution is to focus on an individual's ability to perform all of the essential requirements of the job in question or the academic program in question. Except in health care fields such as medicine, dentistry, and nursing where an individual's HIV infection might pose a significant risk to others, it is difficult to envision an employment or academic situation in which an individual's HIV status would be job- or school-related. Thus, as a general rule, school supervisors and administrators should avoid making inquiries as to an individual's HIV-infection status.

b. Student Health Setting

The federal laws which prohibit discrimination on the basis of handicap do not in any way dictate how a physician should practice medicine. If, in the context of rendering good and complete medical care to students, a physician deems it necessary or appropriate to inquire about HIV infection, then that inquiry should be made. With limited exceptions, medical information obtained by a student health physician should be treated as confidential medical information and not shared with other college or university administrators.

III. STATE LAWS

In addition to the Rehabilitation Act of 1973 and the Americans with Disabilities Act, most states have state laws which prohibit discrimination on the basis of handicap or disability in employment settings.

A. Florida

Florida has a state statute which specifically prohibits discrimination on the basis of AIDS, ARC, and HIV. Paragraphs (2) and (3) of Section 760.50 of the Florida Statutes state as follows:

(2) Any person with or perceived as having acquired immune deficiency syndrome, acquired immune deficiency syndrome related complex, or human immunodeficiency virus shall have every protection made available to handicapped persons.

(3) (a) No person may require an individual to take a human immunodeficiency virus-related test as a condition of hiring, promotion, or continued employment unless the absence of human immunodeficiency virus infection is a bona fide occupational qualification for the job in question.

B. Maryland

Maryland has a state statute which prohibits discrimination on the basis of handicap. Maryland Annotated Code, Art. 49B, Section 16(a) (1) provides as follows:

(a) It shall be an unlawful employment practice for an employer:
(1) To fail or refuse to hire or to discharge any individual, or otherwise to discriminate against any individual with respect to his compensation, terms, conditions, or privileges of employment, because of such individual's . . . physical or mental handicap unrelated in nature and extent so as to reasonably preclude the performance of the employment.

C. New York

New York has a state statute which prohibits discrimination because of disability. Section 296.1 of Article 15 of the New York Human Rights Law (Consolidated Laws Service) provides as follows:

It shall be an unlawful discriminatory practice:
(a) For an employer . . . , because of the . . . disability . . . of any individual, to refuse to hire or employ or to bar or to discharge from employment such individual or to discriminate against such individual in compensation or in terms, **conditions, or privileges of employment.**

———— **BOX 17.2** (*continued*) ————

D. Pennsylvania

Pennsylvania has a state statute which prohibits discrimination of the basis of handicap. Section 955 of Chapter 17 of Title 43 of the Pennsylvania Statutes reads as follows:

It shall be an unlawful discriminatory practice, unless based upon a bona fide occupational qualification . . .

(a) For any employer because of the . . . non-job related handicap or disability of any individual to refuse to hire or employ, or to bar or to discharge from employment such individual, or to otherwise discriminate against such individual with respect to compensation, hire, tenure, terms, conditions or privileges of employment, if the individual is the best able and most competent to perform the services required.

(***Promoting Student Health '91 Legal Issues***. Peter H. Ruger, Leslie Chambers Strohm, The Washington University, St. Louis, Missouri. Outline prepared for the New Jersey Collegiate Summer Institute for Health in Education held July 28–August 2, 1991.)

---

confidential medical information on individuals' HIV status (Dickens, 1989). It is felt that new laws that apply directly to the confidentiality of HIV information should be passed to protect people from social bias. Such new laws were passed in a number of states in 1988 (e.g., California, Florida, Massachusetts, New York, and Vermont.) In Florida, the person to be tested, or the parents of a child to be tested, are given the following statement on confidentiality to read:

Confidentiality

You should be aware that there is some risk associated with letting others know about your test results. It is advised that you keep this information very private and inform only your physician/dentist. It is also advised that you inform your sexual or needle-sharing contacts that they may have been exposed to the virus that causes AIDS and recommend that they be tested.

Parents of children taking the test should be aware that there may be some risk associated with letting others know about their child's test results. It is advised that parents keep this information very private and inform only their child's physician/dentist or foster home. In each of the above cases, using test results as grounds for discrimination in insurance or employment is prohibited in some states. However, the burden of proof is on the persons discriminated against.

Every effort is made to ensure the confidentiality of the test results. Any information that may identify the individual is kept in his or her medical records at the health department and available only to a limited number of people who have a "need-to-know." The "need-to-know" refers to **Allowable Disclosure** (see Box 17.3). These people are the person's physician, nurse, or counselor. In some states, laws prohibit the release of HIV-antibody test information without the individual's written consent.

Many people want new laws that require the tracking and reporting of HIV carriers and their partners. It is doubtful that a single law can be so constructed that it will please everybody. In 1988, there was a fierce battle between opposing forces concerning the Dannemeyer-Gann AIDS Initiative, or Proposition 102 on the California ballot. If this proposition had passed, it would have eliminated confidentiality for people taking the HIV test. Physicians would have had to report names and addresses of those who tested positive and those they reasonably believed to be infected. Failure to report a case would have meant a fine of $250. In addition, the infected would have been required to produce a list of sexual partners to public health officials or be charged with a misdemeanor.

——————— BOX 17.3 ———————

ALLOWABLE DISCLOSURE

Allowable disclosure refers to the special circumstances which justify disclosure of a patient's HIV status without that patient's authorization. The impact of these disclosures may vary greatly. Extreme caution should be taken when making an allowable disclosure; professionals in all areas (health, education, police, and so forth) are advised to consult an attorney before doing so. Typically, the following exceptions to maintain confidentiality are recognized as allowable disclosures:

1. As necessary for health care personnel to proceed with appropriate treatment as determined by physicians.
2. To conduct epidemiological research.
3. To respond to potentially significant exposures of health care or public safety personnel to contaminated blood or body fluids. This exception is applied to discrete exposure incidents, evaluated through risk assessment on a case-by-case basis.
4. As required by law or regulation for reporting child abuse, sexually transmitted diseases, including HIV/AIDS, or cause of death.
5. As required for the welfare of the patient, as in cases of attempted suicide or dementia.
6. As required for the welfare of third parties. This is applicable in cases where third parties are faced with possible harm due to the conduct of a patient or the nature of his or her illness.

   a. There is presently no established **legal** duty for a health care provider to warn sexual or needle-sharing partners of HIV-infected patients, making **duty to warn** one of the most challenging HIV-related determinations for health care providers.
      i. There is no certainty about who must be warned or under what circumstances.
      ii. The more specific the knowledge of who and under what circumstances a third party is at risk, the more compelling the duty to warn that specific third party.
      iii. The legal case most often cited as precedent for disclosure in this type of situation is the *Tarasof* case. [*Tarasof v. Regents of the University of Cali-fornia*, 551 P.2d 334 (CA 1976)] (See Box 17.4.)

(a) The majority legal opinion held that "the protective privilege ends where the public peril begins."
(b) However, the Justices did not state what should be done to adequately warn a potential victim or what constitutes "reasonable efforts to warn."
(c) *Tarasof* may have more bearing on mental health practitioner decisions to warn third parties because they may be held to a somewhat different legal standard than physicians in many jurisdictions.
   iv. Physicians may be absolved of any potential duty to warn by making a statutorily required report to local health department.
   v. Legislation in some states focuses on "privilege to disclose" rather than on duty to warn.
      (a) Under these laws, partner notification is a routinely allowable disclosure and the provider is protected from civil or criminal liability when disclosure is made in good faith.
      (b) **It is important to review state laws affecting these situations**.
   b. Confidentiality may be breached in third-party situations only when all of the following conditions have been met:
      i. It is known that the infected individual will not or cannot carry out the responsibility to warn others known to be at risk;
      ii. Reasonable efforts have failed to persuade the patient to give voluntary disclosure consent;
      iii. There is a high probability both that harm will occur if the confidential information is not disclosed, and that the disclosed information will in fact be used to prevent harm. This is most easily established in the instance of a patient's specific threat of imminent physical violence or harm against a specific person;
      iv. The harm that others at risk would suffer would be serious harm; *and,*
      v. Adequate precautions are taken to guarantee that only necessary information is disclosed, i.e., protecting the identity of the infected person.

The Confidentiality Dilemma

There appears at the moment to be no legal balance between a physician's obligation to his or her patients and the obligation to the public good. **The physician is in a "Catch-22" position:** There does not appear to be a clear moral or legal choice. The following cases help highlight the moral and legal morass confronting physicians in the United States.

Case 1—A physician said he knew that a heart bypass surgery patient was HIV-infected and advised the man against having sex for several weeks after surgery for the sake of his heart. Six months later, the man died of a heart attack. Six months after that, his wife developed AIDS. Was this physician legally obligated to make sure that both the patient and his wife knew of his HIV infection? The wife decided not to sue the physician. Note that the question emphasizes legal obligation. Physicians often fail to exercise their moral obligations when they conflict with the law; especially when lawyers and physicians are groping for mutual agreement on the legality of confidentiality with regard to HIV-infected patients.

Case 2—Key West, Florida (population 30,000) has one of the highest AIDS rates in the United States. Ninety-five percent of AIDS cases are in the homosexual population. It is estimated that one in four people in Key West is homosexual and one in two carries HIV (Breo, 1988).

--------- BOX 17.4 ---------

THE HIPPOCRATIC OATH AND CONFIDENTIALITY

"Whatsoever I shall see or hear in the course of my profession, in my intercourse with men, if it is that which should not be broadcast about, I will never divulge it but consider it a holy secret."

The commitment of a physician to his or her patient has a historical basis. But the commitment of a physician to society is just as strong and historically precedented. The rate at which the AIDS virus is being transmitted worldwide has put the historical debate of confidentiality vs. the public's right to know in a new perspective. Oliver Wendell Holmes wrote that when the public's right to know and an individual's right to privacy come into conflict, the public's right to know comes first.

Harold Schwartz (1988) reported on a 37-year-old bisexual married man whose lover had recently been diagnosed with AIDS. He was worried that he may have acquired the infection and wanted to be tested. After appropriate counseling the test was arranged and he turned out to be HIV-positive. When asked how he planned to bring up this matter with his wife, he said that he had no intention of telling her. She knew nothing about his bisexuality and he would be humiliated and disgraced if she learned of it now.

He promised that he would reduce the number of sexual contacts with his wife, but he could not eliminate them entirely or even rely on safer sex practices because his wife was trying to become pregnant. **What should the physician have done?**

DUTY TO PROTECT WHOM?

When an HIV-infected person behaves in a manner that the physician knows will endanger others, the physician has both a professional and moral obligation to protect the patient's confidentiality and a duty to protect those who may be in danger.

Precedent for the legal obligation to protect those in jeopardy from someone who behaves in a reckless or dangerous manner is the case of *Tarasof vs. Regents of the University of California*. A mentally disturbed psychiatric patient told his psychiatrist the name of a person he was going to kill. The person was not warned. The psychiatrist kept the information confidential and his patient committed murder. The *Tarasof* case is now interpreted with respect to HIV-infected people as the physician's duty to protect people from potential harm.

But individuals in general have an obligation not to harm others. This was made abundantly clear in the case of Marc Christian, age 35, after he initially won 21.7 million dollars from the estate of movie star Rock Hudson. (Hudson died in 1985 of AIDS.) The jury found that Hudson was guilty of outrageous conduct in concealing that he had AIDS from his homosexual lover. The jury ruled that Hudson conspired with his secretary, Mark Miller, to keep secret the actor's disease to induce Christian to continue having high-risk sex with Hudson.

STATE LAWS AND PATIENTS' RIGHTS

Because of the conflict between a patient's right to confidentiality and the public's right to be warned, in 1988, 10 states passed laws authorizing physicians to inform spouses of HIV-infected individuals. The laws absolve the physician from civil or criminal liability so long as he or she informs the patient of the intent to contact the partner in advance of making the actual contact. Ten states established voluntary partner notification programs or programs under which infected individuals can ask public health officials to notify contacts. Through 1996, 40 states and the District of Columbia have passed anti-discrimination laws, 16 states have passed legislation restricting the use of blood tests by insurance companies, and 24 states have made it a felony to willfully or knowingly transmit or expose another individual to HIV.

As of April 1992, 34 states required that HIV infection in people who do not yet meet the criteria for CDC-defined AIDS be reported; these states account for 50% of all AIDS cases reported in the United States (Table 10-5). Twenty-four of the 34 states have enacted legislation or promulgated regulations that require reporting HIV-infected people by name to state or local health departments. These 24 states accounted for 16% of all reported AIDS cases. All 24 states require information to include the person's sex, age, and race/ethnicity; 19 states, mode of transmission; six, clinical status; and three, CD4 T cell count. Sixteen of the 24 states that require reporting by name offer the option of anonymous HIV testing in some circumstances. Thus, patient names are not always provided.

In 12 of the 34 states, *anonymous* individual reports of HIV infection must be provided to the state health department; these 12 states account for 22% of all reported AIDS cases. Eleven of the 12 states require reporting only sex and age; nine, only race/ethnicity; and six, mode of transmission. None of the 12 requires reports on clinical status or CD4 T cell count (*MMWR*, 1991).

A 1988 Florida law requires all testing sites to provide pre- and post-test counseling and stipulates that anyone offering post-test counseling must have special training that includes recognition of suicidal behavior.

California requires that people convicted of first-time prostitution must complete an AIDS education course. Washington and Florida require most health care providers to complete an educational course on HIV and AIDS as a condition of licensure. By the end of 1988, 32 states had laws requiring that health care workers, primarily emergency medical personnel and funeral directors, be notified if the patient or deceased was HIV-infected.

The wife of the owner of Sloppy Joe's Saloon died of AIDS. After the memorial service for his wife, his pregnant girlfriend filed a suit wherein her attorney asked that the Monroe County Health Department and the Florida Department of Health and Rehabilitative Services (HRS) release the bar owner's medical records. The order was granted allowing her personal physician to view the medical file. The judge prohibited further disclosure of the records by either the pregnant woman or her physician.

The lawsuit provoked anger and unrest in Key West and caught private physicians and public health officials in the middle of how to balance the rights of individual patients against the rights of those who may become infected.

The wife had told her physician that both she and her husband tested HIV-positive at out-of-state laboratories. They were both counseled extensively, in particular about the risk of transmitting the virus to others. After the lawsuit was filed, the counseling physician was outraged. He said "I knew that he had understood what I had told him because he told me, 'Well, Doc, this little bugger is a bastard of a virus and there's nothing we can do to beat it so we have to be careful.' "

Should the husband and wife's treating physician have been permitted to warn those whom the carriers might have exposed? Should public health officials be empowered with emergency sanctions to override patient confidentiality? Are such powers needed?

Justice Abbott Goldberg (1989) carefully and precisely defines the legal issue of confidentiality, particularly concerning physician charting on AIDS patients. He states his position: "Physicians are liable if they fail to disclose that a patient has AIDS and this non-disclosure subsequently harms someone. The questions are not whether, but when, to whom, and for how much physicians may be liable for concealing the fact that a patient is infectious for AIDS." Thus, the intentional breach of confidentiality is legally expected from physicians who care for patients with AIDS. This stems, Goldberg argues, from two sources: case law establishing that physicians ". . . [have] both the authority and the duty to violate a patient's confidence in order to protect those persons to whom the patient may communicate a disease" and from the professional view that physicians ". . . have a duty to keep accurate patient records on which they know other providers may rely."

From a legal standpoint, these points are hardly arguable (Murphy, 1989). Justice Goldberg is saying that confidentiality ends where public peril begins. The precedent for Justice Goldberg's interpretation of the current confidentiality laws may have come from the ruling by the California Supreme Court in the case of *Tarasof v. Regents of the University of California* (1976). In this case, the defendants argued that a legal obligation of confidentiality prevented warning a person who was known to be in danger of being attacked by a psychiatric patient. The Court observed, "We recognize the public interest in supporting effective treatment of mental illness and in protecting the rights of patients to privacy, and the consequent public importance of safeguarding the confidential character of psychotherapeutic communication. Against this interest, however, we must weigh the public interest in safety from violent assault."

In prioritizing confidentiality and safety, the Court concluded, "The public policy favoring protection of the confidential character of patient–psychotherapist communications must yield to the extent to which disclosure is essential to avert danger to others. The protective privilege ends where the public peril begins" (Dickens, 1989).

POINT OF INFORMATION 17.2

A PENALTY FOR VIOLATING PATIENT CONFIDENTIALITY

In 1988, an orthopedic surgeon settled out of court to end a suit for breach of patient confidentiality. The surgeon was charged with violating a provision of the California Health and Safety Code that prohibits disclosure of a patient's HIV status without the patient's written consent.

The surgeon stated that in late 1985, a few months after the confidentiality statute went into effect, a patient informed him that he was infected with HIV. The patient was scheduled for surgery and the surgeon was concerned about the possible risk of becoming infected.

The patient verbally agreed that his HIV status could be revealed to members of the surgical team to lessen their chances of becoming infected. The surgeon subsequently entered HIV status into the medical record.

The patient later sued the surgeon for breach of confidentiality under the new law. He asserted that by entering his HIV status in the medical record, the surgeon had violated his privacy and statutory rights.

The suit was ultimately settled, in part because of the patient's reluctance to pursue a public trial. This case illustrates the tug-of-war in the era of AIDS between the obligation to protect patient privacy and the need for physicians and other health professionals to share medical information about their patients.

Under *Tarasof*, physicians are obligated to inform a third party when they have reason to believe that he or she may be endangered by the actions of a patient. Based on the *Tarasof* decision, physicians may assume that if a patient's sexual partners are in danger, they should be notified. There must, however, be a specific target involved. In addition, the physician may be obligated to notify others, including the employer if a patient is involved in an occupation where job responsibilities could put others at increased risk of infection (Hirsh, 1988).

LEGAL ASPECTS OF HIV/AIDS AND HEALTH CARE WORKERS

HIV/AIDS is preventable. Therefore people must be educated on how to prevent HIV infection. They need to be taught how to protect themselves. According to national polls, the United States is doing a reasonably good job in educating the general public about the virus, its transmission, and how to avoid it. However, because thousands of health care workers (HCWs) are known to be HIV-infected or to have AIDS, the public has raised questions concerning the possibility that their doctors, nurses, dentists, and other HCWs might be HIV-infected. They began to ask whether or not they had a right to know the HIV status of their health care professionals. At the same time, doctors, nurses, and other medical professionals, in fear for their own safety, began to raise questions about testing their patients prior to treatment, especially prior to invasive surgery. But **it took the transmission of HIV from dentist David Acer of Stuart, Florida to his patient Kimberly Bergalis in 1987 and the publicity of that case to bring the concerns, fears, and liability of both patients and health care professionals to national debate**.

Following numerous reports, much publicity, and pressure from its members over the Bergalis case, the American Dental Association sent out the following 1991 news release:

The recent case of possible HIV transmission from dentist to patient has raised some uncertainty about the risk of transmission from health care provider to patient. While there is evidence that this dental practice did not consistently adhere to all recommended guidelines for prevention of disease transmission, the precise mechanism of transmission in this case remains unknown. This uncertainty leads to the conclusion that the foremost concern of the dental profession must continue to be protection of the patient. Thus, until the uncertainty about transmission is resolved, the ADA believes that HIV-infected dentists should refrain from performing invasive procedures or should disclose their seropositive status.

In addition to the American Dental Association's news release of January 16, 1991, the American Medical Association issued a January 17, 1991 news release regarding its position on HIV-infected physicians. The statement says:

The American Medical Association believes that physicians who are HIV-positive and who must restrict their normal professional activities have a right to continue their career in medicine in a capacity that poses no identifiable risk to their patients. The American Medical Association pledges its support and protection of these physicians and believes the profession and the public have a need and an obligation to ensure that they continue to be productive as long as they practice medicine safely and responsibly.

The positions of the CDC and the major medical/dental professional associations are constantly shifting. Since issuing its July 27, 1990 report, "Possible Transmission of Human Immunodeficiency Virus to a Patient During an Invasive Dental Procedure," the CDC has issued at least two updates on the Florida situation (January 18, 1991 and June 14, 1991). On July 12, 1991, the Centers for Disease Control and Prevention published its recommendations for preventing HIV and hepatitis B virus (HBV) transmission to patients during exposure-prone invasive procedures.

——————— BOX 17.5 ———————

CENTERS FOR DISEASE CONTROL AND PREVENTION GUIDELINES

The Centers for Disease Control and Prevention (CDC) has emphasized that there is no risk of transmitting HIV in the vast majority of medical treatments. The Department of Health and Human Services stated that the guidelines are aimed at those procedures in which blood exposure could cause transmission, either to a patient from a health care worker or to a health care worker from a patient.

CONTROL GUIDELINES

- Health care workers infected with HIV or the more virulent form of hepatitis B virus (HBV) should not perform "exposure-prone" medical procedures in which the worker might be cut or injured and the worker's blood contact a patient's body cavity, subcutaneous tissues, or mucous membranes.
- Dentists, physicians, and other health care workers who perform exposure-prone procedures should ascertain the HIV or HBV status.
- The CDC does not recommend mandatory testing of health care workers for HIV or HBV antibodies. According to the CDC, the risk of exposure is too low to justify the cost of a mandatory testing program.
- Institutions can improve compliance through education, training, and appropriate confidentiality safeguards.
- Any person infected with HIV or the most virulent form of hepatitis B should not perform

exposure-prone procedures unless they have obtained permission and guidance from special review committees that would require, at a minimum, that potential patients be informed of the worker's HIV or HBV status.

- All health care workers must follow universal precautions against infection, including appropriate use of hand washing, protective barriers, equipment sterilization, careful handling and disposal of needles and other sharp instruments, and the use of gloves.
- Increased use of hepatitis B vaccine should be encouraged for health care workers who are likely to be exposed to blood.
- Research designed to identify modifications of medical, surgical, and dental procedures and of equipment to reduce the risk of injury to health care workers and resultant exposure of patients should be encouraged.
- Whenever possible, health care workers whose practices are modified because of their HIV or HBV status should be provided opportunities to continue patient care activities.

In 1991, Congress enacted a law requiring states, as a condition of federal funding, to adopt the CDC guidelines or their equivalents restricting the practice of HIV-infected health care workers. Beginning 1997, 46 states have adopted the CDC guidelines or their equivalents.

HIV/AIDS: A DOUBLE-EDGED SWORD FOR THE PRACTICING PHYSICIAN AND OTHER HEALTH CARE WORKERS

Questions have been raised concerning the legal obligation of health care personnel to treat HIV/AIDS patients. In November 1987, the Council on Ethical and Judicial Affairs of the American Medical Association issued a statement saying that a physician may not ethically refuse to treat patients who are infected with

the virus. It called on physicians who are infected to act in such a manner that transmission of the virus to patients is not possible. Clearly this statement says that physicians may not refuse to treat HIV/AIDS patients if the physician is qualified to treat such patients. Physicians do have legal obligations to their patients, including those who have HIV/AIDS. Physicians who refuse to treat HIV/AIDS patients may be accused of violating the New Americans with Disabilities Act. This law specifies that a physician's office is a public accommodation and HIV infection, HIV disease, and AIDS are recognized as disabilities. Refusing to treat a disabled person would, in the opinion of most lawyers, be a violation.

HIV Transmission from Physician to Patient and Vice Versa

Communicability of HIV is an important liability issue for personnel involved in the care of HIV/AIDS patients. Those who come into contact with bodily fluids, blood, blood products, or who receive accidental needle pricks are at risk for infection, and they can also spread the virus to other patients. Lawrence Gostin (1989a) wrote that physicians involved in medically invasive procedures have claimed the right to know whether their patients are HIV-infected. Yet that information is of limited value because: (1) the physician should be using **universal precautions** which dictate that all patients be treated as though they were HIV-infected (this may be true, but many people believe that no matter how careful a physician is, if he knew someone had HIV disease/AIDS, he or she would be more careful); and (2) physicians have a professional, if not legal, responsibility to treat infected patients.

Patients also claim the legal right to know if their physician is HIV-infected or has AIDS. If this information were available, especially to those who were to have invasive surgery, which includes intra-abdominal, colon or rectal, thoracic, cardiac, orthopedic, gynecologic, Caesarean section, oral surgery, and so forth, many would opt for an HIV-free surgeon. Withholding seropositive information from a patient who then becomes HIV-infected may make the physician and the hospital liable for damages.

In November 1991, Texas became the first state to pass a bill that puts into law the Centers for Disease Control and Prevention guidelines calling for health care workers with HIV to stop performing "exposure-prone procedures" unless they obtain consent from a peer review group and the patient. Failure to comply could result in disciplinary action by the State Board of Medical Examiners. It may also be used by attorneys to file charges of malpractice on behalf of a client who was not in-

formed. The bill broadly defines an HIV exposure-prone procedure as one that poses a direct and significant risk. The procedures listed in the bill are:

- Any surgical entry into tissue, cavities, or organs
- Repair of major traumatic injuries in an operating or delivery room, emergency department, or outpatient setting
- Vaginal or Caesarean delivery or other invasive obstetric procedure during which bleeding may occur
- Cardiac catheterization or angiography
- Cutting of oral or perioral tissues where bleeding may occur

Although the Texas legislature passed the bill, physicians may have the final word on how the law is applied, since physicians will decide which invasive procedures are "exposure-prone."

Lawrence Gostin (1989a) does not argue for the physician's or the patient's right to be informed of HIV/AIDS status, rather he makes the case that the risks inherent in invasive medical procedures are sufficient for the medical profession to hold patient safety from HIV, hepatitis, and other pathological organisms in high regard.

Gostin writes that professional guidance is required to identify when and where the physician should withdraw from performing an invasive procedure. This is the position the AMA supports.

AMERICAN BAR ASSOCIATION LEGAL DIRECTORY

A comprehensive listing of programs and organizations that provide free legal services to people with HIV/AIDS is available. The 368-page publication was compiled by the American Bar Association's AIDS Coordination Project.

The Directory of Legal Resources for People with AIDS and HIV is organized by state, and each listing includes name, address, telephone number, and a brief description of the project. It also has information on national and state organizations.

A PATIENT'S RIGHT TO KNOW A SURGEON'S HIV STATUS

A recent example of a patient's right to know the HIV status of a physician performing an invasive medical procedure is cited in: *Application of The Hersey Medical Center,* Pennsylvania Superior Court, July 30, 1991. In this case Dr. "John Doe," an obstetrician/gynecologist was cut by a member of the operating team. Although it was unlikely that Dr. Doe's blood was transferred to the patient, Dr. Doe voluntarily took the HIV test. He was HIV-positive. Dr. Doe notified the two hospitals in which he worked and took a leave of absence. The hospitals notified 447 patients who may have had invasive procedures by Dr. Doe. The hospitals further filed petitions with the court alleging that it was their duty to inform potentially exposed patients and a limited number of physicians who worked with Dr. Doe, who could in turn inform their patients. Dr. Doe responded to the petition by asserting his right to privacy and that a compelling need, as required under the Confidentiality of HIV-Related Information Act, did not exist.

The county court authorized disclosure of Dr. Doe's identity and HIV status to the obstetrics and gynecology attending and resident staffs, and to any physician authorized by a patient for whom Dr. Doe participated in a surgical procedure; and an anonymous description of the situation was ordered for the media and all patients identified on the hospital's list.

The appellate court upheld the lower court's order to disclose. The appellate court stated that a "compelling need" was met. On Dr. Doe's right to privacy, the court held that his medical problem was not solely his. It became a public concern the moment he became involved in the invasive procedure. The court held that the public's right to be informed in these situations is compelling and far outweighs a practicing surgeon's right to keep information regarding his or her disease confidential (Landwirth, 1992).

For information on the AIDS Coordination Project or to obtain copies of *The Directory,* contact ABA AIDS Coordination Project, 1800 M Street N.W., Washington D.C., 20036, (202) 331-2248.

OTHER LEGAL HELP SOURCES

AIDS Policy and Law
Buraff Publications
1350 Connecticut Avenue, NW
Washington, DC 20036
800-331-1291
Biweekly report on AIDS law and policy developments

AIDS Project
132 W. 43rd Street
New York, NY 10036
212-944-9800, Ext. 545
Affiliates in almost every state. Discrimination, confidentiality, public health policy, and access to care.

AIDS Policy Center
George Washington University
2021 K Street, NW, Suite 800
Washington, DC 20006
202-872-1445
Gathers, analyzes, and disseminates information on state AIDS policy legislation. Since 1983, maintains collections of summaries of all state laws related to HIV/AIDS.

SUMMARY

This chapter is **not** an exhaustive treatment on HIV/AIDS and the law and ethics. Many excellent papers have not been included because of space limitations. Papers that are included were selected based on the advice of practicing attorneys, members of the medical profession, and colleagues.

HIV/AIDS law has had a mixed record across the United States. Many states have come to accept research that has shown the remarkable efficacy of well-targeted education and counseling. There has also been wide acceptance of the importance of confidentiality and guarantee of anti-discrimination. Ensuring the privacy and equal treatment of people with HIV/AIDS is essential to the success of epidemiologic studies, testing, outreach programs, and treatment for injection drug users. Public health officials will not gain the confidence and cooperation of infected individuals if these individuals are not legally protected from stigma and irrational prejudice (Gostin, 1989a,b).

While legislatures have responded well to health service research, they have also been susceptible to the attitude that the primary modes of HIV transmission are immoral, even criminal. Federal and state statutes, by requiring special emphasis on abstinence from extramarital sex and drug use, ignore the fact that these behaviors have persisted unabated throughout history.

There is political pressure on legislators to use the coercive powers of the state to combat the epidemic. Legislation for compulsory screening, isolation, and criminalization has proceeded despite evidence that these measures are not efficacious and often contradict advice from the Public Health Service. The use of coercive powers, far from impeding the epidemic, may well fuel it (Gostin, 1989a,b).

REVIEW QUESTIONS

(Answers to the Review Questions are on page 581.)

1. What is the confidentiality dilemma in medicine?

2. With respect to the HIV testing confidentiality controversy, what do you think is more important: A person's right to privacy or the public's right to know?

For Discussion:

1. A female physician specializing in emergency medicine at an urban hospital learns that she is HIV-positive. Should any of her patients be informed of her HIV status? If so, when? Before, during, or after treatment? Refer back to

Chapter 15 for additional information on HIV-infected physicians— it may help you formulate an opinion.

2. A 13-year-old runaway female who has exchanged sex for drugs or money enters a drug and rehabilitation program. She reveals her recent lifestyle to a counselor. Should this counselor advise the agency that is providing food, clothing, and shelter to this girl about her lifestyle?

REFERENCES

ALBERT, J., et al. (1993). Forensic evidence by DNA sequencing. *Nature*, 361:595–596.

BREO, DENNIS. (1988). Patient confidentiality: With AIDS where do you draw the line. *Am. Med. News*, 31:3–7.

DICKENS, BERNARD. (1988). Legal rights and duties in the AIDS epidemic. *Science*, 239:580–586.

DICKENS, BERNARD. (1989). Legal limits of AIDS confidentiality. *JAMA*, 259:3449–3451.

DUCKETT, MELVIN J., et al. (1989). AIDS related migration and travel policies and restrictions: AgGlobal survey. *AIDS*, 3:S231–S252.

FLUSS, SEV S., et al. (1989). AIDS, HIV, health care workers: Some international legislation perspectives. *Maryland Law Rev.*, 48:77–92.

GILMORE, NORBERT, J., et al. (1989). International travel and AIDS. *AIDS*, 3:S225–S230.

GOLDBERG, ABBOTT. (1989). Physicians' notes can be deceptive—or revealing. *Consultant*, 29:69–72.

GOSTIN, LAWRENCE O. (1989a). Public health strategies for confronting AIDS. *JAMA*, 261: 1621–1630.

GOSTIN, LAWRENCE O. (1989b). The politics of AIDS: Compulsory state powers, public health and civil liberties. *Ohio State Law J.*, 49:1017–1058.

GOSTIN, LAWRENCE O. (1990a). The AIDS Litigation Project. A national review of Court and Human Rights Commission decisions. Part I: The social impact of AIDS. *JAMA*, 263:1961–1970.

GOSTIN, LAWRENCE O. (1990b). The AIDS Litigation Project. Part II: Discrimination. *JAMA*, 263: 2086–2093.

HIRSH, HAROLD. (1988). Patient confidentiality: New legal risks emerge. *Phys. Manage.*, 28:37–41.

KIRBY, MICHAEL. (1996). Human rights and HIV/AIDS: Upholding human dignity and defending principles. *EXCHANGE*, 1:1–16.

LANDWIRTH, JULIUS. (1992). Courts look at disclosure of physician's HIV status. *Infect. Dis. News*, 5:13.

LUMSDON, KEVIN. (1992). HIV-positive health care workers pose legal, safety challenges for hospitals. *Hospitals*, 66:24–32.

MARINER, WENDY. (1996). AIDS phobia, public health warnings and lawsuits: Deterring harm or rewarding ignorance? *Am. J. Public Health,* 85:1562–1567.

McCORMICK, BRIAN. (1992). HIV-related discrimination lawsuits on the rise. *Am. Med. News,* Feb. 3:9.

Morbidity and Mortality Weekly Report. (1991). Publicly funded HIV counseling and testing—United States, 1990. 40:666–675.

Murphy, Dale P. (1989). Confidentiality and the AIDS patient: the true dilemma. *Consultant,* 29:3.

PALMA, LYNNE L. (1992). Americans with Disabilities Act (ADA): Take the first steps now. *AIDS Newslink: Mountain Plains Regional AIDS Education and Training Center,* 3:8–10.

ROTHSTEIN, MARK A. (1989). Medical screening: AIDS, rights, and health care costs. *Natl. Forum,* 99:7–10.

SCHULMAN, DAVID. (1988). Remembering who we are: AIDS and law in a time of madness. *AIDS Public Policy J.,* 3:75–77.

SCHWARTZ, HAROLD I. (1988). AIDS: Confidentiality versus the duty to warn. *Med. Asp. Human Sexuality,* 22:13.

SHERER, RENSLOW. (1990). AIDS policy into the 1990s. *JAMA,* 263:1972–1974.

SLACK, JAMES D. (1991). *AIDS and the Public Work Force.* Tuscaloosa: University of Alabama Press.

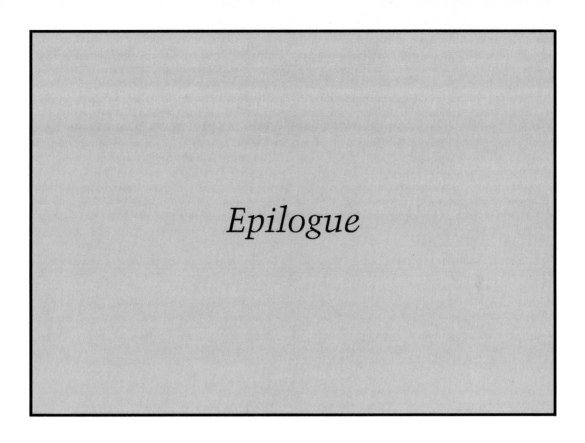

Epilogue

While the achievements of the global response to date should not be underestimated, neither should the challenge ahead. HIV disease/AIDS is a catastrophe in slow motion, and it is essential that the world community pace itself for the long haul. The task ahead calls for clear vision, renewed will, and greatly increased resources. But it also calls for greater determination to use the resources in the interest of everyone: HIV disease or AIDS must not be allowed to join the list of problems, like poverty and hunger, that this world has learned to live with because the powerful have lost interest, and the powerless have no choice.

In the United States, as of June 1998, through 17 years of the HIV/AIDS epidemic, we can reflect on the fact that we have learned a lot about this new disease but there is a long way to go. While it is easy to criticize, condemn, ridicule, and find mistakes in the way the HIV/AIDS pandemic has been handled, society should not lose sight of the outstanding scientific and social achievements made since HIV/AIDS was discovered.

Excellent progress has been made in understanding the biology of the virus, its transmission, therapy, and its relationship to the progression of AIDS. If the 1980s are to be remembered as the period of AIDS violence, hatred, and irrational fears, the 1990s will hopefully be remembered as the time of optimism. HIV disease has become a more treatable illness wherein the quality and duration of life are being extended. Promising antiviral treatments are now in use and vaccines for the prevention of HIV infection are in field trials. HIV/AIDS education will soon reach every grade school, high school, and workplace in the United States. Courts have affirmed the rights of HIV-infected/AIDS patients to a public education and to remain at their jobs.

Two areas of concern that have **not** improved significantly are HIV/AIDS discrimination based on fear and obtaining insurance coverage. Moving through the 1990s, although legislation may help, these two problems may remain.

There is great hope that at some point during the 1990s, the diagnosis of HIV infection will *not* indicate the almost certain destruction of the immune system, the onset of AIDS, and death. It is hoped that before the 1990s are out, HIV will be just another controllable viral infection.

The divisiveness that has marked the 1980s has been too costly, the human toll too great. We can spend the present debating the past but we must look to the future—we must go forward from where we are. Let history be history—learn from it and move on! The way for us to get through this crisis is hand in hand.

Humans shall overcome HIV!

Answers to Review Questions

CHAPTER 1

1. Acquired Immune Deficiency Syndrome

2. No. AIDS is a syndrome. A syndrome is made up of a collection of signs and symptoms of one or more diseases. AIDS patients have a collection of opportunistic infections and cancers. Collectively they are mistakenly referred to as the AIDS disease.

3. In 1983 by Luc Montagnier

4. 1981

5. LAV

6. Five; 1982, 1983, 1985, 1987, and 1993

7. The ARC or AIDS Related Complex definition was a middle ground used before AIDS was better understood. It became meaningless after the 1985 expanded definition listed organisms and symptoms which indicated that two states existed: HIV infection and progression to AIDS.

8. It allows HIV-infected persons earlier access into federal and state medical and social programs.

CHAPTER 2

1. The unbroken transmission of infection from an infected person to an uninfected person.

2. The answer to both questions is unknown at this time.

CHAPTER 3

1. Because it contains RNA as its genetic message and a reverse transcriptase enzyme to make DNA from RNA

2. GAG-POL-ENV; at least six

3. Because HIV has demonstrated an unusually high rate of genetic mutations; (1) the reverse transcriptase enzyme in HIV is highly error prone (makes transcription errors), and (2) a variety of HIV mutants have been found within a single HIV-infected individual.

4. The reverse transcriptase enzyme is highly error prone, making at least one, and in many cases more than one, deletion, addition, or substitution per round of proviral replication.

CHAPTER 4

1. Not really, because there is no way as yet to remove the provirus from the cell's DNA.

2. A physiological measurement that serves as a substitute for a major clinical event.

3. March; December; 11

4. 5

5. Zidovudine, didanosine, zalcitabine, stavudine, lamivudine.

6. Becoming incorporated into DNA as it is being synthesized, thereby stopping reverse transcriptase from attaching the next nucleotide.

7. (a) Clinical biological side effects; (b) the selection of drug-resistant HIV mutants.

8. (a) The number of copies of HIV RNA present in the plasma; (b) this number indicates the reproductive activity of HIV at the time and, if therapy is being used, the effect of the therapy on the reproductive ability of the virus.

9. Saquinavir, ritonavir, indinavir, nelfinavir

10. Indinavir, because either as a monotherapy or in combination, it is the most successful at dropping the viral load.

11. They physically interact with the reverse transcriptase enzyme and interfere with its function.

12. To suppress HIV replication, thereby reducing the number of mutant RNA strands produced.

13. A

14. B

CHAPTER 5

1. T4 helper cells; because T4 cells are crucial for the production of antibodies, a depletion of T4 cells results in immunosuppression which results in OIs.

2. CD4 is a receptor protein (antigen) secreted by certain cells of the immune system, for example, monocytes, macrophages, and T4 helper cells. It becomes located on the exterior of the cellular membrane and happens to be a compatible receptor for the HIV to attach and infect the CD4-carrying cell.

3. The question of true latency after HIV infection has not been settled. Most HIV/AIDS investigators currently believe there is a latent period, a time of few if any clinical symptoms and low levels of HIV in the blood. Other scientists, currently the minority, believe there is no true latency. The virus hides out in the lymph nodes slowly reproducing, and slowly killing off the T4 cells. The virus is always present, increasing slowly in numbers over time.

4. True

5. False

6. True

7. False

8. False

9. True

10. False

11. True

12. True

13. True

CHAPTER 6

1. OI is caused by organisms that are normally within the body and held in check by an active immune system. When the immune system becomes suppressed, for whatever reason, these agents can multiply and produce disease.

2. *Pneumocystis carinii*; lungs, pneumonia

3. *Isospora belli*

4. *Mycobacterium avium intracellulare*

5. False. HIV has not been found in KS tissue. KS is believed to develop as a result of a suppressed immune system and not the virus *per se*.

6. Classic KS, as described by Moritz Kaposi; and KS associated with AIDS

7. False. KS normally affects gay males. It is highly unusual to find KS in hemophiliacs, intravenous drug users and female AIDS patients.

8. True

9. True

CHAPTER 7

1. The 6-stage Walter Reed System and the 4 group CDC system

2. About 30%; about 90%

3. AIDS dementia complex

4. Skin—Kaposi's sarcoma
   Eyes—CMV retinitis
   Mouth—thrush or hairy leukoplakia
   Lungs—pneumocystis pneumonia
   Intestines—diarrhea

5. True

6. False. The average time is 6 to 18 weeks.

7. False. HIV infection leads to HIV disease. AIDS is the result of a weakened immune system that allows opportunistic infections to occur.

8. False. The average length of time is about 11 years.

CHAPTER 8

1. False. The United States currently reports most of the world's AIDS cases.

2. Cases of AIDS-related death, according to the CDC definition, can be traced back to 1952 in the United States and to the mid-1950s in Africa. In addition, studies since 1902 indicate that non-African men have been diagnosed with an aggressive form of Kaposi's sarcoma, a criterion for AIDS in homosexual males.

3. HIV-1 and HIV-2 show a 40% to 50% genetic relationship to each other.

4. False. HIV-1 and HIV-2 are both transmitted via the same routes. HIV-2 is spreading globally in similar fashion to HIV-1.

5. True. All scientific and empirical evidence to date indicates that HIV is not casually transmitted.

6. Through sexual activities: exchange of certain body fluids—blood and blood products, semen and vaginal secretions; and from mother to fetus or newborn by breast milk.

7. False. There is n ot a single documented case of HIV infection caused by deep kissing. HIV has been found in the saliva of infected people in very low concentration, and saliva has been shown to have anti-HIV properties.

8. True; but this assertion has been proven to be untrue. Insects, in particular mosquitoes, have not been shown to transmit HIV successfully.

9. False. According to studies involving the sexual partners of injection drug users and hemophiliacs, HIV transmission from male to female is the more efficient route. This is believed to be due to a greater concentration of HIV found in semen than in vaginal fluid.

10. The answer may be True or False. There have been cases in which a single act of intercourse has resulted in HIV infection. However, the majority of surveys on the sexual partners of injection drug users and hemophiliacs indicate that the number of sexual encounters may increase the risk of HIV infection but does not guarantee infection. Sexual partners of infected people have remained HIV-free after years of unprotected penis–vagina intercourse.

11. The percentage of fetal risk varies widely in a number of hospital studies. At the moment, the risk as reported without zidovudine therapy, varies from less than 30% to over 50%. The figures most commonly used are 30% to 50%. With the use of zidovudine therapy, the risk has been cut to about 8%.

12. D, all of the above

13. True

14. True

15. True

16. True

17. True

18. False

19. True

20. True

21. False

22. True

23. False

CHAPTER 9

1. Latex condoms. They are known to stop the transmission of viruses. This may not be true for animal intestine condoms.

2. Water-based lubricants. Oil-based lubricants weaken the later rubber causing them to leak or break under stress.

3. Safer sex is having sexual intercourse with an *uninfected* partner while using a condom.

4. The answer may be True or False. There have been cases where a single act of intercourse resulted in HIV infection. However, the majority of surveys completed by sexual partners of injection drug users and hemophiliacs indicate that the number of sexual encounters may increase the risk of HIV infection but does not guarantee infection. Sexual partners of infected persons have remained HIV-free after years of unprotected penis-vagina intercourse.

5. No. IDUs exist between "fixes." They lose things, they may not care to pick up new equipment—they need the "fix" now, it may be easier to share. Circumstances vary considerably among the IDU. Just giving them free equipment is no assurance that they will use it.

6. Between 1 in 39,000 and 1 in 200,000.

7. Have several students read their answers for promoting class discussion. Compare their response to that given in the text (that they should be punished).

8. Because attenuated HIV may mutate to a virulent form causing an HIV infection; there is no absolute guarantee that 100% of HIV are inactivated.

9. Because at no time will a whole HIV be present in the vaccine. Only a specific subunit of the HIV will be present in pure form so the vaccine should be free of any contaminating proteins that might prove toxic to one or more persons receiving the vaccine.

10. It is a situation wherein HIV antibodies might predispose the host to become more easily HIV-infected. For whatever reason, it appears that the HIV antibody complex enters the cell more easily than HIV alone.

11. Because of the severe forms of social ostracism that occur when it is learned that someone is HIV-positive or belongs to a high-risk group (gay, injection drug user, bisexual).

12. Universal precautions are a list of rules and regulations provided by the CDC to help prevent HIV infection in health care workers.

13. False

14. False

15. True

16. True

17. True

18. False

19. False

CHAPTER 10

1. The CDC said for each AIDS case there are from 50 to 100 HIV-infected people in the population. They got the 1 to 1.5 million figure using the 50 HIV-infected/AIDS cases; 1986; they are believed to be within plus or minus 10%.

2. Because their social and sexual behaviors and medical needs place these people at a greater risk for HIV exposure than those not practicing these social and sexual behaviors or who do not need blood or blood products.

3. False. Studies show that the time for progression from HIV infection to AIDS is the same regardless of parameters.

4. 52%

5. 30% to 50%

6. 99%

7. Two per 1,000 students; more: the rate for military personnel is 1.4 per 1,000.

8. College students 2/1,000, general population 0.02/1,000; this means the rate of HIV infection on college campuses is about 10 times higher than in the general population.

9. One in 20 to 300

10. Needlestick injuries

11. 3.5%

12. Hepatitis B virus

13. Montana, North and South Dakota, and Wyoming. It probably implies that HIV infection in the heterosexual population in these states is lower than in other states. This would translate into fewer HIV-infected women and few, if any, pediatric cases.

14. GAO—300,000 to 485,000

   CDC—270,000

15. Student's answer; text says no. People most often do not tell the truth—much depends on where, when, why, and who is doing the survey. There are just too many variables involved to believe sexual surveys.

16. About 440,000

17. 60%

CHAPTER 11

1. Approximately 16.4 million

2. About 52%

3. Injection drug use, being a sexual partner of an IDU, and through heterosexual contact.

4. IDU

5. 18 million; 3 million

6. Leading; 25 and 34; fifth; white; 25 and 44; leading; 25 and 44

7. An estimated 90,000 to 100,000

8. North Dakota and Wyoming

9. About 95%

10. (1) maternal viral load; (2) route of delivery, and (3) duration of early membrane rupture.

11. Most orphaned AIDS children have mothers who are IDUs and are themselves HIV-infected. They are AIDS orphans because (1) their par-

ents abandon them due to illness or death; and (2) these children are HIV-infected or demonstrate AIDS and therefore no one wants them.

12. Over 50%

13. Two

14. 28 million

15. 60%

16. 25%

17. About 500,000

18. 1-800-234-8336

CHAPTER 12

1. 26 HIV infections per minute

2. Heterosexual; heterosexual

3. France and Italy, in that order

4. The number of reported AIDS cases is doubling every 11 months.

5. IDUs—the frequency of new HIV infections appears to be leveling off in all other risk categories.

6. Mexico; Cuba; Soviet Union and Pakistan

7. Italy and Spain

CHAPTER 13

1. ELISA; enzyme linked immunosorbent assay

2. That the body will produce antibody against antigenic components of the HIV virus after infection occurs

3. No; a positive antibody result must be repeated in duplicate and if still positive, a confirmatory test is performed prior to telling people they are HIV-infected.

4. No; AIDS is medically diagnosed after certain signs and symptoms of specific diseases occur.

5. Western blot

6. Indirect immunofluorescent assay

7. By a color change in the reaction tube; the peroxidase enzyme oxidizes a clear chromogen into color formation. This occurs if

the HIV antibody–antigen enzyme complex is present in the reaction tube.

8. False. Some newborns receive the HIV antibody passively during pregnancy. About 30% to 50% of HIV-positive newborns are truly HIV-positive; it is unknown whether all HIV-positive newborns go on to develop AIDS. Not all have been discovered and it has not been determined whether 100% of HIV-infected adults or babies will develop AIDS.

9. They are not 100% accurate.

10. Determining that positive and negative tests are truly positive and negative and not falsely positive or negative.

11. Using either too high or too low cutoff points in the spectrophotometer and the presence of cross-reacting antibodies

12. The percentage of false positives will increase as the prevalence of HIV-infected people in a population decreases.

13. It is a screening test value that represents the probability that a positive HIV test is truly positive; because screening tests are not 100% accurate.

14. Western blot

15. There is no standardized WB test interpretation. Different agencies use different WB results (reactive bands) to determine that the test sample is positive.

16. Because the PCR allows for the detection of proviral DNA in cells before the body produces detectable HIV antibody; PCR reactions can be used to determine if high-risk (or anybody) antibody-negative people are HIV-infected but not producing antibodies and whether newborns are truly HIV-positive or passively HIV-positive.

17. True. The FDA approved two home-use HIV antibody test kits in 1996.

18. Between 6 and 18 weeks after HIV infection.

19. As early as 2 weeks after infection.

20. (1) Changes in their lifestyles that reduce stress on their immune systems may delay the onset of illness.

   (2) They can practice safer sex and hopefully not transmit the virus to others.

(3) The earlier the detection, the earlier they can enter into preventive therapy.

21. Mandatory with confidentiality; voluntary with confidentiality, anonymous and blinded.

22. For anonymous testing no personal information is given; in blind tests, the name is deleted but the demographic data remain.

23. Because there are many example of breaches of confidence, which destroys trust and subjects people to social stigma.

24. False

25. True

CHAPTER 14

1. Education, counseling, and signing the test consent form

2. Directive and nondirective counseling

3. To give the test results and counsel the person based on the outcome of those results

4. Denial; anger, bargaining, depression, and acceptance

5. D

6. B

7. A

8. True

9. True

10. False

CHAPTER 15

1. Newspapers, TV, radio, magazines, etc.

2. Barring children from public schools, police wearing rubber gloves during arrests, not going to a restaurant because someone who works there has AIDS, firing AIDS employees, etc.

3. Syphilis

4. Use of tobacco products, alcohol, drugs; nonuse of seat belts and motorcycle helmets, etc.

5. The ways by which one can become HIV-infected and how not to become HIV-infected.

6. Because most of the new cases of HIV infection and AIDS occur in high-risk groups that will not or cannot change sexual and drug practices.

7. Because a larger percentage of teenagers are sexually active with more than one partner, use drugs, use alcohol, and think that they are invulnerable to infection and death.

8. According to the AMA, No. Physicians may not refuse to care for patients with AIDS because of actual risk or fear of contracting the disease.

9. The CDC and AMA feel that a patient's right to that information should be determined on a case-by-case basis where surgery will be performed. There is no legal requirement for physicians to tell their patients of their HIV status.

10. Worker information sessions that explain how the virus can and cannot be transmitted.

CHAPTER 16

1. About $69,000; No, the cost of health care for a number of chronic diseases comes to about $69,000.

2. Indirect costs are the costs of lost productivity due to premature death. They are about five times higher per patient than direct costs.

3. Those who need insurance most are not insurable.

4. If they were to underwrite all the HIV-infected people, it would bankrupt the system, leaving everyone else without insurance.

5. **YOU**

CHAPTER 17

1. There does not appear to be a legal balance between a physician's duties to his or her patients and duties to public health in general. The physician is in a "Catch-22" position.

2. Class discussion topic or student essay on why they take their position:
   (1) The late Justice Oliver Wendell Holmes said that the public's right to know comes first.
   (2) Justice Goldberg (1989) said that the public's right to know is first.
   (3) 72% of Americans oppose the confidentiality of HIV tests.

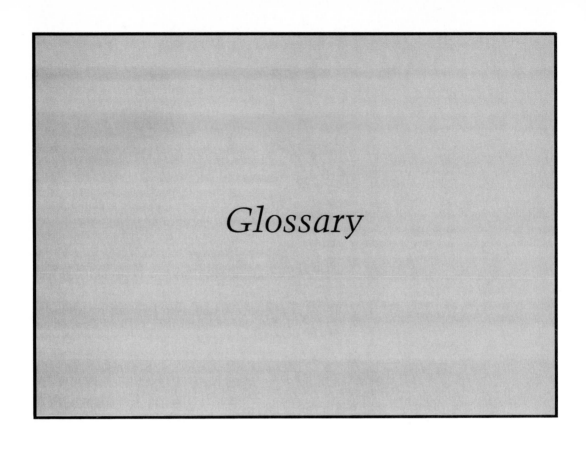

Glossary

ACRONYMS

ACTG AIDS clinical trial group

AIDS acquired immunodeficiency syndrome

ARV AIDS-related virus

AZT azathioprine (this is not zidovudine or azidothymidine)

CD4 a protein imbedded on the surface of a T lymphocyte to which HIV most often binds—a T4 cell.

CD8 a protein imbedded on the surface of a T lymphocyte suppressor cell—a T8 cell.

CDC Centers for Disease Control and Prevention (part of PHS)

3TC Lamivudine; nucleoside analog

CTS Counseling and Testing Services

DHHS Department of Health and Human Services

DNA deoxyribonucleic acid

d4T stavudine; nucleoside analog

ddC dideoxycytosine; nucleoside analog

ddI dideoxyinosine; nucleoside analog

FDA Food and Drug Administration (part of PHS)

HTLV-I human T cell lymphotropic virus, type I

HTLV-II human T cell lymphotropic virus, type II

HTLV-III human T cell lymphotropic virus, type III

IDU Injection Drug User

LAV lymphadenopathy-associated virus

NCI National Cancer Institute (part of NIH)

NEI National Eye Institute (part of NIH)

NIAID National Institute of Allergy and Infectious Diseases (part of NIH)

NIDA National Institute on Drug Abuse (part of PHS)

NIH National Institutes of Health (part of PHS)

OTA Office of Technology Assessment (part of U.S. Congress)

PCR (polymerase chain reaction) a very sensitive test used to detect the presence of HIV

PHS Public Health Service (part of DHHS)

RNA   ribonucleic acid

ZDV   Zidovudine major drug in treating HIV/AIDS persons; nucleoside analog

For the newest anti-HIV drugs, names and use, see Chapter 4.

TERMS

Acquired immunodeficiency syndrome (AIDS):   A life-threatening disease caused by a virus and characterized by the breakdown of the body's immune defenses. (See AIDS.)

Active immunity: Protection against a disease resulting from the production of antibodies in a host that has been exposed to a disease causing antigen.

Acute: Sudden onset, Short-term with severe symptoms.

Acyclovir (Zovirax):   Antiviral drug for herpes 1 and 2 and herpes zoster.

AIDS (acquired immunodeficiency syndrome):   A disease believed to be caused by a retrovirus called HIV and characterized by a deficiency of the immune system. The primary defect in AIDS is an acquired, persistent, quantitative functional depression within the T4 subset of lymphocytes. This depression often leads to infections caused by opportunistic microorganisms in HIV-infected individuals. A rare type of cancer (Kaposi's sarcoma) usually seen in elderly men or in individuals who are severely immunocompromised may also occur. Other associated diseases are currently under investigation and will probably be included in the final definition of AIDS.

AIDS dementia: Neurological complications affecting thinking and behavior; intellectual impairment.

Allergic reaction: A reaction that results from extreme sensitivity to a drug or agent and is not dependent on the amount of drug given. These may be classified into two types, immediate and delayed, based on the time it takes for the reaction to occur.

Analog (analogue):   A chemical molecule that closely resembles another one but which may function differently, thus altering a natural process.

Anemia: Low number of red blood cells.

Anorexia: Prolonged loss of appetite that leads to significant weight loss.

Antibiotic: A chemical substance capable of destroying bacteria and other microorganisms.

Antibody: A blood protein produced by mammals in response to a specific antigen.

Antigen: A large molecule, usually a protein or carbohydrate, which when introduced into the body stimulates the production of an antibody that will react specifically with that antigen.

Antigen-presenting cells: B cells, cells of the monocyte lineage (including macrophages and dentritic cells) and various other body cells that 'present' antigen in a form that T cells can recognize.

Antiserum: Serum portion of the blood that carries the antibodies.

Antiviral: Means against virus; drugs that destroy or weaken virus.

ARC: AIDS-related complex.

Arthritis: Inflammation of the joints and the surrounding tissues.

Arthropod: An insect-like animal.

Aspiration: The removal of fluids by suction.

Asymptomatic carrier: A host which is infected by an organism but does not demonstrate clinical signs or symptoms of the disease.

Asymptomatic seropositive: HIV-positive without signs or symptoms of HIV disease.

Ataxia: Inability to coordinate movement of muscles.

Atrophy: The wasting away or decrease in size and function of a body part.

Attenuated: Weakened.

Atypical: Irregular; not of typical character.

Autoimmunity: Antibodies made against self tissues.

Autoinoculation: A secondary infection originating from an infection site already present in the body.

B lymphocytes or B cells: Lymphocytes that produce antibodies. B lymphocytes proliferate under stimulation from factors released by T lymphocytes.

B- and T-cell lymphomas: Cancers caused by proliferation of the two principal types of white blood cells—B and T lymphocytes.

Bacterium: A microscopic organism composed of a single cell. Many but not all bacteria cause disease.

Blood count: A count of the number of red and white blood cells and platelets.

Bone marrow: Soft tissue located in the cavities of the bones. The bone marrow is the source of all blood cells.

Cancer: A large group of diseases characterized by uncontrolled growth and spread of abnormal cells.

Candida albicans: A fungus; the causative agent of vulvovaginal candidiasis or yeast infection.

Candidiasis: A fungal infection of the mucous membranes (commonly occurring in the mouth, where it is known as Thrush) characterized by whitish spots and/or a burning or painful sensation. It may also occur in the esophagus. It can also cause a red and itchy rash in moist areas, e.g., the vagina.

Capsid: The protein coat of a virus particle.

Carcinogen: Any substance that causes cancer.

Carcinoma: A form of skin cancer that occurs in tissues that cover or line body organs, e.g., intestines, lungs, breasts, uterus, etc.

Cardiovascular: Pertaining to the heart and blood vessels.

CXCR4 (FUSIN): Receptor for human chemokines and a necessary receptor for HIV entrance into T4 cells.

CC-CKR-5 (CKR-5): Receptor for human chemokines and a necessary receptor for HIV entrance into macrophage.

CD: Cluster differentiating type antigens found on T lymphocytes. Each CD is assigned a number: CD1, CD2, etc.

CD4(T4): White blood cell with type 4 protein embedded in the cell surface—target cell for HIV infection.

CD8: Suppressor white blood cell with type 8 protein embedded in the cell surface.

Cell-mediated immunity: The reaction to antigenic material by specific defensive cells (macrophages) rather than antibodies.

Cellular immunity: A collection of cell types that provide protection against various antigens.

Central nervous system (CNS): The brain and spinal cord.

Cerebral spinal fluid (CSF): The fluid which surrounds the brain and spinal cord.

Chain of infection: A series of infections that are directly or immediately connected to a particular source.

Chemokines: Chemicals released by T cell lymphocytes and other cells of the immune system to attract a variety of cell types to sites of inflammation.

Chemotherapy: The use of chemicals that have a specific and toxic effect upon a disease-causing pathogen.

Chlamydia: A species of bacterium, the causative organism of *Lymphogranuloma venereum*, chlamy-

dial urethritis and most cases of newborn conjunctivitis.

Chromosomes: Physical structures in the cell's nucleus that house the genes. Each human cell has 22 pairs of autosomes and two sex chromosomes.

Chronic: Having a long and relatively mild course.

Clade: Related HIV variants classified by degree of genetic similarity; nine are known for HIV.

Clinical latency: Infectious agent developing in a host without producing clinical symptoms.

Clinical manifestations: The signs of a disease as they pertain to or are observed in patients.

CMV: See cytomegalovirus

Cofactor: Factors or agents which are necessary or which increase the probability of the development of disease in the presence of the basic etiologic agent of that disease.

Cohort: A group of individuals with some characteristics in common.

Communicable: Able to spread from one diseased person or animal to another, either directly or indirectly.

Condylomata acuminatum (venereal warts): Viral warts of the genital and anogenital area.

Congenital: Acquired by the newborn before or at the time of birth.

Core proteins: Proteins that make up the internal structure or core of a virus.

Cross-resistance: Development of resistance to one agent as an antibotic, that results in resistance to other, usually similar agents.

Cryptococcal meningitis: A fungal infection that affects the three membranes (meninges) surrounding the brain and spinal cord. Symptoms include severe headache, vertigo, nausea, anorexia, sight disorders and mental deterioration.

Cryptococcosis: A fungal infectious disease often found in the lungs of AIDS patients. It characteristically spreads to the meninges and may also spread to the kidneys and skin. It is due to the fungus *Cryptococcus neoformans*.

Cryptosporidiosis: An infection caused by a protozoan parasite found in the intestines of animals. Acquired in some people by direct contact with the infected animal, it lodges in the intestines and causes severe diarrhea. It may be transmitted from person to person. This infection seems to be occurring more frequently in immunosuppressed people and can lead to prolonged symptoms which do not respond to medication.

Cutaneous: Having to do with the skin.

Cytokines: Powerful chemical substances secreted by cells. Cytokines include lymphokines produced by lymphocytes and monokines produced by monocytes and macrophages.

Cytomegalovirus (CMV): One of a group of highly host-specific herpes viruses that affect humans and other animals. Generally produces mild flu-like symptoms but can be more severe. In the immunosuppressed, it may cause pneumonia.

Cytopathic: Pertaining to or characterized by abnormal changes in cells.

Cytotoxic: Poisonous to cells.

Cytotoxic T cells: A subset of T lymphocytes that carry the T8 marker and can kill body cells infected by viruses or transformed by cancer.

Dementia: Chronic mental deterioration sufficient to significantly impair social and/or occupational function. Usually patients have memory and abstract thinking loss. They may have impairment of more specific higher cortical functions. Frequently progressive and irreversible.

Dendritic cells: White blood cells found in the spleen and other lymphoid organs. Dendritic cells typically use threadlike tentacles to "hold" the antigen, which they present to T cells.

Dermatitis: Inflammation of the skin.

Diagnosis: The identification of a disease by its signs, symptoms and laboratory findings.

Didanosine: Also known as videx; see ddI-inhibits HIV Replication.

Direct transmission: A manner of transmitting disease organisms in which the agent moves immediately from the infected person to the susceptible person, as in person-to-person contact and in droplet contact.

Disease intervention specialist (DIS): A person who performs STD patient interviewing/counseling and field investigation.

Dissemination: Spread of disease throughout the body.

DNA (deoxyribonucleic acid): A linear polymer, made up of deoxyribonucleotide repeating units. It is the carrier of genetic information in living organisms and some viruses.

DNA viruses: Contain DNA as their genetic material.

Dysentery: Inflammation of the intestines, especially the colon, producing pain in the abdomen and diarrhea containing blood and mucus.

Efficacy: Effectiveness.

ELISA test: A blood test which indicates the presence of antibodies to a given antigen. Various ELISA tests are used to detect a variety of infections. The HIV ELISA test does not detect AIDS but only indicates if viral infection has occurred.

Endemic: Prevalent in or peculiar to community or group of people.

Enteric infections: Infections of the intestine.

ENV: HIV gene that codes for protein gp160

Envelope proteins: Proteins that comprise the envelope or surface of a virus, gp120 and gp41.

Enzyme: A catalytic protein that is produced by living cells and promotes the chemical processes of life without itself being altered or destroyed.

Epidemic: When the incidence of a disease surpasses the expected rate in any well-defined geographical area.

Epidemiologic studies: Studies concerned with the relationships of various factors determining the frequency and distribution of certain diseases.

Epidemiology: The study of the factors that impact on the spread of disease in an area.

Epitopes: Characteristic shapes of antigens found on an organism or virus.

Epivir: See 3TC.

Epstein-Barr virus (EBV): A virus that causes infectious mononucleosis. It is spread by saliva. EBV lies dormant in the lymph glands and has been associated with Burkitt's lymphoma, a cancer of the lymph tissue.

Etiologic agent: The organism which causes a disease.

Etiology: The study of the cause of disease.

Extracellular: Found outside the cell wall.

Exudate: To produce liquid in response to disease.

Factor VIII: A naturally occurring protein in plasma that aids in the coagulation of blood. A congenital deficiency of Factor VIII results in the bleeding disorder known as hemophilia A.

Factor VIII concentrate: A concentrated preparation of Factor VIII that is used in the treatment of individuals with hemophilia A.

Fallopian tube: A slender 4-inch-long tube extending from the ovary to the uterus. Eggs released during ovulation pass through this tube to reach the uterus.

False negative: Failure of a test to demonstrate the disease or condition when present.

False positive: A positive test result caused by a disease or condition other than the disease for which the test is designed.

Fellatio: Oral sex involving the penis.

Follicular dendritic cells: Found in germinal centers of lymphoid organs.

Fomite: An inanimate object that can hold infectious agents and transfers them from one individual to another.

Fulminant: Rapid onset, severe.

Fungus: Member of a class of relatively primitive organisms. Fungi include mushrooms, yeasts, rusts, molds and smuts.

Fusin: See CXCR4

Gammaglobulin: The antibody component of the serum.

Ganciclovir (DHPG): An experimental antiviral drug used in the treatment of CMV retinitis.

Gene: The basic unit of heredity; an ordered sequence of nucleotides. A gene contains the information for the synthesis of one polypeptide chain (protein).

Gene expression: The production of RNA and cellular proteins.

Genitourinary: Pertaining to the urinary and reproductive structures; sometimes called the GU tract or system.

Genome: The genetic endowment of an organism.

GP41: Glycoprotein found in envelope of HIV.

GP120: Glycoprotein found in outer level of HIV envelope.

GP160: Precusor glycoprotein to forming gp41 and gp120.

Giardiasis: Infection of the intestinal tract with *Giardia lamblia* (a protozoan) which may cause intermittent diarrhea of lengthy duration.

Globulin: That portion of serum which contains the antibodies.

Glycoproteins: Proteins with carbohydrate groups attached at specific locations.

Glycosylation: The attachment of a carbohydrate molecule to another molecule such as a protein.

Gonococcus: The specific etiologic agent of gonorrhea discovered by Neisser and named *Neisseria gonorrhoeae.*

Granulocytes: Phagocytic white blood cells filled with granules containing potent chemicals that allow the cells to digest microorganisms. Neutrophils, eosinophils, basophils and mast cells are examples of granulocytes.

Hemoglobin: The oxygen-carrying portion of red blood cells which gives them a red color.

Hemophilia: A hereditary bleeding disorder caused by a deficiency in the ability to synthesize one or more of the blood coagulation proteins, e.g., Factor VIII (hemophilia A) or Factor IX (hemophilia B).

Hepatitis: Inflammation of the liver; due to many causes including viruses, several of which are transmissible through blood transfusions and sexual activities.

Hepatosplenomegaly: Enlargement of the liver and spleen.

Herpes simplex virus I (HSV-I): A virus that results in cold sores or fever blisters, most often on the mouth or around the eyes. Like all herpes viruses, it may lie dormant for months or years in nerve tissues and flare up in times of stress, trauma, infection or immunosuppression. There is no cure for any of the herpes viruses.

Herpes simplex virus II (HSV-II): Causes painful sores on the genitals or anus. It is one of the most common sexually transmitted diseases in the United States.

Herpes varicella zoster virus (HVZ): The varicella virus causes chicken pox in children and may reappear in adulthood as herpes zoster. Herpes zoster, also called shingles, is characterized by small, painful blisters on the skin along nerve pathways.

High-risk behavior: A term used to describe certain activities that increase the risk of disease exposure.

High-risk groups: Those groups of people that show a behavioral risk for exposure to a disease or condition.

Histoplasmosis: A disease caused by a fungal infection that can affect all the organs of the body. Symptoms usually include fever, shortness of breath, cough, weight loss and physical exhaustion.

HIV (human immunodeficiency virus): A newly discovered retrovirus that is said to cause AIDS. The target organ of HIV is the T4 subset of T lymphocytes, which regulate the immune system.

HIV-positive: Presence of the human immunodeficiency virus in the body.

Homophobia: Negative bias towards or fear of individuals who are homosexual.

Human leukocyte antigens (HLA): Protein markers of self used in histocompatibility testing. Some HLA types also correlate with certain autoimmune diseases.

Humoral immunity: The production of antibodies for defense against infection or disease.

Hybridoma: A hybrid cell created by fusing a B lymphocyte with a long-lived neoplastic plasma cell, or a T lymphocyte with a lymphoma cell. A B-cell hybridoma secretes a single specific antibody.

Idiotypes: The unique and characteristic parts of an antibody's variable region, which can themselves serve as antigens.

Immunity: Resistance to a disease because of a functioning immune system.

Immune complex: A cluster of interlocking antigens and antibodies.

Immune response: The reaction of the immune system to foreign substances.

Immune status: The state of the body's natural defense to diseases. It is influenced by heredity, age, past illness history, diet and physical and mental health. It includes production of circulating and local antibodies and their mechanism of action.

Immunoassay: The use of antibodies to identify and quantify substances. Often the antibody is linked to a marker such as a fluorescent molecule, a radioactive molecule or an enzyme.

Immunocompetent: Capable of developing an immune response

Immunoglobulins: A family of large protein molecules, also known as antibodies.

Immunostimulant: Any agent that will trigger a body's defenses.

Immunosuppression: When the immune system is not working normally. This can be the result of illness or certain drugs (commonly those used to fight cancer).

Incidence: The total number of new cases of a disease in a given area within a specified time, usually 1 year.

Incubation period: The time between the actual entry of an infectious agent into the body and the onset of disease symptoms.

Indinavir: Crixivan, a protease inhibitor drug.

Indirect transmission: The transmission of a disease to a susceptible person by means of vectors or by airborne route.

Infection: Invasion of the body by viruses or other organisms.

Infectious disease: A disease which is caused by microorganisms or viruses living in or on the body as parasites.

Inflammatory response: Redness, warmth and swelling in response to infection; the result of increased blood flow and a gathering of immune cells and secretions.

Injection drug use: Use of drugs injected by needle into a vein or muscle tissue.

Innate immunity: Inborn or hereditary immunity.

Inoculation: The entry of an infectious organism or virus into the body.

Integrase: HIV enzyme used to insert HIV DNA into host cell DNA.

Interferon: A class of glycoproteins important in immune function and thought to inhibit viral infection.

Interleukins: Chemical messengers that travel from leukocytes to other white blood cells. Some promote cell development, others promote rapid cell division.

Intracellular: Found within the cell wall.

In utero: In the uterus

In vitro: "In glass"—pertains to a biological reaction in an artificial medium.

In vivo: "In the living"—pertains to a biological reaction in a living organism.

IV: Intravenous.

Kaposi's sarcoma: A multifocal, spreading cancer of connective tissue, principally involving the skin; it usually begins on the toes or the feet as reddish blue or brownish soft nodules and tumors.

Keratin: A waterproofing protein in the skin.

Lamivudine: Nucleoside analog inhibits HIV replication.

Langerhans cells: Dendritic cells in the skin that pick up antigen and transport it to lymph nodes.

Latency: A period when a virus or other organism is still in the body but in an inactive state.

Latent viral infection: The virion becomes part of the host cell's DNA.

Lentiviruses: Viruses that cause disease very slowly. HIV is believed to be this type of virus.

Lesion: Any abnormal change in tissue due to disease or injury.

Leukocyte: A white blood cell.

Leukopenia: A decrease in the white blood cell count.

Log: 10-fold difference.

Lymph: A transparent, slightly yellow fluid that carries lymphocytes, bathes the body tissues and drains into the lymphatic vessels.

Lymph nodes: Gland-like structures in the lymphatic system which help to prevent spread of infection.

Lymphadenopathy: Enlargement of the lymph nodes.

Lymphadenopathy syndrome (LAS): A condition characterized by persistent, generalized, enlarged lymph nodes, sometimes with signs of minor illness such as fever and weight loss, which apparently represents a milder reaction to HIV infection. LAS is also known as generalized lymphadenopathy syndrome.

Lymphatic system: A fluid system of vessels and glands which is important in controlling infections and limiting their spread.

Lymphocytes: Specialized white blood cells involved in the immune response.

Lymphoid organs: The organs of the immune system where lymphocytes develop and congregate. They include the bone marrow, thymus, lymph nodes, spleen and other clusters of lymphoid tissue.

Lymphokines: Chemical messengers produced by T and B lymphocytes. They have a variety of protective functions.

Lymphoma: Malignant growth of lymph nodes.

Lymphosarcoma: A general term applied to malignant neoplastic disorders of lymphoid tissue, not including Hodgkin's disease.

Lytic infection: When a virus infects the cell, the cell produces new viruses and breaks open (lyse) releasing the viruses.

Macrophage: A large and versatile immune cell that acts as a microbe-devouring phagocyte, an antigen-presenting cell and an important source of immune secretions.

Macule: A discolored spot or patch on the skin which is not raised or thickened.

Major histocompatibility complex (MHC): A group of genes that controls several aspects of the immune response. MHC genes code for self markers on all body cells.

Malaise: A general feeling of discomfort or fatigue.

Malignant tumor: A tumor made up of cancerous cells. The tumors grow and invade surrounding tissue, then the cells break away and grow elsewhere.

Medicaid: This program is state operated and administered but has federal financial participation. Within certain broad federally determined guidelines, states decide who is eligible; the amount, duration, and scope of services covered; rates of payment for providers; and methods of administering the program. Medicaid provides health care services for certain low-income persons. Medicaid does not provide health services to all poor people in every state. It categorically covers participants in the Aid to Families with Dependent Children program and in the Supplemental Security Income program. In most states it also covers certain other people deemed to be medically needy. The program was authorized in 1965 by Title XIX of the Social Security Act.

Medicare: This is a nationwide health insurance program providing health insurance protection to people 65 years of age and over, people entitled to social security disability payments for 2 years or more, and people with end-stage renal disease, regardless of income. The program was enacted July 30, 1965, as Title XVIII, *Health Insurance for the Aged* of the Social Security Act, and became effective on July 1, 1966. It consists of two separate but coordinated programs, hospital insurance (Part A) and supplementary medical insurance (Part B).

Messenger RNA (mRNA): RNA that serves as the template for protein synthesis; it carries the information from the DNA to the protein synthesizing complex to direct protein synthesis.

Microbes: Minute living organisms including bacteria, viruses, fungi and protozoa.

Microorganisms: Microscopic plants or animals.

Molecule: The smallest amount of a specific chemical substance that can exist alone. To break a molecule down into its constituent atoms is to change its character. A molecule of water, for instance, reverts to oxygen and hydrogen.

Monocyte: A large phagocytic white blood cell which, when it enters tissue, develops into a macrophage.

Monokines: Powerful chemical substances secreted by monocytes and macrophages. They help direct and regulate the immune response.

Morbidity: The proportion of people with a disease in a community.

Morphology: The study of the form and structure of organisms.

Mortality: The number of people who die as a result of a specific cause.

Mucosal immunity: Resistance to infection across, mucous membranes.

Mucous membrane: The lining of the canals and cavities of the body which communicate with external air, such as the intestinal tract, respiratory tract and the genitourinary tract.

Mucous patches: White, patchy growths, usually found in the mouth, that are symptoms of secondary syphilis and are highly infectious.

Mucus: A fluid secreted by membranes

Mutant: A new strain of a virus or microorganism that arises as a result of change in the genes of an existing strain.

Natural killer cells (also called NK cells): Immune cells that kill infected cells directly within 4 hours of contact. NK cells differ from other killer cells, such as cytotoxic T lymphocytes, in that they do not require contact with antigen before they are activated.

Neisseria gonorrhoeae: The bacterium that causes gonorrhea.

Neonatal: Pertaining to the first 4 weeks of life.

Neoplasm: A new abnormal growth, such as a tumor.

Neuropathy: Group of nerve disorders—symptoms range from tingling sensation, numbness to paralysis.

Nevirapine: Non-nucleostide analog inhibits HIV replication.

Nodule: A small node which is solid and can be detected by touch.

Notifiable disease: A notifiable disease is one that, when diagnosed, health providers are required, usually by law, to report to state or local public health officials. Notifiable diseases are those of public interest by reason of their contagiousness, severity, or frequency.

Nucleic acids: Large, naturally occurring molecules composed of chemical building blocks known as nucleotides. There are two kinds of nucleic acid, DNA and RNA.

Nucleoside analog: Synthetic compounds generally similar to one of the bases of DNA.

Nucleotide of DNA: Made up of one of four nitrogen-containing bases (adenine, cytosine, guanine or thymine), a sugar and a phosphate molecule.

Oncogenic: Anything that may give rise to tumors, especially malignant ones.

Opportunistic disease: Disease caused by normally benign microorganisms or viruses that become pathogenic when the immune system is impaired.

p24 antigen: A protein fragment of HIV. The p24 antigen test measures this fragment. A positive test result suggests active HIV replication and may mean the individual has a chance of developing AIDS in the near future.

Parenteral: Not taken in through the digestive system.

Parasite: A plant or animal that lives, grows and feeds on another living organism.

Pathogen: Any disease-producing microorganism or substance.

Pathogenic: Giving rise to disease or causing symptoms.

Pathology: The science of the essential nature of diseases, especially of the structural and functional changes in tissues and organs caused by disease.

Perianal glands: Glands located around the anus.

Perinatal: Occurring in the period during or just after birth.

Phagocytes: Large white blood cells that contribute to the immune defense by ingesting microbes or other cells and foreign particles.

PID (pelvic inflammatory disease):   Inflammation of the female pelvic organs; often the result of gonococcal or chlamydial infection.

Placebo: An inactive substance against which investigational treatments are compared to see how well the treatment worked.

Plasma: The fluid portion of the blood which contains all the chemical constituents of whole blood except the cells.

Plasma cells: Derived from B cells, they produce antibodies.

Platelets: Small oval discs in blood that are necessary for blood to clot.

PLWA: Persons Living With AIDS.

Polymerase chain reaction: Method to detect and amplify very small amounts of DNA in a sample.

Poppers: Slang term for the inhalant drug amyl nitrate.

Positive HIV test: A sample of blood that is reactive on an initial ELISA test, reactive on a second ELISA run of the same specimen and reactive on Western blot, if available.

***Pneumocystis carinii* pneumonia (PCP):**   A rare type of pneumonia primarily found in infants and now common in patients with AIDS.

Prenatal: During pregnancy.

Prevalence: The total number of cases of a disease existing at any time in a given area.

Primary immune response: Production of antibodies about 7 to 10 days after an infection.

Prophylactic treatment: Medical treatment of patients exposed to a disease before the appearance of disease symptoms.

Protease: Enzyme that cuts proteins into peptides (breaks down proteins).

Protense inhibitors: Compounds that inhibit the action of protease.

Proteins: Organic compounds made up of amino acids. Proteins are one of the major constituents of plant and animal cells.

Protocol: Standardization of procedures so that results of treatment or experiments can be compared.

Protozoa: A group of one-celled animals, some of which cause human disease including malaria, sleeping sickness and diarrhea.

Provirus: The genome of an animal virus integrated into the chromosome of the host cell, and thereby replicated in all of the host's daughter cells.

Pruritis: Itching.

Race: Beginning in 1976 the federal government's data systems classified individuals into the following racial groups: American Indian or Alaskan Native, Asian or Pacific Islander, black, and white.

Rate: A rate is a measure of some event, disease, or condition in relation to a unit of population, along with some specification of time.

Receptors: Special molecules located on the surface membranes of cells that attract other molecules to attach to them. (For example CD4, CD8, and CC-CKR-5)

Recombinant DNA: DNA produced by joining pieces of DNA from different sources.

Recombinant DNA techniques: Techniques that allow specific segments of DNA to be isolated and inserted into a bacterium or other host (e.g., yeast, mammalian cells) in a form that will allow the DNA segment to be replicated and expressed as the cellular host multiplies.

Rectum: The end part of the large intestine through which feces are excreted from the body.

Remission: The lessening of the severity of disease or the absence of symptoms over a period of time.

Retroviruses: Viruses that contain RNA and produce a DNA analog of their RNA using an enzyme known as reverse transcriptase.

Reverse transcriptase: An enzyme produced by retroviruses that allows them to produce a DNA analog of their RNA, which may then incorporate into the host cell.

Ritonavir: Novir, a protease inhibitor drug.

RNA (ribonucleic acid):   Any of various nucleic acids that contain ribose and uracil as structural components and are associated with the control of cellular chemical activities.

RNA viruses: Contain RNA as their genetic material.

Salmonella: A bacterium that may cause diarrhea with cramps and sometimes fever.

Sarcoma: A form of cancer that occurs in connective tissue, muscle, bone and cartilage.

Saquinavir: Invirase, a protease inhibitor drug.

Secondary immune response: On repeat exposure to an antigen, there is an accelerated production of antibodies.

Sensitivity: The probability that a test will be positive when the infection is present.

Septicemia: A disease condition in which the infectious agent has spread throughout the lymphatic and blood systems causing a general body infection.

Seroconversion: The point at which an individual exposed to the AIDS virus becomes serologically positive.

Serologic test: Laboratory test made on serum.

Serum: The clear portion of any animal liquid separated from its more solid elements, especially the clear liquid which separates in the clotting of blood (blood serum).

Shigella: A bacterium that can cause dysentery.

Specificity: The probability that a test will be negative when the infection is not present.

Spirochete: A corkscrew-shaped bacterium; e.g., *Treponema pallidum.*

Spleen: A lymphoid organ in the abdominal cavity that is an important center for immune system activities.

Squamous: Scaly or plate-like; a type of cell.

Stavudine: Also known as Zerit; See d4T—inhibits HIV replication.

Sterilizing immunity: Immune response that completely prevents an infection.

STD (sexually transmitted disease):   Any disease which is transmitted primarily through sexual practices.

Subclinical infections: Infections with minimal or no apparent symptoms.

Subunit vaccine: A vaccine that uses only one component of an infectious agent rather than the whole to stimulate an immune response.

Suppressor T cells: A subset of T cells that carry the T8 marker and turn off antibody production and other immune responses.

Surrogate marker: A substitute; a person or agent that replaces another, an alternate.

Surveillance: The process of accumulating information about the incidence and prevalence of disease in an area.

Susceptible: Inability to resist an infection or disease.

Symptomatology: The combined symptoms of a disease.

Syndrome: A set of symptoms which occur together.

Systemic: Affecting the body as a whole.

T cell growth factor (TCGF, also known as interleukin-2):   A glycoprotein that is released by T lymphocytes on stimulation by antigens and which functions as a T cell growth factor by inducing proliferation of activated T cells.

T Helper cells (also called T4 cells):   A subset of T cells that carry the T4 marker and are essential for turning on antibody production, activating cytotoxic T cells and initiating many other immune responses.

T lymphocytes or T cells: Lymphocytes that mature in the thymus and which mediate cellular immune reactions. T lymphocytes also release factors that induce proliferation of T lymphocytes and B lymphocytes.

T8 cells: A subset of T cells that may kill virus-infected cells and suppress immune function when the infection is over.

Thrush: A disease characterized by the formation of whitish spots in the mouth. It is caused by the fungus *Candida albicans* during times of immunosuppression.

Thymus: A primary lymphoid organ high in the chest where T lymphocytes proliferate and mature.

Titer: Level or amount.

Tolerance: A state of nonresponsiveness to a particular antigen or group of antigens.

Toxic reaction: A harmful side effect from a drug; it is dose dependent, i.e., becomes more frequent and severe as the drug dose is increased. All drugs have toxic effects if given in a sufficiently large dose.

Toxoplasmosis: An infection with the protozoan *Taxoplasma gondii*, frequently causing focal encephalitis (inflammation of the brain). It may also involve the heart, lungs, adrenal glands, pancreas and testes.

Transcription: The synthesis of messenger RNA on a DNA template; the resulting RNA sequence is complementary to the DNA sequence. This is the first step in gene expression.

Translation: The process by which the genetic code contained in a nucleotide sequence of messenger RNA directs the synthesis of a specific order of amino acids to produce a protein.

Treponema pallidum: The bacterial spirochete that causes syphilis.

Tropism: Involuntary turning, curving, or attraction to a source of stimulation.

Tumor: A swelling or enlargement; an abnormal mass that can be malignant or benign. It has no useful body function.

Urethra: The tube conveying urine from the bladder out of the body.

Urethritis: Inflammation of the urethra.

Uterus: The womb; a pear-shaped, muscular organ which holds the fetus during pregnancy.

V3 loop: Section of the gp120 protein on the surface of HIV; appears to be important in stimulating neutralizing antibodies.

Vaccine: A preparation of dead organisms, attenuated live organisms, live virulent organisms, or parts of microorganisms that is administered to artificially increase immunity to a particular disease.

Vagina: The canal which leads from the external female genitalia to the cervix.

Vector: The means by which a disease is carried from one human to another.

Venereal warts: Viral *Condylomata acuminata* on or near the anus or genitals.

Vesicle: A small blister on the skin.

Viral load: The total amount of virus in a person's body.

Viremia: The presence of virus in the blood.

Virulence: The ability on the part of an infectious agent to induce, incite or produce pathogenic changes in the host.

Virus: Any of a large group of submicroscopic agents capable of infecting plants, animals and bacteria; characterized by a total dependence on living cells for reproduction and by a lack of independent metabolism.

Vulva: The external parts of the female genitalia including the labia majora, labia minora, mons pubis, clitoris, perineum and vestibulum vagina.

Western Blot: A blood test used to detect antibodies to a given antigen. Compared to the ELISA test, the Western Blot is more specific and more expensive. It can be used to confirm the results of the ELISA test.

X-ray: Radiant energy of extremely short wavelength used to diagnose and treat cancer.

Zalcitabine: Also known as HIVID; see ddC—inhibits HIV replication.

Zidovudine: Also known as Retrovir; see ZDV—inhibits HIV replication.

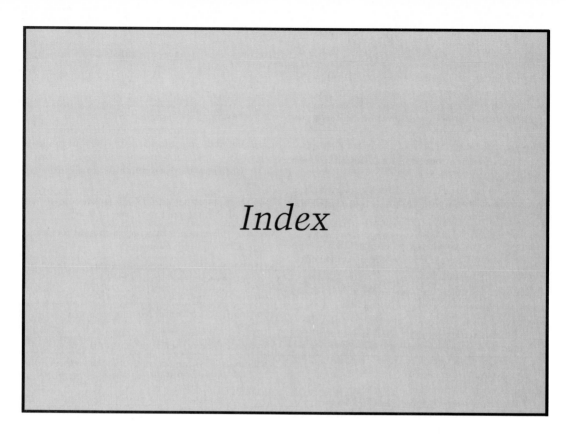

Index

Note: Italicized letters *f* and *t* following page numbers indicate figures and tables, respectively.

Cell-to-cell transmission of HIV, 202, 204f, 206, 207f
  by adhesion, 206, 207f
  by fusion, 206
Cellular immunity, 108
Censorship, of AIDS educational materials, 493-494
Centers for Disease Control and Prevention (CDC), 249
  budget of, 524f
  classification of HIV-related diseases, 176-177, 179t, 180f
  condom ad campaign of, 259-260
  counseling guidelines of, 451t
  and definition of AIDS, 31, 32t
  first report on AIDS, 27-28
  formula for determining number of HIV-infected cases, 302
  and HIV contaminated blood scandal, 210-211
  name change of, 28
  position on HIV-infected health care workers, 568
  precautions recommended by, 279, 279t
  prevention programs supported by, 440
  preventive guidelines for health care workers, 568t, 569
  and screening of health care workers, 214
  testing guidelines of, 451t
Central dogma of molecular biology, 50
Central nervous system (CNS)
  HIV infection of, 181-184, 183f
    clinical manifestations of, 182t
  lymphoma, cost of treatment, 516t
Cerebrospinal fluid, HIV in, 202
Cervical cancer
  human papillomavirus and, 7
  invasive
    AIDS cases with, 33
    in definition of AIDS, 32-33, 33f
Cervical dysplasia, in HIV-infected women, 341-342
Cesarean delivery, and HIV transmission, 348-349
Chancroid
  global incidence of, 236f
  and HIV transmission, 234-235
  risk for, 215
Chemical barrier protection
  against HIV infection, 265-267
  against sexually transmitted diseases, 265-267
Chemokines, 21, 108
  _, as suppressors of HIV infection, 115
  receptors, 14, 53f
    and HIV entry in cell, 115-116, 116f
Chickenpox, attenuated vaccine for, 288
Chickens, cancer in, 50
Childbirth, HIV transmission in, 348-349
Children. See also Newborns
  deaths from AIDS, 12
  disclosing HIV status to, 463

in families affected by HIV, 461-464
with HIV/AIDS. See also Pediatric HIV/AIDS
  discrimination against, 13
  of HIV-infected mothers, 236-240
  infectious diseases affecting, 11
  long-term survivors among, 184
  opportunistic infections in, 184
  orphaned, AIDS and, 346-348
  Pneumocystis carinii pneumonia (PCP) in, 138-139
  rotavirus infection in, 3-6
  sexual assault of, 231-232
  transmission of HIV to mothers, 384
China
  flu virus in, 9
  HIV/AIDS in, 390-391
  HIV-contaminated blood scandal in, 213
Chlamydia infection
  in adolescents, 354
  global incidence of, 236f
  and risk for HIV infection, 215-216, 235
  symptoms of, 146t
Cholera, 4t, 9, 286
Chronic stage of HIV disease, 167, 167f
  heterogeneity in, 60
Church
  attitude toward HIV/AIDS, 487, 490-491
  reaction to condoms, 264
Ciprofloxacin, 134t, 145-146
CKR-5. See CC-CKR-5
Clarithromycin (Biaxin), 134t, 145-146
Class distinctions, in HIV/AIDS treatment, 97
Class I proteins, 102, 111
Class II proteins, 111-112
Clindamycin, for opportunistic infections, 134t
Clinical conditions, in HIV/AIDS, 31-33, 32t 33t
Clinical drug trials, 98, 341
Clinical incubation, 163, 173
Clinical latency. See also Asymptomatic stage of HIV/AIDS
  definition of, 163
  HIV production during, 122-124
Clinton Administration, 429
  and AIDS vaccine, 285
  immigration policy for HIV-positive people, 200
Clofazimine, 134t, 145-146
Clotrimazole (Mycelex Troches), 134t, 137
Cluster differentiation antigens. See CD antigens
CMV. See Cytomegalovirus
Cocaine abusers, and HIV infection, 230
  in women, 337
Coccidioides immitis, 134t
Coccidioidomycosis, 33t, 135
Cocktails, AIDS. See Combination drug therapy

Cofactor
  definition of, 195
  in HIV infection, 119-120
College students
  AIDS cases among, 311-313
  perceptions about HIV/AIDS, 496
Columbia, HIV-contaminated blood scandal in, 213
Combination drug therapy, 74, 76-79, 85, 326
  advantages of, 76
  cost of, 95
  current problems/limitations using, 75, 89-91, 94
  guidelines on, 89
  and opportunistic infections, 131
  premature optimism about, 93
  protease inhibitors in, 93
  success of, 78, 178
  social implications of, 85-86
Commercial sex workers. See Prostitutes
Communicable diseases, 189
  and immigration policy, 200
  laws regarding, 559-561
Computer sites, AIDS-related, 23
Conception, male-to-female HIV transmission during, 345
Condoms
  advertisements for, 258f, 259-260
  animal-derived, 258
  church reaction to, 264
  controversy over promotion of, 256
  cultural attitudes towards
    in Africa, 370-373
    in Brazil, 381
  efficacy of, 255-256, 261-262, 262t
  female, 259f, 262-264, 263f
    questions and answers about, 266
  free distribution of, 260
  history of, 257
  lubricants for, 264-265, 265t
  male, 257-258
  as medical devices, 256-257
  polyurethane (plastic), 257-258, 262
  and prevention of HIV transmission, 251, 254-256
  and prevention of sexually transmitted diseases, 146
  proper placement of, 255
  quality of, 261
  reluctance to use, gender-specific, 448
  risk for HIV infection using, 225, 225t
  in Thai prevention program, 390
  use in World War I and World War II, 254
  varieties of, 257, 259f
Confidentiality
  breach of, 566
  definition of, 556
  dilemma of, 564-567
  Hippocratic oath and, 564
  in HIV testing, 431-434
  laws regarding, 556-562, 566-567
  questions about, 545
  statement on, 562

compared to other diseases, 525-526

Health care system
  discrimination against HIV-infected people in, legal remedies for, 539-541
  inadequacies of, 149-150

Health care worker(s)
  adolescents' concerns about, 356-357
  definition of, 315
  duties of, 502-503
  fear of HIV/AIDS, 502-509
  HIV-infected, 315-316
    CDC guidelines for, 568, 568t, 569
    discrimination against, 554-555
    legal issues regarding, 567-568
    and transmission to patients, 206-215
      precautions against, 206-215
      risk for, 206-215, 504-506
  HIV transmission to, 195-196
    cases of, 507-511
    legal remedies for, 550
    prevention of, 196, 253t, 278-282, 279t
    risk for, 202, 280-281
  legal issues involving, 553
  mandatory testing policy for, impact of, 428
  mistreatment of AIDS patients by, 149-150
  proposed screening for HIV, 214
  refusal to treat AIDS patients, legal implications of, 568-569
  rights of, 545, 570
  transmission of hepatitis B to, 316
  rise in, 202

Health Education AIDS Liaison (HEAL), 38

Health insurance
  for AIDS patients, 531-534
    denial of, 550-551
    screening procedures, 536-538, 537t
    variation by stage of illness, 533
  availability of, 534
  costs of, 534
  laws regarding, 538
  people without, 533-535
  right to, 536
  rising costs of, 531
  risk classification for, 535, 537t

Heckler, Margaret M., 283, 285

Hellinger, Fred, 528

Helper T cells. See T4 cell(s)

Hemophiliacs
  AIDS cases among, 12, 192f193f, 311, 320t
  cost of treating, 525
  HIV transmission to, 40, 210-213
  and public reaction, 277

Hepatitis B virus
  deaths from, 10, 10t, 11
  dose necessary to cause infection, 201
  and liver cancer, 7
  transmission in health care settings, 201-202

transmission to health care workers, 316
universal precautions against, 279
vaccine for, 293

Heroin
  HIV/AIDS among users of, 230
  immunological suppressive effect of, 120

Herpes virus (HHV-8), 154
  and Kaposi's sarcoma, 154

Herpes simplex virus (HSV). See also Genital herpes
  blindness caused by, 142-143
  clinical manifestation of, 134t
  as cofactor in immune deficiency, 120
  in definition of AIDS, 33t
  in HIV-infected women, 341
  and risk for HIV infection, 215
  suppression of immune system response by, 104
  symptoms of, 146t
  therapeutic vaccine for, 287
  treatment of, 134t
  type I, 141
  type II, 141
    perianal and rectal ulcers, 143f
  in U.S., 233-234

Herpes zoster virus (HZV), 143

Heterogeneity of HIV, 58, 60

Heterosexual transmission, 216, 333
  in Africa, 369, 372
  in anal intercourse, 218-219
  in Asia, 64, 379, 385
  in Canada, 377
  cases of, 33-34, 192f193f, 310-311, 320t
    first, 12
    rise in, 321-323
  differences in rate of, 64
  geographic patterns, 200
  global statistics, 362
  risk estimates for, 224-225
  in Thailand, 389

HGPV-16. See Human papillomavirus-16

HHV-8. See Herpes virus

Highly active antiretroviral therapy (HAART), side effects of, 131

Hijras, 388

Hill-Burton Act, 541

Hispanics, HIV/AIDS cases in, 33-34, 308f
  adult/adolescent, 305-307, 355
  among women, 333-334, 335f
  pediatric, 238, 345f

Histoplasma capsulatum (histoplasmosis)
  anal, 136f
  clinical manifestation of, 134t
  in definition of AIDS, 31, 32t, 33t
  geography and risk for, 135
  signs and symptoms of, 135, 136f
  treatments of, 134t

HIV, 27
  agents effective against, 251t
  assembly, 88f
  attachment to T4 cell, 114
  budding, 56f
  as cancer trigger, 155, 156f

as cause of AIDS
  arguments against, 36-39
  evidence for, 39-42
  characteristics of, 47-50
  clearance rate, 170
  core of, 53f, 114
  danger of spreading, 216
  dimensions in Angstroms, 103f
  discovery of, 28-30
  dose necessary to cause infection, 201
  dynamics, implications of, 170
  entry in T4 cells, 115-116, 116f
  free/mature, 56f
  formation of, 88f
  genetic makeup of, 46
  genetic mutation of, 58-60. See also Drug-resistant mutants
  genetic recombination in, 60-65
  genetic resistance to, 116-118
  genome of, 54f, 54-59, 55t
  immunity and, 114
  as lentivirus, 47
  life cycle of, 49, 53f
  lifetime in plasma, 84
  meaning of term, 44-45
  naming of, 29-30
  origin of, 36-45
  pathological uniqueness of, 291
  point of saturation for, 302
  production of, 78f
  protection from antibodies, 114
  replication, mathematical model of, 84
  replication rate, 124
    implications of, 125, 169-170
  reproduction, genes controlling, 56
  reproductive cycle for, 52f
  as retrovirus, 12
  strains of, 12, 29-30
    identified, 3
  structure of, 48f49f
  subtypes of, 60
    B, 64
    D, 64
    E, 60, 63-64
    G, 60
    global distribution of, 62f, 63-64
    group M, 62f, 63
    group O, 62f, 64
    mysteries of, 64
  theories about creation of, 40
  transmission of. See Transmission of HIV

HIV-1, 12, 115-116, 116f
  origin of, 43
  transmission of, 193-194

HIV-2, 12, 29
  origin of, 43
  and SIVsm, 43
  transmission of, 193-194

HIV/AIDS
  distinguishing characteristics of, 11
  impact of, 326
  increase in number of cases, 171
  overview of, 10-12
  progression, classification of, 174
  use of term, 27

Roques, Pierre, 178
Rotaviruses, 3
Rous, Peyton, 50
Rous sarcoma virus, 50
RT. *See* Reverse transcriptase enzyme
Rumors, about HIV/AIDS,
  destructive effects of, 499-501
Russia, HIV/AIDS in, 60, 191, 385
  incidence of, 382t, 383-385
  nosocomial transmission, 232-233
  prevalence of, 365*f*
  spread of epidemic, 384
Rwanda
  HIV/AIDS in, 364, 369
    female-to-male ratio, 332
    prostitution and, 371
    prevalence of HIV genotype in, 64
    sexual practices in, 370
Ryan White CARE Act (1990), 485
Ryan White Reauthorization Act
  (1996), 429

Saag, Michael, 60
Sabia virus, 5-6
Safer sex practices, 252-256
  guidelines for, 252-256, 254t
  importance for adolescents, 353-
    356
  resistance to, gender differences
    in, 448
Saint-Fleur, Henri-Claude, 39
Saliva
  HIV in, 189, 202, 204-206
  and HIV transmission, 197t
  inhibition of HIV infectivity by,
    205
Saliva HIV test, 411-413
Salk, Jonas, 288
Salk vaccine, 288
Salmonella, symptoms of, 146t
Salmonella septicemia, in definition
  of AIDS, 33t
San Francisco, California
  HIV infection in, 217
  homosexual men with HIV in, 217
San Francisco Young Mens Health
  Study, 295
San Marino, HIV/AIDS in, 382t
Saquinavir (Invirase), 74t, 86
  genetic alterations associated with,
    78t
  side effects of, 92
Scarlet fever, epidemics, 4t
Schizophrenia, viruses in, 7
School dropouts, HIV/AIDS in, 356
Schools. See also Education
  HIV/AIDS education in, 13, 248
    Gallup Poll results on, 13t
Screening, of blood and blood
  products, 276-277, 427
Screening tests, 399-406, 408-411
  premarital, 427
Second wave of infections, 75
Self-proteins, 111-112
Semen
  components facilitating HIV
    infection, 217
  HIV in, 202
  HIV-infected cells in, 203-205
Sentinel, 413

SEPs. *See* Syringe exchange programs
Septicemia, in HIV-infected infants,
  184
Septra. *See* Trimethoprim-
  sulfamethoxazole
Seroconversion, 162, 164*f*-165f, 171-
  172, 180*f*
  failure, 174
  timing of, 167f, 172, 180*f*
  vaccine-induced, 295
Seronegativity, 349
Serum, 79
Sex, AIDS cases by, 304, 306f, 307t
  adolescent, 355
  adult, 199t
  in Canada, 380*f*
  in Latin America, 378*f*
Sex education
  adolescents' comments on, 356
  on AIDS prevention, 190
  in counseling, 445
  impact of, 495
Sexual abstinence, and prevention of
  HIV, 251-254
Sexual abuse, female-to-male ratio,
  231
Sexual activity, and risk for HIV
  transmission, 223t
Sexual assault
  of children, 231-232
  HIV transmission via, 228, 231-232
Sexual intercourse. See also Anal
  intercourse; Vaginal
  intercourse
  HIV transmission via, 189, 215-226
    global statistics, 362
    incubation period, 173
    number of sexual encounters
      and, 219-223
  safer sex practices, 248
Sexually transmitted diseases (STDs)
  and acceleration of HIV infection,
    119, 215
  AIDS as, 12
  among adolescents, 354, 495
  chemical barriers against, 265-267
  in childhood victims of sexual
    abuse, 231
  as cofactor in immune deficiency,
    120
  control of, contact tracing in, 282
  in developing nations, 237
  in females, 333
  and HIV transmission, 233-236,
    235t, 238*f*
  prevention of, condoms use as,
    254-255
  and risk for HIV infection, 216
  spermicides against, 259
  successful treatment of, 75
  in United States, 233-235
    geographical distribution, 234*f*
Sexual needs, impact of HIV on, 459
Sexual preference, establishing in
  counseling, 446-447, 447t
Sex under the influence (SUI), 448
Shalala, Donna, 212
Sheep, viruses affecting, 47
Shigella, symptoms of, 146t
Shilts, Randy, 20, 21*f*

Shingles, 220
SI HIV. *See* Syncytium-inducing HIV
  strains
Silent mutations, 58
Simian immunodeficiency virus
  (SIVsm), 43, 47
Single exposure categories, AIDS
  cases in, 302, 303t
Single-use diagnostic system (SUDS),
  411
SIVsm. *See* Simian immunodeficiency
  virus
Slim's disease, 6
Slovak Republic, HIV/AIDS in, 382t
Slovenia, HIV/AIDS in, 382t
Slow progressors, 172
Smallpox
  as biological weapon, 2
  deaths from, 9
  epidemics, 2-3, 4t
  eradication of, 7
  vaccine against, 286, 290
Smallpox virus, 4t
Social issues in HIV/AIDS, 484-485
  in Africa, 369-373
  blame-placing, 480-481
  public backlash, 532-533
  public hysteria, 481-483
Social Security Administration
  (SSA), determination of
    eligibility for disability, 31-32,
    34
Social Security Disability (SSD), 517
Social service providers, advanced
  AIDS medication and, 95
Socioeconomic factors
  for HIV infection, 10
    in Africa, 373-375
  for opportunistic infections, 133-
    135
South America. *See* Latin America
Soviet Union. *See* Russia
Spain, HIV/AIDS in, 382, 382t
Species, genetic stability of, 57-58
Sperm, HIV in, 204-205
Spermicides, 254-256
  efficacy of, 258-259
Spleen, 105*f*
Sporanox. *See* Itraconazole
Sports, and HIV/AIDS, 220-222
Spread of HIV/AIDS, 11
  danger of, 216
  global, 363-364
  mobility and, 199
  pattern of, 190
  social changes and, 44
  in U.S., 193, 194*f*
SSA. *See* Social Security
  Administration
SSD. *See* Social Security Disability
SSI. *See* Supplemental Security
  Income
State disability, 517
State laws, 565
  AIDS-related, 541, 561-562
  prohibiting discrimination, 541
Stavudine (d4T; Zerit), 73, 74t
  in combination therapy, 79
  genetic alterations associated with,
    78t

vaccine-induced antibodies fail to neutralize HIV. Subsequently HIV/AIDS vaccine field trails for 1994 are canceled.

June 1994: FDA approves anti-HIV drug, d4T or stavudine (zerit). 3TC or lamivudine has compassionate use approval. ■ National Institutes of Health Advisory Committee recommends against proceeding with phase III prophylactic vaccine trails in the United States. The World Health Organization approves phase III trials in developing countries.

July 1994: United States HIV/AIDS researchers begin announced push of "back to basics science" to get answers to many questions about HIV.

August 1994: Announcement that the annual International Conference on AIDS will be held every 2 years because of lack of progress against the disease. **■ A defining moment in the history of the AIDS pandemic: AIDS Clinical Trial Group protocol 076 data revealed a 68% reduction in prenatal transmission through the use of zidovudine during late pregnancy and in the newborn.**

October 1994: The federal government opens a toll-free number to provide treatment information by telephone or computer to people with AIDS, their families, and health care providers. The number is 1-800-448-0440, Monday through Friday. English, Spanish, and deaf access are included.

November 1994: Patricia Fleming replaces Kristine Gebbie as the new National AIDS Policy Director.

December 1994: Elizabeth Glaser, a crusader in the fight against AIDS, dies of the disease at age 47. She presented the 1992 Democratic National Convention with an account of her family tragedy. ■ Jocelyn Elders, Surgeon General of the United States and advocate for broad-based sex education in the public schools, is forced to resign. ■ Representatives from 42 nations meet at the first AIDS summit of political leaders. They promise a unified effort to fight HIV disease. ■ Peter Piot is named to head the new United Nations program on HIV/AIDS (UNAIDS). The new program merges six former HIV/AIDS programs into one.

January 1995: First 1 million worldwide AIDS cases *reported* **to the World Health Organization. ■ Scientists George Shaw and David Ho, working independently, show for the first time that from the time of infection, HIV replication is rapid and continuous, and within 2 to 4 weeks the infecting HIV** strain is replaced by drug-resistant mutants. ■ At least 1,200 AIDS cases have been acquired through the United States blood supply.

February 1995: Olympic diver Greg Louganis, who won four gold medals, reveals during a television interview with Barbara Walters that he has AIDS.

March 1995: Two HIV/AIDS investigators report on the first documented case of an HIV-positive newborn male who cleared the virus from his body without external intervention. The child is now 5 years old, healthy, and remains HIV-negative.

April 1995: Michael Merston leaves UNAIDS. Sefano Bertozzi becomes the new Executive Director.

May 1995: U. S. Department of Health and Human Services suspends all blinded HIV testing of newborns because newly-introduced legislation threatens the rights of pregnant women not to know their own HIV status.

June 1995: First National HIV Testing Day, June 27.

July 1995: Institute of Medicine issues its report, **"HIV and the Blood Supply,"** indicating that if clinical, corporate, and government authorities had acted differently, HIV in the blood supply could have been avoided. ■ Twelve cases of HIV infection in women from artificially inseminated donor semen now known. Thirty recipients of semen from HIV-infected donors refuse testing. ■ U.S. Public Health Service publishes guidelines for annual prenatal HIV counseling and volunteer HIV testing of 4 million American women who become pregnant.

AIDS DEATH TOLL REACHES 300,000.

October 1995: New York is first state in nation where physicians must advise new mothers that they can know the outcome of their babies' HIV tests. **■ As of October 1, 501,310 AIDS cases are reported in the United States (first half million cases) and 311,381 have died.**

November 1995: FDA approves the use of lamivudine (3TC) for all HIV-infected persons.

December 1995: Eighth World AIDS Day, December 1, honored in 190 countries. ■ FDA approves the **first** protease inhibitor saquinavir (trade name Inverase) to be used in combination with other drugs to slow HIV reproduction. Standard anti-HIV therapy to this point in time is the use of two nucleoside reverse transcriptase inhibitors. ■ Bill Clinton is the first United States President to hold an all-day White House AIDS summit meeting. There were 250 participants. ■ Jeff Getty, age 38, HIV-infected for 15 years with few measurable T4 cells, is given the first-ever transplantation of baboon bone marrow on December 14. Baboons are not susceptible to HIV. The mixture of baboon and human bone marrow might reconstitute his immune system. Many scientists are sharply divided on the benefit–risk potential of this xenotransplant. **The transplant fails.**

January 1996: Donna Shalala's 1994 National Task Force, the "Dream Team," on AIDS drug development is disbanded, falling far short of any significant achievement.

February 1996: President Clinton signs a defense bill authorizing the mandatory honorable discharge of all 1,049 HIV-positive men/women in the United States military (**repeal pending**). ■ Tommy Morrison, heavyweight boxing contender, age 27, announces, just hours before his fight, that he is HIV-positive. Nevada is one of only a few states that requires HIV testing of boxers.

March 1996: The protease inhibitors ritonavir and indinavir are FDA approved for use in persons who are in the advanced stages of AIDS. FDA approval occurs in a record 72 and 42 days, respectively. ■ Maryland joined eight other states requiring professional fighters and kickboxers licensed by the state to have an HIV test. ■ FDA approves first-ever vaccine against HIV made from DNA (Apollon Inc.). ■ FDA approves nationwide trials of a vaccine (Remune) containing "inactivated" HIV in HIV-infected persons.

May 1996: A second receptor to CD4, named FUSIN, located on the T4 cell is found and believed to be necessary for HIV entry into the T4 cell. ■ Reauthorization of Ryan White CARE Act, through the year 2000, is signed into law. FDA approves the first HIV home testing kit (CONFIDE).

June 1996: On June 5, 1996, the United States AIDS pandemic becomes 15 years old. ■ FDA approves first commercial HIV RNA test, Hoffman-LaRoche's Amplicor. ■ FDA approves the board-scale marketing of Orasure, a saliva-based HIV test. ■ AIDS researchers report a third receptor, a chemokine receptor (CC-CKR-5), a cofactor protein necessary for HIV to enter macrophages. ■ On June 26, New York becomes the first state in the nation to pass legislation mandating HIV testing of all newborns and disclosure of test results to the mother and physicians. ■ **FDA approves nevirapine (Viramune),** the **first** non-nucleoside HIV reverse transcriptase inhibitor.

July 1996: Eleventh International Conference on AIDS held in Vancouver, British Columbia: 14,275 people from 125 countries are in attendance. ■ Reports of newly infected patients on multidrug therapy whose viral loads dropped to undetectable levels suggest that the virus can be held in check. ■ FDA approves second HIV home test kit, HOME ACCESS.

August 1996: FDA approves first human urine test for HIV. ■ Discovery of a 32-nucleotide deletion in the CC-CKR-5 gene that confers resistance to HIV infection in those who are homozygous for this gene deletion (both genes are missing).

November 1996: David Kessler, FDA Chief, resigns. ■ Tommy Morrison becomes the first HIV-infected boxer to enter the ring. He won the fight in Japan in 1 minute, 38 seconds of the first round—**no blood was shed.**

December 1996: Ninth World AIDS Day. ■ **According to the United Nations AIDS program, the death toll has reached 6.4 million. An additional 22.6 million people are infected with the virus.** ■ David Baltimore, Nobel biologist, accepts directorship in the National Institutes of Health $129 million HIV/AIDS vaccine program. ■ U.S. interagency task force releases a 40-page strategy to guide the AIDS policy of the Clinton administration. This is the **first** time that the U.S. Government has developed a comprehensive strategy covering all federal agencies and providing a blueprint for the years ahead. ■ Triple-drug anti-HIV therapy—at least one protease inhibitor—becomes a standard therapy. ■ **David Ho,** *Time Magazine's* **selection for "Man of the Year–1996."**

AIDS DEATH TOLL PASSES 350,000.

January 1997: Worldwide reported AIDS cases from 194 countries reach 1,760,000. By the end of 1997, the number of reported AIDS cases will be over 2,500,000. Estimated 9 million AIDS cases worldwide. About 8 million have died from AIDS.

February 1997: Patricia Fleming, National AIDS Policy Director, resigns. ■ CDC first-time-ever announcement of a marked (23%) decline in AIDS-related deaths for 1996 in the United States.